LIBRARY

College of Physicians and Surgeons
of British Columbia

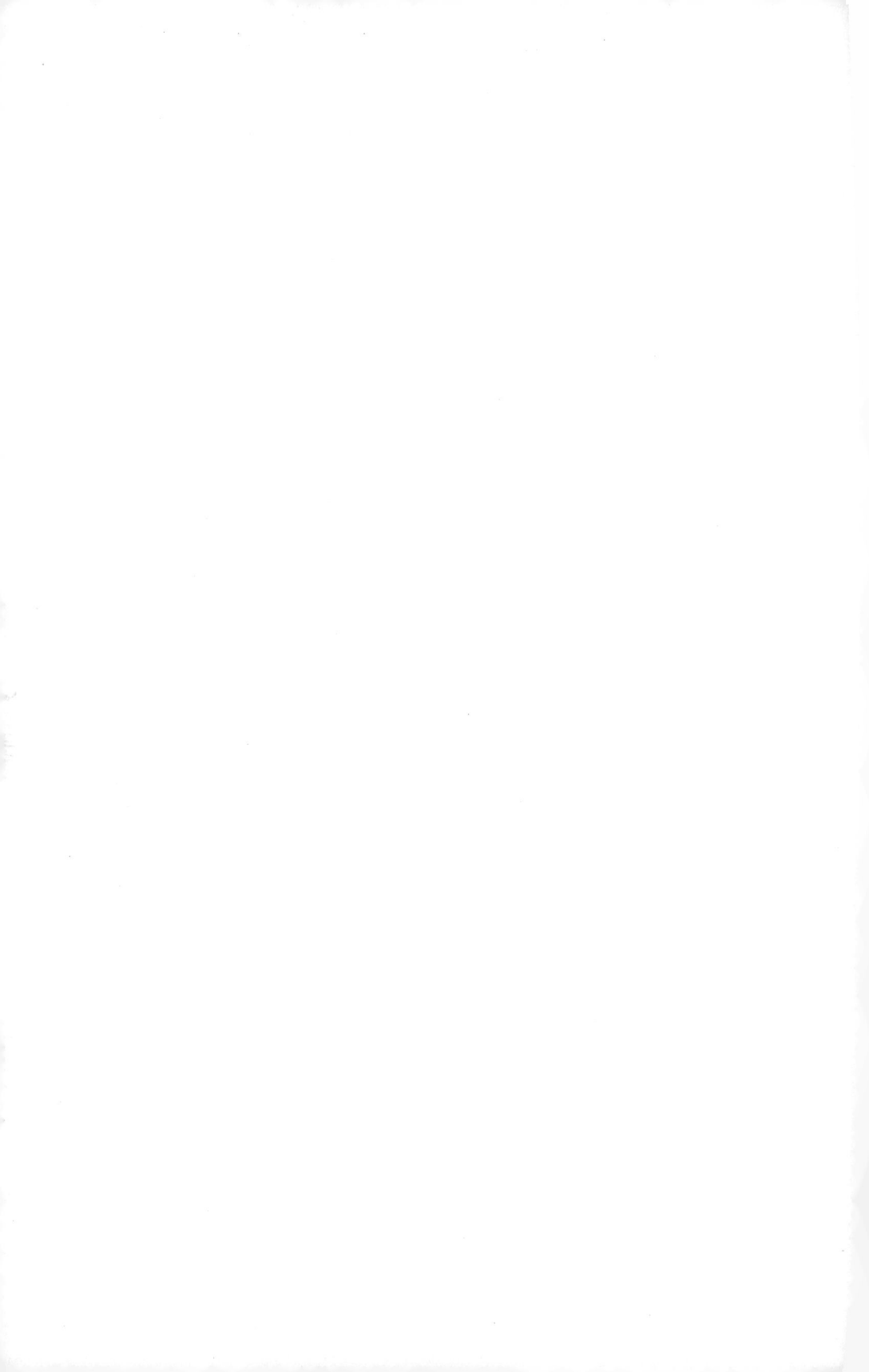

Contemporary Surgical Management *of* Liver, Biliary Tract, *and* Pancreatic Disease

Contemporary Surgical Management *of* Liver, Biliary Tract, *and* Pancreatic Disease

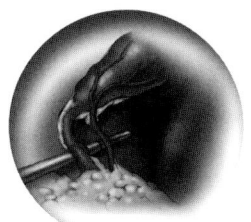 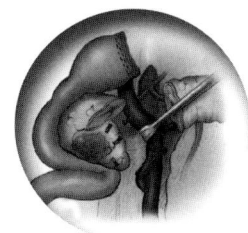 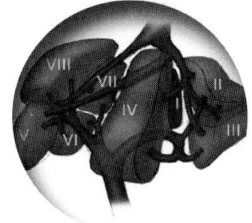

Editors

Dan G Blazer III
Duke University, USA

Paul C Kuo
Loyola University Chicago, USA

Theodore Pappas
Duke University, USA

Bryan M Clary
Duke University, USA

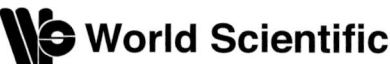

NEW JERSEY · LONDON · SINGAPORE · BEIJING · SHANGHAI · HONG KONG · TAIPEI · CHENNAI

Published by

World Scientific Publishing Co. Pte. Ltd.
5 Toh Tuck Link, Singapore 596224
USA office: 27 Warren Street, Suite 401-402, Hackensack, NJ 07601
UK office: 57 Shelton Street, Covent Garden, London WC2H 9HE

British Library Cataloguing-in-Publication Data
A catalogue record for this book is available from the British Library.

CONTEMPORARY SURGICAL MANAGEMENT OF LIVER, BILIARY TRACT, AND PANCREATIC DISEASE

Copyright © 2014 by World Scientific Publishing Co. Pte. Ltd.

All rights reserved. This book, or parts thereof, may not be reproduced in any form or by any means, electronic or mechanical, including photocopying, recording or any information storage and retrieval system now known or to be invented, without written permission from the publisher.

For photocopying of material in this volume, please pay a copying fee through the Copyright Clearance Center, Inc., 222 Rosewood Drive, Danvers, MA 01923, USA. In this case permission to photocopy is not required from the publisher.

ISBN 978-981-4293-05-1

Typeset by Stallion Press
Email: enquiries@stallionpress.com

Printed in Singapore by Fulsland Offset Printing (S) Pte Ltd Singapore

CONTENTS

Contributing Authors   ix

Section 1   Liver Disease   1

1   Liver anatomy and anatomic variants   3
Shuja Ahmed and Janet E. Tuttle-Newhall

2   Imaging of the liver   21
Nestor Villamizar Ortiz and Bryan M. Clary

3   Hepatic abscess   35
Georgia Beasley and Dan G. Blazer III

4   Cystic disease of the liver   47
Marcus Darrabie and Carlos E. Marroquin

5   Benign liver lesions   65
Immanuel Turner and Paul C. Kuo

6   Primary hepatic malignancies   77
Andrew S. Barbas and Rebekah R. White

7   Surgical treatment of hepatic metastases   91
Nicole de Rosa, Dan G. Blazer III, and Bryan M. Clary

8   Cirrhosis and portal hypertension   109
Keshava Rajagopal and Carlos E. Marroquin

9   Technical management of ascites   127
Carlos E. Marroquin and Bridget M. Marroquin

10   Variceal therapies   145
Carlos E. Marroquin

11	Liver failure Valentino Piacentino, Deborah L. Sudan and Janet E. Tuttle-Newhall	159
12	Liver transplantation Katia Papalezova, Carlos E. Marroquin, Bradley H. Collins, Janet E. Tuttle-Newhall and Paul C. Kuo	173
13	Embolization of liver tumors Leo Villegas and Paul V. Suhocki	191
14	Radiofrequency ablation Syamal Bhattacharya and Carlos E. Marroquin	199
15	Regional therapies for hepatic malignancy Lindsay Talbot and Dan G. Blazer III	209
16	Hepatic resection Michael E. Barfield and Bryan M. Clary	217
17	Surgical techniques: Liver procurement and transplantation Deepak Vikraman and Carlos E. Marroquin	237

Section 2 Biliary Disease — **251**

18	Biliary anatomy Asvin Ganapathi and Sandhya A. Lagoo-Deenadayalan	253
19	Imaging of the biliary tree Asad A. Shah, Theodore N. Pappas	263
20	Benign gallbladder disease: Cholelithiasis, polyps, gallstone ileus Kelley Hutcheson, Dan G. Blazer III	273
21	Benign gallbladder disease: Cholecystitis Ryan Turley, Kelley Hutcheson and Lisa Pickett	283
22	Benign gallbladder disease: Bile duct injuries Dawn M. Elfenbein and Mark Shapiro	295
23	Benign gallbladder disease: Postcholecystectomy syndrome and stricture Judson B. Williams and Sandhya A. Lagoo-Deenadayalan	305

24	Benign gallbladder disease: Choledocholithiasis and cholangitis *Loretta Erhunmwunsee and Aurora D. Pryor*	311
25	Gallbladder cancer *Asad A. Shah, Srinevas K. Reddy, Dan G. Blazer III and Bryan M. Clary*	323
26	Choledochal cysts *Brian R. Untch and Abigail E. Martin*	333
27	Primary biliary cirrhosis and primary sclerosing cholangitis *Vanessa Teaberry and Alastair Smith*	343
28	Bile duct cancer: Peripheral and hilar cholangiocarcinoma *Melissa Danko and Dana Portenier*	353
29	Interventional biliary techniques *Nicholas D. Andersen, and Paul V. Suhocki*	363
30	Surgical techniques: Lap/open cholecystectomy *Sean Lee and Aurora D. Pryor*	369
31	Surgical techniques: Bile duct injury repair *Sapan Desai and Dan G. Blazer III*	377
32	Surgical techniques: Common bile duct exploration *Sebastian G. de la Fuente, Aurora D. Pryor and Theodore N. Pappas*	385
33	Surgical techniques: Bile duct resection/reconstruction *Sarah Evans and Carlos E. Marroquin*	393
34	Surgical techniques: Transduodenal techniques *Sean Lee and Katia Papalezova*	405
Section 3	**Diseases of the Pancreas**	**411**
35	Pancreas anatomy and anatomic variants *Mani A Daneshmand and Eugene P. Ceppa*	413
36	Imaging of the pancreas *Kristy Rialon, Courtney Coursey and Rendon C. Nelson*	417
37	Acute pancreatitis *Mayur B. Patel and Theodore N. Pappas*	435

38	Chronic pancreatitis *Jack Haney and Eugene P. Ceppa*	457
39	Cystic neoplasms of the pancreas *Eugene P. Ceppa and Douglas S. Tyler*	469
40	Periampullary cancer *Diana L. Diesen and Theodore N. Pappas*	491
41	Pancreatic neuroendocrine tumors *Tamarah Westmoreland and John Olson*	511
42	Unusual pancreatic neoplasms *James Padussis and Douglas S. Tyler*	523
43	Pancreas and islet cell transplantation *Keri E. Lunsford and Bradley H. Collins*	533
44	Interventional techniques *Stephen Philcox and Paul Jowell*	557
45	Surgical techniques: Whipple *Rebekah R. White and Eugene P. Ceppa*	577
46	Surgical techniques: Palliative surgery *Jeffrey Nienaber and Theodore N. Pappas*	591
47	Surgical techniques: Distal pancreatectomy *Jin S. Yoo and Aurora D. Pryor*	607
48	Surgical techniques: Enucleation procedures and central pancreatectomy *Elisabeth Tracy and Theodore N. Pappas*	621
49	Surgical techniques: Chronic pancreatic procedures *John C. Haney and Eugene P. Ceppa*	631
50	Surgical techniques: Pancreas transplantation *Errol L. Bush, Kadiyala V. Ravindra and Bradley H. Collins*	639

Index 647

CONTRIBUTING AUTHORS

Shuja Ahmed, MD
Department of Surgery
Wake Forest University School of Medicine
Winston-Salem, North Carolina, USA

Nicholas D. Andersen, MD
Department of Surgery
Duke University Medical Center
Durham, NC, USA

Andrew S. Barbas, MD
Department of Surgery
Duke University Medical Center
Durham, NC, USA

Michael E. Barfield, MD
Department of Surgery
Duke University Medical Center
Durham, NC, USA

Georgia Beasley, MD
Department of Surgery
Duke University Medical Center
Durham, NC, USA

Syamal D. Bhattacharya, MD
Department of Surgery
Duke University Medical Center
Durham, NC, USA

Dan G. Blazer III, MD
Department of Surgery
Duke University Medical Center
Durham, NC, USA

Errol L. Bush, MD
Division of Cardiothoracic Surgery
University of California-San Francisco Medical Center
San Francisco, CA, USA

Eugene P. Ceppa, MD
Department of Surgery
Indiana University School of Medicine
Indianapolis, Indiana, USA

Bryan M. Clary, MD
Department of Surgery
Duke University Medical Center
Durham, NC, USA

Bradley H. Collins, MD
Department of Surgery
Duke University Medical Center
Durham, NC, USA

Courtney Coursey, MD
Department of Radiology
Emory University School of Medicine
Atlanta, GA, USA

Melissa Danko, MD
Department of Surgery
Vanderbilt University School of Medicine
Nashville, TN, USA

Mani A. Daneshmand, MD
Department of Surgery
Duke University Medical Center
Durham, NC, USA

Marcus Darrabie, MD
Department of Surgery
Duke University Medical Center
Durham, NC, USA

Sapan S. Desai, MD, PhD, MBA
Department of Surgery
Duke University
Durham, North Carolina, USA

Diana L. Diesen, MD
Department of Surgery
UT Southwestern Medical Center
Dallas, TX, USA

Dawn M. Elfenbein, MD
Department of Surgery
University of Wisconsin
Madison, WI, USA

Loretta Erhunmwunsee, MD
Department of Surgery
Duke University Medical Center
Durham, NC, USA

Sarah Evans, MD
Department of Surgery
University of Cincinnati
Cincinnati, OH, USA

Sebastian G. de la Fuente, MD
Department of Surgery
Center for Specialized Surgery
Orlando, FL, USA

Asvin Ganapathi, MD
Department of Surgery
Duke University Medical Center
Durham, NC, USA

Jack Haney, MD
Department of Surgery
Duke University Medical Center
Durham, NC, USA

Kelley Hutcheson, MD
Department of Surgery
Washington University School of Medicine
St Louis, Missouri, USA

Paul S. Jowell, MD
Division of Gastroenterology
Duke University Medical Center
Durham, NC, USA

Paul C. Kuo, MD, PhD
Department of Surgery
Loyola University-Chicago
Maywood, IL, USA

Sandhya A. Lagoo-Deenadayalan, MD, PhD
Department of Surgery
Duke University Medical Center
Durham, NC, USA

Sean Lee, MD
Department of Surgery
Duke University Medical Center
Durham, NC, USA

Keri E. Lunsford, MD, PhD
Department of Surgery
UCLA Medical Center
Los Angeles, CA, USA

Bridget M. Marroquin
University of Rochester
Rochester, New York, USA

Carlos E. Marroquin, MD
Department of Surgery
University of Rochester
Rochester, New York, USA

Abigail E. Martin, MD
Department of Surgery
Duke University Medical Center
Durham, NC 27710 USA

Rendon C. Nelson, MD
Department of Radiology
Duke University Medical Center
Durham, NC, USA

Jeffrey Nienaber, MD
Nebraska Heart Institute
Lincoln, NE, USA

John A. Olson, MD, PhD
Department of Surgery
The University of Maryland School of Medicine
Baltimore, MD, USA

Nestor Villamizar Ortiz, MD
Department of Surgery
Brigham and Woman's Hospital
Boston, MA, USA

James Padussis, MD
Department of Surgery
University of Pittsburgh Medical Center
Pittsburgh, PA, USA

Katia Papalezova, MD
Department of Surgery
Montefiore/Albert Einstein College of Medicine
Bronx, New York, USA

Theodore N. Pappas, MD
Department of Surgery
Duke University Medical Center
Durham, NC, USA

Mayur B. Patel, MD
Department of Surgery
Vanderbilt University School of Medicine
Nashville, TN, USA

Stephen Philcox, MD
John Hunter Hospital
New Lambton Heights NSW, Australia

Valentino Piacentino, MD, PhD
Department of Surgery
University of Connecticut
Hartford, CT, USA

Lisa Pickett, MD
Department of Surgery
Duke University Medical Center
Durham, NC, USA

Dana Portenier, MD
Department of Surgery
Duke University Medical Center
Durham, NC, USA

Aurora D. Pryor, MD
Department of Surgery
Stony Brook School of Medicine
Stony Brook, NY, USA

Nicole de Rosa, MD
Department of Surgical Oncology
MD Anderson Cancer Center
Houston, TX, USA

Kadiyala V. Ravindra, MD
Department of Surgery
Duke University Medical Center
Durham, NC, USA

Keshava Rajagopal, MD, PhD
Department of Surgery
University of Maryland Medical Center
Baltimore, MD, USA

Srinevas K. Reddy, MD
Department of Surgery
University of Maryland Medical Center
Baltimore, MD, USA

Kristy Rialon, MD
Department of Surgery
Duke University Medical Center
Durham, NC, USA

Asad A. Shah, MD
Department of Surgery
Duke University Medical Center
Durham, NC, USA

Mark Shapiro, MD
Department of Surgery
Duke University Medical Center
Durham, NC, USA

Alastair Smith, MD
Division of Gastroenterology
Duke University Medical Center
Durham, NC, USA

Debra L. Sudan, MD
Department of Surgery
Duke University Medical Center
Durham, NC, USA

Paul V. Suhocki, MD
Department of Radiology
Duke University Medical Center
Durham, NC, USA

Lindsay Talbot, MD
Department of Surgery
Duke University Medical Center
Durham, NC, USA

Vanessa Schroder, MD
Department of Surgery
Duke University Medical Center
Durham, NC, USA

Elisabeth Tracy, MD
Department of Surgery
Duke University Medical Center
Durham, NC, USA

Ryan Turley, MD
Department of Surgery
Duke University Medical Center
Durham, NC, USA

Immanuel Turner, MD
Department of Surgery
University of Michigan
Ann Arbor, MI, USA

Janet E. Tuttle-Newhall, MD
Department of Surgery
Saint Louis University School of Medicine
St. Louis, Missouri, USA

Douglas S. Tyler, MD
Department of Surgery
Duke University Medical Center
Durham, NC, USA

Brian R. Untch, MD
Department of Surgery
Memorial Sloan-Kettering Cancer Center
New York, NY, USA

Deepak Vikraman, MD
Department of Surgery
Duke University Medical Center
Durham, NC, USA

Leo Villegas, MD
Sacred Heart Health System
Pensacola, FL, USA

Tamarah Westmoreland, MD, PhD
Department of Surgery
Nemours Children's Clinic
Orlando, FL, USA

Rebekah R. White, MD
Department of Surgery
Duke University Medical Center
Durham, North Carolina, USA

Judson B. Williams, MD
Department of Surgery
Duke University Medical Center
Durham, NC, USA

Jin S. Yoo, MD
Department of Surgery
Duke University Medical Center
Durham, NC, USA

Section 1: Liver Disease

LIVER ANATOMY AND ANATOMIC VARIANTS   1

Shuja Ahmed* and
Janet E. Tuttle-Newhall[†]

INTRODUCTION

From the first liver resection by A. Luis in 1886[1] to modern day liver transplantation, hepatobiliary surgery has witnessed major advancements over the last century. Much of this technical achievement has been attained on the back of progressively improved understanding of the liver anatomy and its potential variant. From Cantlie to Couinaud, many anatomists contributed towards this modern-day understanding of the liver anatomy. The liver, by virtue of its friability and propensity to bleed from rich vascularization, continues to be a surgical challenge for today's surgeon despite access to modern instruments and equipment. Good working knowledge of the hepatic anatomy with its variants is therefore an important prerequisite to successful hepatobiliary surgery and the only way to minimize associated complications.

This chapter reviews the anatomy of the liver in some detail. All functional components of the liver, including arterial supply, venous outflow, biliary tree and lymphatics, are sequentially reviewed.

---

*Wake Forest University School of Medicine, Winston-Salem, North Carolina
[†]Saint Louis University School of Medicine, Department of Surgery, St. Louis, Missouri.

FUNCTIONAL SURGICAL ANATOMY

The functional anatomy of the liver has been a subject of much debate and research over the last century and even till today among surgical scholars. The internal liver structure has been clarified.[2-4,5-8] This "functional anatomy" describes liver architecture in terms of hepatic segments based on the distribution of portal pedicle and location of hepatic veins. Essentially, the three main hepatic veins divide the liver into four sectors, each of which receives a portal pedicle with an alternating arrangement of hepatic vein and portal pedicle.

According to Couinaud's landmark description,[7] the liver parenchyma overlying the hepatic veins is termed a scissura. Thus, the main portal scissura (better known as Cantlie's line) contains the middle hepatic vein and extends from the middle of the gallbladder anteriorly to the left of the vena cava posteriorly. This imaginary line divides the liver into right and left lobes and has been used by surgeons to delineate the lobes as such. Of clinical significance, the left and right lobes of the liver are independent in terms of portal and arterial vascularization and of biliary drainage. This anatomical divide is important in determining types and extent of resections.

Subsequently, the right and left lobes are further subdivided into two sectors each by two other portal scissurae. The right portal scissura divides the right lobe into *anteromedial* and *posterolateral* sectors. The right hepatic vein runs in the right scissura. Each of these sectors is further subdivided into *segments*. The anteromedial sector contains segment V anteriorly and segment VIII posteriorly. The posterolateral sector contains segment VI anteriorly and segment VII posteriorly. The left portal scissura containing the left hepatic vein divides the left lobe into *anterior* and *posterior* sectors. Of note, the left portal scissura is not within the umbilical fissure but located posterior to the ligamentum teres. The umbilical fissure overlies a portal pedicle and thus divides the anterior sector into segment III and IV (quadrate lobe). The posterior sector is only composed of segment II.

The *caudate lobe* is referred to as segment I. It lies posteriorly in close proximity to the inferior vena cava and segment IV. Functionally, it is an autonomous segment as it receives its blood supply from both the right and left branches of the hepatic artery and portal vein. Also, its venous drainage is directly into the inferior vena cava instead of the hepatic vein. This is important in setting of Budd-Chiari syndrome. Obstructed hepatic veins cause hepatic outflow to be directed through a hypertrophied caudate lobe into the inferior vena cava.

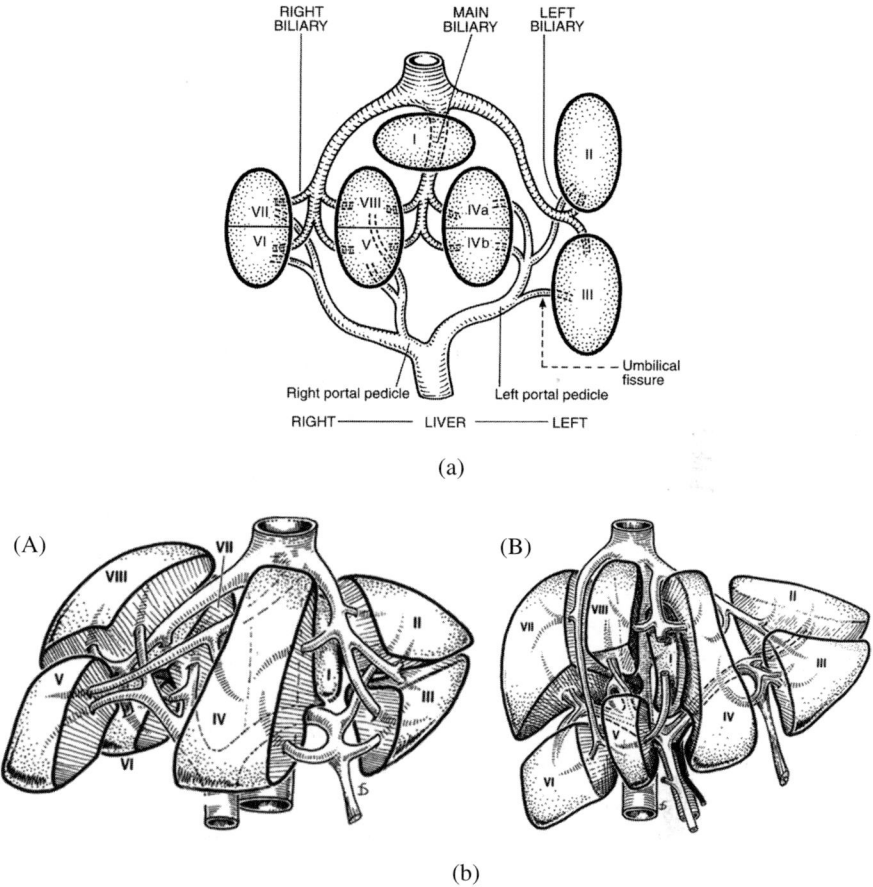

Figure 1. Schematic representation of functional anatomy of liver. Used with permission from *Surgery of the liver, biliary tract and pancreas*. Volume 1. (4th Edition) LH Blumgart.

CLINICAL SIGNIFICANCE

Knowledge of the functional anatomy is important to undertake various types of partial hepatectomies such as lobectomy, and segmentectomies. Understanding the anatomy is less important when planning wedge or "nonanatomic" liver resections. Good working knowledge of the vasculature and bile ducts allows accurate resection with a lower chance of biliary complications, including leaks. Knowledge of the anatomy can also ensure that the post-resected liver remains viable with normal arterial inflow and venous outflow to allow prompt regeneration.

LIVER BLOOD SUPPLY

The liver normally receives 25% of the total cardiac output and is unique in that it receives its blood supply from two main sources: the hepatic artery and portal vein. The hepatic artery provides about 25% of the hepatic blood flow and 50% of the oxygen supply. The portal vein contributes about 75% of the blood flow and 50% of oxygen supply. Mixing of the arterial portal blood occurs in the sinusoids which are drained by the hepatic veins into the inferior vena cava (IVC).

HEPATIC ARTERY

The anatomy of the hepatic artery and its variants has been described in the literature.[9-13] The arterial patterns are of importance in planning and performance of all hepatic surgeries.

Aberrant hepatic arteries are found in 45% of population, based on postmortem examinations. An aberrant artery is *accessory* if it supplies a segment of the liver that also receives blood supply from a normal hepatic artery. It is a *replacing* artery if it is the only blood supply to such lobe or segment.

The common hepatic artery originates from the celiac trunk in 86% of the population. Other sources are superior mesenteric artery (2.9%), aorta (1.1%) and, very rarely, left gastric artery.[14] After its origin, the common hepatic artery runs horizontally along the upper border of the head of the pancreas and gives off the gastroduodenal (GDA) artery posterior and superior to the duodenum. The supraduodenal artery and right gastric artery originate just distal to the GDA. The continuation of the hepatic artery beyond the origins of these vessels is known as the hepatic artery proper (HAP). It turns upwards to ascend in the lesser omentum, enveloped by the hepatoduodenal ligament, in front of the epiploic foramen of Winslow. Within the hepatoduodenal ligament, the HAP lies to the left of the common bile duct and anterior to the portal vein. Together, the hepatic artery proper, the common bile duct and the portal vein form the *portal triad*. Within the ligament, the hepatic artery proper divides into right and left hepatic arteries.

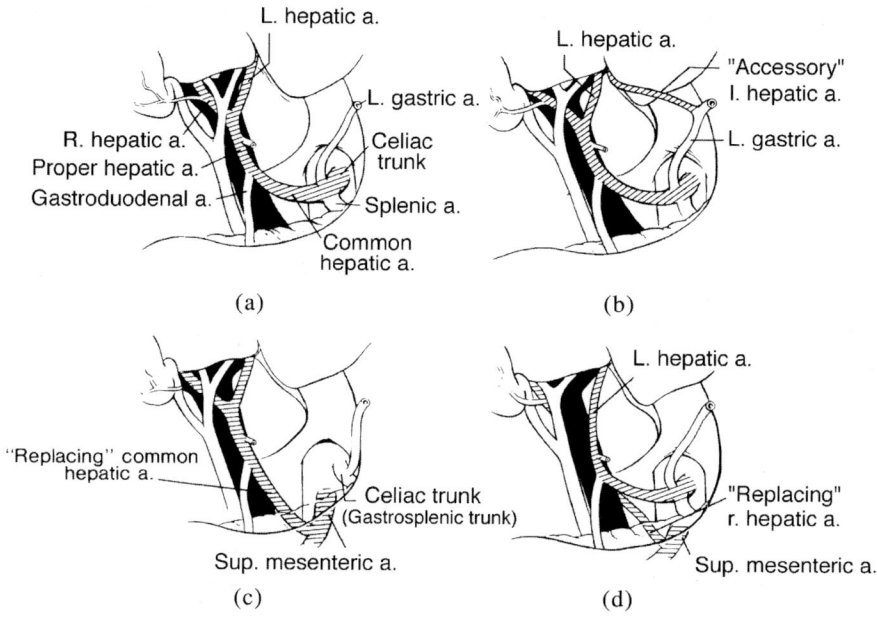

Figure 2. (A) Normal hepatic artery from celiac trunk. (B) Accessory left hepatic artery from left gastric artery. (C) Replacing common hepatic artery arising from superior mesenteric artery. (D) Replacing right hepatic artery arising from superior mesenteric artery. *Hepatic Surgical Anatomy.* Surg Clin N Am 84 (2004) 413–415; used with permission.

The right hepatic artery is a branch of the hepatic artery proper in the majority of the population; however, in 17% of subjects, it arises from the superior mesenteric artery.[14] A "replaced" right hepatic artery is more common than an "accessory" right hepatic artery. Inadvertent ligation of a replaced right hepatic artery, especially where it crosses the junction of the cystic duct and common bile duct, during cholecystectomy, deprives blood supply to the right lobe of the liver and can lead to significant complications. In contrast, ligation of an accessory right hepatic artery that derives from superior mesenteric artery has less significant consequences. At the porta hepatis, the right hepatic artery normally passes to the right behind the hepatic duct and anterior to the portal vein to enter the *Calot triangle* formed by the cystic duct, the hepatic duct and the liver. In 15% of individuals, however, it may pass anterior to the hepatic duct. This variation is worth remembering during exploration of the common bile duct or routine cholecystectomies.

Before entering the liver, the right hepatic artery gives off the cystic artery. Within the liver, the right hepatic artery divides into anterior and posterior segmental arteries which divide further into superior and inferior arteries to supply the respective subsegments. An artery for the caudate lobe also originates and supplies the caudate process and the right side of the caudate lobe. These arteries are found under the respective bile duct branches.

The left hepatic artery usually originates from the HAP. An aberrant left hepatic artery originating from the left gastric artery occurs in 30% of patients.[15] In this variant form, the left hepatic artery is a replaced versus accessory artery in a ratio of 1:1. If replaced, only the right hepatic artery comes off from the celiac axis, whereas, in the presence of an accessory vessel, the common hepatic artery takes its usual course and supplies a right and a left hepatic artery. Ligation of a replaced left hepatic artery, such as during gastrectomy or laparoscopic Nissen fundoplication, would compromise the blood supply to the left lobe of liver. In addition, an accessory left hepatic artery may also come from the right hepatic artery.

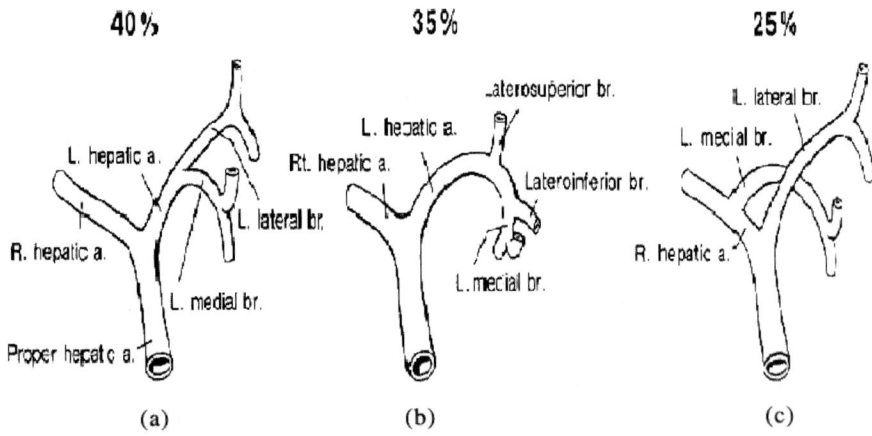

Figure 3. Variations in branching of left hepatic artery. (A) Bifurcation into medial and lateral segmental arteries. (B) Division of lateral segmental artery into laterosuperior and lateroinferior branches. (C) The left medial segmental artery arises from right hepatic artery. *Hepatic Surgical Anatomy.* Surg Clin N Am 84 (2004) 413–415; used with permission.

After its origin, the left hepatic artery supplies the entire left lobe of liver in 40% of patients by dividing into medial and lateral segmental arteries. Interestingly, in 25% of patients, the left hepatic artery supplies only the left lateral segmental; the left medial segment being supplied by a branch of the right hepatic artery crossing the midline. The left hepatic artery also gives off a branch for the caudate lobe supplying its left side.

PORTAL VEIN

The portal vein forms behind the head of the pancreas at the level of L2 through a confluence of the superior mesenteric and splenic veins. It runs behind the first portion of the duodenum and then along the right border of the lesser omentum — as part of portal triad — for a length of 8–10 cm. In its upward course, the portal vein receives the *coronary vein*, which is a continuation the left gastric vein and the esophageal venous plexus. At the liver hilum, it divides into right and left branches to the respective lobes.

The right branch of the portal vein is shorter of the two branches and is located anterior to the caudate process. Near its origin, it gives off a branch for the caudate lobe and then divides into anterior and posterior segmental branches, which further subdivide into superior and inferior subsegmental branches for respective parenchymal subsegments.

The left portal vein is smaller and longer than its counterpart. It also gives off a caudate lobe branch at its origin following which it divides into medial and lateral branches. The medial vessel contains a dilatation, the pars umbilicus, which represents the orifice of the obliterated embryonic ductus venosus.

Portal Vein Variations and Anomalies

Historically, shunt procedures for portal hypertension have created considerable interest in the anatomy of the portal vein. Of note, however, the portal vein system has fewer anatomic variants than the hepatic arterial system. The usual anatomic description of the formation of portal vein is found in 50% of patients. In the other half, the inferior mesenteric vein enters the junction of the splenic and superior mesenteric veins, or it joins the superior mesenteric vein. Rarely, the portal vein may lie anterior to the head of the pancreas and duodenum.

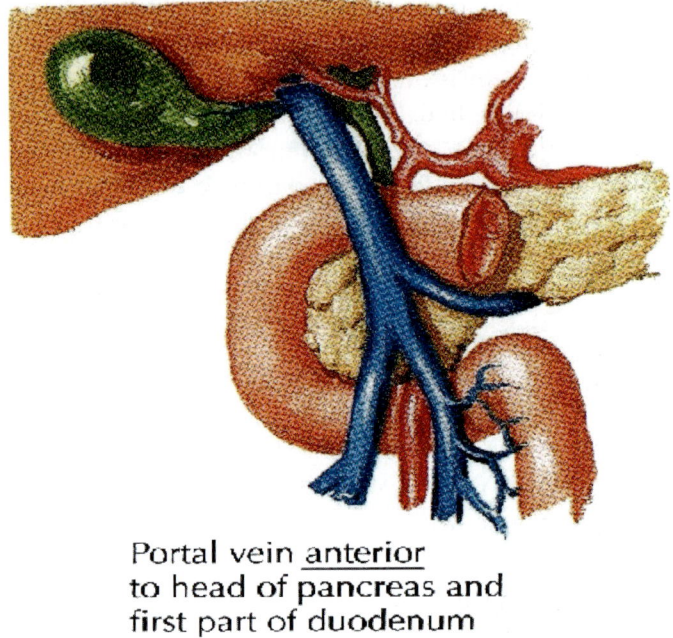

Portal vein anterior to head of pancreas and first part of duodenum

Figure 4. Portal vein lying anterior to pancreas. Used with permission from *Netter's gastroenterology*. Martin H Floch.

Relationship Between Hepatic Artery and Portal Vein Blood Flow

Hepatic arterial blood flow is unique in that it is not determined by the oxygen demand of liver parenchymal cells. Instead, portal blood flow is the major intrinsic regulator of hepatic arterial tone. The *hepatic arterial buffer response*[16] causes changes in hepatic arterial blood flow in response to any portal inflow alterations thus tending to regulate total hepatic blood flow at a constant level. This mechanism depends on portal blood flow removing local concentrations of adenosine. With decreased portal vein inflow, less adenosine is washed out, causing its concentration to rise, thereby resulting in arterial dilatation and increased arterial blood flow.

HEPATIC VEINS

Outflow of the liver is facilitated by the hepatic veins. Three main hepatic veins and many smaller veins drain blood from the liver into IVC. As mentioned previously, the hepatic veins are found intraparenchymally and form the bases for sectors and segments of the liver.

The right hepatic vein is the largest of the three veins. It lies in the right scissura and drains both posterior segments and anterosuperior segment. Together, this constitutes segments V, VI, VII and part of VIII.

The middle hepatic vein serves the left lobe of the liver together with the left hepatic vein. It lies in the median scissura and drains segments IV, V, and part of VIII.

The left hepatic vein lies in the upper portion of the left scissura and drains the segments II, III and part of segment IV. In 60% of cases, the left and middle veins unite to enter the IVC as a single vein. This anatomical confluence is often used for implantation in the caval preservation of technique during the liver transplant. Formal clamping of the vena cava can be avoided by creating a common orifice of the middle and left hepatic veins and clamping the confluens using that common orifice for the upper caval anastomoses of the allograft.

ANATOMY OF BILIARY TREE

The next anatomic system to be discussed in liver anatomy is the biliary system. In order to prevent biliary complications after liver surgery, anatomical knowledge of biliary ductal system is of vital importance.

The bile ducts commence by small passages in hepatocytes which communicate with canaliculi termed *intercellular biliary passages*. Bile flows from canaliculi through ductules into interlobular bile ducts found in portal pedicles. In segmental and subsegmental pedicles surrounded by a Glissonian sheath, bile ducts are found alongside the hepatic artery and portal vein. The segmental bile ducts join to form the right and left hepatic ducts which come together to form the common hepatic duct. As mentioned previously, the common hepatic duct runs along the hepatic artery and portal vein which together form the portal triad.

The right hepatic duct is formed by the union of the anterior and posterior branches at porta hepatis. Each branch is further bifurcated into superior and inferior branches to drain the four segments of the right lobe. These include segments V, VI, VII, VIII. This pattern is usually present in 72% of patients. In the remainder, the anterior, or sometimes posterior, branches empty into the left hepatic duct. The left hepatic duct is formed by the medial and lateral branches converging together. Each branch is formed by superior and inferior branches of the respective segments.

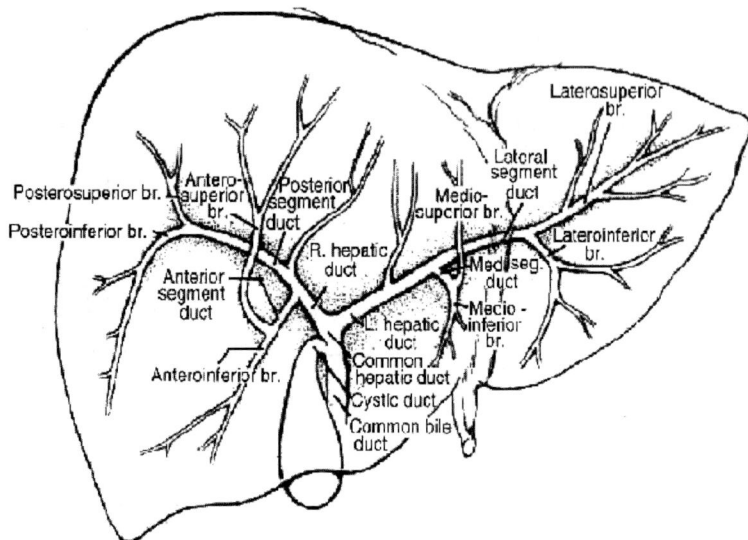

Figure 5. Intrahepatic distribution of bile duct. *Hepatic Surgical Anatomy.* Surg Clin N Am 84 (2004) 413–415; used with permission.

Overall, the left hepatic duct drains segment II, III and IV of the liver. Again, this arrangement is present in 67% of patients.

The caudate lobe (segment I) is unique in that its biliary drainage enters both the right and left hepatic duct systems in 80% of the population. In 15% of patients, it drains only in the left hepatic duct and in the remaining 5% of cases drains only into the right hepatic system.

Gallbladder and Cystic Duct

The gallbladder is a reservoir of bile located on the undersurface of the right lobe of the liver within the cystic fossa and separated from the hepatic parenchyma by the cystic plate. Sometimes it may be deeply embedded in the liver.

Anomalies of the gallbladder are numerous. These include bilobar gallbladders with a single cystic duct but two fundi, duplication of the gallbladder with two cystic ducts, double cystic duct draining unilocular gallbladder. Congenital diverticulum of the gallbladder with a muscular layer has also been described. The cystic duct arises from the infundibulum

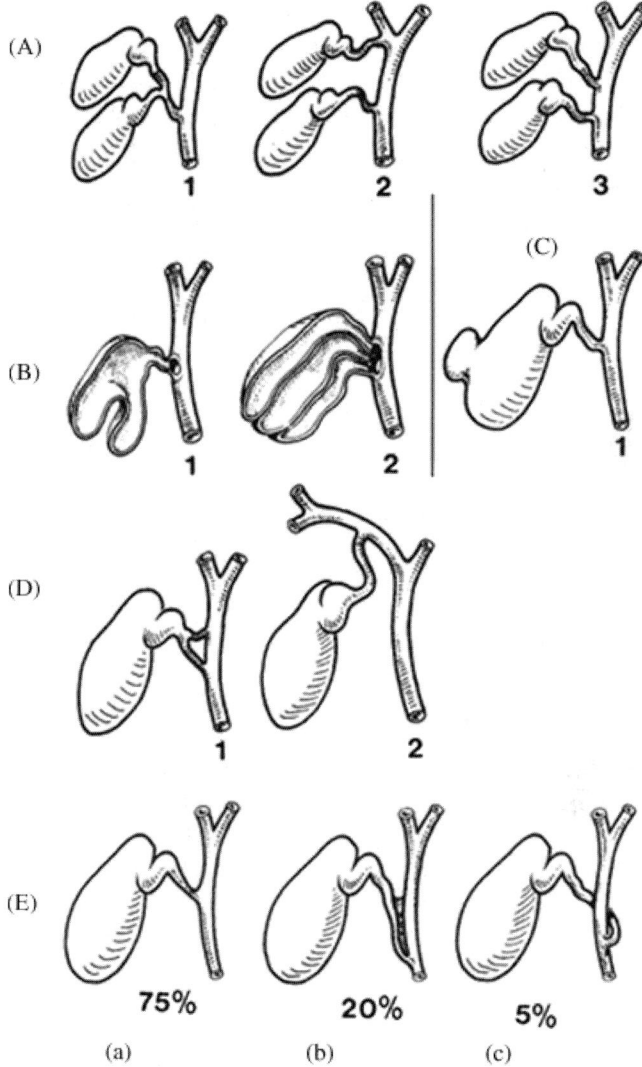

Figure 6. Main variations in gallbladder and cystic duct anatomy: (A) duplicated gallbladder, (B) septum of the gallbladder, (C) diverticulum of the gallbladder, (D) variations in cystic ductal anatomy, (E) Different types of union of the cystic duct and common hepatic duct: (a) angular union, (b) parallel union, (c) spiral union. Used with permission from *Surgery of the liver, biliary tract and pancreas.* (4th Edition) Volume 1. LH Blumgart.

of the gallbladder and joins the common hepatic duct at an angle to form the common bile duct. The cystic duct usually measures 2–4 cm in length and contains prominent concentric folds known as the spiral valves of Heister. The cystic duct frequently exhibits a tortuous or serpentine course. The normal diameter of the cystic duct is variable, ranging from 1–5 mm.

Congenital anatomic variants of the cystic duct are common occurring in 18%–23% of patients.[17] The cystic duct inserts into the middle one-third of the extrahepatic bile duct in 75% of cases and into the distal one-third in 10%. It most commonly inserts from a right lateral position but may have an anterior or posterior spiral insertion, low lateral insertion with a common sheath enclosing the cystic duct and common bile duct, proximal insertion, or low medial insertion at or near the ampulla of Vater.

The level of cystic duct insertion may vary, with an abnormal proximal or distal union accounting for 55% of biliary ductal anatomic variants.[17] The cystic duct may join the right hepatic duct, the left hepatic duct (rarely), or the common hepatic duct high in the porta hepatis. It empties into the proximal common hepatic duct or into the right hepatic duct in 0.3% of cases. The insertion may be low in the intrapancreatic or intraduodenal portion or at the level of the ampulla of Vater. Rarely, the cystic duct inserts directly into the duodenum.

A cystic duct that parallels the common hepatic duct is found in 20% of patients. This anatomy may be problematic at cholecystectomy. Ligation of the cystic duct too close to the common hepatic duct may result in stricture of the latter. Similarly, mistaking the cystic duct for the bile duct can result in iatrogenic injury such as inadvertent ligation or transection of the extrahepatic bile duct.

LIVER HISTOLOGY

The structural and functional organization of the liver has been described by hepatic lobule and hepatic acinus models respectively.

The *lobule* model describes the liver as being organized into lobules which take the shape of irregular polygonal prisms. At the corners between adjacent lobules is the portal triad containing the hepatic artery, portal vein and bile duct. Along the central axis of each lobule runs a central vein which is a branch of the hepatic vein. Occupying the bulk of lobules are hepatocytes arranged into cords separated by sinusoids. The sinusoids are

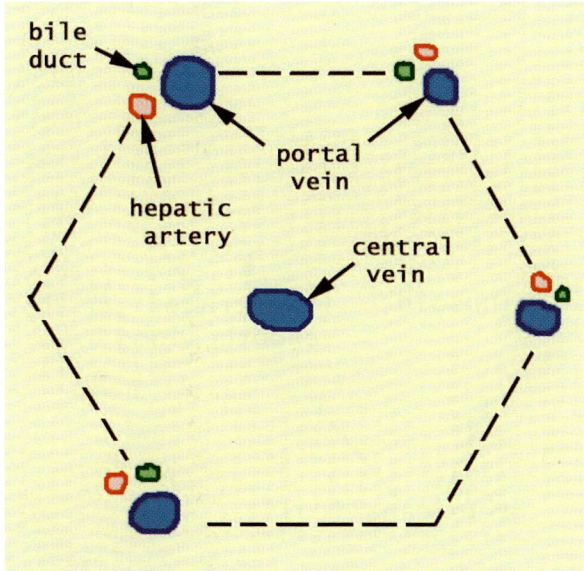

Figure 7. Lobule model of liver organization.

structurally different in that they are lined by fenestrated endothelium which has no underlying basement membrane. Therefore, fenestrations allow blood plasma to flow easily over the exposed surface of hepatocytes in the space of Disse (space between endothelium and hepatic cords). Bile canaliculi formed by apical surfaces of adjacent hepatocytes form a tiny network of passages contained within each cord.

Blood enters the sinusoids from the terminal portal venules. End arterioles of the hepatic arteries also drain into terminal portal venules allowing mixing of the blood. The large sinusoidal volume permits this blood to associate intimately with the hepatocytes, allowing transfer of substances across the hepatocyte membranes. Kupffer cells are associated with the sinusoids allowing destruction of bacteria.

The liver *acinus* encompasses the liver tissue that is served by a single terminal branch of the hepatic artery. These small vessels extend out from portal areas, along the boundaries between adjacent lobules. An acinus is typically diamond-shaped in cross section, with a hepatic arteriole crossing the center and with central veins at the two opposite corners. The acinus includes triangular portions of two adjacent lobules.

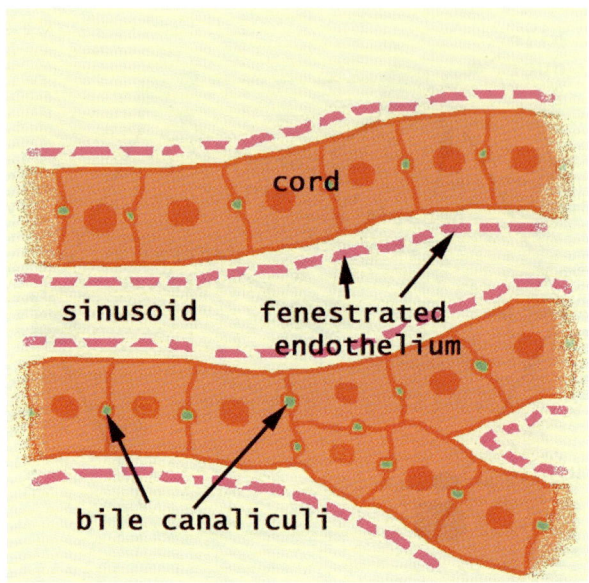

Figure 8. Relationship of hepatocytes with sinusoids.

LYMPHATICS OF THE LIVER

The lymphatic system of the liver is divided into superficial and deep systems and has a different organization from the vasobiliary system. It is important to know the anatomy of the lymphatic system when assessing the spread of malignancies to locoregional lymph nodes.

The superficial system drains in four directions:

1. Vessels that drain the coronary and right triangular ligaments enter the thoracic duct.
2. Vessels of the porta hepatis, close to the falciform ligament, enter the hepatic nodes from which they gain access to celiac nodes and then to the intestinal trunk.
3. Vessels in the posterior part of the left lobe pass through the esophageal opening to enter the pericardia lymph nodes.
4. Vessels which drain the rest of the right lobe enter the celiac nodes.

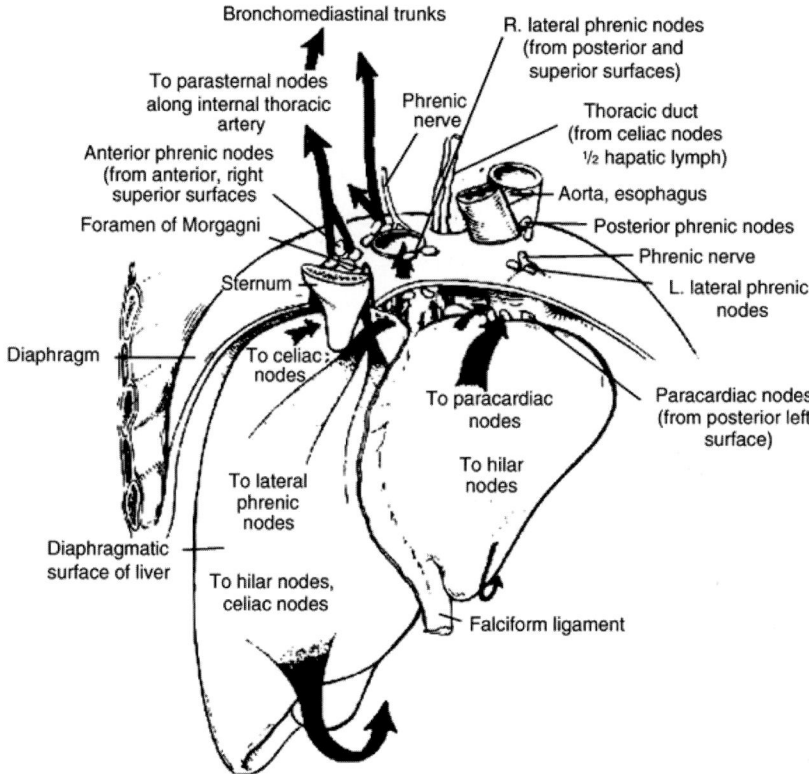

Figure 9. Superficial lymphatic drainage of the liver. *Hepatic Surgical Anatomy.* Surg Clin N Am 84 (2004) 413–415; used with permission.

The deep system is the system with greater lymphatic flow. It forms ascending and descending trunks. The ascending trunk ends in nodes close to IVC in the mediastinum. The descending trunk leaves the porta hepatis and enters the hepatic nodes.

All the vessels (except the paracardial and the ascending trunk, which end in the nodes of the inferior vena cava) enter into the celiac node. From these nodes, they pass into the intestinal lymph trunks, which then enter the cisterna chyli or the abdominal confluence of lymph trunks. The cisterna chyli drains into the thoracic duct. The exceptions enter the bronchomediastinal trunk to reach the right jugulosubclavian junction or the right lymph duct.

CONCLUSION

The rapid evolution of hepatobiliary surgery with performance of radical operations such as trisegmentectomies and split liver transplantation makes knowledge of hepatic anatomy even more imperative for today's surgeon compared to any other era. A clear understanding of the relationships between major anatomic structures in the liver allows surgeons the ability to mitigate risk of surgery and ensure their patients receive the highest quality of care.

REFERENCES

1. Tanabe KK. The past 60 years in liver surgery. *Cancer* 2008; 113(7):1888–1896.
2. McIndoe AH, Counseller VX, 1927: A report on the bilaterality of the liver. *Arch Surg* 15:589.
3. Ton That Tung. La vascularisationveineuse du foieetses applications aux résectionshépatiques. *Thése* Hanoi, 1939.
4. Hjörstö CH. The topography of the intrahepatic duct systems. Acta Anat 1931 11:599–615.
5. Healey JE, Schroy PC. Anatomy of the biliary ducts within the human liver: analysis of the prevailing pattern of branchings and the major variations of the biliary ducts. *Am Med Assoc Arch Surg* 1953 66:599–615.
6. Goldsmith NA, Woodburne RT. Surgical anatomy pertaining to liver resection. *Surg Gynecol Obstet* 1957 195:310–318.
7. Couinaud C. *Le foie: etudes anatomiques et chirurgicales.* Paris, Masson, 1957.
8. Bismuth H. Surgical anatomy and anatomical surgery of the liver. *World J Surg* 1982; 6:3–9.
9. Haller A. *Icones Anatomicae in quibus praecipae partes corporis humani delineate proponuntur et arteriarum potissimum historia continetur.* Gottingen. Vandenhoeck, 1756: VIII 270.
10. Tiedmann F. Tabularumarteriarumcorporushumani. In: Koerpers, Carlsruhe, Muller CF, eds. *Abbildungen der Pulsadern des menschlichen,* 1822:1–250.
11. Adachi B. *Arterien system der Japaner.* Kyoto: Kerkyusha, Tokyo Press 1928: Band II 46–60.
12. Flint ER. Abnormalities of the right hepatic, cystic and gastroduodenal arteries and of the bile duct. *Brit J Surg* 1923;10:509–519
13. Michels NA. *Blood supply and anatomy of the upper abdominal organs.* Philadelphia JB Lippincott Co, 1955:1–581.

14. Van Damme JP, Bonte J. The branches of the celiac trunk. *Acta Anat* 1985;122:110–114.
15. Michels NA. Newer anatomy of the liver and variant blood supply and collateral circulation. *Am J Surg* 1966;112(3):337–347.
16. Lautt WW. Mechanism and role of intrinsic regulation of hepatic arterial blood flow: hepatic arterial buffer response. *Am J Physiol* 1985;249(5 Pt 1):G549–556.
17. Turner MA, Fulcher AS. The cystic duct: normal anatomy and disease processes. *Radiographics* 2001;21(1):3–22.

IMAGING OF THE LIVER 2

Nestor Villamizar Ortiz* and Bryan M. Clary[†]

In the case of liver pathology, the combination of clinical history, tumor markers and appropriate imaging studies can reveal the correct diagnosis in the majority of patients without the need of biopsy.[1] Thus, it is important to know the characteristic features of different focal liver lesions in the most commonly used imaging modalities.

GENERAL CONSIDERATIONS

B mode ultrasound (US) is often the first line of investigation in liver disease; however, confirmatory studies are usually needed. The accuracy of US examination can be improved by using contrast-enhanced ultrasound (CEUS), which provides an assessment of contrast enhancement patterns of liver lesions in real-time. Transabdominal US is inferior in sensitivity for liver metastases compared to either CT or MRI. In contrast, intraoperative US (during which the transducer is placed directly upon the liver surface) is the most sensitive imaging technique for diagnosing liver metastases.[2] Intraoperative US can be helpful in assessing patency of the hepatic blood supply and delineating the extent of disease and vascular landmarks during hepatic resection. Endoscopic ultrasound (EUS) with fine needle aspiration (FNA) biopsy can establish the diagnosis of hepatocellular carcinoma (HCC) and has the potential to improve accuracy of staging compared with CT and MRI.

---

*Brigham and Woman's Hospital, Boston, MA 02115 USA
[†]Duke University Medical Center 3247, Durham, NC 27710 USA

Multidetector row helical computed tomography (MDCT) allows multiple passes through the liver in different vascular phases following bolus contrast injection. The "triple-phase" technique includes an early arterial phase, a late arterial phase, and a portal venous-dominant phase. Hypervascular liver lesions are best appreciated in the late arterial phase. With delayed- or equilibrium-phase scans, cysts can be readily characterised as well. However, when a lesion is indeterminate on contrast-enhanced CT, a dynamic contrast-enhanced MRI with gadolinium chelates is appropriate for lesion characterisation. Most examinations include a T1-weighted in-phase/out-of-phase spoiled gradient echo sequence (T1) and one or more T2-weighted sequences (T2). In addition, the use of MRI tissue-specific contrast agents, including extracellular agents, hepatocyte-specific agents and reticuloendothelial system-specific agents, allows improved detection and characterization of liver tumors. MRI is also useful for delineating vascular involvement and identifying additional intra-abdominal lesions. Helical CT scanning remains the favored technique by most radiologists because of the high cost of MRI, and the long duration required to obtain standard MRI images. Positron emission tomography (PET) has the advantage over cross-sectional anatomical imaging of providing whole body imaging, allowing the detection of multifocal and metastatic disease.[3,4]

BENIGN LESIONS

Lesions smaller than 1 cm found incidentally in imaging studies of the liver are usually benign and, in most cases, represent cysts, hemangiomas and biliary hamartomas.

Symple Cysts

Cysts are the most common focal liver lesion and their incidence increases with age.[5]

Study	Characteristics
US	Well-defined thin wall, hyperechoic
CT	Noncontrast: Very sharply demarcated wall and near water density in the cyst. Contrast: No enhancement (Figure 1).
MRI	T2: Well-defined, very hyperintense. Contrast: No enhancement. **More specific for very small lesions than CT or US.**

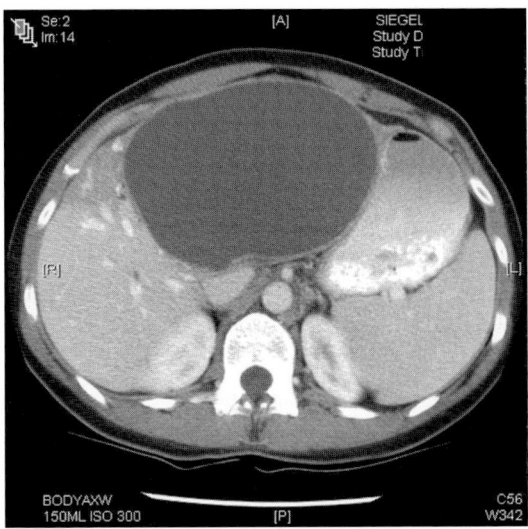

Figure 1. CT scan image of simple liver cyst.

Cystadenoma

Study	Characteristics
US	Hypoechoic, thickened irregular walls and occasional internal echoes representing debris and wall nodularity.
CT	Hypodense, thickened and/or irregular wall, uni- or multilocular, may have septations (Figure 2).

Cystadenocarcinomas are usually multilocular and resemble cystadenomas.

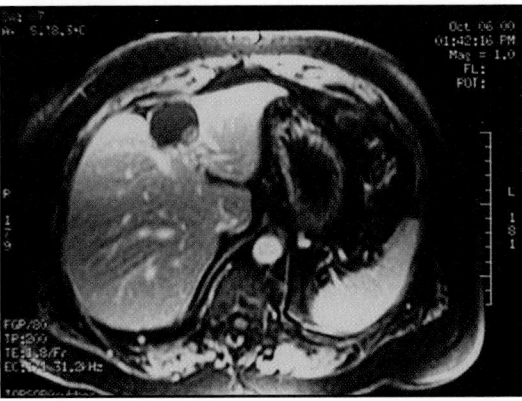

Figure 2. CT scan image of liver cystadenoma.

Cavernous Hemangioma

Study	Characteristics
US	Well-demarcated, homogeneous, hyperechoic. Its appearance overlap with that of HCC and hepatic metastases.
CT	Noncontrast: Well-demarcated, hypodense. Contrast: Peripheral nodular enhancement in the early phase, followed by "filling in" during the late phase. Classically opacify after a delay of 3 or more minutes and remain isodense or hyperdense on delayed scans (Figure 3).
MRI	T1: Smooth, well-demarcated, hypointense, homogeneous. T2: Hyperintense. Contrast: Gadolinium diethylenetriaminepentaacetic acid (Gd-DTPA) results in early peripheral discontinuous nodular or globular enhancement on arterial phase with progressive "filling-in" on delayed scans.

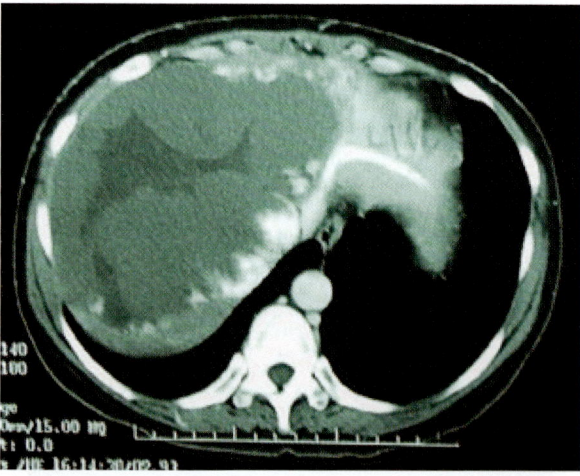

Figure 3. CT scan image of cavernous hemangioma of the liver.

Other radiologic studies

Technetium-99m pertechnetate-labeled red blood cell pool study

Initial hypoperfusion during arterial flow followed by a gradual increase of tracer peaking at 30–50 minutes. The best use of 99mTc-RBC SPECT is for lesions >2 cm to confirm a suspected hemangioma seen as a hyperechoic lesion in ultrasound and to clarify the diagnosis when CT findings are unclear.

Angiography

Reserved for atypical tumors that cannot be diagnosed definitively after multiple non-invasive imaging tests.

Hepatic Adenoma

Study	Characteristics
US	Usually hyperechoic with a central hypoechoic region, which corresponds to hemorrhage. Often large and in the right lobe of the liver.[6]
CT	Noncontrast: Often have central changes consistent with hemorrhage. Contrast: Absence of punctate enhancement of the central scar during the arterial phase, which differentiates them from focal nodular hyperplasia (Figure 4).
MRI	T1: Hyperintense as a result of lipid, and central hemorrhage. T2: Heterogeneous appearance.

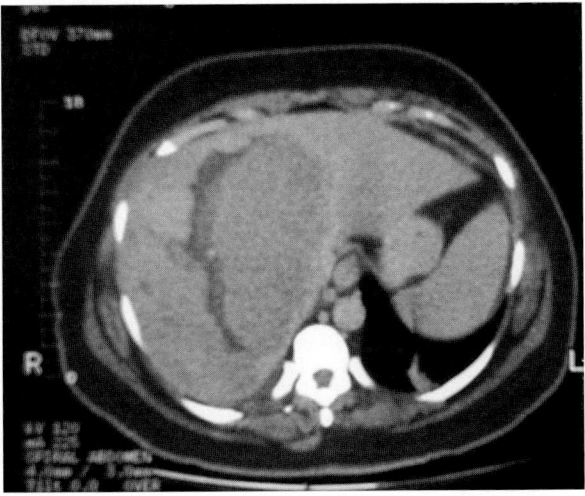

Figure 4. CT scan image of liver hepatic adenoma.

Other radiologic studies

Technetium-99m (99mTc) sulfur colloid scanning

Rarely used. Hepatic adenoma (HA) is seen as a "cold" spot in liver because most adenomas do not take up the sulfur colloid, in contrast to focal nodular hyperplasia (FNH).

Angiography

Rarely used. Approximately one-half of adenomas have the typical features of a hypervascular well-circumscribed tumor with increased peripheral vascularity, in contrast to the central vessel seen in FNH.

Focal Nodular Hyperplasia

Study	Characteristics
US	Variably hyper-, hypo-, or isoechoic.
CT	Noncontrast: Hypo- or isodense. Central scar identified in one-third of patients.
	Contrast: Hyperdense during the hepatic arterial phase due to the arterial origin of its blood supply, and is generally isodense during the portal venous phase, although the central scar may become hyperdense as contrast diffuses into the scar. While characteristic of FNH, a central scar may be present in the fibrolamellar variant of HCC.
MRI	T1: Isointense
	T2: Isointense to slightly hyperintense. The scar is typically hyperintense due to vessels or edema within it.
	Contrast: Hyperintense on early films and more isointense on delayed images (Figure 5).

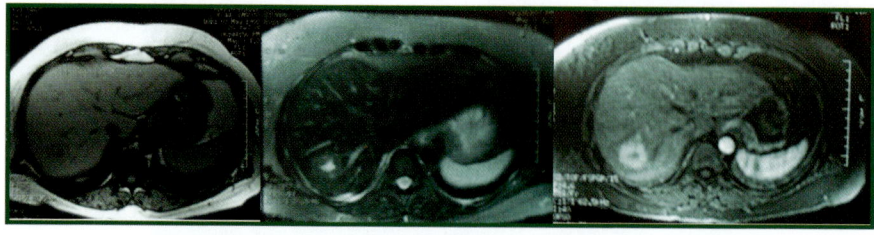

Figure 5. MRI image of focal nodular hyperplasia of the liver.

Other radiologic studies

Technetium sulfur colloid scanning

A characteristic of focal nodular hyperplasia (FNH) is that it usually contains Kupffer cells. Thus, 80% of lesions will show active uptake of technetium sulfur colloid on nuclear medicine scanning, whereas HA and HCC, which lack Kupffer cells, generally will not.

Pyogenic and Amebic Abscess

Pyogenic liver abscess cannot be distinguished from amebic abscess by imaging studies. Most amebic abscesses occur in the right lobe of the liver.

Study	Characteristics
US	Hypoechoic. Single or multiple, round or oval.
CT	Rounded areas that do not enhance, surrounded by a rim-like area of inflammation with increased enhancement.

Other radiologic studies

Chest X-Ray

Fifty percent of patients show an elevated right hemidiaphragm, right basilar infiltrate or right-sided pleural effusion.

MALIGNANT LESIONS

Malignant tumors of the liver are more common than benign lesions.

Metastatic Tumors

In Western countries, metastatic liver tumors are the most common malignant hepatic neoplasm.

Study	Characteristics
US	Findings are variable. As a general rule, metastases from adenocarcinoma are multiple and hypoechoic.[7] Hypoechoic rims and internal heterogeneity also distinguish metastases from most other masses.
CT	Metastatic liver lesions from the colon, stomach, and pancreas are usually hypodense,[8] (Figure 6). Hypervascular metastases, such as those from neuroendocrine tumors (Figure 7), renal cell carcinoma, breast carcinoma, melanoma, and thyroid carcinoma, appear as rapidly enhancing lesions visible on the arterial phase.
MRI	T1: Hypointense T2: Hyperintense Contrast: Because the volume of contrast is much lower than that of CT, better separation of arterial and portal phases can be achieved, improving detection of hypervascular lesions.

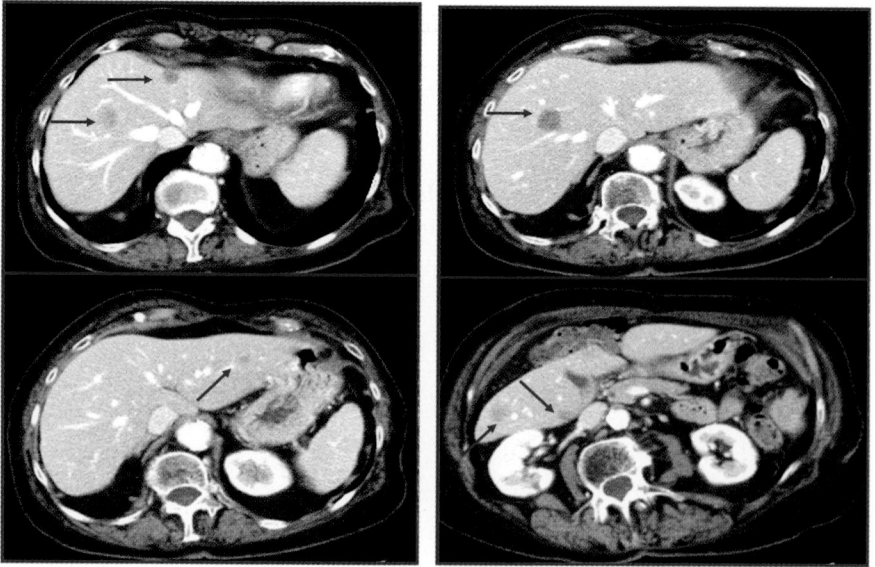

Figure 6. CT scan image of metastatic colon cancer of the liver.

Neuroendocrine Metastasis-CT scan

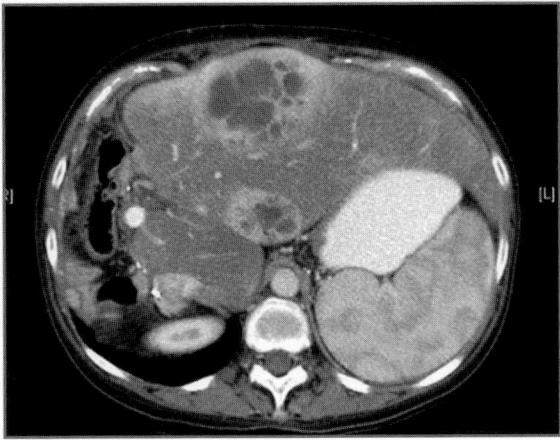

Figure 7. CT scan image of metastatic neuroendocrine tumor of the liver.

Hepatocellular Carcinoma

It can be challenging to distinguish hepatocellular carcinoma (HCC) from regenerative or even dysplastic nodules in patients with cirrhosis. MRI is currently the modality of choice in such settings since distinctions can sometimes be made based upon the enhancement pattern and the presence of iron in regenerative nodules.

Study	Characteristics
US	Sensitivity: 60% (95% CI 44–76%)
	Specificity: 97% (95% CI 95–98%)
	Poorly defined margins and coarse, irregular internal echoes. Small tumors are often hypoechoic. As the tumor grows, the echo pattern tends to become isoechoic or hyperechoic.
CT	Sensitivity: 68% (95% CI 55–80%)
	Specificity: 93% (95% CI 89–96%)
	The arterial phase of enhancement allows for the detection of hypervascular HCCs as small as 3 mm. Some tumors are isoattenuating on both arterial and portal phase imaging, and may be missed. The addition of delayed phase imaging (triple phase helical CT) may improve detection of these tumors (Figure 8).
MRI	Sensitivity: 81% (95% CI 70–91%)
	Specificity: 85% (95% CI 77–93%)
	T1: Hypointense
	T2: Hyperintense

Hepatocellular Carcinoma-CT scan

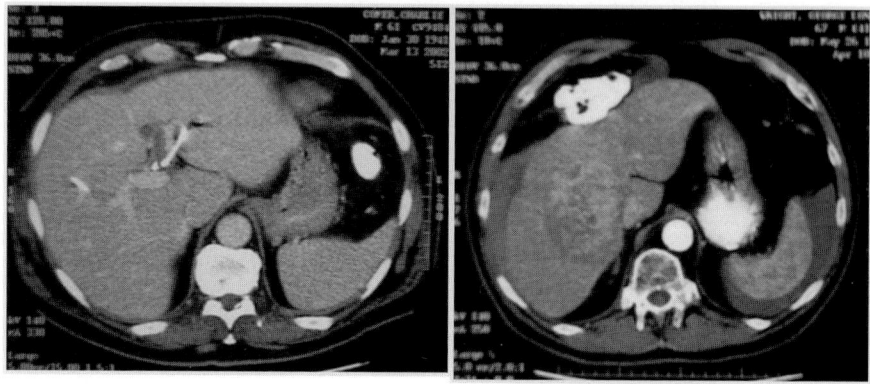

Figure 8.   CT scan image of hepatocellular carcinoma.

Other radiologic studies

Angiography

Indicated for chemoembolization of tumors and to control bleeding from ruptured HCC.

CT hepatic arteriography and arterial portography

Involves injection of contrast dye intraarterially (usually in the superior mesenteric, hepatic, or splenic artery) immediately prior to CT or MRI, and obtaining images during the arterial and portal venous phases. It is uncommonly used in the United States because it is invasive and does not appear to be more accurate.

Experimental imaging modalities

Technetium-99m (99mTc)-labeled anti-alpha-fetoprotein (AFP) Fab' imaging kit may have a role in the detection of HCC.

PET scanning

Its place in the diagnostic and staging evaluation of HCC remains uncertain. HCCs accumulate [^{18}F]fluorodeoxyglucose (FDG) to varying degrees, limiting the sensitivity of PET for primary tumors. A new tracer, [^{11}C]acetate, may improve sensitivity and specificity when used in conjunction with ^{18}F-FDG PET, but is not yet commercially available in the United States.

Cholangiocarcinoma

Study	Characteristics
US	Intrahepatic cholangiocarcinomas appear as a mass lesion. Perihilar and extrahepatic cancers may not be detected, especially if small, but indirect signs (ductal dilatation throughout the obstructed liver segments) may point toward the diagnosis. Papillary tumors appear as polypoid intraluminal masses.
	Nodular cholangiocarcinomas appear as discrete smooth masses with associated mural thickening.
CT	Tumors are globally hypodense during the portal venous phase 70% hyperattenuated on delayed images.[9] Ductal dilatation in both hepatic lobes with a contracted gallbladder or nonunion of the right and left hepatic ducts with or without a visibly thickened wall suggests a Klatskin tumor. Dilatation of the ducts within an atrophied hepatic lobe, in conjunction with a hypertrophic contralateral lobe (the atrophy-hypertrophy complex) suggests invasion of the portal vein. The relationship of the tumor to the vessels and surrounding organs is more easily evaluated on CT as opposed to MRI.
MRCP	T1: Hypointense.
	T2: Hyperintense. May also show central hypointensity corresponding to areas of fibrosis.
	Contrast: Peripheral enhancement followed by progressive and concentric filling in of the tumor. Pooling of contrast on delayed images.

Other radiologic studies

Cholangiography

Indicated if the suspected level of obstruction is distal, or if preoperative drainage of the biliary tree is needed.

Endoscopic ultrasound

Can visualize the local extent of the primary tumor and the status of regional lymph nodes for distal bile duct lesions.

PET scan

The bile duct epithelium has high glucose uptake. In addition, acute cholangitis can cause a false-positive study. Thus, the place of PET scanning in the evaluation of these patients remains unresolved.

Angiography

It can accurately document vascular encasement or thrombosis of the portal vein and hepatic artery. However, with the advent of multiphasic CT and MRCP, it is rarely necessary before surgery.

REFERENCES

1. Torzilli G, Minagawa M, Takayama T, *et al.* Accurate preoperative evaluation of liver mass lesions without fine-needle biopsy. *Hepatology* 1999; 30(4): 889–893.
2. Hagspiel KD, Neidl KF, Eichenberger AC, *et al.* Detection of liver metastases: comparison of superparamagnetic iron oxide-enhanced and unenhanced MR imaging at 1.5 T with dynamic CT, intraoperative US, and percutaneous US. *Radiology* 1995; 196(2):471–478.
3. Ariff B, Lloyd CR, Khan S, *et al.* Imaging of liver cancer. *World J Gastroenterol* 2009; 15(11):1289–1300.
4. Oliva MR, Saini S. Liver cancer imaging: role of CT, MRI, US and PET. *Cancer Imaging* 2004; 4 Spec No A:S42–S46.

5. Gaines PA, Sampson MA. The prevalence and characterization of simple hepatic cysts by ultrasound examination. *Br J Radiol* 1989; 62(736): 335–357.
6. Sandler MA, Petrocelli RD, *et al.* Ultrasonic features and radionuclide correlation in liver cell adenoma and focal nodular hyperlasia. *Radiology* 1980; 135(2):393–397.
7. Sheiner PA, Brower ST. Treatment of metastatic cancer to the liver. *Semin Liver Dis* 1994; 14(2):169–177.
8. Ros PR, Davis GL. The incidental focal liver lesion: photon, proton, or needle? *Hepatology* 1998; 27(5):1183–1190.
9. Valls C, Guma A, Puig I, *et al.* Intrahepatic peripheral cholangiocarcinoma: CT evaluation. *Abdom Imaging* 2000; 25(5):490–496.

HEPATIC ABSCESS 3

Georgia Beasley* and
Dan G. Blazer III*

INTRODUCTION

Hepatic abscess is an increasingly more common intra-abdominal infection that, despite modern management techniques, can still carry considerable morbidity and mortality. The annual incidence of hepatic abscess has been estimated at 2.3 cases per 100,000 and is higher among men than women.[1] Hepatic abscess may be separated into three major categories: pyogenic (bacterial), fungal, and amoebic. Pyogenic abscesses are the most common (approximately 80%), followed by amebic (approximately 10%), then fungal (less than 10 %).[1] In this chapter, the epidemiology, pathogenesis, clinical presentation, and treatment options for each type of liver abscess will be discussed.

PYOGENIC ABSCESS

Epidemiology/Pathogenesis

Pyogenic abscess is by far the most common type of hepatic abscess in industrialized countries primarily resulting from spread of infection via the portal circulation, ascending biliary infection, hematogenous spread of systemic infection, and direct extension. Other than the risks

---

*Duke University Medical Center 3247, Durham, NC 27710 USA

associated with the primary disease process, other risk factors for hepatic abscess include immunosuppressed state, malignancy, diabetes, chronic granulomatous disease, liver transplant and patients receiving chemotherapy. Historically, infection via the portal vein circulation from sources such as appendicitis, diverticulitis, inflammatory bowel disease, or pelvic inflammatory disease represented the most common etiology for pyogenic hepatic abscess. First reported in the landmark paper by Ochsner and Debakey in 1938, appendicitis itself was implicated in a third of all hepatic abscesses.[2] In the modern era, biliary disease is the most common etiology, accounting for 40% to 60% of pyogenic liver abscesses.[1] Sources may include cholecystitis, cholangitis, and instrumentation of the biliary tract. Direct infection may occur from penetrating trauma, perforated viscus, or local tumor ablative techniques such as ethanol injection, radiofrequency ablation, or cryotherapy. Finally, a significant percentage of abscesses (48%) remain cryptogenic despite a thorough search for a cause.[3]

Pyogenic abscesses involve the right lobe of the liver in approximately 70% of cases.[3] While the exact explanation for this observation is unknown, the preferential laminar blood flow to the right lobe of the liver has been postulated as a reason for the increased incidence of hepatic abscesses in the right lobe as opposed to the left lobe of the liver. The right lobe of the liver also has a larger blood supply. The left lobe and caudate lobe are uncommonly involved and bilobar involvement is rare.

A variety of pathogens have been associated with pyogenic abscesses, in part due to the variety of etiologies. A bacterial pathogen is identified in about two thirds of cases. Historically, the most commonly isolated organism was *Escherichia coli* but Klebsiella appears to be emerging as an important pathogen.[3] Generally, most pyogenic liver abscesses are polymicrobial. Mixed facultative and anaerobic species are common, although anaerobes are likely underreported as they are difficult to characterize in the laboratory. Anaerobes are more likely recovered from abscess aspiration[3] as opposed to blood cultures. As such, aspiration is an important diagnostic as well as therapeutic tool.

While mixed infections are most common, abscesses that develop as the result of systemic infections may more commonly be the result of a single organism. When the primary source is outside the abdomen, gram-positive organisms such as *S. aureus* and *S. pyogenes* tend to be more common. The streptococcus milleri group (*S. anginosus, S. constellatus, S. intermedius*) are less frequent causes but have been reported. Other rare pathogens include tuberculous and *Burkholderia pseudomallei* (endemic to South East Asia and Northern Australia.)

An important emerging pathogen noted to cause pyogenic liver abscesses is *Klebsiella pneumoniae*. The clinical entity associated with this infection was first described as an emerging disease in Taiwan in the 1990s.[4] The disease was predominantly reported to affect diabetic, middle-aged individuals and led to serious systemic complications such as endophthalmitis. The visual acuity outcome is poor in patients who develop endophthalmitis despite early and appropriate intervention.[4] An increasing number of reports from the United States suggest that *Klebsiella pneumoniae* should be suspected in patients presenting with hepatic abscesses.[3]

Clinical Presentation/Diagnosis

Clinical diagnosis of hepatic abscess in the absence of appropriate imaging is difficult. Clinical manifestations of pyogenic liver abscesses usually include fever (90%) and abdominal pain (50–75%).[2,5] There is also a broad array of constitutional symptoms that can be found including: malaise, chills, vomiting, cough (from diaphragmatic involvement), nausea, anorexia, weight loss. Jaundice is found about 25% of the time.[5] History of recent travel, diabetes, alcohol use, and immunosuppressed state may raise clinical suspicion. Laboratory abnormalities may include leukocytosis (70–90%), elevated bilirubin or liver enzymes, and elevation of serum alkaline phosphatase.[2,3,5] Blood cultures will be positive in approximately 30–50% of patients.

The definitive diagnosis of hepatic abscess is made by radiographic imaging. Chest radiographs may show an elevated right hemidiaphragm, right basilar infiltrate, or right-sided effusions.[5] Ultrasonographic evaluation may reveal hypoechoic masses with irregularly shaped borders as well as internal septations or cavity debris. The sensitivity of ultrasound is approximately 80–90%.[1] The major benefits of this technique are its portability and diagnostic utility in patients who are critically ill. In the modern era, CT is the most important imaging modality. The sensitivity of CT in diagnosing hepatic abscess is about 95% to 100%.[5] On CT, an abscess appears as a fluid collection with surrounding edema and inflammation that may be loculated with peripheral enhancement when intravenous contrast is given (Figure 1). Gas can also be seen in as many as 20% of lesions.[1,2] CT scan also enables the evaluation for the underlying etiology (e.g. appendicitis, diverticulitis).

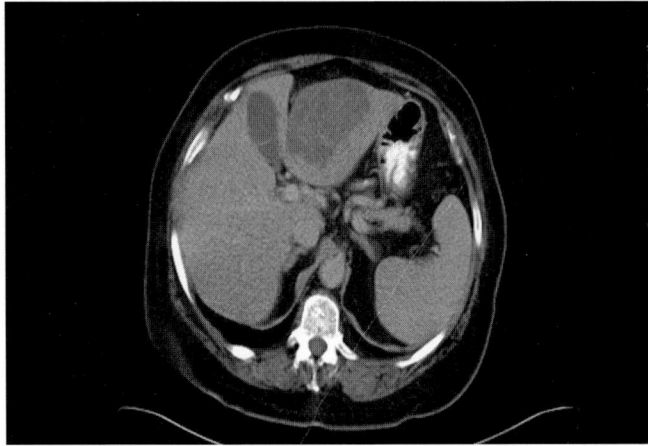

Figure 1. A CT scan demonstrating a hepatic abscess.

Abscesses must be distinguished from tumors and cysts. Tumors generally have a more solid radiographic appearance while cysts appear as fluid collections without localized inflammation. Importantly, pyogenic liver abscesses cannot usually be distinguished from amebic abscesses by imaging studies.

Treatment

With the emergence of more effective antibiotics and percutaneous drainage techniques, the morbidity and mortality from pyogenic hepatic abscesses in the modern era has improved. Prior to their emergence, open surgical debridement was the only treatment that offered a chance for improved survival.

When pyogenic abscess is identified, broad-spectrum antibiotics should be started immediately and percutaneous drainage attempted for culture and potentially definitive therapy. Choice of antibiotics is based upon the probable source of infection and then tailored appropriately based on culture results. Combinations such as (1) ampicillin, an aminoglycoside and metronidazole, (2) a third-generation cephalosporin plus metronidazole (3) a fluoroquinolone plus metronidazole, or (4) monotherapy with a carbapenem are appropriate. There are no randomized controlled trials addressing the duration of antibiotic treatment but antibiotics are usually continued for at least 4 to 12 weeks.[3] Additionally, failure of initial antibiotic treatment should prompt consideration of rare pathogens and pursuit of additional culture data.

Treatment of a pyogenic abscess should also include drainage. Since the mid-1980s, open surgical drainage has been generally reserved for failure of percutaneous drainage. Drainage techniques include CT or ultrasound-guided percutaneous drainage with or without catheter placement. For simple abscesses with a diameter ≤5 cm, needle aspiration may be adequate.[6] For abscesses greater than 5 cm, catheter placement is preferred. If necessary, multiple drains should be placed for adequate drainage. Repeat imaging should be performed to evaluate resolution or progression of the abscess and should be repeated early if the patient is clinically not improving. Percutaneous aspiration/drainage and appropriate antibiotic therapy can be expected to be successful in the majority of cases (nearly 90%).

Open (or laparoscopic) surgical drainage is typically reserved for those cases in which percutaneous drainage has failed. Oschnher and DeBakey first described an extraperitoneal approach to avoid peritoneal or pleural contamination in the pre-antibiotic era. With improvements in techniques and antiobiotics, the transperitoneal approach for drainage of liver abscesses has become standard. The transperitoneal approach allows for adequate visualization and exploration of the entire abdomen for a source of primary infection. Abdominal exploration and potential source control (i.e. resection of perforated viscus) should precede abscess drainage. Drainage of the abscess should include sending fluid for culture and biopsy of the abscess wall. Partial hepatectomy of the involved portion of liver may be required especially in the case of multiple abscesses. Partial hepatectomy can provide an adequate salvage treatment when performed by an experienced surgeon. Closed suction drains should be placed into the abscess cavity and adjacent spaces; the drains will allow for continued drainage and may be used for irrigation. Laparoscopic drainage has been reported and may be appropriate for selected patients.

Finally, therapy should be directed at the underlying cause. The source if intra-abdominal may be identified on abdominal CT scan and the appropriate treatment should follow. Use of ERCP may be important for optimal biliary drainage. If an open approach for abscess drainage is used, surgical exploration of the entire abdomen should be performed including intraoperative cholangiogram and common duct exploration if appropriate.

Historically, mortality from hepatic abscesses was significant but in more modern series, mortality ranges from 2% to 15% with appropriate treatment. The mortality rates for liver abscesses are more likely related to underlying patient co morbidities such as malignancy and not the specific causative pathogen. Results from a recent study, which included 118 patients aged 65 years or older and 221 patients below age 65 years, indicated that age and an Acute Physiology and Chronic Health Evaluation APACHE II score of 15 or greater at hospital admission were risk factors for mortality.[7] A bilirubin level of greater than 3.5 mg/dL, encephalopathy, hypoalbuminemia (i.e. serum albumin level of <2 g/dL), and multiple abscesses are all independent factors that predict poor outcome.[7]

FUNGAL HEPATIC ABSCESS

Fungal hepatic abscesses, primarily Candida species, are rare although they are being recognized with increasing frequency in immunocompromised patients and those with malignant diseases.[8] These abscesses tend to be associated with multiple abscesses. Candida species may also be implicated in mixed infections, most commonly in patients with neutropenia following chemotherapy. Treatment principles for fungal abscesses are similar to that of pyogenic abscesses. Early institution of appropriate antifungal therapy and effective drainage are critical. In patients with hematologic malignancies or other immunocompromised states, who are known to be at risk for fungal infections, amphotericin B treatment should be instituted early. Outcomes in these patients can be poor, especially those presenting with concurrent fungemia.

Hepatic actinomycosis is an even rarer cause of hepatic abscess. Predisposing factors remain largely unknown. Treatment includes prompt percutaneous drainage coupled with long-term intravenous administration of high-dose minocycline and piperacillin.[8] Hepatic actinomycosis should be considered in the differential diagnosis of pyogenic liver abscess, especially in patients that fail to improve with seemingly appropriate therapy.

AMEBIC ABSCESS

Though pyogenic hepatic abscess is much more common in the United States than amebic abscess, amebic abscess should be considered in every patient with hepatic abscess. A travel history should be elicited in all patients. Amebiasis is caused by the protozoan *Entamoeba histolytica*, which is endemic to Mexico, India, Africa, and parts of Central and South America. Approximately 40 to 50 million people are infected annually, with the majority of infections occurring in developing countries due to poorer socioeconomic conditions and sanitation standards.[9] Mortality rates are significant with 40,000 to 110, 000 deaths each year most from severe dehydration secondary to diarrhea. Amebiasis mortality is second only to malaria as cause of death from protozoan parasites.[9,10] In developed countries such as the United States, amebiasis is mainly seen in migrants from and travelers to endemic countries.

Epidemiology/Pathogenesis

Amebic liver abscesses are the most common manifestation of extraintestinal amebiasis. In contrast to pyogenic abscesses, patients with amebic liver abscesses tend to be younger males with a history of travel to an endemic area.[9] Tables 1 and 2 highlight major similarities and differences between pyogenic and amebic liver abscesses.

Hepatic infection occurs when amebae reach the liver through the portal circulation. Entamoeba histolytica is a protozoan that exists in two forms, a cyst stage and a trophozoite stage. Not all strains are considered virulent. Infection is generally via the fecal–oral route, typically through ingestion of contaminated water or vegetables. When cysts are swallowed, they cause infection by excysting (releasing the trophozoite stage) in the digestive tract. The trophozoite stage is readily killed in the environment and cannot survive passage through the acidic stomach to cause infection. Once ingested, the cysts pass into the colon where the trophozoite form is released. The trophozoite form can then invade the intestinal mucosa. The trophozoites then reach the liver through the portal venous system. The

Table 1. Similarities between pyogenic and amebic hepatic abscesses.

Often present with fever and abdominal pain.
More common in patients with immunosuppression.
More common in right hepatic lobe.
CT scan with hepatic fluid collections (may not be able to distinguish abscess type on CT).
Mortality low with proper treatment.

Table 2. Differences between pyogenic and amebic hepatic abscesses.

Pyogenic Abscesses	Amebic Abscesses
Any age	Younger males
Often polymicrobial	Protozoan
Some geographic variability	Endemic areas or h/o travel to endemic areas
Diagnosis with imaging +/− culture	Diagnosis confirmed with serum antibodies
CT with fluid collection and edema	CT with possible rim enhancing lesion
Treatment antiobiotics plus percutaneous drainage	Treatment metronidazole plus luminal agent

trophozoites cause the release of multiple enzymes thus causing localized hepatic necrosis. The necrosis leads to cavity formation in the liver surrounded by a rim of trophozoites.[9,10] The abscess that forms is a result of the liquefaction necrosis of the liver. The consistency of the fluid has the classical description of "anchovy paste". Glisson's capsule is resistant to hydrolysis by the amebae and thus abscesses tend to abut the liver capsule.[9] Secondary bacterial infections are rare but can occur as well.

Clinical Presentation

Clinical symptoms can include fulminant dysentery, bloody diarrhea, weight loss, fatigue, and abdominal pain. Patients with amebic liver abscesses often present with one to several weeks of abdominal pain and fever. Jaundice is a rare presentation and diarrhea occurs in about a third of patients. For travelers returning from an endemic area, presentation will occur within 5 months in 95% of cases.[9,10] Patients with secondary cardiac or pulmonary involvement may present with symptoms primarily due to these complications. Laboratory abnormalities include leukocytosis without eosinophilia, elevated prothrombin time.[9,10] More than 70% of patients with amebic liver abscesses do not have detectable amebae in their stool. As such, a number of different serological tests have been developed over the years to aid in the diagnosis.

Serum antibodies will be detectable in 92–95% of patients at the time of presentation with amebic liver abscess. Eventually 99% of patients will have positive antibody tests, but serological testing may be negative in the first 7 days. Up to 25% of noninfected individuals will also have positive antibodies due to previous infection. An indirect hemagglutination (IHA) has been used with a high sensitivity but again high rates of false positives occur especially in endemic areas. Newer techniques for diagnosis include a rapid enzyme immunoassay with a sensitivity of 93% and a serum antigen detection test that is positive in 75% of patients with amebic liver abscess. These newer techniques may prove to be particularly useful in endemic areas. Antigen tests and polymerase chain reaction (PCR) on aspirated material may also be helpful in establishing the diagnosis.

Finally, similar to pyogenic abscesses, radiologic studies aid in the diagnosis of amebic abscesses. Ultrasound may demonstrate a rounded lesion abutting the liver capsule. Similar to pyogenic abscesses, ultrasound may reveal hypoechoic masses with irregularly shaped borders as well as internal septations or cavity debris. Abdominal CT is likely more sensitive than ultrasound especially in detecting amoebic abscesses. Abdominal CT scan are excellent at detecting amebic abscesses although differentiating amebic from pyogenic abscesses is difficult. CT scan may demonstrate a peripheral rim enhancing liver lesion.

An important difference in the diagnosis of amebic versus pyogenic hepatic abscesses is that diagnostic aspiration is usually not necessary when clinical suspicion in high for an amebic source or laboratory data are confirmatory. In those rare cases when aspiration is necessary, an "anchovy paste" aspirate can be pathognomonic.

Treatment

The primary treatment for amebic abscesses is medical. Metronidazole therapy alone results in a cure rate of more than 90%.[9,10] Metronidazole is well absorbed from the gastrointestinal tract. Clinical improvements are often seen in the first few days following initiation of treatment. Most abscesses heal from the periphery usually in 4 weeks after initiating therapy. The mean time to complete radiologic resolution is 3–9 months with a greater than 50% reduction on liver size within a week.[18] Other nitroimidazoles are also effective. Tinidazole has been approved for the treatment of amebiasis (including amebic liver abscess) by the United States Food and Drug Administration (FDA). Emetine is another effective drug but has major cardiac side effects.

Following therapy for invasive amebiasis with a nitroimidazole (such as metronidazole), treatment with a luminal agent is required, even if stools were negative for organisms. Luminal agents are administered to treat the carrier state. Intraluminal colonization can be treated with agents such as paromomycin or iodoquinol.

Though rarely required for treatment, needle aspiration of amebic abscesses may be necessary, though its role is controversial. A recent review notes that approximately 10% to 15% of patients remain symptomatic despite proper drug treatment and have been been referred for percutaneous drainage.[9,10] Another subgroup of patients thought to potentially benefit from percutaneous drainage are those considered high risk of spontaneous rupture, which carries a higher mortality rate. However, prediction of rupture has been difficult so proper patient selection is difficult. The conclusion of this recent review was that no additional benefit for percutaneous needle aspiration has been definitively proven. Certainly, larger randomized trials are needed to more definitively clarify the role of percutaneous drainage for amebic hepatic abscesses.

As mentioned above, one complication of amebic abscesses is rupture into the peritoneum, pleural cavity, or pericardium. Size of the abscess appears to be the most important risk factor and the incidence of rupture ranges from 3% to 17%.[9,10] Most peritoneal ruptures are contained but rupture may result in fistulization, hollow viscus perforation, or hemorrhage that may not be adequately managed by percutaneous drainage and may require laparotomy. Rupture can increase the mortality of amebic abscesses from 2–4% to 6–30%.[9,10] Similar to pyogenic abscesses, factors associated with poor outcomes include patients that have concurrent chronic illnesses, immunosuppression, and inadequate treatment.

CONCLUSION

Hepatic abscesses can be separated into three categories: pyogenic (bacterial), fungal, and amoebic. Pyogenic abscesses are the most common (80%) in industrialized nations and are usually caused by an infection that has spread from an intra-abdominal or other systemic source although frequently no source is identified. There is a vast array of presenting symptoms and diagnosis is confirmed with CT scan. The mainstay of treatment is appropriate antibiotics and percutaneous abscess drainage with surgical debridment for those failing nonoperative management.

REFERENCES

1. Huang CJ, Pitt HA, Lipsett PA, *et al.* Pyogenic hepatic abscess: changing trends over 42 years. *Ann Surg* 1996; 223:600.
2. Oschner A, DeBakey M, Murray S. Pyogenic abscess of the liver II. An analysis of forty-seven cases with review of the literature. *Am J Surg* 1938; 40:292–319.
3. Rahimian J, Wilson T, Oram V, *et al.* Pyogenic liver abscess: recent trends in etiology and mortality. *CID* 2004; 39:1654–1659.
4. Lederman Edith R, Crum Nancy F. Pyogenic liver abscess with a focus on *Klebsiella pneumoniae* as a primary pathogen: an emerging disease with unique clinical characteristics. *Am J Gastroenterol* 2005; 100:322–331.
5. Branum GD, Tyson GS, Branum MA, *et al.* Hepatic abscess: changes in etiology, diagnosis, and management. *Ann Surg* 1990; 212:655–662.
6. Tan, YM, Chung AY, Chow PK, *et al.* An appraisal of surgical and percutaneous drainage for pyogenic liver abscesses larger than 5 cm. *Ann Surg* 2005; 241:485.
7. Chen SC, Lee YT, Yen CH, *et al.* Pyogenic liver abscess in the elderly: clinical features, outcomes and prognostic factors. *Age Ageing* 2009; 38(3):271–276.
8. Lipsett PA, Huang CJ, Lillemoe KD, *et al.* Fungal hepatic abscesses: characterization and management. *J Gastrointest Surg.* 1997; 1(1):78–84.
9. Haque R, Huston CD, Hughes M, *et al.* Amebiasis. *N Engl J Med* 2003; 348:1565.
10. Maltz G, Knauer CM. Amebic liver abscess: a 15-year experience. *Am J Gastroenterol* 1991; 86:704.

CYSTIC DISEASES OF THE LIVER 4

Marcus Darrabie* and
Carlos E. Marroquin[†]

INTRODUCTION

Liver cysts were initially thought to be rare and incidental findings on surgical exploration. However with the increasing use and refinement of modern imaging modalities, the known incidence has increased to between 3% and 5%. This represents an underestimate as most cysts are unrecognized and asymptomatic. The first reported case of a simple nonparasitic liver cysts occurred in 1856 by Bristowe.[1,2] In contrast, hydatid or parasitic disease has been described since antiquity. Liver cysts are broadly classified as either congenital or acquired and can be subdivided into the following subcategories:

I. Congenital
    a. Simple cyst
    b. Polycystic disease
    c. Choledochal cysts
    d. Bile duct hamartomas
    e. Epidermoid cysts

---

*Department of Surgery, Duke University, Durham, North Carolina
[†]Department of Surgery, University of Rochester, Rochester, New York

II. Acquired
   a. Hydatid diseased (Echinococcal disease)
   b. Neoplastic
      i. Primary: cystadenoma, cystadenocarcinoma, cystic hemangioma, hepatocellular carcinoma
      ii. Secondary: ovary, pancreas, kidney, colon neuroendocrine
   c. False cysts
      i. Intrahepatic abscess or biloma
      ii. Traumatic hematoma

CONGENITAL DISEASE

Simple Hepatic Cysts

Nonparasitic simple cysts are usually asymptomatic and unrecognized. They can be found in 1–5% of the general population with a general 4:1 female predilection. Incidence increases to more than 75% in people older than 70 years of age.[3] They are thought to arise as congenital aberrations during bile duct development. Abdominal ultrasonography demonstrates a well-circumscribed, unilocular or multilocular lesion with internal septae. Cyst dimensions are variable and range from microscopic to lobular. Cyst architecture consists of a dominant cyst that may be accompanied by smaller peripheral cysts. The cysts may be entirely intrahepatic or pedunculated. Histologically, simple cysts are composed of cellular connective tissue lined with cuboidal epithelial cells (Figure 1). Internal analysis of cyst contents demonstrates serous or semisolid organized clot with varying amounts of albumin, mucin, cholesterol, blood, hematoidin, hemosedirin, as well as granular or cellular debris.[1]

Patients with uncomplicated cysts may present with nausea, vomiting, early satiety or obstructive jaundice. A third of these patients have abnormal liver function tests. Large cysts may become symptomatic from mass effect and can be complicated by severe pain, torsion, hemorrhage or infection. Additionally, a bleeding or hemorrhagic cyst may cause rapid enlargement, with rupture leading to peritonitis. Due to a relatively low incidence, no major consensus guidelines have been established. Indications for intervention include symptomatic cysts or rapid enlargement. Several groups have suggested intervention for symptomatic cysts >5 cm and nonsymptomatic cysts >10 cm.[4] Conservative management consists of aspiration, sclerotherapy, or percutaneous drainage. These interventions have demonstrated safety and

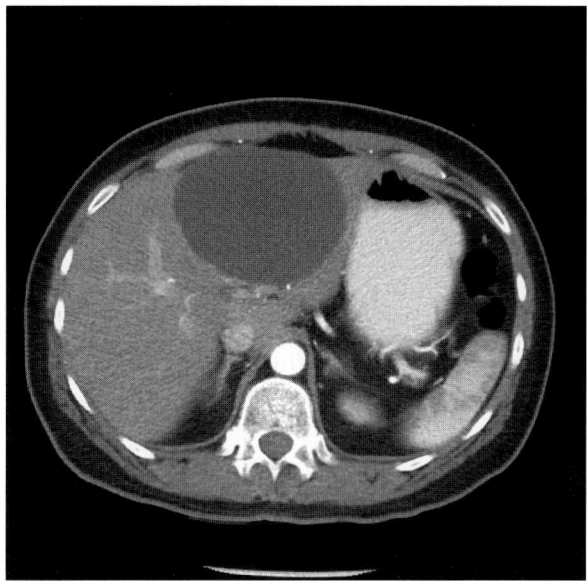

Figure 1. Large simple hepatic cyst.
CT scan demonstrating a large simple hepatic cyst. The usual defining features include thin, smooth wall shape with homogenous and hypoenhancing fluid-filled density and lack of internal septae or structures.

efficacy as an initial step for small simple cysts, though, in general, have high rates of recurrence. Image-guided puncture and aspiration, which can decompress cysts, can be combined with sclerotherapy to limit recurrence.

Prior to the laparoscopic era, hepatic resection was the definitive therapy of simple cysts. Laparoscopic deroofing, first reported in 1991, is now the treatment of choice for simple uncomplicated cysts.5 The decision for open versus minimally invasive surgery depends on the number of cysts, cyst location and potential for malignancy. Large posterior cysts in the right lobe have been particularly prone to recurrence as they are inadequately drained by deroofing and may require Roux-en-Y cystojejunostomy or hand assisted mobilization if attempted laporsocopically. Our preferred approach to these lesions is purely laparoscopically with the patient in the left lateral decubitius position and the bed maximally extended to open the angle between the costal margin and iliac crest. Trocars are placed approximately 5 to 7 cms below the costal margin at the mid-clavicular line, and the anterior and posterior axillary lines. The right triangular ligament is divided with the harmonic scalpel allowing the liver to be mobilized medially. Occasionally, the heptic flexure of the colon must be mobilized, but both of these maneuvers may be performed in a relatively straight forward fashion. Once mobilized, a rigid laparoscopic ultrasound probe is used to identify the cyst and subsequently drain the fluid with suction aspirator. Once drained, the cyst is unroofed with combinations of sharp dissection with the harmonic scalpel and divided with endoscopic staplers. Once unroofed, segments of the cyst wall can and should be sent to pathology and the lining fulgurated with the argon beam. Several large series have demonstrated similar recurrence rates between the two procedures, with slightly lower morbidity and hospital stay in the laparoscopic group.

Polycystic Disease of the Liver

Polycystic liver disease is often associated with polycystic kidney disease and is concurrently associated in almost 50% of reported cases. Autopsy series show a general prevalence of 0.13% to 0.6%. The first significant clinical description was provided by Bristowe in 1856.[2] The inciting process is a failure of intralobular bile duct involution during the developmental process. Cystic proliferation and overgrowth occurs in a setting of abnormal cell arrangements. The genes responsible are inherited in an autosomal dominant fashion and have been identified as PKD1 on chromosome 16 and PKD2 on chromosome 4. Another gene on chromosome 6, PKHD1, has been linked to an autosomal recessive form of the disorder. A classification system has been described on the basis of cyst number, size and presence of nonaffected liver.[8] Type I patients consist of less than 10 large cysts (>10 cm) and limited parenchyma involvement. Type II disease consist of patients with diffuse medium sized cyst involvement with large areas of nonaffected liver involvement. Type III disease consists of widespread, medium and small cysts with minimal sparring of the liver.

Clinical presentation of liver disease has increased due to effective treatment of renal disease. Symptoms are often related to mass effect which can cause a sensation of fullness and dull abdominal pain. In complicated cases, sequelae of severe liver disease can include: ascites, obstructive jaundice, portal hypertension, bleeding varices, cholangitis, or liver abscesses. Progression to fulminant liver disease is rare, though cyst enlargement may lead to the above described symptoms. The diagnosis can be made with

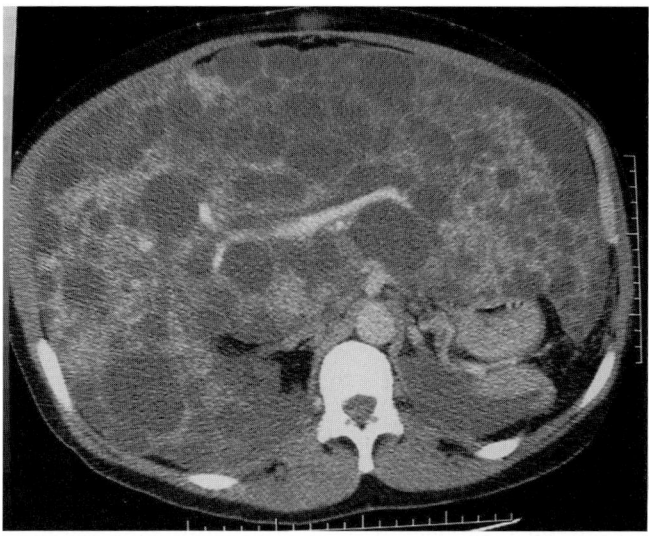

Figure 2. Polycystic liver disease.
CT scan showing polycystic liver disease which can present as multiple diffuse cysts throughout the liver parenchyma. A mixed pattern of large and small, hypoattenuating, thin-walled cysts with resultant hepatomegaly of the liver is shown.

ultrasound or CT scanning (Figure 2). In most cases the diagnosis of polycystic kidney disease is made initially.

As seen in other cystic lesions, treatment is reserved for symptomatic patients. No effective medical therapies exist, however surgical options include cyst aspiration with sclerotherapy, cyst fenestration, laparoscopic and open hepatic resection. In rare cases, transplantation has been performed. Cyst aspiration and sclerotherapy are best suited for inoperable candidates or lesions with minimal cysts. The ultimate goal of therapy is decompression and preservation of normal liver parenchyma. In high risk surgical patients, aspiration and sclerosis is a viable option. While morbidity is low with this procedure, recurrence rates are high. Type I polycystic liver disease candidates are ideally suited for fenestration, which involves deroofing and wide excision of the cyst wall. Laparoscopic fenestration can be performed safely and with minimal morbidity and mortality. The procedure is optimally performed in certain disease profiles as patients with predominant cystic disease in segments VI, VII, VIII as well as deep seated cysts are prone to recurrence from nonvisualized or inadequately fenestrated cysts.[9]

One large series consisting of 44 patients undergoing laparoscopic versus open fenestration demonstrated similar morbidity and mortality with a 13% versus. 11% recurrence rate in the open and laparoscopic groups respectively.[9-10] In several small series, liver transplantation was successfully performed as definitive therapy. Given the resources and requirements for transplantation, the procedure is limited to highly symptomatic patients with extensive disease. Additionally, the risks and benefits of resection must be evaluated in the context of sympatology.[11]

Choledochal Cyst

Choledochal cysts are congenital abnormalities of the bile duct system resulting in cystic dilation of the extrahepatic and intrahepatic biliary tree. The abnormality was first described by Vater and Ezler in 1723. Alonso-Lej *et al.* is credited with an initial three-group classification system which was expanded to the current classification by Todani.[12] Choledochal cysts are rare with a reported incidence of 1 case per 2 million. The etiology is somewhat unclear and likely multifactorial. Defects in the epithelial development and recanalization of the bile ducts during organogenesis result in weakness of the bile duct. Alternatively, a vast majority of patients have been shown to have an anomalous pancreatobiliary junction which predisposes pancreatic secretions and enzymes to reflux into the bile duct causing inflammation and weakening of the bile duct wall.[13]

In general, complications increase with age. Infants or children with disease may be recognized early as biliary obstruction can lead to jaundice or a palpable mass may be identified in the right upper quadrant. Children may develop pancreatitis or cholangitis with histological evidence of hepatocellular inflammation and damage. The most concerning complication is malignant transformation to cholangiocarcinoma, with a reported rate of 9–28%. The risk of malignant transformation increases to as high as 14% after the age of 20. Subclinical inflammation and biliary stasis may go unrecognized for years with symptoms manifesting in adulthood. Adults may present with hepatic abscesses, cirrhosis, and recurrent pancreatitis due to long standing biliary obstruction and cholangitis. A classic triad of abdominal pain, jaundice and palpable right upper quadrant abdominal mass has been described but is only seen in 10–20% patients. Initial workup consists of ultrasound scanning to help establish the initial diagnosis. More precise detail of the duct anatomy can be obtained with CT scanning, percutaneous cholangiography, MRI, or MRCP.

The classification system based on Todani description:

- **Type IA:** Saccular dilation with partial involvement of the extrahepatic bile duct.
- **Type IB:** Saccular dilation involving a limited segment of the CBD.
- **Type IC:** Fusiform dilation involving most or all of the extrahepatic bile duct.
- **Type II:** Isolated diverticulum protruding from the CBD.
- **Type III or choledochocele:** Arise from dilatation of duodenal portion of CBD or where pancreatic duct meets.
- **Type IVA:** Dilatation of both intrahepatic and extrahepatic biliary duct.
- **Type IVB:** Multiple extrahepatic cysts.
- **Type V or Caroli's disease:** Cystic dilatation of intra hepatic biliary ducts.

Type I choledochal cysts are most common of the choledochal cysts representing 80-90%. Type I cysts are dilatations of the entire common bile ducts or portions of the duct. Type II choledochal cysts are diverticula that project from the common bile duct, and Type III choledochal cysts are dilatations of the duodenal portion of the common bile duct; these are also referred to as choledochoceles. Type and IVA and type V or Caroli's disease are special subtypes that extend to the intrahepatic portions of the biliary tree. They are therefore prone to secondary complications such as hepatolithiasis, recurrent cholangitis, and biliary cirrhosis.

The treatment of choice for choledochal cysts is operative therapy. Type I choledochal cyst are managed with complete resection of the cyst with Roux-en-Y hepatico-jejunostomy. Type II choledochal cysts are also managed with resection, and the extent of the defect will determine if it can be repaired primarily over a T-tube or a formal hepatico-jejunostomy is necessary. Treatment of type III choledochal cysts are excised through a transduodenal approach. The choledochocele is enucleated and the common bile duct and pancreatic duct are re-implanted into the duodenum with a mucosal to mucosal approach. Type IVA choledochal cysts are managed with excision of the dilated extrahepatic duct. Biliary and enteric continuity is established in most cases with a Roux-en-Y biliary-enteric anastomosis. Resection of the intrahepatic dilatation is usually withheld, though it is often performed in instances where dilation, with multiple abscesses or hepatolithiasis, is limited to a focal area of the liver. Additionally, transhepatic or transjejunal tubes can be placed to reduce complications and assist in the reduction of intrahepatic stones. Malignant transformation in the residual intrahepatic component is a potential concern, however, is rarely encountered.

Type V choledochal cyst, or Caroli's disease, is characterized by dilatation of the intrahepatic ducts. Despite similar radiographical findings, Caroli's disease has a particularly unique constellation of clinical findings that distinguishes it from other choledochal cysts. It has been linked with several chromosomal abnormalities and is suggested to arise from ductal plate abnormalities. Clinically, patients may present with congenital hepatic fibrosis as well as hepatolithiasis and renal disease. Cholangitis is a common complication and in general there is a 7% risk of cholangiocarcinoma. If dilatation is limited to a single hepatic lobe, usually the left, the affected lobe is resected. Patients who have bilobar disease and signs of biliary cirrhosis, portal hypertension, or liver failure may be candidates for liver transplantation.[14–15]

Laparoscopic techniques have been utilized successfully in the management of choledochal cysts. Angiographic techniques have also been utilized to treat complications of choledochal cysts. One group reported embolization of an actively bleeding artery after the hepatic artery was ruptured by a choledochal cyst.[16] Additionally, ultrasound-guided, percutaneous choledochal cystostomy has been performed in children with severe hepatic dysfunction as a temporizing measure to decompress the biliary system until the infants were ready to undergo surgery.[17]

Bile Duct Hamartoma

Biliary hamaratomas or von Meyenburg complexes are cystic tumors that originate from embryonic bile ducts that fail to involute. They are generally benign and present as incidental findings on imaging or laparotomy. Most lesions are found in children prior to the age of 2. The majority of lesions are found in female and occur in the right lobe of the liver, however may also be present throughout the liver. Histologically, they may appear as gray-white nodular lesions. It may be challenging to distinguish these lesions from metastatic disease or other forms of cystic dilation. The lesions have been described in cirrhotic livers and are often associated with polycystic liver disease. Abdominal imaging demonstrates a well-defined, anechoic, multi or unilocular structure on ultrasound. CT demonstrates a hypovascular mass with a capsule with cystic or solid components. A theoretical malignant potential has been described, however, little to no evidence has been shown to support malignant transformation. Nonetheless, they may enlarge at a rapid rate and become very large. Surgical procedures such as enucleation and marsupialization have been performed, though definitive therapy in symptomatic patients consists of local excision or lobectomy.[18]

Epidermoid Cysts

Epidermoid cysts of the liver are extremely rare. Few cases have been described in the literature. In general, the lesions are benign, asymptomatic and slow growing. They may be unilocular or multilocular. As they become larger in size, obstructive symptoms may appear such as jaundice, abdominal pain, or cyst rupture. Histologically, cysts may contain cuboidal, columnar, squamous or pseudostratified cylindrical epithelial types. In some cases, dysplastic transformations to squamous metaplasia have been demonstrated. The etiology is unknown but it has been suggested that they may originate from accessory foregut remnants that give rise to squamous epithelium similar to the esophagus. Several cases of malignant transformation to squamous cell cancer have been reported.[19] Due to this malignant potential, early diagnosis in suspected cases is suggested and hepatic resection is the standard treatment.[20]

ACQUIRED CYSTS

Pyogenic Abscesses

Pyogenic abscesses are the most common hepatic abscesses in the US. Biliary tract obstruction or cholangitis secondary to cholelithiasis and malignancy accounts for approximately 35% of cases. Portal pyema secondary to diverticulits, inflammatory bowel disease, and perforated appendicitis are also relatively common causes. Fever and abdominal pain are common presenting complaints. Diagnosis is often made with an abdominal ultrasound or CT scan on presentation. There is a predilection for the right lobe involvement. Blood cultures and abscess aspiration can help guide therapy. Empiric antimicrobial coverage should be initiated and subsequently tailored once the organism is identified and sensitivities are reported. Treat parenterally for three to four weeks and complete a total of 8 weeks with oral agents. Repeat CT scan should be performed within one month after stopping therapy to insure adequate resolution.

Complicated cases require operative drainage. This can be performed through laparoscopic or open approaches. Usually after failed percutaneous attempts or in cases of large or multi-loculated abscesses. Patients may present with concurrent abdominal process or a ruptured abscess into peritoneum or pleura. These patients can deteriorate rapidly and mortality can approach 30%.

Amebic Abscesses

Amoebic abscesses are the most common liver abscess world-wide and constitute 10% of all abscesses (figure 3). *Entamoeba histolytica* is prevalent in tropical and sub-tropical climates where sanitation and public health measures are poor. Cysts are ingested in contaminated food stuff and trophocytes are released and multiply in the colon. Fever and abdominal pain are

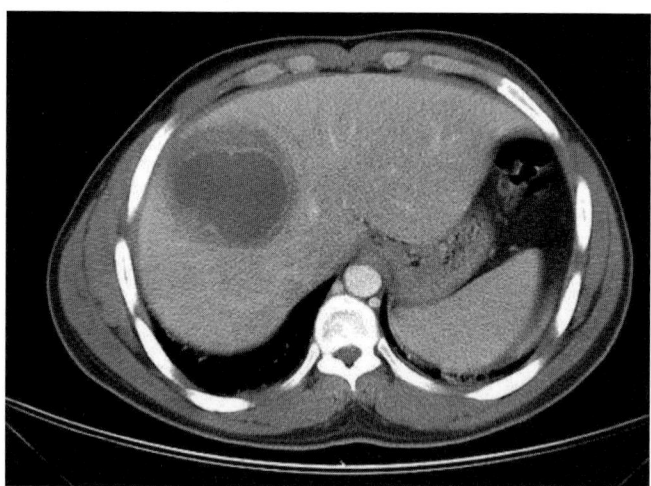

Figure 3. Amebic abscess.

CT scan demonstrating large amebic abscess in the right hepatic lobe. Typical features include an irregular thick wall and peripheral enhancement giving the appearance of a double target sign. Internal contents may consist of necrotic and hemorrhagic tissue.

typical at presentation. The diagnosis can be made with ultrasound or CT scan and a predilection for the right lobe is also found with Amebiasis. An antibody titer for *E. histolytica* should be checked and Flagyl is the treatment of choice. Flagyl, usually, results in clinical improvement in three days. Luminal agents should also be administered (iodoquinol, paromomycin, diloxanide furoate) to treat the asymptomatic colonized state. Failure to treat luminal colonizatioin will lead to an approximate 10% recurrence. Catheter drainage should be considered and may be required in large abscesses (larger than 5 cm) where risk of abscess rupture is real. Similarly, because therapy is usually very effective with Flagyl, failure to respond to therapy after seven days should prompt a more aggressive approach. These patients should be converted to chloroquine and percutaneous drainage should be contemplated.

Hydatid Cysts

Hippocrates indentified the hydatid cyst in the liver as "Jecur aqua repletum" or livers full of water.[21] Hydatid or echinococcal cysts are primarily caused by infection with the parasite *Echinococcus granulosus*. Hydatid disease is endemic in sheep erding areas of the world. Hydatid is Greek for "drop of water" while echinococcosis means "hedgehog berry". Additional species that cause infection include: *Echinococcus multilocularis,Echinococcus oligartus,*and *Echinococcus vogeli*.

The parasite is seen worldwide because of increased travel and immigration. The highest incidence has been reported in the Mediterranean, Middle East, and South America.[22] In 1681, Redi described the worm and in 1833, Sibold described the developmental life cycle of the parasite. The primary host is the dog. Humans may become intermediate hosts when meat is ingested from other domestic hosts.

Upon ingestion, eggs hatch in the duodenum, burrow into the venous supply of the jejunum, and eventually become trapped in the liver. If the larvae are not overcome by the host reaction, a cyst develops. The cyst has three layers: an outer layer that consists of modified host cells that contain dense fibrous protective tissue, a middle laminated membrane that is acellular, and an inner germinal layer that is the active cyst layer where larvae are produced. Echinococcal cysts are classified by a system devised by Gharbi on the basis of ultrasonographic findings[23] in Table 1. An additional classification system has been proposed that takes into account pathology

Table 1. Hydatid cyst classification.

Type 1: Pure fluid collection
Type 2: Fluid collection with a split wall
Type 3: Fluid collection with septa
Type 4: Heterogeneous echo patterns
Type 5: Reflecting thick walls

as well as the natural history of infection.[24] Most patients are asymptomatic; however, complications from infestation include infection, rupture, spread to adjacent structures, or anaphylaxis. In uncomplicated cases, symptoms include abdominal pain, fatigue, fever, nausea or dyspepsia.

Diagnosis can be confirmed by detection of immune complexes and antigens with ELISA which has 90% positivity rate. Ultrasonography is the primary diagnostic method revealing thick walled cysts with calcifications. CT scans are confirmatory and provide information on location, number and depth of cysts. MRI adds little to the diagnosis and may provide additional structural detail. In cases of uncertainty, percutaneous, image-guided fine needle aspiration should only be performed if the serologic workup is equivocal. Medical therapy with the anti-tubulin agents, albendazole or mebendazole can be administered. Indications for medical management include widely disseminated disease, localized disease in poor surgical candidates, ruptured cysts, and as prophylaxis for intraoperative spillage. Medical therapy is also indicated for a period of at least two weeks following drainage to prevent recurrence.

Chemotherapy has been more effective in pulmonary hydatid disease. One large series showed 74.1% of cysts with degenerative changes at the end of an initial treatment cycle.[25] However, treatment is still surgical in nature with pulmonary hydatidosis. In general, chemotherapy is used as a complement to operative treatment to avoid recurrence. Surgery has two objectives: to remove the parasite and to treat the bronchi-pericyst pathology and other associated lesions. Surgery is the primary treatment modality for hepatic infections. General indications for surgery are for noncomplicated cysts with a peripheral location in healthy patients. The spectrum of surgical procedures are defined by radical approaches such as pericystectomy or hepatic resection and conservative approaches such as drainage and obliteration of cyst cavities. Objectives in management are to inactivate scolices (parasitic organs for attachment), prevent spillage of cyst contents, eliminate all viable cyst contents, and management of the residual cyst cavity. Evacuation may be performed with external drainage using the PAIR technique, while obliteration of the cavity can be performed with a sclerosing agent, omentopexy, or approximation of cyst walls with capitonnage, introflexion, or capsulorrhapy. The PAIR technique consists of several sequential steps: After percutaneous aspiration of the hydatid cyst under US or CT guidance, a protoscolicidal agent (20% sodium chloride solution or 95% ethanol) is injected into the cyst cavity; the final step is reaspiration of the cyst contents. The advantage of PAIR is that it is less invasive and in combination with albendazole therapy is an effective and safe alternative to surgery.

In general, operative intervention can occur through open or laparoscopic approaches. Total cystectomy, unroofing, evacuation, and obliteration of the cyst cavity is the objective. The first laparoscopic report was published in 1994 by Bickel. Advantages of laparoscopy include shorter hospital stay and reduced wound complications. Disadvantages are difficulty in controlling spillage and aspiration of cyst fluid which can lead to complications. Preventing leakage or spillage of cyst contents is essential as it may lead to postoperative infection and has been identified as a source of anaphylactic shock and peritonitis. As with other cystic diseases, recurrence is a major issue with rates between 1% and 25%.[26] In a series of 304 patients with hepatic hydatid cysts, surgical intervention was found to have better outcomes and fewer complications. Therefore, external or percutaneous drainage may be better suited for types I and II disease where it can be performed with minimal complications and little to no side effects. No direct studies have compared laparoscopy to open procedures.[11]

Cystic Neoplasms

Primary liver tumors undergo cystic transformation as a result of internal necrosis following rapid tumor expansion and outgrowth of blood supply. Hepatocellular carcinoma and cystic hemangioma are the two most common cystic subtypes. In the case of giant hemangiomas, large hypoechogenic central areas may mimic cystademona. Identifying characteristics include a prominent enhancing rim, centripetal filling, globular vessels as well as a peripheral nodular enhancing patter seen on contrast enhanced CT and MR.

Hepatocellular carcinoma may present as a large hypodense multiseptated mass imitating a cystic lesion on imaging. Other than an appropriate history to suggest underlying liver disease, distinguishing features of hepatocellular carcinoma may be present, such as hypervascularity of the solid parts, a capsule, and vascular or biliary invasion. CT and MR may demonstrate coexisting sequelae of liver cirrhosis such as hypertrophy of the left hepatic lobe, regenerative nodules, splenomegaly, and recanalization of the umbilical vein.

Biliary cystadenomas are rare and indolent cystic tumors. They range in size from 1.5 cm to 35 cm, and occur predominantly in middle-aged women. Cystadenomas are differentiated radiographically from other cystic lesions by the presence of well defined thick walls, papillary projections and prominent internal septae. It is often difficult to distinguish malignant transformation to cystadenocarcinoma as it may appear similar on imaging. Malignant transformation is often accompanied by nodular septae, thick irregular walls and strong contrast enhancement as well as vascular signals on imaging. Histological examination reveals a single layer of mucin-secreting cells lining the cyst wall. The cyst fluid within the tumor can be proteinaceous, mucinous, serous, gelatinous, or hemorrhagic.[27] Ultrasonography and CT imaging, in combination with elevated CA19-9, CEA and presence of mucin on FNA, can differentiate these lesions from hemorrhagic or complicated cysts. Once the diagnosis is established in either cystadenoma or cystadenocarcinoma, surgery should be performed. If at resection the diagnosis is in question, intraoperative biopsy should be performed to determine the extent of resection and to rule out possible cholangiocarcinoma.[28]

Cystic Metastases

Metastases to the liver are common, and may present with partial or incomplete cysts. The most likely tumor is colon cancer, however, the differential diagnosis includes melanoma, carcinoid, breast cancer, renal cancer, and ovarian cancer. Two suggested mechanisms may explain cyst formation in hepatic metastases. Rapid growth of a hypervascular tumor may lead to necrosis and cyst formation as seen in metastases from neuroendocrine tumors, sarcomas, melanomas, and certain subtypes of lung and breast carcinoma. In most cases, contrast-enhanced CT and MR imaging will demonstrate multiple lesions with strong enhancement of the periphery. The borders of the cystic lesions are heterogeneous and poorly defined with amputated vessels. Metastases may lead to segmental dilation of the peripheral bile ducts with mucin casts as in the case of an isolated mucin-producing melanoma or mucinous adenocarcinomas, such as colorectal or ovarian carcinoma.[29]

False Cysts

Intrahepatic hemorrhage may mimic the appearance of a cystic mass; especially in the case of chronic hematomas, which present similar to cystic fluid on imaging. Intrahepatic bleeding is primarily caused by surgery and trauma. In some cases, bleeding from a hepatic mass may be attributed to an intrahepatic adenoma. Symptoms are primarily due to size, location, and duration of bleeding. In cases of trauma, there may be associated injuries such as hepatic lacerations, rib fractures or perihepatic fluid. Imaging of the liver with CT scanning can often determine the cause of bleeding. MRI is the optimal study as it can distinguish the paramagnetic effect of methemoglobin. Hematoma with a concurrent mass is suggestive of malignancy.[29]

Liver abscesses or bilomas may appear as an irregular cystic mass on both CT and MR scanning (Figure 4). These lesions may be intrahepatic or perihepatic and give the appearance of cysts as they are without septa or calcifications. They may occur spontaneously, traumatically, or

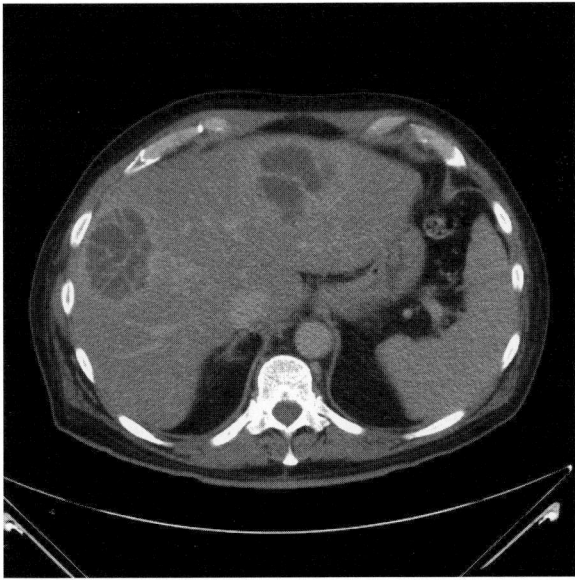

Figure 4. Pyogenic abscess.

CT scan demonstrating a pyogenic abscess. The cystic appearing lesion is thick-wall shaped and often contains internal pyogenic material as well as septations.

iatrogenically from surgery. Extravasation of bile into the liver may cause a reaction and formation of a pseudocapsule.[29]

REFERENCES

1. Munroe HS. Solitary nonparasitic cyst of the liver. *Ann Surg* 1942; 116(5): 751–762.
2. Bristowe F. Cystic disease of the liver associated with similar disease of the kidneys. *Trans Pathol Soc Lond* 1856; 7:229–234.
3. Caremani M, Vincenti A, Benci A,. et al., Ecographic epidemiology of nonparasitic hepatic cysts. *J Clin Ultrasound* 1993; 21(2):115–118.
4. Treckmann JW, Paul A, Sgourakis G, et al., Surgical treatment of nonparasitic cysts of the liver: open versus laparoscopic treatment. *Am J Surg* 2009; 199(6): 776–781.
5. Palanivelu C, Jani K, Malladi V. Laparoscopic management of benign nonparasitic hepatic cysts: a prospective nonrandomized study. *South Med J* 2006; 99(10):1063–1067.
6. Gall TM, Oniscu GC, Madhavan K, et al., Surgical management and longterm follow-up of non-parasitic hepatic cysts. *HPB (Oxford)* 2009; 11(3):235–41.
7. Mazza OM, Fernandez DL, Pekolj J, et al., Management of nonparasitic hepatic cysts. *J Am Coll Surg* 2009; 209(6):733–9.
8. Gigot JF, Jadoul P, Que F, et al., Adult polycystic liver disease: is fenestration the most adequate operation for long-term management? *Ann Surg* 1997; 225(3): 286–94.
9. Russell RT, Pinson CW. Surgical management of polycystic liver disease. *World J Gastroenterol* 2007; 13(38):5052–9.
10. Koperna T, Vogl S, Satzinger U, et al., Nonparasitic cysts of the liver: results and options of surgical treatment. *World J Surg* 1997; 21(8):850–4; discussion 4–5.
11. Balik AA, Basoglu M, Celebi F, et al., Surgical treatment of hydatid disease of the liver: review of 304 cases. *Arch Surg* 1999; 134(2):166–9.
12. Todani T, Watanabe Y, Narusue M, et al., Congenital bile duct cysts: classification, operative procedures, and review of thirty-seven cases including cancer arising from choledochal cyst. *Am J Surg* 1977; 134(2):263–9.
13. Babbitt DP. Congenital choledochal cysts: new etiological concept based on anomalous relationships of the common bile duct and pancreatic bulb. *Ann Radiol* (Paris). 1969; 12(3):231–40.
14. Lal R, Agarwal S, Shivhare R, et al., Type IV-A choledochal cysts: a challenge. *J Hepatobiliary Pancreat Surg.* 2005; 12(2):129–34.

15. Visser BC, Suh I, Way LW, et al., Congenital choledochal cysts in adults. Arch Surg 2004; 139(8):855–60; discussion 60–2.
16. Kirimlioglu V, Yilmaz S, Katz DA, et al., Choledochal cyst spontaneously rupturing the hepatic artery. Dig Dis Sci 2000; 45(3):544–8.
17. Gulati MS, Srivastava DN, Paul SB, et al., Pre-operative management of congenital choledochal cyst with ultrasound-guided percutaneous choledochalcystostomy. Australas Radiol 1999; 43(4):514–6.
18. Murray JD, Ricketts RR. Mesenchymal hamartoma of the liver. Am Surg 1998; 64(11):1097–103.
19. Odemis B, Koksal AS, Yuksel O, et al., Squamous cell cancer of the liver arising from an epidermoid cyst: case report and review of the literature. Dig Dis Sci.2006; 51(7):1278–84.
20. Chiu B, Melin-Aldana H, Superina RA. Management of an epidermoid cyst of the intrahepatic ducts. J Pediatr Surg 2005; 40(12):e31–3.
21. Gourgiotis S, Stratopoulos C, Moustafellos P, et al., Surgical techniques and treatment for hepatic hydatid cysts. Surg Today 2007; 37(5):389–95.
22. Safioleas M, Misiakos E, Manti C, et al., Diagnostic evaluation and surgical management of hydatid disease of the liver. World J Surg 1994; 18(6):859–65.
23. Gharbi HA, Hassine W, Brauner MW, et al., Ultrasound examination of the hydatic liver. Radiology 1981; 139(2):459–63.
24. Lewall DB, McCorkell SJ. Hepatic echinococcal cysts: sonographic appearance and classification. Radiology 1985; 155(3):773–5.
25. Haddad MC, Al-Awar G, Huwaijah SH, et al., Echinococcal cysts of the liver: a retrospective analysis of clinico-radiological findings and different therapeutic modalities. Clin Imaging 2001; 25(6):403–8.
26. Buttenschoen K, Carli Buttenschoen D. Echinococcus granulosus infection: the challenge of surgical treatment. Langenbecks Arch Surg 2003; 388(4):218–30.
27. Sarmiento JM, Nagorney, David M. Management of hepatic cysts (including hydatid disease). Operative Techniques in General Surgery 2002; 4(1):76–87.
28. Teoh AY, Ng SS, Lee KF, et al., Biliary cystadenoma and other complicated cystic lesions of the liver: diagnostic and therapeutic challenges. World J Surg 2006; 30(8):1560–6.
29. Mortele KJ, Ros PR. Cystic focal liver lesions in the adult: differential CT and MR imaging features. Radiographics 2001; 21(4):895–910.

BENIGN LIVER LESIONS 5

Immanuel Turner* and
Paul C. Kuo[†]

INTRODUCTION

With the increase in the technology and use of abdominal imaging, the frequency of finding benign liver lesions has increased.[1,2] The tumors can be broken into categories based on the cell of origin and tumor-like factors. Simple cysts are usually congenital and form after hepatic bile ducts develop with failure to connect to extra hepatic ducts. Mesenchymal tumors include hemangioma, fibroma, lipoma, angiomyolipoma, and lymphangioma. The epithelial cell tumors include the hepatocellular adenoma and bile duct adenoma. The tumor-like lesions include the focal nodular hyperplasia (FNH), nodular regenerative hyperplasia, hammartomas, and inflammatory pseudotumors.

The epidemiology of the benign hepatic tumors has shown an increase in frequency which parallels the recent increase in imaging studies of the abdomen. The simple cyst is the most common benign hepatic lesion. Hemangioma is the second most common and most common solid hepatic tumor at an estimated prevalence of 1–7.4% of the population. Focal nodular hyperplasia occurs in approximately 0.4% of the population and hepatic adenoma in 0.004% of the population.

---

*University of Michigan, Ann Arbor, MI, USA.
[†]Loyola University, Maywood, IL, USA.

CYSTIC TUMORS

Simple Cysts

Pathophysiology

Hepatic cysts are the most common benign hepatic lesion.[1,3] The prevalence in the US is reportedly 5%. Embryological failure of the bile ducts to connect to extrahepatic ducts is thought to contribute to the pathogenesis. Simple cysts usually contain fluid that is similar in composition to serum. There is a strong female predominance. Histologically, they are made up of simple cuboidal epithelium (identical to bile ducts) with a rim of fibrous stroma.

Clinical presentation

Patients are usually asymptomatic. Cysts that become >5 cm may cause mass effect in right upper quadrant. In addition, intracystic hemorrhage or infection may be the initial presentation.

Diagnostic imaging

Simple cysts can be diagnosed on US, CT or MRI with water attenuation, thin wall, no septations, and hyperenhancement if intracystic hemorrhage present.

Management

Most simple cysts are best managed conservatively. The preferred treatment would be US or CT-guided percutaneous aspiration, followed by schlerotherapy with alcohol. Surgical indications include difficulty excluding malignancy, biliary communication, or infection. Laparoscopic fenestration and deroofing has shown to be safe and effective.

MESENCHYMAL TUMORS

Hemangioma

Pathophysiology

The prevalence of hemangioma ranges from 3% to 20%, with a female: male ratio of 5 to 6:1.[1,2,4] Hemangiomas are congenital vascular malformations and comprised of an endothelial lining on a thin fibrous stroma making up blood filled spaces. Some of these tumors have estrogen receptors, and accelerated growth has been associated with high estrogen states including puberty, pregnancy, oral contraceptive use, and androgen therapy. These findings suggest a hormonal influence in pathogenesis.

Clinical presentation

Most common clinical presentation is an incidental finding during ultrasonographic examination of the abdomen. Patients with hemangiomas >5 cm amy present with nonspecific abdominal symptoms. Alternatively, symptoms can also present when there is necrosis, infarction, or thrombosis of the tumor. Kasabach-Meritt syndrome occurs rarely and is characterized by thrombocytopenia and disseminated intravascular coagulopathy associated with giant hemangiomas. The clinical presentation for these patients includes upper abdominal pain and bleeding. Alkaline phosphatase may be slightly elevated

Diagnostic imaging

Hemangiomas usually have characteristic features on imaging (Figure 1). On ultrasound, they appear well defined, lobulated, homogeneous hyperechoic mass with the possibility of hypoechoic components depending on the presence of hemorrhage, fibrosis, or calcification. Ultrasound can establish the diagnosis in 80% of lesions <6 cm in the presence of posterior acoustic enhancement. Hemangiomas are often diagnosed on multiphasic CT. In early enhanced images, peripheral nodular or globular enhancement with centripetal filling is appreciated. In hemangiomas >2 cm, CT is associated with sensitivity and specificity >90% when peripheral nodular enhancement and centripetal filling is seen on delayed images. The most sensitive and specific test for hemangioma is the MRI T1 weighted image with values of 85% and 95%, respectively.

Management

Treatment is not indicated for asymptomatic patients. Hemangiomas <5 cm with established stability at 6-month interval require no intervention. Indications for surgical management include symptoms, complications,

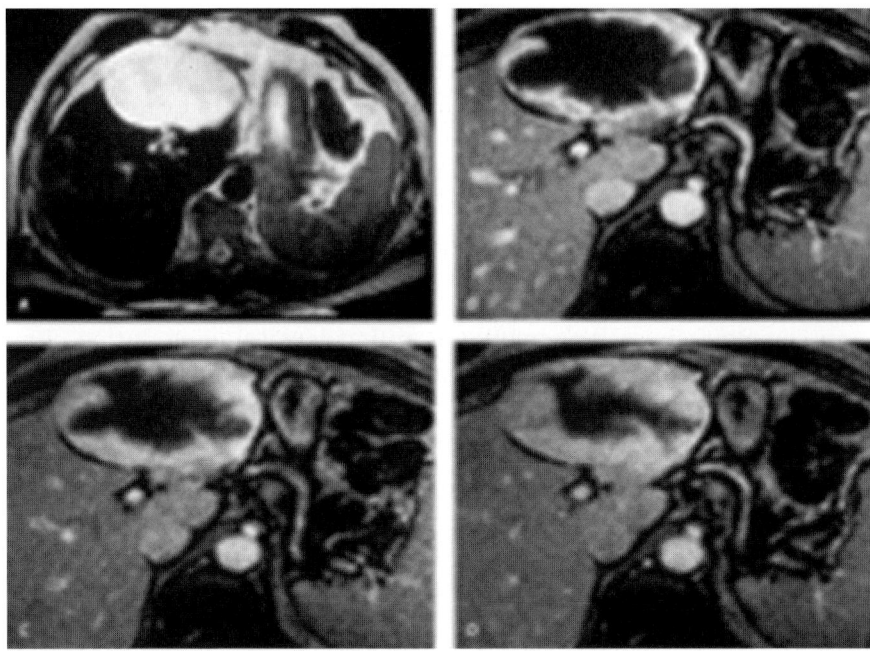

Figure 1. Hemangioma MRI (T2 image).

and inability to exclude malignancy. Transarterial embolization is indicated for symptomatic disease, acute bleeding, and consumption coagulopathy. Surgical resection has been reported in 2% of hemangiomas. Enucleation rather than resection may be used to minimize blood loss and preserve hepatic parenchyma.

Benign Lipomatous Tumors

Pathophysiology

Angiomyolipomas are composed of variable proportions of adipose tissue and smooth muscle with thick- or thin-walled blood vessels.[5] Some tumors have extensive extramedullary hematopoieses and have been termed myelolipoma and angiomyelolipoma. Flow cytometry shows a DNA pattern consistent with a benign lesion.

Diagnostic imaging

On ultrasound, angiomyolipoma is a well-circumscribed, homogeneous, and highly echogenic tumor. Enhanced CT demosntrates a density in Hounsfield units similar to fat (−2 to −115). MRI can also be diagnostic.

Management

Budd–Chiari syndrome related to compression of the hepatic veins has been described. Malignant transformation has not been reported. Indications for surgical intervention include symptomatic lesions and those where diagnosis cannot be confirmed. Operative resection is the management option of choice.

EPITHELIAL TUMORS

Hepatocellular Adenoma (Hepatic Adenoma)

Pathophysiology

Hepatic adenoma is pathologically characterized by the benign proliferation of hepatocytes.[6] It occurs predominantly in women with female: male ratio of 4:1. In addition, the pathogenesis is not completely understood, but a strong association with oral contraceptives has been documented. Macroscopically, these tumors are usually solitary (70–80%) most of the time. They are well-circumscribed, round, and unencapsulated, but may compress adjacent hepatic tissue. Size ranges from 5 to 15 cm with gross intratumor fat, necrosis, and hemorrhage observed commonly. Microscopically, hepatic adenomas comprises plates of cells that resemble normal hepatocytes septated by dilated sinusoids. The sinusoids are then perfused by feeding arteries and contribute to the hypervascularity. There is a noted propensity for rupture secondary to hypervascularity, loose connective tissue, the absence of true capsule and subcapsular location of hepatic adenomas. A key histologic finding is the lack of bile ductules which distinguishes it from FNH.

Clinical presentation

Small and isolated hepatic adenomas are usually asymptomatic. Large lesions may cause a sensation of right upper quadrant fullness or discomfort. The adenomas are of clinical importance because of their tendency to spontaneous rupture and hemorrhage. Rare cases of malignant transformation have been reported with the risk increased with multiple tumors. Work up for determination of malignancy should include serum α-fetoprotein and liver function tests, which are normal in patients with hepatic adenoma,

Diagnostic imaging

On ultrasound, hepatic adenomas have nonspecific mixed echoic patterns. Color Doppler ultrasound can demonstrate peripheral peritumoral and intratumoral blood flow with continuous triphasic waveform. These findings are absent in FNH and can be used to differentiate between the two. On multiphasic CT and MRI, hepatic adenomas show more specific findings. They are heterogenous due to intratumoral hemorrhage, necrosis, and fat components noted on CT. These tumors show early enhancement because of their rich arterial supply, also noted on MRI. Hepatic scintigraphy may show absent or decreased uptake, reflecting the decreased number and function of Kupffer cells.

Management

Secondary to the risk of rupture and malignant transformation, hepatic adenomas must be identified and treated promptly. Surgical resection is the option of choice. However, in the patient with acute hemorrhage at presentation, hepatic arterial embolization should be considered. Laparoscopic operative management has been associated with good outcomes.

Bile Duct Adenoma

Intrahepatic bile duct adenoma is a rare, non-neoplastic tumor most often diagnosed incidentally.[7] Microscopically, they consist of numerous uniform, normal appearing bile duct-like structures that are surrounded by a small amount of fibrous stroma. These lesions can be confused with cholangiocarcinoma or metastatic adenocarcinoma on frozen section analysis. The distinguishing feature is the absence of hyperchromasia, mitotic activity, and vascular invasion. Radiologic imaging is nonspecific. It is usually a well-circumscribed, subcapsular mass with a diameter of <1 cm. Reportedly, the bile duct adenoma is more of a reactive process to a focal injury rather than a true neoplasm or developmental anomaly. No surgical management is indicated.

TUMOR-LIKE LESIONS

Focal Nodular Hyperplasia (FNH)

Pathophysiology

FNH is the second most common benign solid tumor of the liver and makes up 8% of all primary hepatic tumors.[6] The underlying pathophysiology is not well understood. Most recently, it may be considered a non-neoplastic, hyperplastic response to congenital vascular malformation. Histologically, it is defined by benign appearing hepatocytes occurring in liver that is normal. It is encountered in as many as 3% of the general population, with predominance in women of childbearing years (female: male ratio 6–8:1). There is an association with oral contraceptives. The size of the tumor ranges from <5 cm (most common) to 15 cm (rare). Pathology slides show well-circumscribed, globular, lobulated, and unencapsulated tumors. The characteristic histologic features include a dense central stellate scar and septa that radiate from this scar. The scar consists of bile ductules, cholangiolar proliferation, surrounding inflammatory infiltrates, and malformed vessels but no portal veins. The normal hepatic parenchyma between the septa includes hepatic cords of hepatocytes, sinusoids, and Kupffer cells.

Clinical presentation

FNH as large as 10 cm are rarely symptomatic. Clinical symptoms such as epigastic or right upper quadrant pain are found in less than one third of all patients. Spontaneous rupture is rare, and malignant transformation has not been described. Liver function tests are normal. Determination of the diagnosis of FNH is critical because of its benign clinical course.

Diagnostic imaging

The central fibrous scar is the most characteristic finding on imaging studies (Figure 2). FNH is not well demonstrated by simple ultrasound.

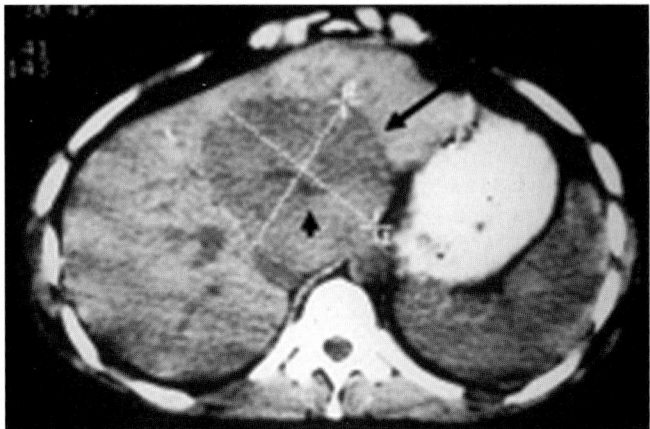

Figure 2. Enhanced CT FNH with hypodense scar.

Color Doppler may be helpful in showing the vascularity suspected with FNH. On multiphasic CT and enhanced MRI, typical features are very characteristic. Multiphasic CT imaging of FNH demonstrates it to be homogenous, iso-attenuating, and in the late arterial phase, bright homogeneous enhancement and hypodense scar is present. In the portal phase, FNH is difficult to detect because it is iso-attenuating. MRI images show the hyperintense central scar on T2 weighted images. On hepatic scintigraphy, FNH may show normal (30%) or increased (30%) uptake, compared to normal liver. Uptake is determined by the size and number of Kupffer cells involved.

Management

Asymptomatic patients are usually followed clinically for development of symptoms and radiographically with ultrasound for enlargement of tumor. The most common indications for operative intervention are undetermined nature of the tumor, presence of symptoms, or suspicion of metastasis. If surgical resection is not feasible, transarterial embolization should be considered. The potential association with accelerated growth in high estrogen states suggests more frequent ultrasounds during pregnancy and the post-partum period.

Nodular Regenerative Hyperplasia (NRH)

Pathophysiology

Nodular regenerative hyperplasia is a rare benign proliferative lesion with references that include nodular transformation and noncirrhotic nodulation.[8] It is characterized by diffuse involvement of the liver with nodules of hyperplastic hepatocytes. Histologic keys include thickened regenerating hepatocytes with centrilobular atrophy. The pathogenesis is thought to be a primary vascular process that leads to obliteration of portal vein, which in turn induces ischemia, atrophy of hepatocytes in the central zone followed by proliferation. Alternative theories discuss a preneoplastic process that leads to NRH secondary to prevalence of hepatocyte dysplasia (20–42%), and HCC found in livers of patients diagnosed. NRH prevalence is reported to be approximately 2–3%.

Clinical presentation

NRH usually causes no symptoms and is frequently discovered incidentally. Some patients can present with portal hypertension, hepatomegaly, and splenomegaly thought to be related to compression of the main portal vein at the hilum. Nonspecific elevation of liver function tests along with hepatic failure, rupture of the liver, and malignant transformation can occur.

Diagnostic imaging

Imaging is not specific and histologic diagnosis is often warranted. On enhanced CT, NRH shows normal findings or hypoattenuating nodules. Hyperattenuation on US or CT represents hemorrhage or aterioportal shunting.

Management

Diagnosis should be confirmed with histologic examination. In asymptomatic patients, no treatment is necessary, but follow-up is recommended for the potentially rare development of HCC. Patients who develop portal hypertension require medical therapy, but endoscopic therapy and portocaval shunt may be useful. Rarely, patients progress to liver failure and require transplantation.

Mesenchymal Hamartoma

Mesenchymal hamartoma is a rare lesion of bile ducts, immature mesenchymal cells, and hepatocytes.[9] The majority of these lesions are diagnosed in childhood. The clinical presentation is nonspecific. The imaging findings reveal solid or multicystic lesions. Diagnosis can be obtained percutaneously, but is most often confirmed after surgical resection.

Inflammatory Pseudotumor

Inflammatory pseudotumor is a rare non-neoplastic hepatic tumor.[10] Its appearance is concerning for a malignant tumor, but the clinical course and histology are benign. The pathogenesis is thought to be related to an underlying infectious process. Clinical presentation is nonspecific with constitutional symptoms of fever, malaise, weight loss or related to mass effect. Biopsy is necessary to make the diagnosis. Histologic examination reveals myofibroblasts, polyclonal plasma cells, and fibrous tissue. Surgical resection has been performed for most reported cases.

REFERENCES

1. Assy N, Nasser G, Djibre A, *et al.* Characteristics of common solid liver lesions and recommendations for diagnostic workup. *World J Gastroenterol* 2009; 15: 3217–3227.
2. Choi BY, Nguyen MH. The diagnosis and management of benign hepatic tumors. *J Clin Gastroenterol* 2005; 39:401–412.
3. Onori P, Franchitto A, Mancinelli R, *et al.* Polycystic liver diseases. *Dig Liver Dis* 2010; 42:261–271.
4. Bahirwani R, Reddy KR. Review article: the evaluation of solitary liver masses. *Aliment Pharmacol Ther* 2008; 28:953–965.
5. Petrolla AA, Xin W. Hepatic angiomyolipoma. *Arch Pathol Lab Med* 2008; 132:1679–1682.
6. Lizardi-Cervera J, Cuellar-Gamboa L, Motola-Kuba D. Focal nodular hyperplasia and hepatic adenoma: a review. *Ann Hepatol* 2006; 5:206–211.

7. Fletcher ND, Wise PE, Sharp KW. Common bile duct papillary adenoma causing obstructive jaundice: case report and review of the literature. *Am Surg* 2004; 70:448–452.
8. Reshamwala PA, Kleiner DE, Heller T. Nodular regenerative hyperplasia: not all nodules are created equal. *Hepatology* 2006; 44:7–14.
9. Siddiqui MA, McKenna BJ. Hepatic mesenchymal hamartoma: a short review. *Arch Pathol Lab Med* 2006; 130:1567–1569.
10. Milias K, Madhavan KK, Bellamy C, *et al.* Inflammatory pseudotumors of the liver: experience of a specialist surgical unit. *J Gastroenterol Hepatol* 2009; 24: 1562–1566.

PRIMARY HEPATIC MALIGNANCIES   6

Andrew S. Barbas* and Rebekah R. White*

The two most common primary hepatic malignancies are hepatocellular carcinoma (HCC) and intrahepatic cholangiocarcinoma (ICC). HCC accounts for 85–90% of primary hepatic malignancies and ICC accounts for the remaining 10–15%. Other rare primary hepatic malignancies include angiosarcoma, epithelioid hemangioendothelioma, and primary lymphoma. Over the last 3 decades, advances in cross-sectional imaging, improved understanding of the segmental anatomy of the liver, and advances in technical aspects of hepatic resection have improved the safety of hepatic resection with perioperative mortality approaching 1–2%. Accordingly, the aggressive surgical management of primary hepatic malignancies has become much more common in the current era.

HEPATOCELLULAR CARCINOMA

Hepatocellular carcinoma (HCC) is the most common primary liver malignancy and the third leading cause of cancer death worldwide. Patients at risk for the development of HCC have disease processes resulting in chronic liver inflammation and injury. Chronic viral hepatitis is by far the most important risk factor for the development of HCC, accounting for approximately 80% of HCC cases. Hepatitis B virus (HBV) makes up

*Duke University School of Medicine, Department of Surgery, Durham, North Carolina.

50–55% of HCC cases and Hepatitis C virus (HCV) accounts for 25–30% of HCC. Other etiologies include alcoholic liver disease, hemochromatosis, primary biliary cirrhosis, Wilson's disease, α1-antitrypsin deficiency, and non-alcoholic steatohepatitis (NASH). Consistent with the worldwide distribution of HBV infection, HCC is most prevalent in southeast Asia and tropical Africa. In the United States, the incidence of HCC has risen steadily over the last 30 years, attributed to the increasing prevalence of HCV infection as well as NASH.

Overall, HCC carries a relatively poor prognosis because it is often diagnosed at an advanced stage. Surveillance strategies have been employed in high-risk patients in an attempt to diagnose HCC earlier and improve treatment outcomes.

Pathogenesis

The epidemiologic link between chronic viral hepatitis and the development of HCC has been well documented. Several hypotheses link chronic viral infection with molecular events leading to cancer development. In the case of HBV infection, insertional mutagenesis of the DNA viral genome into hepatocyte chromosomal DNA is postulated to play a role in the development of cancer. Additionally, the chronic inflammation and fibrosis caused by chronic viral infection is thought to create a milieu favoring the development of dysplasia and subsequent cancer formation. This hypothesis may explain the development of HCC in nonviral etiologies of HCC like NASH, Wilson's disease and primary biliary cirrhosis.

Surveillance and Diagnosis

Most patients with early stage HCC are asymptomatic. By the time clinical symptoms develop, the disease is usually advanced. At the time of presentation, only 30% of patients have disease that is amenable to curative treatment strategies. Accordingly, much emphasis has been placed on the development of surveillance programs for high-risk patients. Patients considered high risk include those with chronic viral hepatitis, alcoholic cirrhosis, hemochromatosis, and primary biliary cirrhosis. Current strategies include liver ultrasound and measurement of serum α-fetoprotein (AFP) at 6- or 12-month intervals in high-risk populations. Liver ultrasound has a sensitivity of 58–78% with a specificity of greater than 90% for HCC.[1] Advantages of this modality include its low cost, noninvasive nature, and avoidance of nephrotoxic contrast agents. Limitations of liver ultrasound as a screening test include less than ideal sensitivity, particularly for detection of tumors in the setting of a cirrhotic nodular liver and in obese patients. Additionally, as with most ultrasound examinations, accuracy is dependent on operator experience.

AFP has a sensitivity ranging from 39–65% and specificity ranging from 76–97%, depending on the cutoff values used to establish diagnosis. AFP levels greater than 20 ng/mL are found in 75% of patients with HCC. However, using this relatively low cutoff level for AFP, false positives may occur in patients with chronic liver inflammation, particularly viral hepatitis. Specificity increases at the expense of sensitivity when higher cutoff levels (200 ng/mL) are employed. An AFP greater than 200 ng/mL combined with cross-sectional imaging demonstrating a hypervascular mass is considered diagnostic for HCC.

If a mass is detected on ultrasound, cross-sectional imaging is obtained for further characterization. Spiral CT and MRI are the primary imaging modalities used to evaluate suspected HCC, and a standard CT protocol should include contrast enhanced images in the arterial, portal-venous, and delayed phases. HCC demonstrates relatively specific imaging characteristics, most notably early uptake of contrast in the arterial phase, reflecting tumor blood supply derived from the hepatic artery. Additionally, early washout in the delayed venous phase is commonly seen, attributed to relatively rapid venous drainage from tumor tissue compared to the surrounding liver parenchyma. CT and MRI are also useful for delineating the extent of disease in terms of peritoneal and nodal metastases, as well as characterizing the relationship of the tumor to the vascular and biliary trees.

Once a diagnosis of HCC is made, evaluation of underlying liver function is critical. Measurement of serum bilirubin, prothrombin time, and albumin can help assess the synthetic function of the liver. The Child–Pugh classification system incorporates these laboratory studies along with clinical parameters (the presence or absence of ascites and encephalopathy) into a score that is used to group patients in one of three categories: Child–Pugh A, B, or C (Table 1). Class A patients have relatively preserved liver function while class C patients have significant liver dysfunction. Child–Pugh class has traditionally also been used to estimate surgical risk for planned hepatic resection and guide treatment decisions. In the absence of any significant comorbidities, Child–Pugh class A patients can safely tolerate hepatic resection while class C patients have a prohibitively high risk of perioperative mortality. These patients are typically

Table 1. Child-Pugh classification of liver disease severity.

Child-Pugh classification of liver disease severity

Parameter	1 point	2 points	3 points
Bilirubin (mg/dl)	<2	2–3	>3
Albumin (g/dl)	>3.5	2.8–3.5	<2.8
Prothrombin time (seconds over control) or	1–3	4–6	>6
INR	<1.7	1.7–2.2	>2.2
Ascites	None	Slight	Moderate
Encephalopathy (grade)	None	I–II	III–IV

Grade A: 5–6, Grade B: 7–9, Grade C: 10–15 points.

only considered for liver transplantation or nonoperative therapies. For Child–Pugh class B patients, determination of therapeutic approach is often made on a case-by-case basis. Additional considerations in the preoperative evaluation include determination of the presence of portal hypertension. Clinical or radiologic evidence of portal hypertension often prompts measurement of the portal-hepatic venous pressure gradient. Values greater than 12 mmHg are indicative of significant portal hypertension which is a relative contraindication to undergoing surgical resection for HCC. In addition to evaluation of liver function and determination of the presence of portal hypertension, major hepatic resection represents a major physiologic stress on the body and necessitates careful evaluation of comorbid conditions.

Staging

Several clinical staging systems have been developed to predict prognosis for individual patients based on pretreatment clinical parameters. In some systems, stratification of patients based on these parameters is also used to select the most effective treatment modality for a particular patient. Each system has its advantages and disadvantages and there is no definite consensus on which system should be used.

The Cancer of the Liver Italian Program (CLIP) classification system consists of Child-Pugh class, tumor morphology (uninodular vs. multinodular and extent of liver involvement), AFP, and the presence or absence of

Table 2. Cancer of the Liver Italian Program (CLIP) classification system.

Parameter	0 points	1 point	2 points
Child-Pugh stage	A	B	C
Tumor morphology	Uninodular and extension ≤50%	Multinodular and extension ≤50%	Massive or extension >50%
AFP (ng/dl)	<400	≤400	
Portal vein thrombosis	No	Yes	

Table 3. The Barcelona Liver Clinic (BCLC) staging system.

BCLC stage	PS	Tumor features	Liver function	Treatment options
A1	0	Single <5 cm	No PH	Surgery, RFA
A2	0	Single <5 cm	PH, normal bili	Surgery, RFA, Transplant
A3	0	Single <5 cm	PH, abnormal bili	RFA, Transplant
A4	0	3 tumors <3 cm	N/A	Transplant, TACE
B	0	Large multinodular	CP A–B	TACE
C	1–2	Vascular invasion or metastasis	CP A–B	Systemic treatment
D	3–4	Any	CP C	Supportive care

CP: Child-Pugh, PH: portal hypertension, PS: Eastern Cooperative Oncology group performance status, RFA: radiofrequency ablation, TACE: transarterial chemoembolization.

portal vein thrombosis[2] (Table 2). A patient is assigned 0, 1, or 2 points for each parameter and the total score is calculated, with a higher score indicating more advanced disease and a worse overall prognosis.

Another widely accepted system of classification is the Barcelona Clinic Liver Cancer (BCLC) system, which incorporates Eastern Cooperative Oncology Group (ECOG) performance status, tumor burden, hepatic function, and the presence or absence of portal hypertension to determine a patient's clinical stage[3] (Table 3). A unique feature of this staging system is that clinical stage is linked to particular treatment modalities and can be used to guide decision-making for clinicians.

Table 4. TNM staging for HCC (AJCC 7th edition).

TNM staging for HCC–AJCC 7th edition	
T stage	
T1	Single tumor without vascular invasion
T2	Single tumor with vascular invasion present Multiple tumors, all < 5 cm
T3a	Multiple tumors, any > 5 cm
T3b	Tumor of any size involving major branch of portal or hepatic vein
T4	Tumor with direct invasion of adjacent organs (other than gallbladder) Tumor perforates the visceral peritoneum
N stage	
N0	No regional lymph node metastasis
N1	Regional lymph node metastasis (hepatic artery, portal vein, hilar, hepatoduodenal ligament, inferior phrenic, and caval lymph node basins)
M stage	
M0	No distant metastasis
M1	Distant metastasis

Table 5. Staging of HCC (AJCC 7th edition).

Stage groupings — HCC, AJCC 7th edition	
Stage I	T1 N0 M0
Stage II	T2 N0 M0
Stage IIIA	T3a N0 M0
Stage IIIB	T3b N0 M0
Stage IIIC	T4 N0 M0
Stage IVA	Any T, N1 M0
Stage IVB	Any T, Any N, M1

In patients having undergone surgical resection, the American Joint Committee on Cancer/International Union Against Cancer (AJCC/UICC) TNM pathologic staging system is also used for HCC (Tables 4 and 5). The TNM system can also be used to guide treatment decisions regarding postoperative adjuvant therapy. However, a significant limitation for the use of TNM pathologic staging in prognostication for HCC is that it does not take into account the patient's underlying liver function, which has been shown to be an important predictor of survival in several published series.

Treatment — Curative Intent

In patients with limited disease, several treatment modalities are available for curative intent including surgical resection, liver transplantation, and tumor ablation. The most appropriate choice for an individual patient is made in a multidisciplinary fashion taking into account a patient's disease burden, presence or absence of portal hypertension, underlying liver function, and comorbid conditions.

Surgical resection is ideally suited for noncirrhotic patients with a technically resectable lesion based on location remote from major vascular structures, unilobar involvement, absence of portal hypertension, and adequate functional hepatic reserve. However, in the United States, only a very small percentage of patients, approximately 5%, satisfy these conditions. Surgical resection can be curative in some patients, with 5-year survival ranging from 20–60% in published series. In general, however, surgical resection is marked by a high rate of recurrence with 50% of resected patients recurring at 3 years and 70% by 5 years.[4] It is unclear whether this relatively poor cure rate is due to true recurrence of the original tumor or the development of new primary tumors in the setting of an abnormal underlying liver that provides a carcinogenic milieu, a phenomenon known as "field effect".

If a patient is not a candidate for surgical resection due to unfavorable tumor location, multicentricity, inadequate functional hepatic reserve, or the presence of portal hypertension, liver transplantation is considered. The Milan criteria established by Mazzaferro and colleagues in 1996 are used to determine whether a patient with HCC qualifies for transplantation.[5] Patients with a single tumor less than 5 cm or up to three tumors smaller than 3 cm are considered candidates for transplantation. Patients who meet these criteria and undergo transplantation have a 5-year survival in excess of 70%. Liberalization of the Milan size criteria to include patients with a single tumor less than 6.5 cm or up to three tumors less than 4.5 cm has been proposed by the University of California San Francisco

(UCSF) group.[6] Using these liberalized criteria, the UCSF group demonstrated 5-year recurrence free survivals of 80% in their transplanted patients. Because most HCC patients are generally in stable medical condition, their Model for End-Stage Liver Disease (MELD) scores tend to be lower than those patients in fulminant hepatic failure on the transplant waiting list. To decrease time on the waiting list and prevent significant progression of disease, patients with HCC are awarded exception points which are added to their MELD score and increase the chances of receiving an organ.

If a patient is not a candidate for either surgical resection or liver transplantation, percutaneous tumor ablation is considered. Ablation can be accomplished by either chemical or thermal techniques. Chemical ablation is accomplished by injecting lesions with ethanol or acetic acid, producing cellular dehydration and tumor necrosis. Percutaneous ethanol injection (PEI) was the first technique introduced clinically and is best suited for tumors smaller than 2 cm, in which it induces necrosis in nearly 100% of tumors. In larger tumors from 3–5 cm, its efficacy drops to approximately 50%.[1] Thermal ablation can be accomplished by radiofrequency energy, microwave energy, or cryoablation, producing local heating (or freezing) of the tumor and cellular death. Radiofrequency ablation (RFA) is the most studied of the thermal techniques and is similarly efficacious as PEI for small tumors less than 2 cm. For larger tumors up to 4 cm, RFA appears to have superior efficacy in terms of local tumor control, recurrence rate, and disease-free survival. Additionally, RFA can be performed effectively in difficult locations, for example in tumors adjacent to large vessels. More recently, strategies involving ablative therapies as a bridge to transplantation have been explored for patients on the transplant waiting list.

Treatment — Palliative

In patients with advanced disease, the goal of treatment is to prolong survival and improve or maintain quality of life. Embolization techniques have demonstrated effective palliation for HCC. In transarterial embolization (TAE), embolizing agents (for example, coils or gelatin sponge particles) are injected directly via the hepatic artery to occlude tumor vasculature. In transarterial chemoembolization (TACE), chemotherapeutic agents, most commonly doxorubicin or cisplatin, are delivered in combination with embolization agents via the hepatic artery. These strategies are best suited for patients with relatively preserved liver function (Child–Pugh class A or B) and with no evidence of portal vein thrombosis to minimize the risk of liver failure. Meta analyses of the published series of TACE have demonstrated significantly improved patient survival and established it as the standard of care for patients with BCLC stage B disease and in select BCLC stage C patients.[7] More recently, radioembolization strategies have emerged involving the delivery of radioactive microspheres via the hepatic artery. This technique has been shown to be safe in carefully selected patients, and further studies are ongoing to determine clinical efficacy.

Systemic chemotherapy has historically been ineffective in the treatment of advanced HCC. Doxorubicin has been evaluated in clinical trials leading to partial responses in only 10% of patients and no demonstrable survival benefit. More recently, the development of targeted therapies have resulted in new agents with activity against HCC. Sorafenib is a small-molecule inhibitor of multiple tyrosine kinases involved in aberrant cell signaling pathways in HCC. In the 2007 phase III Sorafenib HCC Assessment Randomized Protocol (SHARP) trial, patients with advanced HCC randomized to sorafenib therapy demonstrated a significantly longer time to progression and overall survival compared to placebo.[8] This trial helped establish sorafenib as the new standard of care for patients with advanced and metastatic HCC. Ongoing trials are underway to evaluate the use of sorafenib in combination with other treatment modalities like TACE and other molecularly targeted therapies.

Fibrolamellar HCC

Fibrolamellar HCC is a distinct variant of HCC that typically affects young patients in the second and third decades of life with no underlying liver disease. Serum AFP is usually in the normal range and cross-sectional imaging demonstrates a heterogeneous mass with a central scar which can appear similar to focal nodular hyperplasia (FNH). Surgical resection is the mainstay of therapy and outcomes appear to be more favorable in terms of recurrence and overall survival compared to patients with typical HCC. Multiplicity of disease and the presence of nodal metastases are predictors of decreased survival in patients with fibrolamellar HCC.

Summary

HCC continues to be a major worldwide health problem with a poor overall prognosis. At the time of diagnosis, most patients have advanced disease precluding curative therapy. In those patients treated with curative intent, high rates of recurrence lead to suboptimal long-term outcomes. Refinements in surveillance strategies and the continued development of cross-sectional imaging technology will help establish the diagnosis at earlier stages. Moreover, continued development of targeted therapies and incorporation of these agents into neoadjuvant and adjuvant treatment regimens will likely lead to improved outcomes and increased survival over time.

INTRAHEPATIC CHOLANGIOCARCINOMA

Intrahepatic cholangiocarcinoma (ICC) is a primary hepatic malignancy arising from the biliary epithelium of the intrahepatic bile ducts. It is the second most common primary hepatic malignancy after HCC, accounting for 10–15% of primary liver cancers. Risk factors associated with ICC are increasing age, primary sclerosing cholangitis, primary biliary cirrhosis, non-alcoholic fatty liver disease, and viral hepatitis. The incidence of ICC is increasing in the United States, which may in part be related to more accurate diagnosis of the disease in the current era as well as increasing rates of hepatitis C and non-alcoholic fatty liver disease. ICC is categorized as one of three types based on morphologic features: (1) mass-forming, (2) periductal-infiltrating, or (3) intraductal-growth. The mass-forming type is the most common, accounting for more than 85% of tumors.

Diagnosis

Similar to HCC, early stage ICC is usually asymptomatic. Most cases of ICC are discovered incidentally on imaging performed for other indications. In advanced disease, patients may experience abdominal pain and weight loss. In contrast to HCC, ICC lacks clear distinguishing characteristics on cross-sectional imaging and in many instances resembles a hypoattenuating metastatic lesion. As such, a biopsy of the lesion is usually obtained and is found to be consistent with adenocarcinoma. Subsequent investigation for an occult gastrointestinal primary often includes upper and lower endoscopy and positron emission tomography (PET). Serum tumor markers including carbohydrate antigen 19–9 (CA 19–9), carcinoembryonic antigen (CEA), and AFP are commonly checked in addition to these diagnostic modalities. CA 19–9 appears to be the most relevant marker for ICC with a sensitivity of 53% and specificity between 75% and 90%.[9] Dedicated cross-sectional imaging consists of contrast enhanced spiral CT or MRI with fine cuts through the liver.

Treatment — Curative Intent

Surgical resection is the primary therapy for ICC and provides the only meaningful chance for cure. Careful consideration of comorbid conditions is necessary to determine whether patients can tolerate the major surgery commonly required for these tumors. The goals of surgical resection are to completely resect all disease while preserving an adequate functional liver remnant. Because these tumors are often large at the time of diagnosis, obtaining an R0 resection margin can be technically challenging, often requiring an extended hepatectomy or concomitant resection of the extrahepatic bile duct with biliary reconstruction. Clinically involved lymph nodes are removed along with the specimen but routine lymphadenectomy is not performed by most hepatobiliary surgeons.

Staging and Prognosis

Pathologic staging of ICC is based on TNM classification from the AJCC/UICC (Tables 6 and 7). Overall, 5-year survival after surgical resection ranges from 14–40% in published series. In general, the presence of nodal metastases confers a relatively poor prognosis, with 5-year survival after resection ranging from 4% to 11%. Other factors independently associated with poor outcomes include multiplicity of disease, vascular invasion, and positive margins of resection.[10]

Treatment — Palliative

Patients with unresectable disease have a median survival between 5 and 8 months. Systemic chemotherapy remains the mainstay of treatment for unresectable patients. Traditional 5-FU based chemotherapy regimens historically have demonstrated very poor response rates in ICC ranging from

Table 6. TNM staging for ICC (AJCC 7th edition).

	T stage
T1	Solitary tumor without vascular invasion (includes major vascular and microvascular invasion)
T2a	Solitary tumor with vascular invasion
T2b	Multiple tumors, with or without vascular invasion
T3	Tumor perforating the visceral peritoneum or involving local extrahepatic structures by direct invasion
T4	Tumor with periductal invasion (includes periductal-infiltrating or mixed mass-forming and periductal-infiltrating growth patterns)
	N stage
N0	No regional lymph node metastasis
N1	Regional lymph node metastasis (nodal involvement of the celiac, periaortic, or caval lymph nodes is considered M1 disease)
	M stage
M0	No distant metastasis
M1	Distant metastasis (includes nodal involvement of celiac, periaortic, or caval lymph nodes)

Table 7. Staging of ICC (AJCC 7th edition).

Stage I	T1 N0 M0
Stage II	T2 N0 M0
Stage III	T3 N0 M0
Stage IVA	T4 N0 M0
	Any T, N1, M0
Stage IVB	Any T, Any N, M1

10% to 30%. Recent improvements in response rates with significantly increased progression-free and overall survival have been demonstrated with combined treatment regimens consisting of gemcitabine and cisplatin. Additional clinical trials are underway evaluating the efficacy of recently developed targeted therapies in conjunction with conventional chemotherapy.

Summary

ICC is the second most common hepatic primary malignancy after HCC with increasing incidence in the United States. Surgical therapy remains the primary treatment for ICC, but a significant proportion of patients present with advanced disease not amenable to curative resection. Ongoing development of molecularly targeted therapies brings hope for improvements in survival and quality of life in these patients.

REFERENCES

1. Mendizabal M, Reddy KR. Current management of hepatocellular carcinoma. *Med Clin North Am* 2009; 93:885–900, viii.
2. A new prognostic system for hepatocellular carcinoma: a retrospective study of 435 patients: the Cancer of the Liver Italian Program (CLIP) investigators. *Hepatology* 1998; 28:751–755.
3. Llovet JM, Bru C, Bruix J. Prognosis of hepatocellular carcinoma: the BCLC staging classification. *Semin Liver Dis* 1999; 19:329–338.
4. Verslype C, Van Cutsem E, Dicato M, et al. The management of hepatocellular carcinoma. Current expert opinion and recommendations derived from the 10th World Congress on Gastrointestinal Cancer, Barcelona, 2008. *Ann Oncol* 2009; 20 Suppl 7:vii1–vii6.
5. Mazzaferro V, Regalia E, Doci R, et al. Liver transplantation for the treatment of small hepatocellular carcinomas in patients with cirrhosis. *N Engl J Med* 1996; 334:693–699.
6. Yao FY, Ferrell L, Bass NM, et al. Liver transplantation for hepatocellular carcinoma: expansion of the tumor size limits does not adversely impact survival. *Hepatology* 2001; 33:1394–1403.
7. O'Neil BH, Venook AP. Hepatocellular carcinoma: the role of the North American GI Steering Committee Hepatobiliary Task Force and the advent of effective drug therapy. *Oncologist* 2007; 12:1425–1432.
8. Llovet JM, Ricci S, Mazzaferro V, et al. Sorafenib in advanced hepatocellular carcinoma. *N Engl J Med* 2008; 359:378–390.
9. Poultsides GA, Zhu AX, Choti MA, et al. Intrahepatic cholangiocarcinoma. *Surg Clin North Am* 90:817–837.
10. Choi SB, Kim KS, Choi JY, et al. The prognosis and survival outcome of intrahepatic cholangiocarcinoma following surgical resection: association of lymph node metastasis and lymph node dissection with survival. *Ann Surg Oncol* 2009; 16:3048–3056.

SURGICAL TREATMENT OF HEPATIC METASTASES 7

Nicole de Rosa[*], Dan G. Blazer III[†], and Bryan M. Clary[†]

COLORECTAL LIVER METASTASES

Introduction

Colorectal cancer (CRC) is the third leading cause of cancer in the United States and the third leading cause of cancer-related mortality. The liver is the most common site of hematogenous spread of colorectal cancer via the portal vein circulation and, in approximately one-third of patients, represents the only site of metastasis. In 2009, an estimated 147,000 new cases of CRC will be diagnosed and approximately 50% of these patients will develop liver metastases in their lifetime. Synchronous lesions will be present in 15% to 25% of patients, while an additional 20% to 25% will develop metachronous tumors.

The natural history of colorectal liver metastases (CLM) if left untreated is rapid progression to death with median survival times of 7–14 months, and rare 5-year survival. Poor prognostic factors for survival in unresected patients include the extent of the liver disease, the presence of extrahepatic metastases, carcinoembryonic antigen level, and patient age. In unresected patients, the utilization of modern chemotherapeutic agents in the past decade (including oxaliplatin, irinotecan, and targeted

---

[*] Duke University Medical Center 3443, Durham, NC 27710 USA
[†] Duke University Medical Center 3247, Durham, NC 27710 USA

agents against VEGF and EGF) has resulted in an improvement of median survival from 12 to 24 months. Even with these successes, long-term survival remains rare in the absence of local hepatic therapies.

Although randomized trials evaluating the role of hepatic resection do not exist, most would agree that it is critical to the possibility of long-term survival. An extensive number of large retrospective series clearly document the curative potential of resection. Furthermore, contemporary series suggest improvements in outcomes following resection that are likely multifactorial in etiology, but may include advances in imaging, operative technique, and the inclusion of more effective adjuvant and salvage therapies. As such, the cornerstone of treatment in the current era relies upon an aggressive mindset focused on issues of resectability, extent of disease characterization, perioperative care, and systemic adjuvant therapies.

Diagnosis

Carcinoembryonic antigen

Carcinoembryonic antigen (CEA) blood level is a tumor marker commonly used as a prognostic indicator and diagnostic assay to detect recurrences after resection of primary and metastatic colorectal cancers. Preoperatively, a CEA level >5.0 ng/mL in the setting of primary colorectal cancer is a poor prognostic factor. The Eastern Cooperative Oncology Group followed high-risk patients on INT0089 after resection of their primary tumors and determined that CEA measurement was the most cost-effective method of detecting potentially resectable colorectal metastases. Current guidelines from the American Society of Clinical Oncology include serum CEA testing every 2–3 months for 2 or more years after resection in patients with stage II or stage III disease who would be operable candidates for hepatic extirpation. Two documented levels above baseline, regardless of radiographic confirmation, indicate disease progression. It is important to note that mild elevations (false positives) may be seen in the smoking population.

Imaging studies

The proper identification of candidates for hepatectomy relies heavily on a thorough extent of disease evaluation. An appreciation of the common sites of metastatic disease is required in the planning of preoperative imaging. In addition to the site of tumor deposits, preoperative imaging must provide intra- and extrahepatic vascular details that affect resectability and operative planning.

Computed tomography (CT) scanning, given its ease of use and precise anatomical detail of the chest and abdominal cavities, is favored by many hepatobiliary surgeons and medical oncologists in the routine surveillance and preoperative planning of patients with colorectal cancer metastases. Although mild controversy exists regarding the relative merit of a chest CT in comparison to a plain chest radiograph, it is clear that CT can identify and more easily follow small suspected pulmonary metastases in this high-risk population. As the identification of pulmonary metastases often precludes hepatectomy, CT should be strongly considered in all patients undergoing evaluation for hepatic resection. CT provides anatomic details needed for surgical planning including lobar architecture, the relationship of the tumors to vascular and biliary structures, and the ability to measure future liver remnant volumes in patients requiring large volume resections. The typical appearance of a metastasis is that of a hypodense mass on venous phase imaging with peripheral enhancement. A spectrum of appearances can occur though and may be affected by systemic therapies. These may include the presence of calcifications, hypervascularity, or subtlety of the lesion (Table 1). Any intrahepatic lesion that does not fit classic criteria for the common benign lesions (cysts, hemangioma, FNH, etc.) should be viewed as suspicious in patients with a history of colorectal cancer. Historically, the sensitivity of CT was as low as 50% due to the slow acquisition of images and the inability to obtain portal venous phase images in a single run. With the advent of contrast-enhanced helical CT, current sensitivities of 73% to 83% are reported. It is critical to proper operative planning and lesion detection to include intravenous contrast, preferentially with arterial and venous phases. Although patients with mild dye allergies may be properly prophylaxed with preimaging steroids, those with prior life-threatening allergies and/or significant renal impairment require an alternative approach to imaging.

Magnetic resonance imaging (MRI) is another frequently used modality for the characterization of colorectal metastases and in some institutions is the preferred method of cross-sectional imaging of the abdomen. With the current use of contrast agents, such as gadolinium and ferumoxide, the ability to detect CLM has greatly improved with a sensitivity of 80% to 100% and a specificity of 93% to 100%. MRI has

Table 1. Imaging modalities used for the diagnosis of colorectal liver metastases.

Imaging modality	Advantages	Disadvantages	Recommendations
CT	Anatomic information of segmental anatomy vascular and biliary structures. Anatomic information including biliary imaging with MCRP.	Low sensitivity for small (< 1 cm) lesions.	Triphasic protocol. Abdomen, pelvis, chest. Routine usage.
MRI	Especially useful in patients with fatty liver disease from diabetes or chemotherapy.	High cost.	Reserve MRI for patients with equivocal CT lesions.
PET	Functional information. High sensitivity and specificity.	Limited detection of small lesions (< 1 cm) and limited utility after chemotherapy.	PET/CT may be used in lieu of laparoscopy to prevent futile laparotomy.
Colonoscopy			Routine usage. Within 6 months.

utility in the characterization of suspected benign lesions that do not meet classic criteria on CT scanning and additionally is feasible in patients with profound iodinated contrast allergies. Although historically utilized in patients with renal insufficiency (versus CT), the recent association of gadolinium with nephrogenic systemic fibrosis has limited its application to this patient population. An important advantage of MRI over CT is in its ability to readily image the biliary system when needed. Additionally, MRI is particularly useful in imaging patients with fatty liver changes secondary to diabetes or chemotherapy. The detection of small lesions (<1 cm) by MRI is limited with sensitivities of 57% to 63%.

Whole body positron emission tomography (PET) is commonly performed for evaluating patients with metastatic disease. PET relies on the use of a radiopharmaceutical, most commonly 18F-fluorodeoxyglucose (18F-FDG), which is a glucose analogue preferentially taken up by highly metabolic tissues such as cancer cells. Because it is unable to proceed through the glycolytic pathway, 18F-FDG accumulates in these cells, and imaging is subsequently used to localize the pattern of distribution. PET provides functional information at the cellular level, but unlike CT or MRI, the anatomic detail is limited. To address this drawback, PET has been combined with CT to provide anatomic localization of these functional abnormalities. In a prospective trial by Ruers *et al.*, 150 patients were randomized to CT alone or CT plus 18F-FDG PET for preoperative evaluation, to determine the utility of combined PET/CT for surgical planning. This study showed that PET/CT reduced the percentage of nontherapeutic laparotomies by 17%, thereby preventing unnecessary surgery in 1 of every 6 patients. Limitations of PET include the detection of small metastases (<1 cm) and lesions that have been exposed to chemotherapy. In addition, false positives are common; one of the more frequent being that of pelvic avidity in patients with prior resection and radiation. Controversy exists about the routine inclusion of PET scanning in patients being considered for hepatic resection. The data do suggest better patient selection through the exclusion of patients with otherwise occult metastatic disease. Given the expense and issues of false positivity, its use is far from universal.

Although the identification of distant metastatic disease is paramount, it is also important to ensure that patients have had relatively recent colonoscopic evaluation given the possibility of metachronous primaries and anastomotic recurrences.

Treatment

Evaluation of the patient for hepatectomy

Appropriate patient selection is an important factor in reducing operative morbidity and mortality after hepatectomy. The preoperative evaluation should begin with a comprehensive medical history and physical examination. Patient comorbidities including cardiac disease, pulmonary status, history of liver disease, and markers of overall physiologic health, such as the American Society of Anesthesiology (ASA) score, should be determined. Patients with excessive comorbidities and limited functional status are properly excluded from hepatectomy. Although age has long been a concern for perioperative mortality, it has not been shown to be an independent risk factor for increased postoperative death.

Determination of tumor resectability

The definition of "resectable" has undergone significant revision in recent years reflecting improvements in perioperative care and adjuvant therapies as well as a recognition that long-term survival is possible in patients with adverse risk factors. Historical contraindications to hepatic extirpation included patients with >3 metastases, metastasis >5 cm in greatest diameter, bilobar disease, a perceived inability to obtain a 1-cm margin, and the presence of extrahepatic disease. Recent studies demonstrate that long-term survival benefits can be achieved in patients with these characteristics. The importance of a microscopically negative margin remains vital to attaining long-term survival, however the width of the margin does not significantly impact outcomes. Therefore, the choice of a nonanatomic resection in lieu of an anatomic resection should be individualized and based upon the distribution, number, and size of the metastases. In this manner, a curative resection can be performed with maximal preservation of normal liver parenchyma. The number of metastases is no longer considered a contraindication to surgery, and extrahepatic disease should be considered a relative contraindication.

Because of the proven survival benefit in these patient subsets, there has been a shift in the treatment paradigm of CLM. Standards of resectability, once focused on what was to be removed from the liver, have been replaced with contemporary criteria that focus instead on what remains.

The current definition for resectability includes the ability to: (1) resect all disease with a negative microscopic margin, (2) preserve sufficient liver remnant volume (>20% total estimated liver volume in patients with normal parenchyma) in two adjacent liver segments with intact vascular inflow, outflow, and biliary drainage, and (3) attain margin-negative resection of extrahepatic metastatic disease.

Evaluation of future liver remnant

The most important predictors of poor perioperative outcomes following partial hepatectomy include pre-existing hepatic dysfunction, the complexity of the procedure, and the concomitant performance of additional procedures. As such, an assessment of the future liver remnant volume (FLRV) and function is crucial to appropriate patient selection for hepatectomy. Baseline liver function tests should evaluate the presence of active hepatitis, and INR, bilirubin, and albumin levels should be determined. In Western countries, the Child–Pugh score is traditionally used to estimate hepatic functional reserve. Patients with Child–Pugh A designations and who are without portal hypertension, are considered good operative candidates. In patients with normal hepatic parenchyma, a FLRV of 20% is generally adequate whereas in patients with chronic liver disease, the minimal volume requirement increases to 40%. CT and MRI can provide reproducible methods of calculating the future liver remnant volume.

For patients who are felt to be at risk for inadequate liver remnant size, portal vein embolization (PVE) may be incorporated preoperatively. By embolizing the region of the liver to be resected, splachnic venous return is shunted to the FLR, resulting in hypertrophy. PVE is typically conducted 3–6 weeks preoperatively and has been shown to increase volume and function of the liver remnant as measured by bile volume flow and indocyanine green excretion. Increased resectability rates for CLM have been reported between 63% and 84% with 3-year survival in these patients ranging from 35% to 40%. No current evidence indicates a significant improvement in patient outcomes, but some studies have observed a decrease in recurrence rates in patients undergoing hepatectomy with PVE when compared to similar resections without PVE. For patients with bilateral disease requiring large volume hepatectomies, a staged approach may be required in an effort to maintain a suitable liver remnant postoperatively.

Intraoperative assessment

Staging laparoscopy can be used to guide surgical decision-making in patients with a high risk of extrahepatic disease. Laparoscopic evaluation of the liver and abdominal cavity immediately prior to laparotomy has been shown to avoid nontherapeutic laparotomies in 10–25% of patients who were initially determined to have resectable disease by radiography. The likelihood of identifying this occult disease is clearly greater in patients with a significant number of negative prognostic factors (multiplicity, very high CEA levels, known extrahepatic disease, etc.) such that the routine application in low-risk patients is likely unnecessary. Intraoperative ultrasound is critical in the conduct of the operation as it identifies lesions that alter the operative planning in approximately 10% of patients.

Contemporary Outcomes

Mortality and morbidity

In patients with otherwise normal liver parenchyma undergoing metastasectomy for CLM, mortality rates prior to 1980 were approximately 20%. Factors associated with increased perioperative mortality include the presence of underlying liver disease, emergent resection, blood transfusion requirement, extended hepatectomy, and biliary malignancies. With better patient selection, advances in technical expertise, and developments in anesthesia monitoring, the overall mortality of hepatectomy is currently reported to be 3%, and as low as 1% at high volume centers. As the perioperative mortality has decreased, surgeons have taken an increasingly aggressive approach to the management of CLM. Because of this strategy, it is unlikely that mortality rates will further decrease. Therefore, a mortality risk of 3% to 5% is considered acceptable for this potentially curative procedure (Figure 1).

Despite decreased mortality rates, the perioperative morbidity rates associated with hepatectomy remain high at 22%. Postoperative complications associated with hepatectomy include pulmonary infection (11.9%), abdominal abscess with or without biliary fistula (7.1%), hemorrhage (2%), liver failure (1.2%), and kidney failure (0.7%).

Oncologic outcomes

Resection of colorectal liver metastases is required to achieve long-term survival. After hepatic extirpation with curative intent, median survival times are between 20 and 60 months (Figure 1). In large series reported

Author	Year	N	Interval	Mortality (%)	5 yr Survival (%)	Median Survival (mo)
Rees	2008	929	1987-2005	1.5	36	43
Katan	2008	1531	1986-2004	3.5	37	
Reddy	2007	230	1996-2006	2.8	45	42
Fong	2007	792	1991-1998		35	41
Wei	2006	423	1993-2002	1.6	47	53
Pawlik	2005	557	1990-2004	0.9	58	74
Choti	2002	226	1984-1999	0.9	40	46
			1984-1992		31	36
			1993-1999		58	
Cummings	2007	833	1991-2003	4.3	33	45
Robertson	2009	3957	2001-2004	4	25	

Figure 1. Current status of hepatic resection for colorectal liver metastases.

between the 1960s and the mid 1990s, 5-year survival rates were in the range of 33% to 36%. Single and multi-institution data from the late 1990's to the present suggest that the 5-year survival rates are improving with a number of series reporting 5-year survival exceeding 50%. Studies with long-term follow-up have reported 10-year survivals of approximately 20%. Despite R0 resection, 60% to 70% of patients will experience local, regional, or distant recurrence. Major prognostic factors that predict tumor recurrence include the presence of >3 metastases and extrahepatic disease. The median time to recurrence is 10 months and 80% occur within the first 2 years after resection. Untreated recurrent CLM are associated with a median survival time of 8–10 months, similar to the prognosis for untreated CLM at initial diagnosis. Repeat hepatectomy with curative intent is possible in 10% to 15% of patients, with a 5-year overall survival of 15% to 40% in select patients. Therefore, repeat resection for patients who meet the current operative criteria is recommended.

Patient survival after partial hepatectomy has been linked to several clinicopathologic features. Factors that are reliably present as significant in most retrospective series include multiplicity, extrahepatic disease, involved margins, very high CEA levels, and the nodal status of the primary colorectal tumor. In contemporary series, where adjuvant systemic therapy variables are included, many of these factors are secondary to effective adjuvant therapy. In an effort to stratify patients who may benefit from hepatic extirpation, and to provide a system for enrollment in clinical trials, several authors have suggested clinical risk scoring systems. The Clinical Risk Score (CRS) suggested by Fong et al. is the most widely used and has been verified by several independent investigators. A single-institution series of 1001 consecutive patients identified five preoperative criteria that were independent predictors of prognosis. These included: (1) a lymph node positive primary tumor, (2) disease-free interval <12 months, (3) largest tumor diameter >5 cm, (4) greater than 1 liver metastasis, and (5) a preoperative CEA level >200 IU/mL. One point was assigned for each risk factor and patients were organized into three risk groups (low-risk = 0, moderate-risk = 1–2, and high-risk >3). A significant difference in 5-year survival was observed among these groups with low-risk and high-risk 5-year survival rates of 60% and <20%, respectively (see Figure 5).

The CRS may be used to stratify high-risk patients for clinical trials and to guide preoperative diagnostic studies, as high-risk patients more frequently undergo futile laparotomies. The use of the CRS to determine candidacy for liver resection should be cautioned and hepatic resection should be considered in most patients if negative surgical margins can be obtained while leaving an adequate functional hepatic remnant. This strategy remains justified given the inadequacies of non-extirpative approaches.

Chemotherapy

It is well established that systemic therapy is effective in the unresectable population of patients with colorectal metastases. For decades, the only active combinations were 5-flourouracil based. Unresectable patients treated with 5-FU/leucovorin bolus regimens have response rates ranging from 20% to 30% with median survival times of 11.5 months (in comparison with 6–9 months in the absence of therapy). Over the past decade, a number of new cytotoxic and targeted agents have led to improved outcomes in unresectable patients such that the median survival of these patients exceeds 2 years from the diagnosis of metastatic disease.

In 2000, 5-FU/leucovorin was used in combination with irinotecan (FOLFIRI) as first-line treatment for patients with stage IV CRC. The addition of irinotecan, a topoisomerase 1 inhibitor, increased response rates to 39%, extended progression-free survival, and lengthened overall survival to 14.8 months, when compared with 5-FU/leucovorin alone. Another addition to the chemotherapeutic repertoire is the combination of oxaliplatin and 5-FU/leucovorin (FOLFOX). Oxaliplatin is a cisplatin derivative that inhibits DNA synthesis. FOLFOX has similar response rates as FOLFIRI with less severe toxicities. Interestingly, when FOLFOX and FOLFIRI are used sequentially, survival is prolonged.

Contemporary targeted biologic agents have also been used in combinatorial treatments for metastatic colorectal cancer. Bevacizumab (Avastin), an antivascular endothelial growth factor A monoclonal antibody, inhibits angiogenesis and is currently used with infusional chemotherapy as a first-line treatment. Therapeutic combinations containing bevacizumab have increased response rates of 35% to 45% and increased median survival times of 20.3 months. Cetuximab, an anti-epidermal growth factor receptor monoclonal antibody, is currently under investigation for use as a first-line therapy in CRC. The addition of cetuximab to FOLFOX or FOLFIRI increases response rates to approximately 70% and further increases resectability rates by about 7.5%.

Although data demonstrating improvements in overall survival with adjuvant systemic therapy in resected patients with hepatic metastases are currently lacking, there are a number of randomized trials suggesting improvements in progression-free survival. These data and the efficacy in unresectable patients are such that most resectable patients in the current era are approached in a multimodal fashion with the combination of resection and systemic therapy. The excellent response rates of current regimens have also increased the proportion of patients with metastatic disease who are able to undergo resection.

The optimal timing of resection and systemic therapy is a point of controversy in resectable patients. Historically, patients were recommended systemic therapy in advance of hepatectomy as a means of better selecting patients. Some studies suggest that preoperative treatment is associated with a 3% to 16% lower rate of positive surgical margins when compared to surgery alone. Chemotherapy may also be better tolerated in the presence of the entire liver allowing for higher dosages to be used. A randomized trial by the European Organization for the Research and Treatment of Cancer Trial 40983 studied patients receiving surgical therapy alone versus surgical therapy with preoperative and postoperative FOLFOX (6 cycles). This study demonstrated an improvement in 3-year progression-free survival by 9.2% in resected patients, albeit with an increase in perioperative morbidity. Of note, the use of a short course of prehepatectomy chemotherapy did lead to a reduction in the number of patients undergoing hepatic resection. In addition to concerns regarding hepatic toxicity and increased perioperative morbidity, there are a number of additional potential disadvantages to prehepatectomy chemotherapy. These include rendering clinically relevant disease occult at the time of hepatectomy. As such, decisions regarding the timing of therapy involve nuance and require close communication between surgeons and medical oncologists.

Timing of Surgical Treatments for Synchronous Presenters

Synchronous liver metastases are discovered in 15% to 25% of patients with colorectal cancer. The optimal timing of hepatectomy relative to resection of the colorectal primary and to chemotherapy remains unclear. Classically, initial resection of the colorectal primary is completed, followed by 8 to 12 weeks of chemotherapy. If the metastases are resectable and no interval disease progression has occurred, metastasectomy is offered. The rationale for this treatment algorithm is that patients who present with synchronous CLM have poor overall survival times and that the morbidity of simultaneous colorectal and hepatic procedure is assumed to be prohibitive. This approach ensures that: (1) all patients are treated with chemotherapy, (2) unnecessary and morbid hepatic resections are avoided in patients with aggressive disease who will not benefit from the treatment, and (3) the chemotherapy regimen can be tailored by *in vivo* response.

Issues of increased morbidity following hepatectomy in pretreated patients have led to a reassessment of this strategy. A number of series clearly demonstrate that early removal of the asymptomatic primary tumor is not necessary if systemic therapy is required for hepatic tumor downsizing to achieve resection. Furthermore, patients requiring low complexity hepatic and colorectal resections can often undergo these procedures simultaneously. A number of factors influence the feasibility of simultaneous resections including incisions, tumor location, and the complexity of the procedures. As such, a flexible and personalized approach to synchronous patients is required whereby some patients are best approached in a traditional manner and others with attention to the hepatic tumor first.

Regional

An alternative to systemic chemotherapy is hepatic arterial chemotherapy (HAI). HAI was developed with the rationale that CLM rely almost exclusively on the hepatic artery blood supply while normal liver cells rely predominantly on blood from the portal vein circulation. HAI using fluorodeoxyuridine (FUDR) alone improves response rates when compared to systemic chemotherapy in randomized control trials. FUDR infusion in addition to systemic triple agent chemotherapy yields response and resectability rates of 15% to 90% and 0% to 35%, respectively. Furthermore, in patients who have failed first-line neoadjuvant chemotherapy, FUDR infusion combined with systemic irinotecan or oxaliplatin regimens yields response and resection rates of 73% to 88% and 23% to 35%, respectively. Disadvantages of HAI include complications such as pump malfunction, arterial injuries including embolic events and aneurysms, as well as intrahepatic complications such as biliary sclerosing cholangitis and biliary stricture. Recent advances in minimally invasive percutaneous procedures for arterial port implantation may avoid arterial complications associated with an axillary artery approach and may be more advantageous than laparotomy. HAI may be most useful in patients with isolated liver metastases that are not amenable to resection or ablation, or in patients who have failed first-line chemotherapy.

The utility of HAI as an adjuvant to resection of hepatic metastases remains controversial as its efficacy outside of single institution experiences is unclear. The significant toxicity that can occur in addition to the growing experience with contemporary systemic regimens have diminished the enthusiasm for its use in this setting. A recent randomized trial designed to assess the efficacy of HAI in conjunction with contemporary systemic therapy (NSABP C-09) failed to accrue patients and was closed early.

Ablation

In situ tumor destruction can be accomplished with a variety of technologies including radiofrequency (RFA), cryotherapy, microwave (MA), laser, and ultrasonic energy. Over the past decade, there has been a transition from cryoablation to RFA and more recently MA. RFA and MA can be applied percutaneously, laparoscopically, or via open surgical approaches. The largest reported contemporary experiences are with RFA and document a number of important lessons. It is clear that local control with ablation is problematic with lesions greater than 2–3 cm in size and for those lesions in difficult locations where image guidance is difficult or large vessels reside. Thermal ablative technologies are also of limited usefulness for lesions near the hilum given the issues of biliary toxicity. The infusion of cold saline in the biliary tree has been advocated as a means of lessening these risks.

The choice of approach (surgical versus percutaneous, laparoscopic versus open) is largely dependent upon local expertise and tumor location and to a lesser extent on philosophical approaches to the disease. Percutaneous RFA is the least invasive approach and is often performed on an outpatient basis with low complication rates. A disadvantage to this approach is the lack of operative staging given the consideration that 15–20% of patients have additional disease (liver or otherwise) on surgical exploration. Lesions located in the dome of the liver or adjacent to the surface are relative contraindications to the laparoscopic approach. Open RFA likely provides the best visualization and targeting of liver lesions and intraoperative staging, but is associated with higher rates of morbidity. Laparoscopic RFA, although technically more challenging, seeks to balance issues of intraoperative staging and perioperative morbidity. The ability to confidently and accurately place the ablation probes laparoscopically requires extensive experience and as such may be less efficacious in the hands of most surgeons.

Randomized trials comparing thermal ablation to partial hepatectomy have not been conducted in patients with metastatic colorectal cancer. The patient populations undergoing ablation and resection are likely very different with respect to tumor burden and underlying functional status and as such retrospective experiences comparing the two modalities are flawed. Nonetheless, it appears that overall outcomes may be better with partial hepatectomy, which remains the gold-standard in the current era.

Embolization

Intra-arterial embolization is an option for liver-directed therapy in patients with tumors not amenable to resection or ablation. Transarterial chemoembolization (TACE) of liver lesions was first utilized in the treatment of hepatocellular carcinoma. TACE delivers targeted chemotherapy through the hepatic artery while simultaneously embolizing the vascular supply to the tumor. Studies show that TACE is a low durability treatment, with disease progression occuring within months, and has a limited improvement in survival.

An alternative to chemoembolization is selective internal radiation therapy (SIRT) with single-dose 90 yttrium microspheres, also delivered via the hepatic artery. A retrospective review of the Unites States experience with SIRT was published in 2005 and showed that in patients with chemoresistant tumors who had failed both first- and second-line chemotherapy median actuarial survival was 11 months, in comparison to 5 months observed in historic controls. Further studies are needed to define the role of SIRT in combination with standard chemotherapeutic regimens.

NEUROENDOCRINE LIVER METASTASES

The annual incidence of neuroendocrine tumors is estimated to be between 2.5 and 4.5 per 100,000 population per year. Approximately 75% of patients have metastatic disease at their initial presentation. Neuroendocrine liver metastases (NE) comprise almost 10% of liver metastases overall and in 90% of cases are multifocal and bilateral.

Several imaging modalities are used for localizing neuroendocrine tumors including US, endoscopic ultrasonography (EUS), CT, MRI, and somatostatin receptor scintigraphy (SRS). The sensitivities of US, CT, and MRI in detecting NE are 46%, 42%, and 43%, respectively. The combination of SRS and CT/MRI has a sensitivity of 96% and may be the best method for NE detection depending upon the histologic type. One exception to this recommendation is for insulinomas, which due to their downregulated expression of somatostatin receptor subtype-2, are best detected by the use of EUS. As a practical rule, SRS is not routinely utilized given the cost and fact that many neuroendocrine tumors fail to localize. It is important that cross-sectional imaging (MRI, CT) includes an arterial phase as NE liver metastases (NLMs) are often hypervascular and visualized on this phase only.

Similar to outcomes for CLMs, surgical resection of NLMs is favored when possible and, for the most part, decisions about resectability are similar. Long-term survival after complete resection is possible, with 5-year survival rates reported at 61–76%. However, because NLMs are often detected in the setting of extensive tumor burden, complete surgical resection is often not possible. In addition, though these tumors may behave in a more indolent manner from an oncologic perspective, because of the secretion of excess hormones, these tumors may cause significant morbidity as compared to other primary tumors. For this reason, unique to NLMs, incomplete hepatic resection may be justified in patients whose symptoms are refractory to other therapies. Symptom improvement, even in the setting of incomplete resection, can be dramatic.

Other locoregional modalities, such as RFA and TACE, may also offer durable symptom relief and play an important role in the comprehensive care of these complicated patients. Finally, liver transplantation has been explored as a modality for patients with unresectable NLMs. A more thorough review of these modalities in the setting of NLMs was recently published by Reddy *et al.* and is beyond the scope of this chapter.

NONCOLORECTAL NON-NEUROENDOCRINE LIVER METASTASES

The role of partial hepatectomy for noncolorectal non-neuroendocrine tumors (NCRNE) remains controversial given the even smaller amount of supporting literature than for CRM and NE. A number of sizeable retrospective experiences document long-term survival rates in selected patients that are notable for survival outcomes similar to the CRM experience. The improving morbidity profile of partial hepatectomy, introduction of ablative technologies, and the mature experiences in CRM and NE have prompted an increased interest in local management options for these patients.

As a general rule, it is possible to identify broad categories of patients who may or may not benefit from local treatments of liver metastases. For example, patients with genitourinary tumors have quite acceptable outcomes whereas patients with adenocarcinoma of the pancreas, lung, or esophagus with few exceptions should be precluded from local therapies.

In an effort to stratify patients prior to surgical intervention, a prognostic model has been developed by Adam *et al.* Patient clinicopathological factors and long-term outcomes were analyzed in 1452 patients with NCRNE. Five-year and 10-year, overall and disease-free survivals, were 36% and 21% and 23% and 15%, respectively. Factors associated with a poor prognosis included patient age >60 years, nonbreast origin, melanoma or squamous histology, disease-free interval of <12 months, extrahepatic metastases, R2 resection, and major hepatectomy. When patients were organized into three risk groups (low-risk = 0 to 3, mid-risk = 4 to 6, and high-risk ≥7), 5-year survival rates varied significantly at 46%, 33%, and <10%, respectively.

In summary, hepatectomy can be performed safely and can yield long-term survival benefits similar to that for CLM in highly select patients with NCRNE. Delayed liver resection of >6 months and the use of adjuvant chemoradiotherapy in addition to an understanding of the underlying biology of the primary tumor histology may better select patients.

REFERENCES

1. Jemal A, Siegel R, Ward E, *et al.* Cancer statistics, 2009. *CA Cancer J Clin* 2009; 59:225–249.
2. Scheele J, Stangl R, Altendorf-Hofmann A. Hepatic metastases from colorectal carcinoma: Impact of surgical resection on the natural history. *Br J Surg* 1990; 77:1241–1246.
3. Pawlik TM, Choti MA. surgical therapy for colorectal metastases to the liver. *J Gastrointest Surg* 2007; 11:1057–1077.
4. Sharma S, Camci C, Jabbour N. Management of hepatic metastasis from colorectal cancers: An update. *J Hepatobiliary Pancreat Surg* 2008; 15:570–580.
5. Compton C, Fenoglio-Preiser CM, Pettigrew N, Fielding LP. American joint committee on cancer prognostic factors consensus conference. Cancer 2000; 88(7): 1739–1757.
6. Bast RC, Ravdin P, Hayes DF, *et al.* Somerfield MR. 2000 Update of recommendations for the use of tumor markers in breast and colorectal cancer: Clinical practice guidelines of the American Society of Clinical Oncology. *J Clin Oncol* 2001; 19(6): 1865–1878.
7. Bhattacharjya S, Bhattacharjya T, Baber S, *et al.* Prospective study of contrast-enhanced computed tomography, computed tomography during arterioportography, and magnetic resonance imaging for staging colorectal liver metastases for liver resection. *Br J Surg* 2004; 91: 1361–1369.
8. Mainenti PP, Mancini M, Mainolfi C, *et al.* Detection of colo-rectal liver metastases: Prospective comparison of contrast enhanced us, multidetector CT, PET/CT, and 1.5 tesla mr with extracellular and reticulo-endothelial cell specific contrast agents. *Abdom Imaging* 2010; 35(5):511–521.
9. Ruers TJM, Wiering B, van der Sijp JRM, *et al.* Improved selection of patients for hepatic surgery of colorectal liver metastases with 18F-FDG PET: A Randomized Study. *J Nucl Med* 2009; 50(7):1036–1041.
10. Belghiti J, Hiramatsu K, Benoist S, *et al.* Seven hundred forty-seven hepatectomies in the 1990s: An update to evaluate the actual risk of liver resection. *J Am Coll Surg* 2000; 191:38–46.
11. Altendorf-Hofmann A, Scheele J. A critical review of the major indicators of prognosis after resection of hepatic metastases from colorectal carcinoma. *Surg Oncol Clin* N Am 2003; 12(1):165–192.

12. Barbot DJ, Marks JH, Feld RI, *et al.* Improved staging of liver tumors using laparoscopic intraoperative ultrasound. *J Surg Oncol* 1997; 64:63–67.
13. Reddy SK, Barbas AS, Clary BM. Synchronous colorectal liver metastases: Is it time to reconsider traditional paradigms of management? *Ann Surg Oncol* 2009; 16:2395–2410.
14. Fong Y, Fortner J, Sun RL, *et al.* Clinical score for predicting recurrence after hepatic resection for metastatic colorectal cancer: Analysis of 1001 consecutive cases. *Ann Surg* 1999; 230:309–321.
15. Cescon M, Vetrone G, Grazi GL, *et al.* Trends in perioperative outcome after hepatic resection: Analysis of 1500 consecutive unselected cases over 20 years. *Ann Surg* 2009; 249:995–1002.
16. Khatri VP, Chee KG, Petrelli NJ. modern multimodality approach to hepatic colorectal metastases: Solutions and controversies. *Surg Oncol* 2007; 16:71–83.
17. Sutcliffe R, Maguire D, Ramage J, *et al.* Management of neuroendocrine liver metastases. *Am J Surg* 2004; 187:39–46.
18. Reddy SK, Barbas AS, Marroquin CE, *et al.* Resection of noncolorectal nonneuroendocrine liver metastases: A comparative analysis. *J Am Coll Surg* 2007; 204:372–382.
19. Adam R, Chiche L, Aloia T, *et al.* and the Association Francaise de Chirurgie. Hepatic resection for noncolorectal nonendocrine liver metastases: Analysis of 1452 patients and development of a prognostic model. *Ann Surg* 2006; 244:524–535.
20. Reddy SK, Clary BM. Neuroendocrine liver metastases. *Surg Clin North Am.* 2010 Aug; 90(4):853–61.

CIRRHOSIS AND PORTAL HYPERTENSION

8

Keshava Rajagopal* and
Carlos E. Marroquin[†]

INTRODUCTION

Chronic liver disease is estimated to kill 30,000–35,000 people in the United States annually, making it approximately the 10th leading cause of death. Most of these patients have end-stage liver disease, characterized by cirrhosis and its sequelae. Cirrhosis specifically refers to hepatic scarring that results as a consequence of chronic liver disease, with fibrosis and nodular foci of regeneration. Laennec first coined the term in the early 19th century, although cirrhosis and potential etiologic contributors were appreciated at least centuries before Laennec. The term is derived from the Greek "κιρροσ", or tawny, in reference to the color and appearance of the cirrhotic liver at autopsy. In this chapter, we outline the pathophysiology, diagnosis and treatment of cirrhosis and its sequelae.

PATHOPHYSIOLOGY

Cirrhosis functionally is a syndrome, in that many different disease processes yield it as an end-state. Table 1 lists various causes of chronic liver disease that may result in cirrhosis. Due to chronic injury, myofibroblasts

---

*Duke University Medical Center, Durham, NC 27710 USA
[†]University of Rochester, Rochester, New York, USA

Table 1. Etiologies of liver disease.

Viral hepatitis	Alcohol-induced liver disease
Hepatitis A, B, C, D	Autoimmune hepatitis
CMV, EBV, Herpes virus	Systemic disorders
Rubella, adenovirus, enterovirus	Familial amyloidotic polyneuropathy
Cholestatic liver diseases	Sarcoidosis
Primary biliary cirrhosis	Non-alcoholic steato hepatitis
Primary sclerosing cholangitis	(NASH)
In-born errors of metabolism	Circulatory disorders
Hemochromatosis	Budd-Chiari syndrome
Wilson's disease	Veno-occlusive disease
Alpha-1-antitrypsin deficiency	Cryptogenic cirrhosis
Glycogen storage diseases	Fulminant hepatic failure
Tyrosinemia	Acute viral hepatitis
Alagille syndrome	Acute drug-induced hepatitis
Crigler-Najjar type I	Budd-Chiari syndrome
Severe familial hypercholesterolemia	Veno-occlusive disease
Hereditary oxalosis	Wilson's disease
Cystic fibrosis	Primary hepatic malignancy

and stellate cells of Ito in the liver, normally responsible for the synthesis of extracellular matrix components, become hyperactive. Moreover, degradation of matrix proteins by metalloproteinases is inhibited. This imbalance between extracellular matrix production and degradation causes net matrix accumulation within the liver. As chronic liver disease is characterized by loss of functioning hepatocyte mass, the result is a replacement of functional liver tissue with scar. However, unlike other tissues and organs with little if any endogenous functional or proliferative regenerative capacity, functioning hepatocytes are able to re-enter the cell cycle and proliferate. This compensatory response occurs within fibrotic liver architecture, and thus, there exist regenerative foci that form hepatic nodules.

The subcellular and cellular processes characterizing cirrhosis and end-stage liver disease have macroscopic and physiologic sequelae. These sequelae result in increased resistance to portal blood flow in the liver, as the liver becomes progressively more fibrotic, and as the vascular architecture of the liver becomes disrupted. This is compounded by the evolution of increased portal flow secondary to the development of a hyperdynamic state and splanchnic vasodilation. The result of this dynamic interplay is portal hypertension or an elevated portal venous pressure. In the absence of an elevation in the hepatic venous/inferior vena caval pressure, which alone can result in portal hypertension, portal hypertension occurs in the setting of an increase in the pressure difference between the portal vein and the inferior vena cava, and can be simply expressed by a fluid mechanical analogy to Ohm's Law. The ΔP is the transhepatic pressure difference, Q is the portal blood flow and R is the resistance to flow.

$$\Delta P = Q \ x \ R$$

Consequently, it is relatively straightforward conceptually that portal pressures are increased by either an increase in blood flow or by an increase in resistance. The contribution to increasing pressures by the resistance that a stiff, cirrhotic liver generates is intuitive to most and easy to appreciate. However, it is critical to realize that as the degree of liver failure progresses, so does the hyperdynamic state that contributes increasing amounts of gut arterial, and thus, portal venous flow. The contribution from increasing flow exerts a greater influence on the morbidity that develops during later stages of the disease.

Normal transhepatic pressure differences range between 0 and 5 mm Hg. It is crucial to understand that portal hypertension is central to the development of complications from end-stage liver disease. It is the cause of gastroesophageal varices, variceal bleeding, ascites, encephalopathy, hepato-renal syndrome, splenomegaly, hepato-hydrothorax, and hepatopulmonary syndrome. Portal hypertension results in the formation of varices, and can produce disfiguring, painful ascites and lethal variceal hemorrhage when transhepatic pressure differences exceed 12 mm Hg.

Portal hypertension may be divided into three types based on the location of abnormally elevated impedance to portal blood flow: prehepatic, intrahepatic, and posthepatic (Table 2). Prehepatic causes produce extrahepatic portal venous obstruction and manifest no biochemical evidence of liver failure. Intrahepatic causes of portal hypertension are further subdivided according to the anatomic zone of obstruction relative to the sinusoid and according to the hepatic venous catheterization results (see below). The reality is that syndromes that produce a presinusoidal picture at their inception will eventually generate a sinusoidal component with disease progression and the evolution of fibrosis.

Presinusoidal portal hypertension is associated with schistosomiasis, sarcoidosis, and primary biliary cirrhosis. There is a long list of etiologies that produce sinusoidal portal hypertension, with the common denominator being cirrhosis. Postsinusoidal portal hypertension is caused by any etiology of hepatic venous outflow obstruction (Budd–Chiari Syndrome), and

Table 2. Etiology of portal hypertension.

Prehepatic portal hypertension
   Extra-hepatic portal vein obstruction
      Portal vein thrombosis (most common)
      Splenic vein thrombosis
      Extrinsic compression of the portal vein
      Congenital abnormalities

Intrahepatic portal hypertension
   Presinusoidal (Normal hepatic wedge pressure/normal free pressure)
      Schistosomiasis
      Sarcoidosis
      Tuberculosis
      Primary biliary cirrhosis

Sinusoidal (Increased hepatic wedge pressure/normal free pressure)
      Alcoholic cirrhosis
      Viral hepatitis
      Chronic biliary obstruction
      Nodular transformation
      Congenital hepatic fibrosis
      Polycystic disease
      Amyloidosis
      Acute fatty liver of pregnancy
      Hemochromatosis
      Wilson's disease
      α_1- antitrypsin deficiency

Postsinusoidal (Increased hepatic wedge pressure/increased free pressure)
      Veno-occlusive disease
      Central hyaline sclerosis

Posthepatic portal hypertension
   Inferior vena cava obstruction
      Budd-Chiari syndrome
      Congenital malformation of the IVC
      Thrombosis of the IVC
      Malignant IVC obstruction
   Cardiac disease (increased right heart pressures)
      Constrictive pericarditis
      Tricuspid insufficiency
      Cardiomyopathy

right atrial hypertension. Elevated hepatic vascular resistance is common to all types except those with an elevated inferior vena caval/right atrial pressure. As previously mentioned, aggravating the issue of increased resistance to flow secondary to cirrhosis and intrahepatic vascular disruption is an increase in splanchnic blood flow. Splanchnic arteriolar dilatation occurs in the setting of chronic liver disease secondary to the local release of endothelial and humoral vasodilators such as nitric oxide and glucagon.

Chronic liver disease manifests in other clinically relevant ways, both related and unrelated to cirrhosis and portal hypertension. Hepatic dysfunction causes reduced synthesis of plasma proteins, including coagulation factors. Thus, patients with chronic liver disease are hypoproteinemic and coagulopathic and the severity of both of these processes correlates with the degree of hepatic insufficiency. In turn, as quantified by the Starling equation for transcapillary fluid flux, portal venous hypertension and hypoproteinemia cause a net increase in the combined mechanical/oncotic pressure gradient in favor of transudation into the peritoneal space:

$$Q = k \int \nabla P_{net} \cdot dA,$$

in which Q represents fluid flow, k is a constant that expresses permeability or filtration, ∇P_{net} is the net pressure gradient (this is a true gradient, as opposed to a difference), integrated across the surface area for fluid transfer A. In chronic liver disease with portal hypertension, the net pressure gradient increases, and permeability increases as well, thus causing net fluid transudation. This is clinically manifested as ascites.

HISTORY AND PHYSICAL EXAMINATION

The history and physical examination are indispensable in the evaluation of the patient with cirrhosis. This is because historical information and physical examination complement the biochemical parameters that allow one to assess not only the presence, but the severity of liver disease (Table 3). This evaluation has been found to be predictive of short- and long-term morbidity and mortality. Detailed information regarding risk factors for chronic liver disease should be obtained during the history component of the evaluation; risk factors of known of hepatitides (IV drug use, tattoos etc.), alcohol consumption, potential causes of systemic venous hypertension including heart failure, autoimmune diseases, and rare genetic/familial

Table 3. Child-Turcotte-Pugh score.

Clinical and biochemical parameters	Score for increasing abnormality		
	1	2	3
Encephalopathy (grade)	None	1–2	3
Ascites	None	Slight	Moderate
Albumin (g/dL)	>3.5	2.8–3.5	<2.8
Prothrombin time (sec)	1–4	4–6	>6
Bilirubin (mg/dL)	1–2	2–3	>3

Class A = 5–6 points; Class B = 7–9 points; Class C = 10–15 points.

diseases. Patients may provide a history of weakness, fatigue, and confusion. They may report self-identified jaundice, abdominal swelling, and systemic edema. Perhaps most important, detailed questions regarding gastrointestinal bleeding with specific questions of any episodes of hematemesis, increasing abdominal girth, and difficulty concentrating or other clinical evidence of encephalopathy should be asked, as these represent the most direct clinical evidence of advanced portal hypertension.

On physical examination, stigmata of chronic liver disease are often readily apparent, and the more advanced the stage of disease, the more asthenic the patient and apparent the findings. Numerous spider angiomata are often easily observed on the face and chest of patients with advanced liver disease. These represent a central arteriole with multiple small venules radiating from the central arteriole giving the appearance of small "spiders". These are believed to result from estrogen excess due to inadequate hepatic metabolism. Another overt finding in patients with chronic liver disease is the sweet scent of *fetor hepaticus*. This is commonly a late sign of and is likely caused by multiple sources. In addition to portosystemic shunting that allows mercaptans to pass directly into the lungs, the presence of ammonia and ketones in the breath combined with exhaled mercaptans produces the very characteristic scent that is also referred to as the breath of the dead. Jaundice may be identified on examination of the skin, conjunctivae, and other mucous (e.g. oral) membranes.

Although relatively uncommon, some patients with chronic liver disease have pulmonary manifestations that become clinically evident. These pulmonary manifestations of chronic liver disease include: (1) associated parenchymal lung disorders, (2) hepato-hydrothorax, (3) and pulmonary vascular disorders — hepatopulmonary syndrome and portopulmonary hypertension. Parenchymal lung disease can occur in association with primary biliary cirrhosis, α-1-antitrypsin deficiency and sarcoidosis. The pulmonary effects are manifestations of the same disease afflicting the liver. However, only a minority of these patients will be affected by parenchymal involvement. Patients with PBC may develop obstructive (bronchiolitis obliterans) or restrictive lung diseases (pulmonary fibrosis). While patients with α-1-antitrypsin deficiency develop obstructive physiology (emphysema with or without bronchiolitis), patients with sarcoidosis tend to develop a restrictive process secondary to pulmonary fibrosis. Hepatic hydrothorax, or pulmonary ascites, are pleural effusions that occur in the presence of chronic liver disease. These patients may demonstrate clinical respiratory insufficiency. On examination, decreased breath sounds are present most commonly in isolation on the right, i.e. the effusions are more common on the right left or bilateral. Ascites is not only present, but the source of the effusion as it migrates to the pleural space through small diaphragmatic defects. Hepatopulmonary syndrome (HPS) manifests with hypoxemia in the presence of chronic liver disease, and is the result of inappropriate pulmonary vasodilation, that decreases surface area contact between RBCs and the pulmonary vasodilation, that resulting in a diffusion limitation of oxygen and hypoxia. There should be no known cardiac or pulmonary source to account for the hypoxemia. Overt intrapulmonary shunting secondary to dilated pre-capillary and capillary vasculature results in a clinically significant ventilation-perfusion mismatch. Patients with HPS may manifest with dyspnea that is alleviated by lying down (platypnea) and hypoxemia, often exacerbated by an upright position (orthodeoxia). Finally, porto-pulmonary hypertension, in contrast to HPS, is characterized by pulmonary vasoconstriction and chronic vascular pruning and obliteration. Porto-pulmonary hypertension is associated with a mean pulmonary artery pressure greater than 25 mm Hg. Elevated pulmonary vascular resistance, and thus right ventricular afterload, may cause right ventricular diastolic dysfunction and/or failure. Patients are not commonly symptomatic. Since liver disease progresses through a continuum, patients who develop portopulmonary hypertension also tend to progress through a continuum. They are initially asymptomatic but will eventually begin to complain of non-specific discomfort which may ultimately lead to a symptomatic phase characterized by dyspnea. As such, patients who are found to have right ventricular systolic pressures greater than 50 mm He should undergo cardiac catheterization to evaluate the mean pulmonary artery pressures; if greater than 35 mm Hg, these patients are candidates and may respond to therapy.

Ascites is also commonly observed upon abdominal examination, and characteristic findings include the presence of fluid waves and shifting dullness. Portal hypertension may cause the exaggerated development of portal-systemic venous collateral networks (including varices — see Chapter 10), which are often evident on physical examination. Those evident on examination include so-called *caput medusae*, and hemorrhoids. Hepatic encephalopathy may manifest with confusion, altered level of consciousness, and asterixis may be documented during the examination of the extremities — a characteristic wrist tremor induced upon dorsiflexion of the upper extremities. Finally, peripheral edema is often present as a sequela of hypoproteinemia and volume expansion which is often present in cirrhotic patients.

LABORATORY TESTS AND IMAGING STUDIES

Blood tests are essential in the evaluation of patients with cirrhosis and portal hypertension. They are used to determine the severity of each patient's disease and to establish the etiology of their disease. The severity of liver disease is partially assessed by laboratory testing in the CTP system (Table 3), and is entirely based upon laboratory testing in the Model of End-Stage Liver Disease (MELD) system (Table 4). The MELD model was devised originally to assess the survival of patients undergoing transjugular intrahepatic portosystemic shunt placement (TIPS). The model relies on three objective and reproducible parameters. The ability of MELD to predict the 3-month mortality of patients with ESLD was validated in a study at the Mayo clinic. Moreover, MELD was shown to be as good as the CTP classification in terms of its ability to predict survival in patients with ESLD of diverse etiologies. In 2002, the MELD score replaced time on the waiting list as the criteria which would be used to allocate livers to patients with liver disease as it proved a good predictor of the severity of disease. This change in UNOS policy insured that livers would be allocated to the sickest patients. Essential tests to evaluate the severity of liver disease include: complete blood count, coagulation profile, serum albumin and total protein,

Table 4. Model for end-stage liver disease score.

Criteria:
   Bilirubin (mg/dL)
   International normalized ratio (INR) for prothrombin time
   Creatinine (mg/dL)

Formula:
   MELD Score = 11.2 log(INR) + 3.78 log(Bilirubin) + 9.57 log(Creatinine)

Prognosis in hospitalized patients:

Meld Score	3 Month Mortality
<9	4%
10–19	27%
20–29	76%
30–39	83%
>40	100%

and metabolic panel — inclusive of serum bilirubin and creatinine. Additional tests are used to establish the etiology of disease such as a hepatitis panel, CMV DNA, and EBV titers to evaluate viral causes. Other laboratory assays include antimitochondrial antibody levels (primary biliary cirrhosis), antinuclear antibody levels (autoimmune hepatitis), iron studies (hemochromatosis), ceruloplasmin (Wilson's disease), and α1-antitrypsin assay.

Imaging and other diagnostic studies are generally related to evaluating portal hypertension and tumor surveillance. Non-invasive hepatic imaging may provide information regarding the quality of hepatic blood flow. Duplex ultrasonography is the most commonly used of these modalities, and can be used to screen for tumors in addition to assessing flow in the hepatic artery, portal vein, and hepatic veins. An important ultrasonographic finding in the setting of portal hypertension is the reversal of the direction of portal blood flow, such that it is away from the liver (hepatofugal) rather than towards the liver (hepatopetal). Finally, ultrasound screening for the development of hepatoma should be performed every 6 months for patients with established cirrhosis. Once a suspicious lesion is identified, efforts to better characterize the lesion should be undertaken with MRI or CT scans depending on the local radiographic abilities.

Hepatic venous catheterization is the best test to ascertain the existence and severity of portal venous hypertension. Hepatic venous blood pressures are measured via a balloon-tipped catheter, which is then advanced while inflated until a hepatic venous occlusion pressure waveform is obtained; this is approximately equivalent to the portal venous pressure. For antegrade transhepatic venous flow to occur, the mean portal venous pressure must exceed the mean nonocclusion hepatic venous pressure, and for a fixed transhepatic venous flow rate, the difference between the portal venous and hepatic venous pressures is proportional to the hepatic resistance. A hepatic venous pressure "gradient" (this is really a difference, not a gradient in mathematical terms; hepatic venous occlusion pressure minus hepatic venous pressure) of >12 mm Hg is considered substantially elevated, and is the point at which one can begin to observe substantial morbidity associated with advanced liver disease.

NONSURGICAL THERAPIES OF SEQUELAE OF END-STAGE LIVER DISEASE

Hepatic Dysfunction

The treatment of liver dysfunction is supportive, as current approaches cannot delay the progression of, stall, or reverse hepatocyte dysfunction, and the only therapeutic strategy that improves hepatocyte function is replacement in the form of liver transplantation. Broadly, the most important priority in the treatment of liver dysfunction in cirrhosis is to ensure adequate quantities of somatic proteins, particularly those circulating in the bloodstream — e.g. coagulation factors, and albumin, which are deficient in hepatic dysfunction. Protein and caloric supplementation is often beneficial, and is tolerated by most cirrhotic patients. Similarly, cofactors are often deficient, and vitamin/mineral supplementation is beneficial. Notable among these are calcium and zinc. Finally, hyperbilirubinemia is ubiquitous in cirrhosis due to both non-cholestatic and cholestatic etiologies. This often results in pruritus, which can be treated medically using agents such as cholestyramine and ursodeoxycholic acid. In some patients with refractory pruritus, ultraviolet phototherapy or plasmapheresis may be necessary.

Encephalopathy

Hepatic encephalopathy reflects the degree of liver failure and portosystemic shunting on the central nervous system. Neurologic derangement is thought to arise due to impairment of normal portal blood flow and hepatic clearance of metabolites that arise from the gastrointestinal tract. The lack of clearance of GI-derived compounds leads to neurotoxicity and encephalopathy. While ammonia is important in the development of hepatic encephalopathy, it is yet unclear what specific biochemical compound or compounds mediate the neurotoxicity. In cirrhosis, deficient transhepatic portal blood flow and increased flow through portal-systemic collateral networks result in high concentrations of these neurotoxic compounds in the systemic circulations of these neurotoxic compounds. Encephalopathy ensues, and it is important to note that since portal-systemic collateral flow is important in the pathogenesis, portal systemic shunting procedures do not benefit and may initiate or exacerbate encephalopathy. The manifestations of hepatic encephalopathy can range from an inability to concentrate to outright coma with an inability to respond to noxious stimuli and is graded from 0 to 4 (Table 5).

Since the pathogenesis of hepatic encephalopathy can be multifactorial, adequate therapy must attempt to identify precipitating factor or factors that produced the decompensation such as infections or a GI bleed. In addition, treatment of encephalopathy is supportive and focused on the removal and inhibition of production of neurotoxic compounds. Most commonly, lactulose is used to facilitate gut-mediated excretion of these compounds. Oral antibiotics, e.g. neomycin, and more recently, rifaximin, reduce gut levels of ammonia-synthesizing bacteria. Finally, although

Table 5. Grades of hepatic encephalopathy.

Grade	Neurologic manifestation
0	No alteration in consciousness
1	Difficulty concentrating, euphoria or anxiety
2	Lethargy, disorientation, personality change, inappropriate behavior
3	Somnolence, stupor, confusion, responds to noxious stimuli
4	Coma with no response to noxious stimuli

increasingly uncommon, lowering dietary protein intake may be required in a small subset of patients with refractory hepatic encephalopathy.

Hepatorenal Syndrome

In its broadest sense, hepatorenal syndrome (HRS) is renal failure occurring in the setting of hepatic dysfunction. The pathogenesis of HRS emanates from a relative systemic arterial (excluding the splanchnic circulation) hypovolemia that occurs because of extreme splanchnic vasodilation. The relative systemic hypovolemia is sensed by the kidneys and activates the vasoconstricting and salt and water retention mechanisms of the renin–angiotensin system in the kidney. It is critical to evaluate any other potential underlying renal pathology before making a diagnosis of HRS. Renal vasoconstriction and impaired renal perfusion are known to occur, with concomitant gut vasodilation and augmented splanchnic blood flow that results because of release of vasodilators into the splanchnic circulation. Patients with HRS have characteristic stigmata of liver disease (ascites, jaundice etc.) with decreasing renal function marked by decreased urine output and rising creatinine.

Hepatorenal syndrome has been observed to occur in two different varieties, acute and chronic. Type I is acute renal failure that typically occurs within weeks of presentation. It can be observed in the setting of fulminant hepatic failure, and is also seen, not uncommonly, in patients with chronic liver disease after a precipitating event such as a GI bleed with hypotension, infection, decreased circulating volume secondary to dehydration, and iatrogenically after large volume paracentesis. Type II HRS is chronic renal insufficiency that evolves slowly with moderate changes in creatinine over time in the setting of declining liver function. Type II HRS is more amenable to medical management. The morbidity of hepatorenal syndrome is substantial and its development is associated with an increased mortality. This important detail is captured by the MELD score, since serum Cr is included in its calculation and contributes to the MELD's ability to predict 3-month mortality.

The first step in making the diagnosis of HRS is to rule out other potential causes of renal failure such prerenal, renal and postrenal etiologies. Commonly used criteria for diagnosing hepatorenal syndrome include: (1) clinically or objectively determined normal cardiac output and/or euvolemia, and the absence of shock, (2) the absence of known pre-existing renal disease or other renal causes for the decreasing renal function (e.g. glomerulonephritis, ATN, nephrotoxic agents), (3) oliguria (<500 ml/day urine output), (4) urine sodium <10 mEq/L, and (5) Cr clearance <40 ml/min with serum Cr >1.5 mg/dL (6) and no evidence of parenchymal renal disease evidenced by proteinuria with abnormal renal ultrasound.[4]

The treatment of HRS is initially comprised of intravascular volume expansion and the avoidance of diuretic agents. Recent evidence suggests that the judicious use of systemic vasoconstrictors may be helpful by producing vasoconstriciton of the dilated splanchnic vascular bed. Vasopressin has been utilized as it effectively binds the V1 receptors in the mesenteric vascular bed producing greater mesenteric than renal vasoconstriction. Terlipressin is a long-acting analog of vasopressin. It also causes direct vasoconstriction of the systemic arteriolar and splanchnic vasculature to a greater degree than the renal vessels by its greater affinity for the V1 receptor than the V2 receptor in the renal vascular bed. Midrodrine is an α1-adrenergic receptor agonist that has been shown to be effective at reversing HRS when used in combination with albumin and octreotide. In fact, this combination of agents was found to significantly improve short-term survival and renal function in both HRS type 1 and type 2.[6] This strategy may provide a significant benefit as a bridge to liver transplantation in HRS type 1 and may improve the outcomes of liver transplantation by ameliorating post transplant renal insufficiency which is associated with higher mortality rates. Transjugular intrahepatic portosystemic shunts have been shown to have an extremely favorable effect of HRS and the associated mortality. Unfortunately, the use of TIPS is often limited in these patients since it can exacerbate hepatic encephalopathy and precipitate decompensation. Finally, as is the case with Type I patients, liver transplantation is the definitive therapy for Type II hepatorenal syndrome as it corrects both the underlying liver disease and the associated circulatory dysfunction of portal hypertension.

Portal Hypertension — Ascites

The development of ascites is one of the first manifestations of liver disease and a common complication of cirrhosis. Ascites in chronic liver disease has traditionally been viewed as developing from "back-pressure" from increased intrahepatic hydrostatic pressure into the hepatic and splanchnic circulation, and decreased oncotic pressure that results from hypoproteinemia. The splanchnic vasodilation seen with portal hypertension generates greater capillary pressure secondary to higher blood flow rate into the splanchnic capillary bed. This results in a leakage of fluid into the peritoneal cavity. In addition to increasing blood flow through the splanchnic capillary beds, splanchnic vasodilation affects nonsplanchnic systemic arterial pressures, which subsequently results in activation of the renin-angiotensin system. The ultimate effect is a constituitive retention of sodium and water by the kidneys and continuous formation of ascites. The diagnosis is established by history, physical examination, and definitively, by paracentesis and analysis of ascitic fluid. Ascites due to liver disease is generally low protein (<2.5 g/dL), with a high serum albumin-ascites gradient (>1.1 g/dL). In addition, paracentesis may establish the presence of spontaneous bacterial peritonitis, a morbid complication of ascites. A variety of treatments exist for ascites.

Medical therapy is the first-line treatment, and comprises sodium restriction and diuretic usage. Patients should be instructed not to use salt in their food and not to cook with salt. The sodium intake should be restricted to 50 mEq/day. Sodium restriction is critical to the effectiveness of diuretics in controlling ascites. Spironolactone and lasix are the most commonly used diuretics with spironolactone being the principal diuretic. Patients with ascites should be weighed daily and the objective should be half a kilogram weight loss daily. Spironolactone should be started at a dose of 100 mg/day and doubled every other day if no effect is observed up to a dose of 400 mg. Lasix should be started once spironolactone has been maximized. Lasix is started at a dose of 40 mg/day and increased to a maximum dose of 160 mg/day. Once ascites has been effectively controlled, diuretic doses should be reduced to a maintenance dose that effectively prevents the ascites from re-accumulating. If medical management fails to control the development of ascites, patients may develop painful, tense ascites that produces substantial morbidity. Tense ascites can impair systemic venous return (abdominal compartment syndrome physiology) and result in relative and occasionally profound hypotension. Tense ascites can also result in respiratory compromise due to chest wall restriction. When these systemic manifestations are evident, large volume paracentesis can be therapeutic. Finally, peritoneovenous shunts translocate ascites into the systemic venous circulation, and are effective treatments for refractory ascites. The most commonly used peritoneo-venous shunts are the LeVeen and Denver shunts. Both have a unidirectional valve mechanism that maintains unidirectional peritoneal cavity-systemic venous ascitic fluid flow, but the Denver shunt has an additional externally actuated pump, conceived to augment ascitic flow. Other interventions include portal-systemic shunt placement and will be discussed in Chapter 10.

Pulmonary Manifestations

Parenchymal Diseases

As discussed, end-stage liver disease is associated with pulmonary complications. Patients with pulmonary manifestations of PBC may present with clinical manifestations of either obstructive or restrictive lung disease, and clinically their course may progress from an initial lymphocytic pneumonitis, to a bronchiolitis obliterans that is steroid responsive, to pulmonary fibrosis that is steroid unresponsive. In contrast, patients with α1-antitrypsin deficiency will present with clinical manifestations of obstructive lung disease only. While a some of these patients are candidates for α1-antitrypsin supplementation from pooled serum, a small number are cured surgically via combined orthotopic lung (generally bilateral) and liver transplantation. Similarly, patients with sarcoidosis, who tend to develop a restrictive process secondary to pulmonary fibrosis, may be salvaged with a combined lung and liver transplant.

Hepato-Hydrothorax

The majority of these cases are associated with obvious abdominal ascites and are the result of direct migration of peritoneal ascites through small diaphragmatic defect(s) to the pleural space, thereby yielding pleural effusions. Diagnostic evaluation most commonly reveals a unilateral right-sided pleural effusion, although bilateral pleural effusions may be present. The most effective way to deal with a significant pleural effusion is to treat the underlying ascites as outlined earlier. As with all sequelae of end-stage liver diseases, definitive treatment is achieved by liver transplantation.

Hepatopulmonary Syndrome

As discussed earlier, hepatopulmonary syndrome is believed to be caused by nitric oxide-mediated inappropriate pulmonary vasodilatation. In addition, pulmonary arteriovenous malformations may develop. Hypoxemia due to hepatopulmonary syndrome is multifactorial, as discussed, and no reliable treatment other than liver transplantation exists. Moreover, complete resolution typically occurs after transplantation.

Portopulmonary Hypertension

Less than 10% of patients with advanced liver disease will develop clinically significant portopulmonary hypertension. Portopulmonary hypertension is graded as mild (mean pulmonary artery pressure 25–35 mm Hg), moderate (35–50 mm Hg), and severe (>50 mm Hg). Patients are initially suspected of having portopulmonary hypertension during workup on screening transthoracic echocardiography. Patients who are found to have a right ventricular systolic pressure greater than 50 mm Hg should undergo cardiac catheterization to evaluate the mean pulmonary artery pressures for confirmation of the diagnosis and hemodynamic profiling. Pharmacologic therapies comprise pulmonary arteriolar/venular dilators. Importantly only patients with mild disease, or patients whose portopulmonary hypertension is downgraded to a mild level after initiation of medical therapy, are candidates for isolated liver transplantation. In patients with more severe portopulmonary hypertension, combined orthotopic lung (bilateral)- liver transplantation may be reasonable, but long-term results are unclear.

REFERENCES

1. Bosch J, D'Amico G, Garcia-Pagan JC. Portal hypertension and nonsurgical management. In: RE Schiff, MF Sorrell, WC Maddrey (eds). *Schiff's Diseases of the Liver*. 10th edition, Lippincott Williams & Wilkins. 2007.
2. Wiesner R, Edwards E, Freeman R, *et al*. Model for end-stage liver disease (MELD) and allocation of liver donors. *Gastroenterology* 2003; 124(1):91–96.
3. Bruix J, Sherman M. Management of hepatocellular carcinoma. *AASLD Practice Guideline*.
4. Arroyo V, Gines P, Gerbes AL, *et al*. Definition and diagnostic criteria of refractory ascites and hepatorenal syndrome in cirrhosis. International ascites club. *Hepatology* 1996; 23(1):164–176.

5. Arroyo V, Guevara M, Gines P. Hepatorenal syndrome in cirrhosis: pathogenesis and treatment. *Gastroenterology* 2002; 122(6):1658–1676.
6. Skagen M, Einstein M, Lucey MR, *et al.* Combination treatment with octreotide, midodrine, and albumin improves survival in patients with type 1 and type 2 hepatorenal syndrome. *J Clin Gast* 2009; 43(7):680–685.
7. Krowka MJ. Recent pulmonary observations in alpha 1-antitrypsin deficiency, primary biliary cirrhosis, chronic hepatitis C, and other hepatic problems. *Clin Chest Med* 1996; 17(1):67–82.
8. Ramsay MA, Simpson BR, Nguyen AT, *et al.* Severe pulmonary hypertension in liver transplant candidates. *Liver Transpl Surg* 1997; 3(5):494–500.
9. Kuo PC, Plotkin JS, Gaine S, *et al.* (1999) Portopulmonary hypertension and the liver transplant candidate. *Transplantation* 67(8):1087–1093.

TECHNICAL MANAGEMENT OF ASCITES 9

Carlos E. Marroquin*
and Bridget M. Marroquin*

INTRODUCTION

Ascites is the most common manifestation of decompensated liver disease.[1,2] The development of ascites is an important milestone in the natural history of end-stage liver disease as only 50% of these patients go on to survive 2–5 years after developing ascites.[2] Ascites is another manifestation of the systemic effects of portal hypertension. The splanchnic vasodilation seen with portal hypertension generates greater capillary pressure secondary to higher inflow of blood at high pressure into the splanchnic capillary bed. This results in leakage of fluid into the peritoneal cavity. Splanchnic vasodilation decreases the peripheral arterial pressure gradients. The net effect of a decrease in the arterial pressure gradient is the activation of the renin–angiotensin system, and constitutive retention of sodium and water by the kidneys. Constant retention of sodium and water by the kidneys results in continuous formation of ascites. Patients will often indicate they believed they were "out of shape" when they could no longer fit into their clothing because of increasing abdominal girth. Examination reveals the characteristic fluid waves and shifting dullness of ascites.

Most patients will respond initially to medical therapy. Medical therapy is first-line, and comprises sodium restriction and diuretic usage. Patients

*University of Rochester, Rochester, New York, USA

should be instructed not to use salt in their food and not to cook with salt. Sodium restriction is critical to the effectiveness of diuretics in controlling ascites. Spironolactone and lasix are the most commonly used diuretics with spironolactone being the principal diuretic. Spironolactone should be started at a dose of 100 mg/day and doubled every other day if no effect is observed up to a dose of 400 mg. Lasix should be started once spironolactone has been maximized. Lasix is started at a dose of 40 mg/day and increased to a maximum dose of 160 mg/day. Once ascites has been effectively controlled, diuretic doses should be reduced to a maintenance dose that effectively prevents the ascites from re-accumulating.

PARACENTESIS

If medical management fails, tense ascites may develop which has the capacity to produce substantial morbidity. Tense ascites can restrict cardiac preload and result in relative and occasionally profound hypotension. Tense ascites can also result in respiratory compromise. When these systemic manifestations are evident, large volume paracentesis (LVP) can be therapeutic. LVP involves the removal of greater than 5 liters of ascitic fluid. LVP has traditionally been performed with a great deal of trepidation for fear of complications attributed to an acute reduction in intravascular volume. However, Kao et al.[3] have demonstrated that LVP can be performed safely with no significant change in serum sodium, urea nitrogen, hematocrit or postural systolic blood pressure difference 24 or 48 hours after LVP. While LVP is clearly safe and effectively ameliorates symptoms and systemic consequences of tense ascites, it does have potential morbidity. As such, one must always evaluate the risk/benefit of performing LVP. LVP has been associated with mechanical complications such as bleeding from direct puncture/laceration of a mesenteric vessel, a subcutaneous or omental varix with resultant hemodynamic compromise or death.[4] Abdominal paracentesis is also a risk for mechanical perforation of the gastrointestinal tract with peritonitis and sepsis.[5] One can also demonstrate systemic manifestations of paracentesis. While LVP is clearly a safe procedure, it has been associated with activation of the renin–angiotensin system and circulatory alterations. These systemic manifestations are referred to as post-paracentesis circulatory syndrome (PCS).[6-8] Moreover, it has been demonstrated that patients whose plasma renin activity rises above 50% of their basal level experience greater morbidity and mortality.[6,9] PCS may be ameliorated by albumin administration during paracentesis. Once patients begin to require regular paracentesis, one should begin to consider transjugular portosystemic shunt (TIPS) placement for management of the refractory ascites.

TRANSJUGULAR PORTOSYSTEMIC SHUNT

Until the early 1990s, surgical decompression, as will be discussed later, was the mainstay of management of recalcitrant, diuretic unresponsive ascites. With the advent of TIPS,[10] surgical shunts were all but abandoned due to the unacceptably high morbidity and mortality. TIPS is effective and offers the added advantage of being a non-invasive approach in patients who would possibly not tolerate general anesthesia and who could be said to have a hostile abdomen. During the course of performing a TIPS procedure, interventional radiologists create a side-to-side shunt that is generally placed through the right internal jugular vein under local anesthesia. The increased resistance to portal blood flow that develops in the liver parenchyma as the liver becomes progressively stiffer and as the vascular architecture of the liver becomes disrupted is converted to a low-resistance bed between the intrahepatic portion of the portal vein and the hepatic veins by use of an expandable stent (Figures 1–3). Successful TIPS placement results in improved renal function, sodium excretion, and better control of

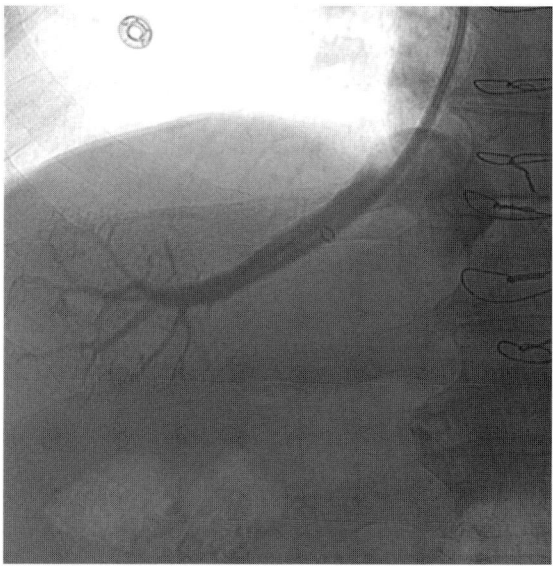

Figure 1. Guidewire in the IVC and the right hepatic vein.

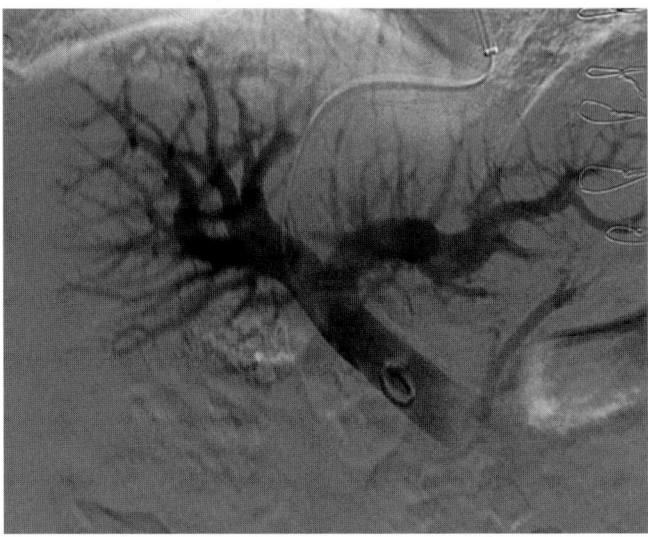

Figure 2. Glidewire in the right portal vein after access is established through the parenchyma.

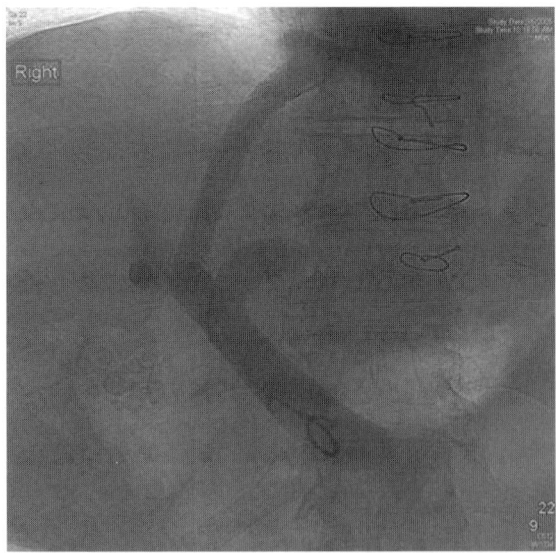

Figure 3. Completion portal venogram demonstrating a patent portal vein and shunt.

ascites. While TIPS was more effective at removing ascites when compared with paracentesis without a significant difference in mortality, gastrointestinal bleeding, infection, or acute renal failure, TIPS patients were found to develop hepatic encephalopathy significantly more often in a Cochrane database analysis.[12] Approximately 25% of patients can develop post-TIPS encephalopathy. These patients will generally respond to therapy with lactulose and conservative management. However, patients who are refractory to supportive care, have a high mortality. Predictors of post-TIPS encephalopathy include pre-TIPS encephalopathy, and age. As such, dense encephalopathy is a contraindication to proceeding with TIPS placement.

The effect of TIPS on the pulmonary circulation is multifactorial and depends on the interaction of the changes in venous return, effective circulating volume, systemic vascular resistance, and myocardial reserve.[13] A known history of congestive heart failure is another contraindication to TIPS as increasing the venous return will precipitate heart failure in patients with known right heart dysfunction and prior episodes of heart failure. Similarly, pulmonary hypertension and hepatopulmonary syndrome is aggravated by the immediate increase in venous return to the heart. Since the outcome is unpredictable, TIPS should not be performed in patients with advanced forms of pulmonary hypertension or hepatopulmonary syndrome. When patients have a dilated biliary tree, whether from an obstructive process or primarily as in Caroli's disease, the risk of perforating a biliary radicle is significant enough to warrant aborting the idea of TIPS in these patients. Similarly, one should not consider placing a TIPS in patients with polycystic liver disease as these patients are also at greater risk of bleeding and infectious complications.[14,15] Hepatic dysfunction should be assessed with the MELD score before placing a TIPS. The MELD score incorporates bilirubin, INR, and creatinine [MELD = $(11.2 \log(INR) + 3.78 \log(bilirubin)) + 9.57 \log(creatinine)$] to assess a given patient's severity of disease. Patients with severe dysfunction are at greater risk of further decompensation and dying after a TIPS procedure. The earliest manifestation of decompensation is encephalopathy followed over time by hemodynamic compromise and progressive multiorgan failure. Progressive encephalopathy is seen in patients with advanced liver disease and tends to occur within the first month. As previously mentioned, most of these cases will respond to conservative management. In cases that do not respond to conservative management, the TIPS can be occluded with embolic therapy by interventional radiology with some recovery. Ultimately, salvage transplantation offers the only meaningful survival for patients who do not respond to conservative treatment.

While we use the MELD score to prognosticate, there are patients whose degree of portal hypertension is greater than the MELD would predict. The 30-day mortality is believed to be on the order of 18% for patients with MELD score between 18 and 23. The mortality increased to 43% if the score was above 25.[13] While many believe portal vein thrombosis presents a contraindication to proceeding with TIPS, it is not an absolute impediment to proper TIPS placement and is only a relative contraindication.[16] Similarly, hepatic vein obstruction, as in Budd-Chiari, and hepatocellular carcinoma only represent relative contraindications to TIPS placement. In some institutions, interventional radiologists have successfully placed direct–intrahepatic portacaval shunts (DIPS) by puncturing through the caudate lobe. This creates a communication between the cava and the portal vein in cases when the hepatic veins are not accessible because of malignancy or some other obstructive process.

Patients require periodic surveillance after a TIPS has been placed. This is usually performed with ultrasound and is done to assess TIPS patency. Thrombosis is not uncommon after insertion and occurs in less than 20% of cases. Stenosis can be seen with greater frequency and often requires revision during the surveillance period. The recurrence of ascites is often the hallmark of a failing shunt and will require revision. While TIPS enjoys a very high technical success rate, it is associated with complications and a less than 1% procedural mortality rate.[13] Hepatic capsule perforation with intraperitoneal bleeding is observed in less than 1% of all TIPS performed and hemobilia is also observed in less than 5% of cases.[17] The initial morbidity from these procedures is relatively minor and permits expectant management. In fact, it is reasonable to assume that a number of these cases never come to clinical significance. During the course of expectant management, one should aggressively correct any degree of coagulopathy with factors. If the patient is thrombocytopenic or has uremia that may predispose to platelet dysfunction, platelets should be infused to correct the thrombocytopenia and adjuncts like DDAVP and premarin should be used to increase platelet adherence that evolves in a uremic environment. Despite these complications, TIPS is associated with great clinical success and very low morbidity. The low morbidity is a direct result of the non-invasive nature of the procedure and the ability to perform the procedure under local without general anesthesia. Two key distinguishing features from the invasive surgical shunts which were popular in the 1970s and 1980s.

Prior to placing a TIPS, patients should be studied with an ultrasound of the neck to assess the patency of the internal jugular veins. In addition, they should have a CT or MRI of the abdomen to evaluate the liver for masses, biliary dilatation, cysts, and hepatic or portal vein thrombosis. Radiologists also prefer to drain any accumulated ascites prior to performing the procedure. The abdomen is prepped and draped in a sterile manner as the paracentesis should be performed under sterile technique. The overlying skin is infiltrated with local anesthetic (~10 cc of 1% lidocaine). Because of the risk of injury to the GI tract, the abdominal cavity is accessed under ultrasound guidance using micropuncture technique. The seldinger technique is subsequently used to dilate the tract with serial catheters until a dialysis catheter is left in the abdomen for LVP. Once the abdomen has been tapped dry, the drainage catheter is removed and a sterile dressing placed at the puncture site. The right neck is prepared and draped in the usual sterile fashion for the next portion of the procedure. After administering local anesthetic (usually 1% lidocaine), the right internal jugular vein is accessed under ultrasound guidance using the micropuncture technique and a guidewire is passed. The needle is subsequently exchanged for a 5 French sheath. The guidewire is passed into the IVC and the sheath is then upsized to 14 French. The wire is passed into the IVC and the right hepatic vein is selected using a vertebral curve catheter (Figure 1). The guidewires are exchanged over which a balloon occlusion catheter is placed and CO_2 venogram performed with right hepatic vein balloon occlusion to demonstrated the right, left and main trunk of the portal vein. The balloon catheter is replaced with a 10 French introducer sheath through which a special needle (Colapinto needle) is passed and used to puncture the right portal vein through the liver parenchyma. A Glidewire is then passed into the main portal vein and the Colapinto needle removed. The intervening parenchymal tract between the hepatic and portal system is dilated. A catheter is subsequently passed over the wire that allows central and portal pressure measurements which are used to determine the pressure gradients. A CO_2 portogram is repeated to verify a patent portal vein (Figure 2). A stent is then passed over the wire through the tract and deployed creating a shunt between the right hepatic and portal veins. A completion portal venogram is then performed which demonstrates a patent portal vein and shunt (Figure 3). Since virtually all of these patients are anticoagulated and thrombocytopenic, one should prepare them by having products on hand and infused if necessary. Moreover, once completed, point pressure should be applied to the internal jugular puncture site until adequate hemostasis is obtained, and sterile dressings applied. Patients are typically admitted for monitoring and support in the event they become unstable and decompensate. TIPS may require revision, as such, they are monitored with surveillance ultrasounds to insure they remain patent and pressure gradients are measured. Finally, clinical follow-up is also crucial as the first sign that a TIPS is failing is the re-accumulation of ascites.

SURGICAL SHUNTS

Since the advent of TIPS, surgical portasystemic shunts are uncommonly performed. While TIPS is the mainstay of therapy for patients with sequelae of portal hypertension, in this case ascites, it is a labor- and resource-intensive procedure that requires maintenance and follow-up. As such, one very real and sound indication for a surgical shunt is in patients who are reasonably compensated and have no realistic means of follow-up care or plausibility of transplantation ever or in the near future. Some of these patients are well compensated such that they do not qualify for a transplant in the near future and do not, or cannot, go through the periodic surveillance necessary for TIPS management. Someone who may not be able to have surveillance ultrasounds performed every 3 to 6 months as a result of their personal disposition or rural residence may do well with a surgical shunt. Shunt procedures are described in terms of selective, partial and nonselective or total portosystemic shunts. In the interest of simplicity, one should think of these surgical procedures as total or selective. They are selective in that some shunts will decompress the esophageal and gastric varices exclusively without affecting the portal flow. The partial shunts are essentially total shunts which attempt to fractionate flow by using small caliber (8–10 mm) synthetic grafts that only divert a portion of the mesenteric flow into the systemic circulation. The reality is that partial shunts will tend to become total shunts because of the lower resistance through the shunt relative to the high resistance within the sinusoidal bed of the liver.

In terms of the application of surgical shunts to the management of ascites, the preferred shunts are the total shunts as they decompress the entire portomesenteric venous system. While our preferred shunt in the management of ascites is the mesocaval shunt with a 20 mm graft (a total shunt), we do consider a side-to-side portacaval shunt with jugular vein and a side-to-side portacaval shunt equivalent procedures that are technically more difficult to perform. The so-called partial shunts (side-to-side portacaval, mesocaval, and mesorenal shunts) with 10-mm grafts are inferior and prone to thrombosis. Moreover, partial shunts are rarely capable of fractionating flow as the portal vein is converted into an outflow tract because of preferential flow from the high resistance sinusoidal bed in the liver towards the low resistance in the newly created shunt. Finally, one would never perform a selective shunt to treat ascites as it would worsen the ascites.

Careful evaluation and planning is critical. In the current era of TIPS and transplantation, one must have compelling reasons to perform a surgical shunt for the management of ascites. These procedures represent high risk medical and surgical procedures. Therefore, we must be relatively comfortable that the patient will tolerate not only the surgical procedure from a technical standpoint, but also from an anesthetic perspective. First, one must be certain the indication is appropriate and hepatic vein wedge pressures are obtained to confirm the diagnosis of portal hypertension if it has not already been performed. Normal portal pressure gradients (PPG) range between 0 and 5 mmHg. While the development of ascites requires a minimal portal pressure gradient of 12 mmHg, it is crucial to understand that other factors contribute to the development of ascites. Although the initial mechanism that contributes to the development of ascites is sinusoidal hypertension, other factors like splanchnic vasodilation generate greater inflow of blood at high pressure into the capillary bed and results in leakage of fluid into the peritoneal cavity. Splanchnic vasodilation decreases the peripheral arterial pressure gradients. As a result, there is a decrease in the arterial pressure gradient and a reflexive activation of the renin–angiotensin system, and constitutive retention of sodium and water which continually fuel the maintenance of ascites. This phenomenon becomes marked at higher PPG (>12 mmHg).

While it is common to perform the hepatic wedge pressures, patients who are not going through the usual TIPS algorithm may not have had pressures measured. An MRI or CT scan of the abdomen with angiographic reconstruction will establish the critical anatomy and vascular relationships and patency. From a medical perspective, as previously discussed, the MELD or Child–Turcotte–Pugh (CTP) score will distinguish the high-risk patients from the low-risk patients. In general, patients selected for a surgical shunt should be relatively well compensated (CTP A/B or MELD < 20) with no access to medical care. Otherwise, relatively well-compensated patients with access to health care and refractory ascites should undergo TIPS. Moreover, patients who are poorly compensated and have access to healthcare should undergo evaluation and transplantation if they are viable candidates. There is an intermediate group of patients with access to healthcare who may undergo TIPS and tolerate the procedure. However, some may not tolerate the procedure and will require a salvage transplant. Finally, some patients are at a prohibitive risk of suffering lethal consequences from TIPS and are also not transplant candidates. We would argue these patients are best managed with symptomatic, palliative approaches.

MESOCAVAL SHUNT

Since it is truly a matter of time before liver failure patients with refractory ascites progress to the point of requiring a liver transplant, our first consideration for the surgical management of ascites is the mesocaval shunt or H-graft. The main reason for this decision is that it does not violate the porta hepatis that will require dissection at the time of transplantation. In addition, it can be managed relatively easily with ligation or simply firing a vascular load across the shunt after the transplant. The technical aspect of performing a mesocaval shunt is relatively straightforward. After adequate exploration and exposure has been optimized, one exposes the root of the transverse mesocolon. Once exposed, a transverse incision is made at the base of the transverse mesocolon (Figure 4). The dissection is carried out while looking for the superior mesenteric vein (SMV) along the midline. Once the SMV is located, it is skeletonized over a length from the first branch point to the level of the pancreas. This requires dissection through the transverse mesocolon. The objective is to clear enough vein to allow placement of a small Satinsky side-bitting clamp. At this point, the

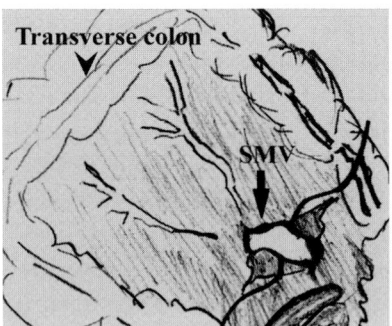

Figure 4. Exposed SMV at the root of transverse mesocolon; a transverse incision at the base of the transverse mesocolon exposes the superior mesenteric vein (SMV) along the midline. Once the SMV is located, it is skeletonized over a sufficient length that will allow placement of a small Satinsky side-bitting clamp.

duodenum is mobilized exposing the inferior vena cava (IVC). The IVC is also skeletonized sufficiently to place a side-bitting clamp. This can be done in a relatively straightforward manner. The one caveat is that the duodenum needs to be retracted with a malleable retractor on a fixed table retractor (Boolwalter retractor) to facilitate this exposure. Efforts to perfect the caval skeletonization with extensive mobilization of the IVC can be hazardous and unnecessary. The vena cava only needs to be cleared anteriorly over a sufficient length to comfortably position a side-bitting clamp. Between the SMV and IVC, one will encounter a swath of the transverse mesocolon (Figure 5). This should be divided. The IVC is controlled with a Satinsky clamp and curved scissors on a right angle (Haimovici or Satinsky scissors) are used to fashion a cavotomy to match the graft. If one is attempting to fashion a partial shunt, the graft should be no larger than a 10-mm graft. Else, one can use an 18- or 20-mm graft to create a total shunt. An end-to-side anastomosis is created with two 5–0 prolene sutures (36 inches on an SH needle). One side of the anatomosis is fashioned first running one end towards the other and meeting in the middle where they are tied. The other side is completed in a similar fashion. Once the anastomosis is completed, a separate clamp is placed on the graft above the

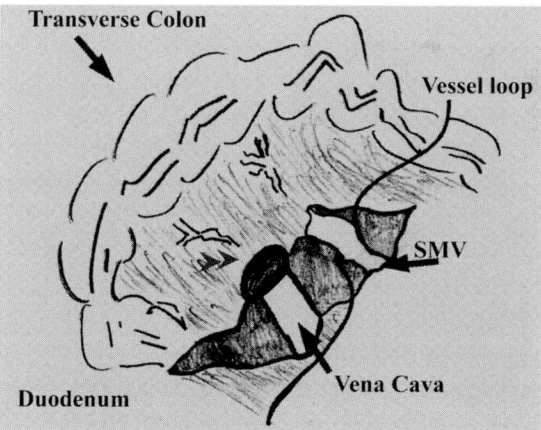

Figure 5. Exposed vena cava and SMV; Once the SMV is located dissection proceeds through the transverse mesocolon. The duodenum (double arrowheads) is mobilized exposing the inferior vena cava (IVC). The IVC is skeletonized sufficiently to place a side-bitting clamp.

anastomosis and the Satinsky removed. This allows one to test the integrity of the anastomosis and reconstitute caval flow. Once the caval anastomosis has been performed, the graft is cut to the appropriate length and orientation. It is critical to orient the anastomosis on the SMV at right angle to the caval anastomosis. Two angled Glover clamps are used to obtain proximal and distal control on the SMV. Any vascular clamp can be used to obtain proximal and distal control on the vein; we prefer the Glover clamps as they allow one to work without obstruction. It is critical to place one clamp on the SMV flush with the pancreatic gland and the second above the first branching vein. This is critical to facilitate the procedure as it allows us to perform the anastomosis on the anterior surface of the SMV as described by Cameron.[18] This is a slight variation from the classic H-shunt which was an interposition mesocaval shunt in which the anastomosis was performed on the undersurface of the SMV. Again, curved scissors are used to fashion a venotomy matching the graft and an end-to-side anastomosis is created using two 5–0 prolene sutures (36 inches on an SH needle) (Figure 6). One side of the anatomosis is fashioned first running one end towards the other and meeting in the middle where they are tied. The other side is

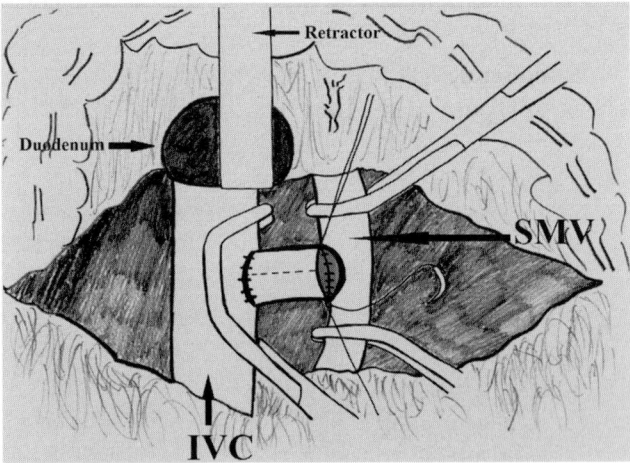

Figure 6. Interposition meso-caval shunt; one side of the anatomosis is fashioned first running one end towards the other and meeting in the middle where they are tied. The other side is completed in a similar fashion. Prior to completing the anastomosis, the clamp is flashed and the graft is allowed to back bleed until one is certain air is flushed through the graft.

completed in a similar fashion. Because the right side of the graft abuts the duodenum, the entire anatomosis should be fashioned form the patient's left sewing the opposing, right side from inside the graft in a running manner. Prior to completing the anastomosis, the clamp is flashed and the graft is allowed to back bleed until one is certain air is flushed through the graft. Alternatively, one can vent the graft, while it is filling, with a needle as described by Cameron. At this point, the sutures are tied and both clamps are completely removed establishing flow through the graft. Capussotti et al. have provided evidence that a partial portacaval shunt using an H interposition graft results in significantly lower encephalopathy rates and improved long-term preservation of liver function than a direct side-to-side portacaval shunt.[19] Since it also avoids manipulation of the porta hepatis, it is our preferred graft as it does not complicate future transplant options.

PORTACAVAL SHUNTS

Another shunt one could use to treat ascites is an interposition portacaval shunt (Figure 7a). This shunt would establish retrograde flow between the portal vein and vena cava and effectively decompress the portamesenteric venous system. The hepatoduodenal ligament is divided and the common bile duct is dissected free and retracted medially with a vessel loop. The portal vein is subsequently exposed from below its bifurcation to the edge of the pancreas. The peritoneum over the cava is opened exposing the anterior surface of the cava as it emerges from the caudate lobe. Extensive dissection is again not advised. Only enough to allow placement of a small Satinsky clamp. An appropriate-sized graft is subsequently selected and the portacaval shunt fashioned in a similar manner as the mesocaval shunt. In a similar fashion, an end-to-side porta-caval shunt (Figure 7b) is created by dividing the portal vein at the level of its bifurcation with a vascular stapler or ligating each branch separately at the bifurcation with a suture ligature utilizing 4–0 prolene. The portal vein is subsequently controlled with a Glover clamp at the edge of the pancreas. A Satinsky is placed on the cava and the portal vein is swung down onto the cava. The staple line is cut away from the portal vein and a cavotomy is made with curved scissors and an end-to-side anastomosis is fashioned using two 5–0 prolene sutures (36 inch on an SH needle). Finally, a side-to-side portacaval (Figure 7c) shunt may be performed to treat ascites. The hepatoduodenal ligament is opened and the CBD is retracted medially to allow access to the PV. The

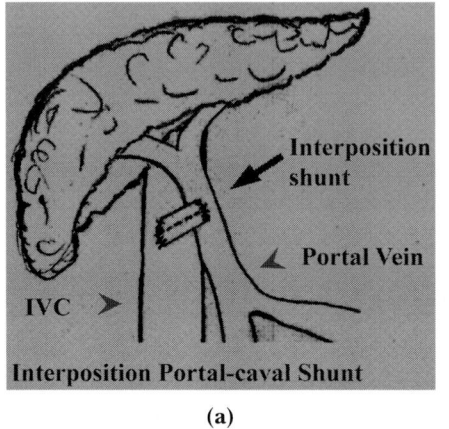
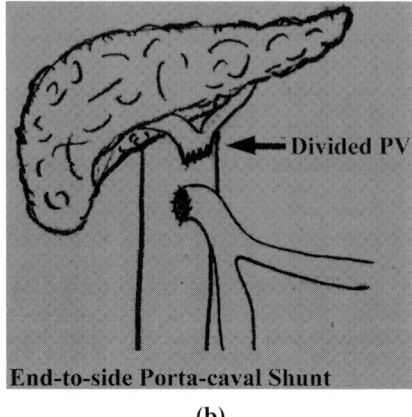

(a) (b)

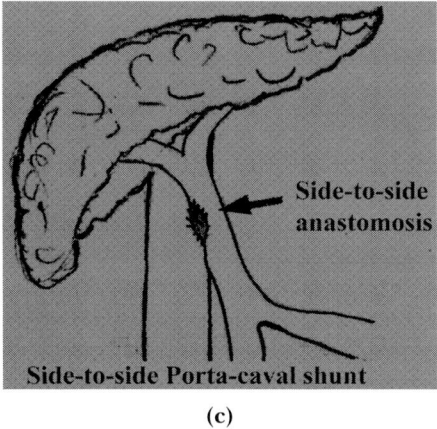

(c)

Figures 7a, 7b, 7c. The portal vein is exposed from below its bifurcation to the edge of the pancreas and the peritoneum over the vena-cava is opened exposing the anterior surface of the vena-cava. An appropriate size graft is used to fashion an interposition porta-caval shunt (figure 7a). An end-to-side porta-caval shunt (figure 7b) equires division of the portal vein at the level of the bifurcation and an end-to-side anastomosis is fashioned using two 5–0 prolene sutures. A side-to-side porta-caval shunt (figure 7c) requires the portal vein and vena-cava are mobilized. The cava is skeletonized circumferentially to allow it to move towards the portal vein and the anastomosis is fashioned with two 5–0 prolene sutures (all require a 36 inch prolene on an SH needle).

portal vein is mobilized extensively down below the edge of the pancreas. In this case, the cava is exposed anteriorly and requires more extensive mobilization than with the other shunts. The cava is skeletonized circumferentially to allow it to move towards the portal vein. The cava is controlled with a Satinsky and the portal vein with two glover clamps. The curved scissors are used to create a cavotomy on the anterior surface of the cava with a slight medial orientation and a venotomy is made on the undersurface of the portal vein. The anastomosis is fashioned with two 5–0 prolene sutures (36 inch on an SH needle).

PERITONEOVENOUS SHUNT

When patients are at a prohibitive risk of suffering lethal consequences from TIPS and if they are not transplant candidates, their survival is limited and they are best managed with symptomatic, palliative approaches. Since tense ascites can make each and every breath painful and exhausting, managing the ascites is an important part of palliation. Since their demise is not always eminent, and since serial large volume paracentesis can be not only harmful, but painful, we believe peritoneovenous shunts can be useful in the palliative setting. The most commonly used peritoneovenous shunts are the LeVeen and Denver shunts. Peritoneovenous shunts translocate ascites into the systemic venous circulation, and can effectively treat refractory ascites. These shunts have fallen out of favor because they can be very morbid. Peritoneovenous shunts have been associated with disseminated intravascular coagulation (DIC), infectious complications, variceal bleeding and lower overall survival. Both the LeVeen and Denver shunts have a unidirectional valve mechanism that maintains unidirectional peritoneal cavity–systemic venous ascitic fluid flow, but the Denver shunt has an additional externally actuated pump, conceived to augment ascitic flow. Before placing either of these shunts, patients should have an ultrasound of their neck to evaluate the patency of their jugular veins. If possible, the procedure should be performed under IV sedation as general anesthesia may not be tolerated by these patients resulting in lethal decompensation. The abdomen, thorax and neck are prepared and draped in the usual sterile fashion with sterile barrier devices. Since an adequate vein may not be available, we like to initiate the procedure by identifying and isolating the internal jugular vein.

An incision is made anterior to the sternocleidomastoid and deepened through the platysma and, subsequently, down onto the carotid sheath. The carotid sheath is opened and we identify the internal jugular vein. The vein is skeletonized and two separate vessel loops are used to control the vein. Once the vein is adequately controlled, we subsequently moved down to the anterior abdominal wall, where a transverse incision is made approximately 2–3 cm below the costal margin at the anterior axillary line. We subsequently spread the external oblique fibers followed by the internal oblique fibers. The transverse abdominus fibers are spread and the peritoneal layer is identified. Two pursestring sutures are placed on the peritoneal layer in two concentric circles, and we subsequently open the peritoneum and pass the peritoneal catheter into the peritoneum. We look for immediate filling of the tubing, valve, and external tube by capillary action. The purse string sutures are secured and we subsequently tunnel along the lateral aspect of the thorax and over the clavicle and come out through the incision anterior to the sternocleidomastoid. An umbilical tape is placed on the tunneler and passed down through the incision. The umbilical tape is fastened to the catheter, which is subsequently pulled up through the incision. At this point, we test the valve for flow through the catheter by pushing the pump several times. Vessel loops are placed on the IJ and controlled proximally and distally. A pursestring is placed on the internal jugular vein and incised centrally. The catheter is passed into the vein, and subsequently secured. Once the catheter is secured, a film is obtained to verify placement and the absence of a pneumothorax. All incisions are closed and clean, dry dressings are applied.

While there are a variety of ways to deal with ascites, one thing is clear, it represents the beginning of the end as it is the most common initial manifestation of end stage liver disease. Once patients develop ascites, they should be temporized with the least morbidity possible with the ultimate goal of referring into a liver transplant program. As will be discussed later, liver transplantation is the only therapy that offers both a durable survival and an exceptional quality of life.

REFERENCES

1. Planas *et al.* Natural history of decompensated hepatitis C virus-related cirrhosis. A study of 200 patients. *J Hepatol* 2004; 40:823–830.
2. Saadeh *et al.* Management of ascites in patients with end-stage liver disease. Rev *Gastroenterol Disord.* 2004; 4(4):175–85.

3. Kao *et al.* The effect of large volume paracentesis on plasma volume–a cause of hypovolemia? *Hepatology* 1985; 5(3):403–407.
4. Arnold *et al.* Acute hemoperitoneum after large-volume paracentesis. *Gastroenterology* 1997; 113(3):978–82.
5. Mallory *et al.* Complications of diagnostic paracentesis in patients with liver disease. *JAMA* 1978; 239(7):628–630.
6. Ginés P, Titó LI, Arroyo V, *et al.* Randomized comparative study of therapeutic paracentesis with and without intravenous albumin in cirrhosis. *Gastroenterology* 1988; 94:1493–502.
7. Panos MZ, Moore K, Panayiotis V, *et al.* Single total paracentesis for tense ascites: Sequential hemodynamic changes and right atrial size. *Hepatology* 1990; 11:662–7.
8. Pozzi M, Osculati G, Boari G, *et al.* Time course of circulatory and humoral effects of rapid total paracentesis in cirrhotic patients with tense ascites. *Gastroenterology* 1994; 106:709–19.
9. Ginés A, Fernández-Esparrach G, Monescillo A, *et al.* Randomized trial comparing albumin, dextran 70, and polygeline in cirrhotic patients with ascites treated by paracentesis. *Gastroenterology* 1996; 111:1002–10.
10. Ferral *et al.* Refractory ascites: Early experience in treatment with transjugular intrahepatic portosystemic shunt. *Radiology* 1993; 189(3):795–801.
11. D'Amico *et al.* Uncovered transjugular intrahepatic portosystemic shunt for refractory ascites: a meta-analysis.*Gastroenterology* 2005; 129(4):1282–1293.
12. Saab *et al.* TIPS versus paracentesis for cirrhotic patients with refractory ascites. *Cochrane Database Syst Rev* 2006; (4):CD004889.
13. Darcy M. Technique of transjugular intrahepatic portosystemic shunt placement. In: LH Blamgart (ed). *Surgery of the Liver, Biliary Tract, and Pancreas.* 4th edition, Elsevier Health Sciences. 2006.
14. Suhocki *et al.* Treatment of TIPS/biliary fistula-related endotipsitis with a covered stent. *J Vasc Interv Radiol* 2008; 19(6):937–939.
15. Jawaid *et al.* Biliary-venous fistula complicating transjugular intrahepatic portosystemic shunt presenting with recurrent bacteremia, jaundice, anemia and fever. *Am J Transplant* 2003; 3(12):1604–1607.
16. Perarnau *et al.* Feasibility and long-term evolution of TIPS in cirrhotic patients with portal thrombosis. *Eur J Gastroenterol Hepatol* 2010; 22(9): 1093–1098.
17. Marroquin CE, Marroquin BM, Management of bleeding from the biliary tree. In: Aurora (ed). *Management of Gastrointestinal Tract Bleeding.* 1st edition, Springer, New York.

18. Cameron and Sandone. Interposition mesocaval shunt. In: BC Decker (ed). *Atlas of Gastrointestinal Surgery.* 2nd edition, pp. 193–203. 1992.
19. Capussotti *et al.* Liver function and encephalopathy after partial vs. direct side-to-side portacaval shunt: A prospective randomized clinical trial. *Surgery* 2000; 127(6):614–612.

VARICEAL THERAPIES 10

Carlos E. Marroquin

INTRODUCTION

The liver has a dual blood supply that provides a total blood flow of approximately 1500 ml/min; approximately 1000 ml/min through the portal vein and 500 ml/min through the hepatic artery. Despite a fairly robust flow, the vast anastomotic vascular network of the liver has an intrinsically low resistance. Normal portal pressure is on the order of 6–8 mmHg, and normal hepatic vein pressure is approximately 2–4 mmHg. As the architecture of the liver remodels into regenerative nodules and a bridging scar that characterizes a stiff, shrunken cirrhotic liver, the vascular network of the liver also becomes disrupted. One direct consequence of these changes is an increase in the resistance to blood flow through the liver. This is compounded by the evolution of increased portal flow secondary to the development of a hyperdynamic state and splanchnic vasodilation. The result is portal hypertension which is formally defined as an increase in the pressure gradient between the portal vein and the inferior vena cava.

As the resistance to flow rises, collateral circuits (varices) with lower resistance to flow begin to develop to decompress the portal pressures through four well-established vascular networks which include the esophageal venous plexus, the cardiac venous plexus of the stomach, the retroperitoneal–umbilical venous plexus, and the hemorrhoidal venous plexus of the rectum. These naturally occurring portasystemic shunts form spontaneously throughout the body as the portal pressure gradient rises to 10 mmHg (Table 1). By the time patients are diagnosed with end-stage liver disease or

Table 1. Porta-systemic venous shunts.

- Caput medusae via the umbilical vein
- Esophageal varices via the coronary vein, short gastric veins, and azygous vein
- Gastric varices via the coronary vein, gastroepiploic vein and short gastric veins
- Hemorrhoids via superior hemorrhoidal vein, and hemorrhoidal veins
- Retroperitoneal varices via superior mesenteric vein, and inferior mesenteric vein
- Splenorenal shunt via splenic vein

cirrhosis, varices are present in approximately 30% of well-compensated patients and up to 60% of decompensated patients. While there are many complications of portal hypertension, the most acutely lethal complication is gastrointestinal bleeding from esophageal varices. Patients are at risk of variceal bleeding once the portal pressure gradient exceeds 12 mmHg. Some 30–50% of patients with known varices bleed within 1 year and approximately 80% of those with large varices bleed within 2 years. Once a patient with Childs C cirrhosis has experienced their first variceal hemorrhage, approximately 30% will re-bleed within 6 weeks and approximately 40% will die within 6 weeks. Nearly two-thirds of Child C cirrhotics will die within 12 months of their initial bleed.

Once patients are found to have esophageal varices by endoscopic surveillance, prophylaxis is appealing. It is not surprising that variceal size and intravariceal pressures are predictive of the risk of bleeding. Garcia-Tsao et al. found that the mean hepatic vein pressure gradient (HVPG) was significantly higher in patients who had bled from varices than in patients who had not. They also found that patients with large varices were more likely to bleed.[1] Similarly, red wale signs and deteriorating liver function are also predictive of the risk of bleeding. As such, great emphasis is placed on prevention.

PRIMARY PROPHYLAXIS/PREVENTING THE FIRST BLEED

While there is no evidence that demonstrates that any therapy can prevent variceal formation, there is good data to support prophylaxis starting when small varices are detected. β-Blockers reduce splanchnic blood flow. As such, they are capable of reducing pressures by approximately 20%. Unfortunately, the effect of nonselective β-blockade (NSBB) are variable, unpredictable, and are associated with many side effects. Nevertheless, many anecdotal reports indicate that there is a 40–50% reduction in bleeding. Merkel *et al.* demonstrated that β-blocker prophylaxis of variceal bleeding in patients with compensated cirrhosis should be started when small esophageal varices are present.[2] β-Blocker prophylaxis with Nadolol resulted in less growth of varices, and the cumulative probability of variceal bleeding was also lower in patients randomized to nadolol. Therefore, as long as patients do not develop dose limiting toxicities, NSBB is clearly beneficial. NSBB is best utilized in young patients without cardiovascular disease and well-preserved hepatic function.

Controlled trials have been conducted to evaluate the effectiveness of prophylaxis. Since the majority of patients undergo surveillance with endoscopy, it makes sense that endoscopic means would be practical in primary prophylaxis or preventing the first bleed. Although sclerotherapy is not recommended for prophylaxis, variceal banding was found to be more effective and was also associated with less complications. As such, esophageal banding is applied in the prophylactic setting. However, these procedures are invasive, and despite their benefits, they are associated with morbidity. While the majority of studies to date have found no difference in mortality or rates of bleeding between band ligation and nonselective β-blockers,[3] recent data have demonstrated that carvedilol may be more effective than endoscopic therapy.[4] However, further studies are required to assess whether carvedilol is a better option than standard NSBBs. Either may be used as primary prophylaxis in high-risk esophageal varices.[5] Independent of the strategy that is employed, it is clear that preventing the first bleed is possible with either esophageal band ligation at the time of the surveillance endoscopy or exclusively in patients who do not tolerate β-blockade therapy.

MEDICAL MANAGEMENT OF PATIENTS WITH BLEEDING VARICES

While preventing the first bleed should be the focus of our practice, it is not uncommon to encounter a patient for the first time during an acute bleed. The first and most important objective during an acute bleed is insuring adequate access for resuscitation. Two 16 gauge IVs in the antecubital fossa are generally sufficient. Otherwise, central access is necessary. A foley catheter should be placed and patients should be admitted to an ICU and an arterial line should be placed to allow monitoring and frequent laboratory sampling. If there is any question whether the patient is at risk

Table 2. Initial therapies for esophageal bleeding.

- Balloon tamponade
- Octreotide
- Sclerotherapy/Band Ligation
- TIPS
- Surgical Therapy
- Liver transplantation

of aspirating or unable to protect their airway because of an underlying encephalopathy, they should undergo elective endotracheal intubation while their esophageal bleeding is resolved. In terms of resuscitation, use blood products liberally to correct coagulopathies and replete their oxygen carrying capacity. In addition to blood products, pharmacologic adjuncts may assist in stopping the blood loss. Vasopressin constricts splanchnic flow which helps decrease portal pressures and variceal pressure head. Vasopressin is administered intravenously and is started with a 20-U bolus and an IV drip at 0.4 Units/minute. Vasopressin is 50–70% effective at stopping the blood loss, but is associated with very high re-bleeding rates. Another adjunct that is utilized is octreotide. Octreotide, which is a somatostatin analog, also reduces splanchnic blood flow and portal pressures. It is administered intravenously and is initially infused at 10–20 µg/hr. It is subsequently titrated up to 50 µg/hr as long as the systemic pressures tolerate the increasing rates. Octreotide is also used to prevent early bleeding after sclerotherapy or band ligation. It is also 50–70% effective with the advantage of a minimal side effect profile and our preferred agent. Once patients are resuscitated, characterized by stabilization of vital signs and appropriate urine output, upper endoscopy with variceal banding should be performed. Variceal banding is 85–90% effective in acute setting and should be used in conjunction with adjunctive medical management, preferably octreotide.

MECHANICAL TAMPONADE WITH SENGSTAKEN-BLAKEMORE TUBE

On rare occasions, we may be confronted by a patient who is difficult to resuscitate and impossible to band because their variceal hemorrhage is secondary to ruptured varices. In these cases, direct tamponade is necessary to control the hemorrhage. Control of ruptured varices by direct compression with gastric and esophageal balloons was proposed by Sengstaken and Blakemore[6] in the late 1940s. Residents and ICU personnel should be familiar with the storage location, placement and management of a Sengstaken–Blakemore (S-B) tube. Since these tubes are used so infrequently, and because they have the potential of being life-saving; a standard lecture on their use should be part of every ICU rotation. Sengstaken and Blakemore designed a triple lumen tube with esophageal, and gastric balloons, and a gastric suction port. The Minnesota tube is a modification of an S-B tube that includes a fourth port above the esophageal balloon for suctioning oral and esophageal secretions.

While one may be able to place an S-B tube without intubating the patient, control of the airway should be performed prior to placement of an S-B tube. Endotracheal intubation helps control a combative patient and facilitates placement of the S-B tube and may be protective against aspiration.[7] Balloon tamponade is temporarily effective in 80% of patients. Once the S-B tube has been placed, the gastric balloon is inflated with 50 cc of air. It is critical to verify placement of the balloon within the stomach with a KUB. Once confirmed, the gastric balloon is inflated with 250–500 cc of air. Traction is placed on the tube with the objective of pulling the gastric balloon tightly against the gastroesophageal junction. The S-B tube is held in place by securing it to a football helmet or a catcher's mask which should be provided with the kit. Alternatively, a pulley with traction should be fixed to the bed. Both gastric and esophageal aspiration ports are placed to low intermittent suction. If bleeding does not stop, blood will continue to drain through the esophageal port. If bleeding continues, inflate the esophageal balloon to 35mmHg. If bleeding continues, the gastric balloon may be inflated to a maximum of 500 cc of air. After bleeding has been controlled, reduce the pressure in the esophageal balloon by 5mmHg every 3 hours until 25mmHg is reached without bleeding; this pressure is generally maintained for the next 12–24 hours. If bleeding is controlled, deflate the esophageal balloon for 5 minutes every 6 hours to help prevent esophageal necrosis. Ideally, the balloons are not disturbed for 24 hours. Over the next 24 hours, the esophageal balloon is deflated first. The gastric balloon is deflated and the S-B tube removed 24 hours later.

S-B tubes are 90% effective in the primary control of variceal hemorrhage. They are associated with a 37% rate of recurrent bleeding and a wide range of major complications ranging from 9%–45%. S-B tubes are associated with aspiration, esophageal laceration, esophageal rupture, and asphyxiation from laryngeal obstruction. They are also associated with a mortality of 2–22%. Aspiration is the most commonly encountered complication.[8] Aspiration is directly associated with massive volumes of blood that emanate from the ruptured varix. Esophageal perforation or rupture occurs when improperly positioned gastric balloon is inflated in the esophagus. Esophageal necrosis secondary to excessive or prolonged inflation of the esophageal balloon is also reported.[9] Finally, asphyxiation has also been reported with the S-B tube and is the result of displacement of the tube.[10,11]

IMPROVED SURVIVAL AFTER INITIAL BLEED

The majority of esophageal bleeding cases do not progress to the placement of an S-B tube. In fact, mortality has improved over the last two decades for patients with esophageal hemorrhage and the use of the S-B tube has decreased substantially.[12] In a review of their patients admitted with variceal bleeding during the years 1980, 1985, 1990, 1995, and 2000, the Mayo clinic found that while balloon tamponade was the first-line treatment in 1980, patients treated in 2000 received a vasoactive agent, endoscopic treatment, and an antibiotic prophylaxis in 90% to 100% of cases. During the study time period, in-hospital mortality decreased threefold over the 2 decades. The improved survival was associated with lower re-bleeding rates (from 47% in 1980 to 13% in 2000) and lower bacterial infection rates (from 38% to 14%). These improved outcomes were found to be due to earlier use of pharmacologic and endoscopic therapies in conjunction with short-term antibiotic prophylaxis.

TRANSJUGULAR INTRAHEPATIC PORTACAVAL SHUNT

Given the high mortality among patients who re-bleed following medical and endoscopic therapy, early transjugular intrahepatic portacaval shunt (TIPS) has effectively reduced the re-bleeding rate and mortality. Monescillo et al. studied the effect of early decompression of portal hypertension with TIPS on the outcome of variceal bleeding.[13] They found that increased portal pressure estimated by early HVPG measurement is a determinant of treatment failure and survival in variceal bleeding. Moreover, early TIPS placement was found to reduce treatment failure and mortality in high risk patients defined by hemodynamic criteria as a HVPG greater than or equal

Table 3. Complications of TIPS.

Hemoperitoneum	
Capsular hematoma	
Hemobilia	<5%
Portal vein thrombosis	
Bacteremia	
Fever	5–10%
Re-bleeding	
Hepatic encephalopathy	15–25%
Shunt occlusion	25%–100%

to 20 mmHg. In a separate study, early TIPS was also found to significantly reduce mortality in high risk groups. Garcia-Pagan *et al.* randomized high risk cirrhotic patients with acute esophageal bleed who received standard medical therapy (vasoactive drugs plus esophageal band ligation [EBL]) to undergo TIPS, within the first 72 hours after admission or to continue on vasoactive drugs plus EBL. In the control group, TIPS was used as a salvage therapy for patients who failed standard medical therapy. Standard medical and endoscopic therapy failed to control the variceal bleed. Standard therapy also failed to prevent re-bleeding. Moreover, the survival was markedly better in the TIPS group leading to the conclusion that early treatment with TIPS is associated with significant reductions in re-bleeding and mortality in high-risk cirrhotic patients with acute esophageal bleeding.[14]

While TIPS has been traditionally used as a salvage therapy in patients who failed combined medical and endoscopic therapy, we believe early application of TIPS will yield the greatest benefits in terms of re-bleeding, transfusion requirement and survival. TIPS decompression is an intrahepatic shunt. The expected re-bleeding rates after TIPS are up to 5% in the short-term and up to 50% in the long-term. The greatest advantage of TIPS is that no general anesthesia is required and is relatively non-invasive. It is associated with a very high technical success rate and does not derail a transplant option. The disadvantages of TIPS include an up to 30% incidence of encephalopathy and an approximately 50% occlusion rate by one year necessitating frequent surveillance. TIPS is also associated with other technical complications (Figure 3). The technical aspects of TIPS placement was discussed in the previous chapter.

Management of patients with portal hypertension has changed dramatically over the last decade and continues to evolve rapidly. As we have discussed previously, patients with portal hypertension and esophageal varices are managed with medical therapy with the goal to prevent the initial bleed. Once patients develop bleeding esophageal varices, they are managed with vasoactive drugs and endoscopic variceal banding. Despite data that support earlier use of TIPS, patients with acute bleeding are managed with tips after they have failed medical therapy. Since its introduction, the use of TIPS has grown exponentially and has served as an effective bridge to transplantation. This increased use of tips has virtually eliminated the need for emergency portasystemic shunting.

PORTASYSTEMIC SHUNTS FOR BLEEDING VARICES

While exceedingly small, there is a group of patients with portal hypertension and bleeding varices that cannot be controlled adequately with standard medical therapy and still possess sufficient hepatic reserve and synthetic capacity that they are not yet candidates for liver transplantation. There is also a subgroup of patients who may not, can not, or will not comply with the requisite surveillance required after a TIPS procedure. These patients may be candidates for portasystemic shunts. The first step in considering a portasystemic shunt, is to evaluate the patient's underlying hepatic reserve. While there are many tools to perform this evaluation, our preferred is the Child–Pugh classification (Table 4). It incorporates two clinical parameters and three biochemical parameters to assess a given patient's operative mortality. The operative mortality of a Child C cirrhotic is prohibitive and these patients should only be considered for either transplantation or palliative care. There is a subgroup of patients who appear to be well or relatively well compensated (Child A or B cirrhotics) who have other stigmata of advanced portal hypertension (thrombocytopenia, splenomegally, retroperitoneal varices, etc.). These patients need to be approached with a great deal of caution as they are less well compensated than a cursory evaluation would predict. As such, their outcomes will be worse than expected.

Shunt procedures should be thought of, conceptually, as total or selective. They are selective in that some shunts will decompress the esophageal and gastric varices exclusively without affecting the portal flow. Total shunts decompress the entire portal mesenteric venous system. There are many authors who describe partial shunts. The partial shunts are, anatomically, total shunts which attempt to fractionate flow by using small caliber (8–10 mm) synthetic grafts that only divert a portion of the mesenteric flow into the systemic circulation. These partial shunts tend to become total

Table 4. Evaluating operative risk according to the Child's classification.

Parameter	Points		
	1	2	3
Albumin (g/dL)	>3.5	2.8–3.5	<2.8
Total bilirubin (mg/dL)	<2	2–3	>3
INR	<1.7	1.71–2.24	>2.25
Ascites	None	Controlled	Refractory
Encephalopathy (grade)	None	I–II	III–IV

Child's classification	Points
A	5–6
B	7–9
C	10–15

Operative mortality according to Child's classification

	A	B	C
Emergent	20–30%	40–50%	75–100%
Urgent	10–20%	20–40%	50–75%
Elective	0–10%	15–20%	30–50%

Table 5. Outcomes according to shunt type.

	Re-bleed rates	Ascites	Enceph.	Degree of difficulty
TIPS	<5% short-term <50% longterm	Reasonable	20–30%	0
Total P-S Shunt	0–5%	Good	30–40%	3
Partial P-S Shunts	5–10%	Reasonable	20%	1
Selective shunts	10–15 %	Poor and may ppt	Least	5

shunts because of the lower resistance through the shunt relative to the high resistance within the sinusoidal bed of the liver.

In terms of the application of surgical shunts to the management of variceal bleeding, the preferred shunts are the total shunts as they decompress the entire portamesenteric venous system with excellent results with regards to bleeding and ascites formation (Table 5). Our preferred total shunt is the mesocaval shunt with a 20-mm graft (described in Chapter 9). We prefer this shunt as it effectively deals with the problem at hand, esophageal bleeding, and preserves the possibility of transplantation for those patients whose underlying liver disease continues to progress. However, the results with a side-to-side interposition portacaval shunt with vein or PTFE, and a side-to-side portacaval shunt are equivalent as they all effectively decompress the entire portamesenteric system (described in Chapter 9). The total shunts have a very acceptable variceal re-bleeding rate on the order of less than or equal to 5%. While they also provide better control of ascites, they are total shunts that divert all of the portal circulation resulting in higher rates of encephalopathy (up to 30% and 40% in some series).

The partial shunts (side-to-side portacaval, mesocaval, and mesorenal shunts) are constructed in an anatomically similar fashion to total shunts but differ in that they utilize small, 10-mm grafts with the objective of fractionating portal flow. They are reasonably effective at controlling the hemorrhage with a 5–10% re-bleeding rate. The disadvantage of partial shunts is that they are prone to thrombosis. In those cases in which they effectively divide the flow between the portal and systemic circuits, they are associated with lower rates of encephalopathy (~20%). Realistically, partial shunts are rarely capable of fractionating flow as the portal vein is converted into an outflow tract because of preferential flow from the high resistance sinusoidal bed in the liver towards the low resistance in the newly created shunt. Lastly, selective portasystemic shunts are anatomically selective in that they decompress the esophageal and gastric varices without affecting the portal flow. The distal splenorenal shunt or Warren shunt is the most commonly utilized selective shunt.[15,16] The re-bleeding rates are on the order of 10% to 15% and the rates of encephalopathy are the least because there is no interruption of the portal flow. One significant problem with the splenorenal shunt is that it handles ascites very poorly and may, infact, precipitate the accumulation of ascites where there once was none. It is also a technically demanding procedure that requires mobilization of the pancreas and dissecting the splenic vein away from the pancreas while ligating and dividing the small perforating branches from the pancreas to the splenic vein. The left renal vein must also be exposed in the retroperitoneum. Selective decompression is achieved through ligation and division of the splenic vein at the portal vein confluence with anastomosis of the distal end of the splenic vein to the left renal vein. This allows decompression of the gastroesophageal varices through the short gastric. In addition,

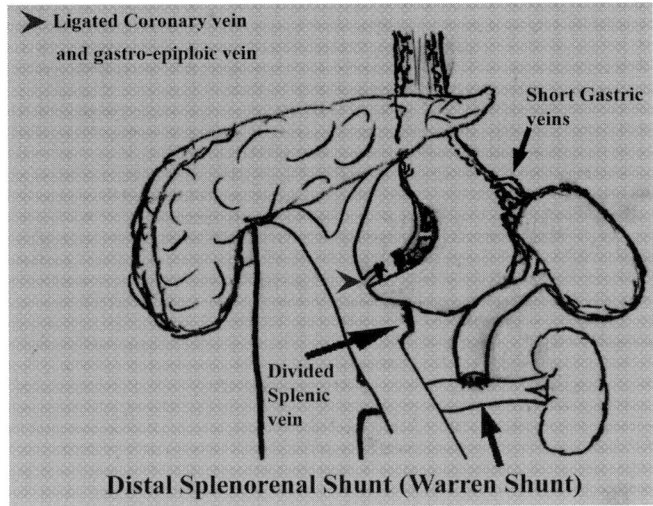

Figure 1. The distal splenorenal shunt or Warren shunt is the most commonly utilized selective shunt. The pancreas is mobilized sufficiently to allow dissection of the splenic vein away from the undersurface of the pancreas. The left renal vein is also exposed in the retroperitoneum and selective decompression is achieved through ligation and division of the splenic vein at the portal vein confluence with anastomosis of the distal end of the splenic vein to the side of left renal vein. This allows decompression of the gastroesophageal varices through the short gastric. In addition, the coronary vein, and the gastroepiploic veins, must be dissected free and ligated.

the coronary vein, and the gastroepiploic veins, must be dissected free and ligated (Figure 1). Ligation of the portosystemic collaterals like the coronary vein will increase the portal pressures and sinusoidal pressures resulting in worsening ascites.

DEVASCULARIZATION/SUGIURA PROCEDURE

In cases of acute variceal hemorrhage where no shuntable options are present, specifically in cases of splanchnic thrombosis where no shunt can be constructed, a devascularization procedure may be considered. Dr. Sugiura developed an aggressive surgical approach for patients who failed conservative management and who were not candidates for a shunt in 1973.[17] Devascularization procedures have the components of splenectomy and devascularization of the greater and lesser curves of the stomach as well as the distal 7 cm of the esophagus. The main role is control of the acute bleed. The Sugiura procedure was popularized in Japan. It involves gastroesophageal devascularization, splenectomy, and esophageal transection with vagotomy and pyloroplasty. Devascularization procedures are not justified in shuntable patients. In addition to controlling the acute variceal bleed, liver perfusion is preserved and it is associated with low portosystemic encephalopathy rates. Complications associated with the procedure include liver failure, re-bleeding, anastomotic leak, pleural effusion, portal vein thrombosis, ascites, pancreatitis, subphrenic abscess, encephalopathy, and esophageal strictures.

The initial Sugiura procedure involved a two-step procedure. A thoracotomy was performed first followed by a laparotomy. In some cases, the laparotomy was performed weeks later. Dr. Sugiura reported excellent results with low rates of re-bleeding and low morbidity and mortality.[18] Inokuchi[19] reported a large series with over 3000 patients with re-bleeding rates of 7%, operative mortality of 9%, and incidence of encephalopathy of 5%. However, his results have been difficult to reproduce in the United States or other parts of the world. As such, a modified Sugiura procedure has been adopted by surgeons who perform the procedure.[20] The procedure includes a splenectomy followed by devascularization of the upper two-thirds of the lesser and greater curvature of the stomach including 6–10 cm of the distal esophagus. The distal esophageal devascularization is performed through the diaphragmatic hiatus. The left gastric (coronary) vein was carefully preserved to allow drainage into the azygous system. This is critical as the Sugiura procedure is based on the principle of dividing the perforating veins of the esophagus and the stomach while maintaining the plexus of collaterals that connect the coronary vein to the azygous system.[17] A gastrotomy is subsequently made through which an EEA (end-to-end anastomosing) autosuture stapling device (Ethicon, Somerville, NJ) is introduced into the distal esophagus. The EEA is fired 4–6 cm above the gastroesophageal junction effectively transecting and reanastomosing the esophagus. The anastomotic staple line is reinforced with 3–0 silk lembert sutures. Esophageal transection divides the intramucosal venous plexus which is what effectively controls the bleeding. Finally, since the vagus nerve is sacrificed, a pyloroplasty is performed to assist gastric emptying. The modified Sugiura was found to be very effective in a series that was performed at Duke University.[16] With the modified Sugiura, the Duke series demonstrated comparable outcomes to the Japanese with a 7% re-bleeding rate, 7% encephalopathy rate, and an overall mortality of 7%.

Esophageal variceal bleeding is associated with a mortality rate of 30–70%. Consequently, various therapies are used to treat patients with bleeding esophageal varices. Prophylaxis is critical and is best employed once patients develop varices. The most effective medical therapy is use of a nonselective β-blocker, which has been shown to reduce the incidence of first bleeding episodes and bleeding-related mortality. Because side effects limit the usefulness of medical therapy, endoscopic therapies are employed very effectively. The combination of medical and endoscopic therapies adds degrees of success. However, because even combinations of therapies fail to control the bleeding in some cases, progressively more invasive and morbid procedures are required to treat esophageal hemorrhaging. The greatest good can be accomplished by an early and thorough referral to a quarternary facility that offers not only medical interventions, but a vast array of therapies that will bridge patients to their best chance of a meaningful and durable survival, transplantation!

REFERENCES

1. Garcia-Tsao *et al.* Portal pressure, presence of gastroesophageal varices and variceal bleeding. *Hepatology* 1985; 5(3):419–424.
2. Merkel *et al.* A placebo-controlled clinical trial of nadolol in the prophylaxis of growth of small esophageal varices in cirrhosis. *Gastroenterology* 2004; 127(2): 476–484.
3. Bosch *et al.* Pharmacological versus endoscopic therapy in the prevention of variceal hemorrhage: and the winner is ... *Hepatology* 2009; 50(3):674–767.
4. Tripathi *et al.* Randomized controlled trial of carvedilol versus variceal band ligation for the prevention of the first variceal bleed. *Hepatology*. 2009; 50(3):825–833.
5. Gluud *et al.* Banding Ligation *Versus* beta-blockers as primary prophylaxis in esophageal varices: systematic review of randomized trials Am J gastroenterol. 2007; 102(12):2842–2848; quiz 2841, 2849. Review.
6. Balloon Tamponage for the control of hemorrhage from esophageal varices Robert W. Sengstaken and Arthur H. Blakemore *Ann Surg.* 1950; 131(5):781–789.
7. Edlich RF, Landé AJ, Goodale RL, *et al.* Prevention of aspiration pneumonia by continuous esophageal aspiration during esophagogastric tamponade and gastric cooling. *Surgery.* 1968; 64(2):405–408.

8. Panes J, Teres J, Bosch J, *et al.* Efficacy of balloon tamponade in treatment of bleeding gastric and esophageal varices. Results in 151 consecutive episodes. *Dig Dis Sci.* 1988; 33(4):454–459.
9. Pinto-Marques P, Romaozinho JM, Ferreira M, *et al.* Esophageal perforation — associated risk with balloon tamponade after endoscopic therapy. Myth or reality?. *Hepatogastroenterology* 2006; 53(70):536–539.
10. Collyer TC, Dawson SE, Earl D. Acute upper airway obstruction due to displacement of a Sengstaken-Blakemore tube. *Eur J Anaesthesiol.* 2008; 25(4): 341–342.
11. Agarwal R, Aggarwal AN, Gupta D. Endobronchial malposition of Sengstaken-Blakemore tube. *J Emerg Med.* 2008; 34(1):93–94.
12. Carbonel *et al.* Improved survival after variceal bleeding in patients with cirrhosis over the past two decades. *Hepatology* 2004; 40(3):652–659.
13. Monescillo *et al.* Influence of portal hypertension and its early decompression by TIPS placement on the outcome of variceal bleeding. *Hepatology.* 2004; 40(4):793–801.
14. Garcia-Pagan *et al.* An early decission for PTFE-TIPS improves survival in high risk cirrhotic patients admitted with an acute variceal bleeding. *A Multicenterrct Hepatology* 2008; Suppl; 373A–374A. abstract
15. Warren *et al.* Selective distal splenorenal shunt. Technique and results of operation. *Arch Surg* 1974; 108(3):306–314.
16. Warren *et al.* Selective trans-splenic decompression of gastro-oesophageal varices of distal splenorenal shunt. *Ann Surg* 1967; 166(3):437–455.
17. Sugiura *et al.* A new technique for treating esophageal varices. *Thoracic Cardiovasc Surg* 1973; 66(5):677–685.
18. Sugiura M, Futagawa S. Results of six hundred-six esophageal transections with paraesophagogastric devascularization in the teatent of esophageal varices. *J Vasc Surg* 1984; 1:254–260.
19. Inokuchi *et al.* Japanese research society for portal hypertension: a nationwide survey of 3588 patients. *World J Surg* 1985; 9:171–182.
20. Selzner *et al.* Current indication of a modified surgical procedure in the management of variceal bleeding. *J Am Coll Surg* 2001; 193(2):166–73.

LIVER FAILURE 11

Valentino Piacentino*, Deborah L. Sudan* and Janet E. Tuttle-Newhall[†]

INTRODUCTION

In the United States, chronic liver disease is ranked as the 12th most common cause of death and is responsible for 25,000 deaths annually. Liver disease can occur from multiple etiologies and progress to liver dysfunction or failure with considerable variability in rate of onset and associated complications. The estimated prevalence of cirrhosis in the United States has been reported between 115,000 and 2.4 million, if one takes into account the burden of hepatitis C, estimated at 3.9 million Americans, and that 59% have evidence of liver dysfunction and cirrhosis.[1] The international impact of viral hepatitis and mortality is even greater than in the United States, with liver disease ranked 1st as the most common cause of death in China. Currently, 16,224 patients diagnosed with end-stage liver failure and deemed adequate candidates await liver transplantation in the United States.[2] The majority of patients with cirrhosis liver failure decline over months to years due to progression of chronic disease; however, acute (or fulminant liver failure, by definition, leads to severe liver dysfunction within weeks of the onset of symptoms. Acute liver failure may require urgent liver transplantation for the patient to survive if their own liver

---

*Duke University Medical Center, Durham, NC 27710 USA.
[†]St Louis University Hospital and Cardinal Glennon Medical Center, St Louis, MO 63110 USA

does not recover from the acute injury, as there are no other effective methods of liver supportive therapy currently available. Advances in nonsurgical and surgical treatment and hepatic transplantation over the past decade have improved survival in patients with acute and chronic liver failure. This chapter will detail the epidemiology, associated symptoms, diagnostic modalities and treatment options available to patients with liver failure.

LIVER FAILURE EPIDEMIOLOGY AND ETIOLOGIES

Table 1 depicts the most common causes of acute and chronic liver failure. The most common hepatic virus leading to chronic liver disease in the United States is currently hepatitis C; however, worldwide hepatitis B remains the most common cause of chronic liver disease and contributor to complications of liver disease including hepatocellular carcinoma. Hepatitis C is the cause for over 50% of adult liver transplants in the United States.[3] Both hepatitis B and C lead to hepatocyte death and can cause progressive fibrosis of the liver parenchyma that ultimately leads to cirrhosis, portal hypertension and its complications as well as eventual impairment of the synthetic capabilities of the liver unless successfully treated. In addition, alcoholic liver disease causes fat infiltration into the liver and loss of hepatocytes due to repeated direct toxicity. It is a common cause of cirrhosis and subsequent liver failure. Non-alcoholic fatty liver disease (NAFLD) is an increasing cause of liver disease due to it s relation of type II diabetes mellitus and obesity. It is thought to be the most common cause of incidental liver disease currently in the United States. Approximately 10% of NAFLD patients develop a severe form of liver, non-alcoholic steatohepatitis (NASH). NASH is related to fat in the liver, inflammation leading to eventual fibrosis and liver dysfunction.[4]

Cholestatic and metabolic diseases make up the remainder of the majority of cases of chronic liver disease in the United States.[3] Cholestatic liver diseases include primary biliary cirrhosis (PBC) and primary sclerosing cholangitis (PSC) in adults, and biliary atresia in children. PBC is a chronic liver disease that is characterized by inflammation and progressive destruction of the small bile ducts. The majority of patients with PBC are women, between the ages of 30 and 60. PSC is an uncommon, chronic progressive disorder that leads to scarring and inflammation of the medium and large bile ducts of the liver. Both diseases lead to progressive

Table 1. Etiologies of liver failure.

Non-cholestatic liver disease	Biliary atresia
Alcoholic cirrhosis	Metabolic diseases
Autoimmune hepatitis	Alpha-1 antitrypsin deficiency
Viral hepatitis (A, B and C)	Hemochromatosis
Cryptogenic cirrhosis	Alagile's syndrome
Cholestatic liver disease	Wilson's disease
Primary biliary cirrhosis	Malignant neoplasm
Primary sclerosing cholangitis	Hepatocellular carcinoma (usually as a component of chronic liver disease)
Acute hepatic necrosis	Hepatoblastoma
Hepatitis B (Surface Antigen +)	Fibrolamellar hepatocellular carcinoma
Hepatitis C	Other
Drug ingestions	Cystic fibrosis
Unknown causes	Budd–Chiari

Based on liver diagnostic categories of the Organ Procurement and Transplant Network (OPTN).

destruction and blockage of the bile ducts and inability of the liver to secrete bile out of the biliary systems. When this occurs, progressive scarring of the liver occurs which leads to cirrhosis. Both disorders are thought to have an autoimmune origin.

With development of cirrhosis, both outflow resistance of the portal vein and the function of the liver are compromised. The result of portal hypertension is ascites, splenomegaly, varices formation and encephalopathy. The result of hepatic cellular dysfunction is a decrease in hepatic metabolism leading to increased risk for medication toxicity, and decreased protein synthesis leading to malnutrition, coagulopathy and hypoalbuminemia. These derangements can mimic other diseases such as cancer (cachexia and muscle wasting) and heart disease (fatigue, ascites and peripheral edema) and cause delay in diagnosis. Although all of these symptoms may occur in acute liver failure, the onset is more rapid (over days or weeks) and most often associated with elevated liver enzymes, coagulopathy, marked jaundice and encephalopathy in severe cases.

Acute liver failure (or fulminant hepatic failure, FHF) is defined by abrupt loss of liver function due to drug toxicity, acute viral infection, presentation of autoimmune hepatitis, Wilson's disease or other unknown causes within 8 weeks of the onset of symptoms or laboratory abnormalities. One of the more common causes of FHF is acetaminophen overdose and this usually presents as hyperacute liver failure (within 1 week of injury) and can be highly lethal. Large ingestions of Tylenol can be associated with severe coagulopathy, coma and renal failure.[5] Other idiosyncratic medication reactions and viral infections may present as *FHF* (onset within 8–28 days) or *subacute* liver failure (onset of liver failure within 4–12 weeks). The majority of cases of FHF were fatal before liver transplantation. Approximately 5% of liver transplant in the United States necessitate urgent liver transplant work up as a result of FHF.[2]

SYMPTOMATOLOGY AND PHYSICAL EXAMINATION FINDINGS

The history and physical examination is essential in assessing the liver disease patient. Questions in the history should include asking the patient and their caregivers, knowledge of previous diagnosis of liver disease, history of encephalopathy, ascites, previous (if any) endoscopies for varices, previous gastrointestinal bleeding episodes, risk factors for hepatitis (such as tattoos, history of blood transfusions, previous transplants prior to 1995), and medications as well as any allergies they may have.

On physical examination, confusion, lethargy, tremor, and even mood change, can occur with encephalopathy. Patients with encephalopathy may exhibit asterixis (flapping tremor upon arm extension, digit abduction, and wrist dorsiflexion) and the mental status change may range from mild confusion to coma. Ability to protect their airway must be part of the assessment in patients with dense encephalopathy. In patients with new onset of encephalopathy, an underlying cause such as infection or gastrointestinal luminal bleeding must be ruled out. There are additional physical examination findings that can assess presence of portal hypertension. Given the associated portal and mesenteric anatomy, and the consequences of cirrhosis on that circulatory pathway, there are many presentations physically. On the skin, chest wall and abdomen, the presence of small telangectasias and subcutaneous venous collaterals can be present. These dermal manifestations of liver disease are thought to be due to abnormal cutaneous blood flow regulation and abnormal estrogen levels.[6] Also, petechiae may be found when the patient is thrombocytopenic. Hyperbilirubinemia, sometimes associated with liver dysfunction, can be assessed with the presence or absence of icteric sclera and darkening/yellowing of the skin. A lung examination may reveal the presence of a right pleural effusion, common with ascites and portal hypertension. Palpation of the abdomen may reveal a fluid wave with ascites and splenomegaly. In patients with PSC and PBC, a large liver edge may be palpable as well. Engorged paraumbilical veins may be seen on the abdominal wall in some patients, classically described as a caput medusa and may or may not be associated with an umbilical hernia. Anorectal varices can be found and the rectal examination gives the examiner the opportunity to check the patient's stool for gross or occult blood. Arm and facial muscle wasting may also be present, and often, in the presence of ascites, patients may have large amounts of dependent peripheral edema in the lower extremities.

Of note, infections in patients with liver disease are often hard to diagnose as classic symptoms of fever, and leukocytosis may be absent. Encephalopathy and fluid retention (increased ascites and peripheral edema) may often be the only signs of infected abdominal fluid (spontaneous bacterial peritonitis, or SBP), pneumonia, urinary tract infection, or bacteremia. In addition, bleeding events may be sporadic in nature and intensity, and can range from minimal bleeding such as with tooth brushing to hypovolemic shock due to large volume luminal blood loss. A clinician may find blood on the teeth and gums and/or blood on rectal examination in a confused liver patient who cannot give an accurate history.

DIAGNOSTIC MODALITIES

Laboratory Workup

In patients suspected of having liver dysfunction, laboratory tests are useful to determine causes of liver disease, severity of hepatic dysfunction, and may be reflective of portal hypertension. Serological testing for hepatitis A, B and C need to be performed to determine not only cause of any hepatic dysfunction, but whether or not the viral infections are treatable. Other tests, such as antinuclear antibody titers, serum copper, iron panels including transferrin, may be reflective of other causes of liver disease such as autoimmune hepatitis, Wilson's disease, and hemochromotosis. Standard liver "function" tests, such as alanine transaminase (ALT or SGPT) and aspartate transaminase (AST or SGOT) are only reflective of hepatocyte death and are relatively nonspecific for degree of liver impairment. Elevations of conjugated bilirubin, alkaline phosphatase and gamma-glutamyl transpeptidase (GGT), are associated with biliary obstructive diseases. The only true "function" test is that of prothrombin time (PT) international normalized ratio (INR) and in most cases is elevated due to poor production of clotting factors. Albumin levels are generally decreased as well, but albumin may be decreased not only due to liver disease but other forms of catabolic stress and/or fluid resuscitation. In addition, leucopenia and thrombocytopenia are common in the presence of portal hypertension and splenomegaly.

Ultrasound

Imaging of the liver by ultrasound is non-invasive, and if done by the right operator, provides rapid assessment of hepatic anatomy, surface contour and size, and patency of the inflow (hepatic artery and portal vein) and outflow (hepatic veins) vessels. An ultrasound can often discern biliary duct size with some certainty. In addition, hepatic tumors can often be visualized, when present. Ultrasound plus serum testing for α-fetoprotein (AFP) is used as the test of choice for routine screening for tumors in patients with chronic liver disease. Nodules found in patients with cirrhosis that are greater than 1 cm should be considered a positive screening result and mandate further investigation.[7] Ultrasound is also useful for guiding bedside percutaneous liver biopsies.

CT and MRI

A triphasic CT scan of the abdomen or contrast-enhanced MRI with gadolinium have become the standard for evaluation of suspected liver tumors found on ultrasound or screening, and following tumors in patients listed for liver transplant. CT and MRI offer the benefit of non-invasive staging that enhance any interventional plan for diagnosis, or treatment. Often, CT or MRI imaging characteristics may offer diagnostic clues to whether the tumor is benign or malignant, and may even obviate need to intervention. Hypervascularity on contrast imaging with subsequent contrast "washout" in the early or later venous phase, is characteristic of hepatocellular carcinoma (HCC). Using these radiological characteristics for diagnoses, the need for a tissue diagnosis via biopsy can be obviated. Using these guidelines and imaging that is state-of-the-art, strategies of treatment can be devised with detailed imaging and computer-based anatomical reconstructions of the imaging data. Sequential studies can evaluate response to treatment or maintenance of transplant eligibility.[7]

Endoscopy

Endoscopy is warranted in patients with suspected portal hypertension. On endoscopy, varices can be found in the upper and lower GI tract. In asymptomatic patients, these varices can be treated medically with nonselective β blockers to prevent bleeding in more than 50% of patients with medium to large varices. Intervention such as banding may be helpful as well to prevent bleeding from large varices or in those patients who have smaller varices that have bled through β blockage. In the decompensating liver patient with a GI bleed, endoscopy is mandatory as part of therapy to confirm the site of bleeding as well as providing a basis for therapeutic intervention. Luminal bleeding in a patient with liver disease may be from varices, but other causes such as peptic ulcer disease must be excluded as well when considering treatment options.[8]

MANAGEMENT OPTIONS

FHF

For acute liver disease, there are treatment options available. Once a diagnosis is made or suspected, those patients, require movement to an ICU for monitoring and support. The cause of FHF is often not known; however, if testing reveals an acute viral infection or drug toxicity, there may be medical therapies available. The capacity of the liver to recover from an acute injury is usually based on any underlying liver impairment such as associated with alcohol use, or presence of NAFLD. In acetaminophen toxicity, there are treatments available such as N-acetylcysteine, that can potentially improve liver recovery by augmenting hepatic glutathione reserves and together with glutathione, bind to toxic metabolites produced by acetaminophen degradation. There are also specific guidelines for patients with and without acetaminophen toxicity developed to predict recovery or need for urgent transplantation. These are the King's College guidelines and can be found in Table 2.[5] Currently, extracorporeal liver assist devices to support the patient while the liver recovers, are in development but have

Table 2. King's College Guidelines for acute acetaminophen toxicity and non-acetaminophen toxicity.

The King's College Criteria identify two groups of patients that have a poor prognosis with acetaminophen induced liver failure:

Arterial pH < 7.3

Or those with all of the following:

- A PT INR of greater than 6.5,
- Serum creatinine of greater than 3 mg/dl
- Evidence of encephalopathy

For patients with non-acetaminophen–induced liver failure
The presence of encephalopathy (of grade III or IV).

INR greater than 6.5; or,

Three of the following five criteria:

- Patient age of less than 11 or greater than 40;
- Serum creatinine of greater than 3 g/dl
- Time from onset of jaundice to the development of coma of greater than 7 days;
- INR greater than 3.5; or,
- Drug toxicity, regardless of whether it was the cause of the acute liver failure.

not been approved for human use, except on a clinical trial basis. There have been attempts to use xeno-livers from pigs to provide *ex vivo* support for patients with liver failure as well; however, the risk of zoonosis has limited this practice as well.

There are limited options for treatment in patients with FHF. Good ICU care, with attention to presence and progression of encephalopathy, early and aggressive airway protection when indicated with waning mental status, ulcer prophylaxis, and medications for any underlying cause are often the only options in some cases.[9] The decision for transplant candidacy should be made early in the patient's course. The transplant workup including psychiatric examination for patients with drug ingestions, may become difficult once the patients are intubated. The use of biopsies may be helpful to discern underlying causes (i.e. autoimmune hepatitis) and the degree of necrosis. While the biopsy itself is a poor predictor for the need of transplant; it can be used in the overall clinical assessment to determine whether a patient should be listed for transplantation or not, if they are eligible. Eligibility for transplant is determined by whether or not the patient has no significant medical comorbidities that would preclude survival from surgery long term (such as severe cardiovascular disease, COPD) and the psychosocial support to be compliant with postoperative medications, clinic appointments, and to care for a transplanted organ. Once the determination is made that the patient is a candidate for transplant, the assessment of whether or not the patient's liver can recover without transplant can, in some circumstances, be difficult. Certainly, serial coagulation profiles and the measurement of sequential clotting factor measurements such as Factor V and VII can be useful. Correction of the PT INR must be approached cautiously as the PT is a direct reflection of liver function, and as such of recovery or failure. The degree of hepatocyte injury can be manifested by a rise in the AST and ALT; however, falling levels may be more reflective of hepatocyte loss as opposed to the liver recovery. Mental status changes are key to determining whether or not a patient will recover or not. The use of any sedating medications such as narcotics, benzodiazepines, or phenothiazenes are to be avoided. Agitation is often a sign of waning mental status. When intubating patients with FHF, it is important to use limited amounts of short acting medications that are not hepatically cleared such that frequent neurological evaluations can be performed. Increased intracranial pressure is a complication of FHF and if present, can only be reversed by liver transplantation. If the decision has been made to perform a transplant, there are some centers that advocate the use of intracranial pressure monitoring devices. The risk of implantation of these devices, must be weighed against the benefit of knowing the intracranial pressure in the coagulopathic FHF patient. FHF patients are given priority on the UNOS waiting list, and there are now larger geographical sharing areas to prevent patients with FHF from dying due to lack of organ availability.

Once transplanted, outcomes after liver transplant are excellent with the 1-year survival of over 90%. For those patients not eligible for transplant, if the liver does not recover with maximum support care, their lifespan is limited. Death ensues from infections, luminal bleeding, and brain herniation from increased ICP or cardiovascular collapse.

Chronic Liver Disease

For patients with chronic liver disease, the severity of the liver disease and its complications determine the strategies of management options.

Historically, the Child's Pugh classification has been used to gauge severity of a patient's liver disease, predict patients survival from surgical interventions and was once used as the platform for liver allocation in the United States. The Child's Pugh Turcotte score is based on several subjective clinical parameters including severity of ascites, and encephalopathy. Currently, the Model for End-Stage Liver disease (MELD) is the severity of liver dysfunction scoring system that depends on objective parameters such as PT INR, serum bilirubin and serum Creatinine levels. It is a proven predictor of survival of patients after transhepatic portacaval shunting (TIPS) and elective general surgery procedures.[10,11] One criticism of the MELD scoring system, is that it does not reflect the degree of portal hypertension that a patient with liver disease has present and it is the complications of portal hypertension that lead to the majority of patients morbidity and mortality with chronic liver disease.

The only known cure for end-stage liver disease is transplantation. Any decision regarding therapy of chronic liver disease and its complications, must be made after the decision regarding the patients candidacy for transplantation as the natural history is variable in terms of progression to end organ failure determined by underlying disease. Each transplant center has its own set of inclusion and exclusion criteria; however, generally, the exclusion criteria focus on comorbid conditions that would affect the potential candidates survival and their ability to care for a transplanted organ. The discussion of determination of candidacy for transplant is beyond this chapter; however, while caring for patients with chronic liver disease, the need for transplant should be determined early and referral made to a center that performs transplant made, to facilitate the patient's care if the need arises. In order to be listed for transplant, a patients MELD score must be greater than 10; in order to be allocated an organ, the MELD score must be greater or equal to 15. For patients with liver tumors as a complication of their end-stage liver disease, the tumor must be within the liver and not outside of the Milan criteria Table 3 for additional tumor points. Each UNOS region assigns points to limit time for patients with tumors on the waiting list to less than 6 months in order to facilitate their transplant while the tumor is within criteria. Most patients with chronic liver disease are medically managed for the complications of portal hypertension including varices, ascites, and encephalopathy during the course of their disease whether they are candidates for transplant or not.

Table 3. Eligibility for UNOS Tumor Points: Milan Criteria.[2]

T1 1 nodule less than 2 cm
T2 1 nodule 2–5 cm; 2 or 3 nodules, all less than 3 cm

Varices

Portal hypertension is a progressive complication of chronic liver disease. The gastroesohageal collaterals are the most relevant as their rupture results in variceal bleeding, the most common lethal complication of end-stage liver disease. Their presence and severity are reflective of the severity of liver disease and are present in over 50% of patients with cirrhosis. As discussed previously, endoscopy is the test of choice to diagnose varices. In patients with varices who have not bled, there are data to support using nonselective β blockers to prevent bleeding episodes. In patients with larger varices at risk for rupture, endoscopic banding can be used on a regular basis to decrease the risk of rupture. Banding can also be used emergently to control variceal bleeding in some cases. If bleeding is suspected or occurs, monitoring in an ICU setting, antibiotic prophylaxis, use of pharmacological therapies such as somatostatin, should be started as soon as possible. If bleeding cannot be controlled by pharmacological or endoscopic measures, balloon tamponade may be a temporizing measure until the decision for rescue therapies can be determined. Historically, patients with medical refractory acute variceal hemorrhage have been treated surgically with portal decompression procedures such as total shunts (portacaval) or selective shunts (distal splenorenal); however, these procedures have generally been replaced in the emergent setting with a TIPS. Distal splenorenal shunts are reserved for patients with favorable anatomy and used electively in patients with medically refractory varices that are not candidates for TIPS.[8]

Ascites

Ascites is the most common complication of cirrhosis and is associated with a poor quality of life, increased risk of infections, renal failure, and a poor long-term outcome. Patients with ascites have a poor 5-year survival, 30–40%, and should be evaluated for transplantation. The pathophysiology of ascites is multifactorial but is a related to perturbations in splanchnic vasodilatation. Increased hepatic resistance to portal flow due to cirrhosis, gradual development of portal hypertension with subsequent collateral vein formation, and shunting of blood to the systemic circulation. Disturbances in increasing arterial flow lead to increased retention of fluid in the peritoneal cavity due to increased intestinal permeability.[12] Fluid retention and impaired renal function may lead to dilutional hyponatremia.

General management of ascites involves dietary sodium restriction, fluid restriction, and low dose diuretics. Lasix at 20–40 mg a day facilitates dieresis but must be used under close supervision to avoid over dieresis and renal impairment. In patients with severe ascites, aldactone and paracentesis may be used as well. The need for large volume paracentesis portends a limited survival and must be used with caution. In patients with medical refractory ascites, which occurs in 5–10% of patients, a TIPS may be used to relieve the accumulation of fluid in the abdomen and relieve portal hypertension. TIPS, however, can be associated with increased risk of encephalopathy, right heart failure, and renal failure. An assessment of the patients heart function by echocardiogram and liver reserve by calculating MELD must be made prior to any decision to place a TIPS. The use of TIPS is controversial in those patients not candidates for liver transplant due to the complication rate, need for close surveillance and restenosis rate of the shunt requiring invasive interventions. In a third of patients with ascites, the ascites itself will become infected. Spontaneous bacterial peritonitis (SBP) is diagnosed by a diagnostic paracentesis with the findings of 250 white blood cells per cc. The infection of the ascites is also related to decreased integrity of the intestinal barrier such that gut flora organisms are the most common pathogens. Once initial treatment with antibiotics is completed, antibiotic suppression with oral agents is effective in preventing recurrent infections. SBP is also associated with hepatorenal syndrome (HRS). Prognosis with HRS is poor and the diagnosis can be made by measuring urinary sodium. Due to the underlying vasoconstriction in renal circulation, the kidney is unable to retain sodium.

Encephalopathy

Encephalopathy is also a very common complication of chronic liver disease. In the presence of chronic liver disease, it represents hepatic decompensation. The true pathophysiology of encephalopathy is not clearly defined; however, it is thought to be related to the lack of clearance of substances normally metabolized by the liver. Encephalopathy may range from mild confusion to dense coma. Serum ammonia levels may be helpful in discerning the diagnosis, but a true relationship with levels of serum ammonia and level of encephalopathy has not been proven. Encephalopathy is often the presenting symptom of underlying infection in patients with chronic liver disease, and may be the only sign of SBP; a thorough investigation of underlying causes (and other causes of mental status changes) must be undertaken. If an underlying cause such as SBP is found as the inciting cause of encephalopathy, it is reversible with treatment. Other causes of encephalopathy in patients with chronic liver disease include luminal bleeding and medication use (such as sedatives or narcotics) and a urine toxicology screen in mandatory in new onset mental status changes. Treatment of encephalopathy is based on the correction of any underlying cause, and the use of cathartics such as lactulose, and non-absorbable antibiotics such as neomycin.[13] Care must be taken in using lactulose and other cathartics, to avoid voluminous diarrhea and electrolyte abnormalities.

CONCLUSION

Liver disease is a common cause of mortality and morbidity currently in the United States. Familiarity with acute liver and chronic liver disease and their complications will facilitate quality patient care and improve outcomes. Early decision for transplantation in the management of these patients is paramount in their care.

REFERENCES

1. Xu J, Kochanek KD, Murphy SL, *et al.* Deaths: final data for 2007. *National Vital Statistics Report* 2010; 19:1–2.
2. http://optn.transplant.hrsa.gov/data. June 23, 2011.
3. Kim, WR, Brown RS, Terrault NA, *et al.* Burden of liver disease in the United States. *Hepatology* 2002; 36(1):227–242.
4. Pascale A, Pais R, Ratzui V. An overview of non alcoholic steatohepatitis: past, present and future. *J Gastro Lvr Ds* 2010; 19(4):415–423.
5. O'Grady J, Alexander G, Hayllar K, *et al.* Early indicators of prognosis in fulminant hepatic failure. *Gastroenterology* 1989; 97 (2):439–445.

6. Li CP, Lee FY, Hwang SJ, *et al.* Spider angiomas in patients with liver cirrhosis: role of alcoholism and impaired liver function. *Scand J Gastroenterol* 1999; 34 (5):520–523.
7. Bruix J Sherman. AASLD practice guideline: management of hepatocellular carcinoma. *Hepatology* 2005; 42(5):1208–1236.
8. Garcia-Taos G, Sanyal AJ, Grace N, *et al.* Prevention and management of gastro esophageal varices and variceal hemorrhage in cirrhosis. *Hepatology* 2007; 46(3):922–938.
9. Polson J, Lee W (2005). AASLD position paper: the management of acute liver failure. *Hepatology* 2005; 41(5):1179–1197.
10. Malinchoc M, Kamath PS, Gordon FD, *et al.* A model to predict poor survival in patients undergoing transjugular intrahepatic portosystemic shunts. *Hepatology* 2000; 31(4):864–871.
11. Befeler AS, Palmer DE, Hoffman *et al.* The safety of intra-abdominal surgery in cirrhotics: MELD is superior to Child-Turcotte-Pugh in predicting outcome. *Arch. Surg* 2005; 140:650–654.
12. Gines P, Cardenas A, Arroyo V, *et al.* Management of cirrhosis and ascites. *N Engl J Med* 2005; 350:1646–1654.
13. Ferenci P, Lockwood A, Mullen K, *et al.* Hepatic encephalopathy — definition, nomenclature, diagnosis, and quantification: final report of the working party at the 11th World Congresses of Gastroenterology, Vienna, 1998. *Hepatology* 2002; 35(3):716–721.

LIVER TRANSPLANTATION 12

Katia Papalezova*, Carlos E. Marroquin[†],
Bradley H. Collins[‡], Janet E. Tuttle-Newhall[§]
and Paul C. Kuo[¶]

INTRODUCTION

Today, liver transplantation is a lifesaving procedure for patients with chronic end-stage liver disease and acute liver failure.[1-3] The indications and contraindications for liver transplantation have become well-established. In the pretransplantation era, liver failure was nearly universally fatal, with mortality from fulminant hepatic failure of 80–90%, and 1-year mortality from decompensated cirrhosis of more than 50%. Dr. Thomas Starzl performed the first three human liver transplants at the University of Colorado in 1963, but did not achieve 1-year survival until 1967. With the implementation of cyclosporine-based immunosuppression in the late 1970s and early 1980s, the 1-year survival doubled to 30%.[40] In 1983, these improved outcomes led to the decision at a National Institutes of Health Consensus Development Conference that liver transplantation was no

---

*Montefiore/Albert Einstein College of Medicine, Bronx, New York, USA
[†]University of Rochester, Rochester, New York, USA
[‡]Duke University Medical Center, Durham, NC 27710 USA
[§]St Louis University Hospital and Cardinal Glennon Medical Center, St Louis, MO 63110 USA
[¶]Address correspondence and requests for reprints to: Paul C. Kuo, M.D., M.B.A. Duke University Medical Center 110 Bell Bldg, Box 3522 Durham, NC 27710 Phone: (919) 668-1856 FAX: (919) 684-8716 E mail: kuo00004@mc.duke.edu

longer an experimental procedure and deserved broader application in clinical practice.[4] This meeting initiated the modern era of liver transplantation. Over the last three decades, there have been significant improvements in recipient selection, donor management, operative technique, immunosuppression, and postoperative management of liver recipients which have led to 1-year survival for adult and pediatric deceased donor liver transplantation (DDLT) of 85%, and 5- and 10-year survival of 70% and 60%, respectively.[5–8]

A significant number of patients with end-stage liver disease (ESLD) die of disease-related complications. Once individuals develop ESLD, liver transplantation offers the only effective therapy. Although the vast majority of liver transplants are performed for ESLD secondary to viral hepatitis and alcoholism, there are a variety of etiologies of liver failure with a common set of indications for liver transplantation. Herein we will review the variety of causes of liver failure, the indications for liver transplantation, and the means by which these organs are allocated.

CAUSES OF LIVER FAILURE

Liver failure can result from a heterogeneous group of etiologies. These can range from acute fulminant failure to chronic dysfunction which evolves over years. Both acute and chronic liver failure result from a variety of causes (Table 1). The most common are viral hepatitis and alcohol-induced cirrhosis.

Viral Hepatitis

Viral hepatitis refers to infection of the liver by a group of hepatotropic viruses. The hepatitis A virus[9] (HAV) generally produces a benign, self-limited disease. It is spread through the fecal–oral route. Although HAV rarely progresses to ESLD, in a rare instant (<0.1%), HAV has the capacity to induce fulminant hepatic failure.

HBV is spread through parenteral routes — most commonly through blood transfusions, and intravenous drug use — and through the exchange of body fluids. Infection with hepatitis B can result in an asymptomatic carrier state, an acute hepatitis with complete recovery, or chronic hepatitis with progression to cirrhosis. Additionally, a small minority of infections with HBV can progress rapidly to fulminant failure with poor outcomes in

Table 1. Indications for liver transplantation.

Viral hepatitis	**Systemic disorders**
Hepatitis A, B,C, D	Familial amyloidotic polyneuropathy
Alcohol-induced liver disease	Sarcoidosis
Auto-immune hepatitis	Non-alcoholic steatohepatitis (NASH)
Cholestatic liver diseases	
Primary biliary cirrhosis	**Circulatory disorders**
Primary sclerosing cholangitis	Budd-Chiari syndrome
	Veno-Occlusive disease
In-born errors of metabolism	
Hemochromatosis	**Cryptogenic cirrhosis**
Wilson's disease	**Fulminant hepatic failure**
Alpha-1-antitrypsin deficiency	Acute viral hepatitis
Glycogen storage diseases	Acute drug induced hepatitis
Tyrosinemia	Budd-Chiari syndrome
Alagille syndrome	Veno-Occlusive disease
Crigler-Najjar type I	Wilson's disease
Severe familial hypercholesterolemia	Primary hepatic malignant
Hereditary oxalosis	
Cystic fibrosis	

the absence of an emergent liver transplant. Finally, HBV is probably the most common carcinogen worldwide given a strong predisposition to the evolution of hepatocellular carcinoma.

Persistent infection and chronic hepatitis are the hallmarks of hepatitis C virus (HCV) infection.[10] Transmission is parenteral accounting for the vast majority of transfusion-associated hepatitis. A large number of individuals infected with HCV will progress to chronic disease (~85%) and eventually develop cirrhosis and ESLD requiring transplantation.

Hepatitis D virus (HDV) is a defective virus and only capable of infection in the presence of hepatitis B viral infection.[11] Acute coinfection with HDV and HBV can result in mild hepatitis which has the potential of degenerating into fulminant hepatitis. Similarly, superinfection of chronic HBV with HDV can convert into a chronic state that terminates in cirrhosis and ESLD or can cause the deterioration of a chronic HBV infection into a fulminant hepatitis with hepatic necrosis.

Alcohol Induced Liver Disease

Alcoholic hepatitis accounts for 10–20% of individuals listed for transplantation in the United States. Some of these individuals have a combined history of alcoholic and viral hepatitis but only about 10% have a pure diagnosis of Laennec's cirrhosis.

AUTOIMMUNE DISORDERS

Autoimmune hepatitis is seen less frequently. This is often a diagnosis of exclusion in the presence of high immunologic titers. This disease process affects mainly women. The first steps in making the diagnosis is a negative viral workup, a negative search for other possible etiologies, followed by finding an elevation in the serum immunoglobulin G (IgG) levels against antinuclear antibodies (ANA), anti-smooth muscle antibodies (SMA), and antimitochondrial antibodies. Three types of autoimmune hepatitis are recognized.[12,13] Type 1 is the prototypical form with positive ANA or SMA, or both. Type 2 is seen in the pediatric population and is characterized by antibodies against liver and kidney microsomal antigens (anti-LKM-1). Type 3 is characterized by antibodies against soluble liver antigen (anti-SLA) or liver pancreas antigen (anti-LP) or both. These patients tend to respond favorably to steroids and antiproliferative agents early in their disease state, and liver transplantation is reserved for those who progress to cirrhosis and decompensated liver disease.

CHOLESTATIC LIVER DISEASES

Primary biliary cirrhosis (PBC) is a chronic disorder characterized at the outset by destruction of the intrahepatic bile ducts, and portal inflammation. After a prolonged clinical course, these patients progress to cirrhosis and liver failure. The disease progression requires 2 to 3 decades before the development of signs and symptoms. The pathophysiology of PBC involves an autoimmune mechanism. Ninety percent of patients with PBC have antimitochondrial antibodies. Patients with PBC require liver transplantation for end-stage disease.

Primary sclerosing cholangitis (PSC) leads to a progressive destruction of the intra- and extrahepatic bile ducts. Localized and multifocal strictures can be seen in association with segments of dilated intrahepatic and extrahepatic bile ducts. PSC is seen more commonly in middle-aged men, and it is seen in association with ulcerative colitis. A small percentage (5–15%) of patients with PSC will develop cholangio-carcinoma. The etiology of PSC is not clear, but genetic and immunological mechanisms are believed to play a role. The median survival from diagnosis to death is about 12 years. The combination of ursodeoxycholic acid with endoscopic dilatation offers symptomatic relief, but progression to cirrhosis and failure is the rule. End-stage disease requires transplantation.

IN-BORN ERRORS OF METABOLISM

Some causes of liver failure are the result of metabolic disorders. Hemochromatosis can be genetic or acquired. Hereditary hemochromatosis is a recessive trait passed on through Mendelian genetics. Acquired or secondary hemochromatosis is the result of iron overload from iatrogenic or surreptitious sources which lead to multiple systemic complications. The genetic defect in patients with hemochromatosis involves an uncontrolled absorption of iron which results in iron overload and subsequent tissue damage from direct iron toxicity of solid organs (liver, pancreas, heart, and endocrine glands). When diagnosis is made early, treatment with regular phlebotomy allows a normal life. However, if untreated, lethal outcomes are the result of hepatic and cardiac complications.

Wilson's disease is the result of a genetic defect on chromosome 13 which results in an autosomal recessive disorder of copper metabolism.[14] Hepatolenticular degeneration occurs from toxic accumulation of copper in the liver, brain and eye. These individuals exhibit normal copper absorption with altered hepatic excretion. Although controversial, there are effective medical therapies for Wilson's disease.[5] Therefore, these individuals rarely require transplantation.

α1 Antitrypsin deficiency is an autosomal recessive disorder that results in sub-physiologic levels of α1 antitrypsin. α1 Antitrypsin is a protease inhibitor which is synthesized predominantly by the liver. This impairs hepatic secretion and results in accumulation of α1 antitrypsin within the hepatocyte endoplasmic reticulum and subsequent hepatocellular damage. These individuals develop active inflammation with cholestasis that can progress to cirrhosis. Treatment for severely affected individuals consists of liver transplantation.

Glycogen storage diseases (GSD) or glycogenoses comprise a variety of inherited disorders arising from abnormalities of the enzymes that regulate the synthesis or degradation of glycogen.[15] Although there are a variety of enzymatic abnormalities or deficiencies that result in hepatic glycogen storage diseases, there are two that occasionally require liver transplantation.[16] One of these enzymatic deficiencies involves glucose 6-phosphatase (also known as glycogen storage disease I or von Gierke disease) which catalyzes the conversion of glucose 6-phosphate into glucose and inorganic phosphate in hepatocytes and renal epithelial cells.[15] The second form of enzymatic deficiency involves glycogen-debranching enzyme or type III glycogen storage disease. This is also known as Cori disease which results in an inability to release glucose from glycogen stores and limit dextrin-like glycogen accumulates in the liver. Occasionally, these patients do not respond to medical therapy and they develop serious complications of their glycogen storage disease which may lead to cirrhosis. When this occurs, liver transplantation offers a viable alternative. Twenty-two to seventy-five percent of patients with GSD I and approximately 25% of patients with GSD III develop hepatic adenomas.[16,17] They have the capacity of malignant transformation which is the second indication for liver transplantation in this population.

Tyrosinemia type I or hepatorenal tyrosinemia produces profound pathologic changes involving the liver, kidney and nervous system. There are three types of tyrosinemia syndromes described,[18] but only type I has necessitated liver transplantation. Alagille syndrome is a dominantly inherited multisystem disorder occurring approximately once in every 100,000 live births. Alagille syndrome is a cholestatic liver disease that is associated with vertebral, cardiovascular, ophthalmologic, endocrine and nervous system disorders. Although some patients have an asymptomatic natural history, others progress to liver failure requiring liver transplantation.[19] Finally, Crigler–Najjar type I, severe familial hypercholesterolemia, hereditary oxalosis, and cystic fibrosis are nonhepatic manifestations of metabolic diseases whose genetic defect is expressed in the liver and may be corrected with liver transplantation.

SYSTEMIC DISORDERS

Familial amyloidotic polyneuropathy (FAP) is a rare disorder transmitted as an autosomal dominant trait, and is associated with the production of a mutant protein known as transthyretin (TTR).[20] The disease progression is varied and may progress from a peripheral neuropathy to death approximately 10 years after the onset of the disease. Although FAP does not produce cirrhosis and liver failure, liver transplantation is life saving because TTR is produced by the liver.

Sarcoidosis is a granulomatous disease of unknown etiology. The characteristic lesion is a noncaseating granuloma that can involve most any tissue. Although granulomas are found on liver biopsies, hepatic dysfunction is not common. In the extreme, sarcoidosis may produce liver failure with associated portal hypertension and variceal bleeding. These patients rarely require liver transplantation, although recurrence is a real concern.[21–24]

Given the increasing trend toward obesity in the United States and western cultures. Non-alcoholic steatohepatitis (NASH) is becoming a recognized form of liver failure with greater frequency. The main risk factors associated with NASH are obesity, hypertension, hyperlipidemia and insulin resistance.[25,26] NASH represents a stage within the spectrum of nonalcoholic fatty liver diseases. NASH is defined by the absence of alcohol consumption in association with diffuse steatosis on liver biopsy with lobular inflammation and hepatocyte degeneration.[27] Sustained liver injury in these individuals leads to progressive fibrosis. Ultimately, liver failure can ensue. In extreme cases of failure, liver transplant is the only treatment.

CIRCULATORY DISORDERS

Budd–Chiari syndrome is characterized by thrombotic occlusion of the hepatic veins. Budd–Chiari typically develops in the presence of hypercoagulability.[28] Although not always progressive, the onset of symptoms involves the evolution of abdominal pain from hepatomegaly and ascites. Continued decline is the result of hepatic decompensation owing to obstruction of blood flow. Centrilobular necrosis is followed by the onset of fulminant hepatic failure in acute and subacute cases. Fibrosis is the end result of chronic cases.

The management of Budd–Chiari syndrome is supportive in self-limited cases. In cases of progressive decline, biopsies should be obtained of both lobes of the liver (to avoid sampling errors). If the biopsies indicate the injury is reversible, management should proceed towards re-establishing hepatic vein patency with thrombolytics or angioplasty with stenting.[28] Patients with diffuse disease and portal hypertension should be managed with portal or mesenteric venous shunting. Patients who present in fulminant failure or progress to fibrosis secondary to chronic failure should be treated with a liver transplant.[29]

Veno-occlusive disease (VOD) can be confused with Budd–Chiari syndrome and is an iatrogenic cause of portal hypertension due to occlusion of small hepatic veins. The initial lesion is zone III necrosis with progression to hepatic congestion and fatal liver failure in some patients. VOD is seen in the setting of malignancy after bone marrow transplantation[30] following intensive therapy with an incidence of 4–22%[31] and may also be seen during the course of systemic therapy with cytotoxic agents and in association with radiation therapy.[32] VOD generally presents acutely with the onset of jaundice, abdominal pain, hepatomegaly, and ascites. The mainstay of therapy is supportive. Liver transplantation could be life saving, but should only be considered in patients undergoing therapy for benign disease.

CRYPTOGENIC DISORDERS

Cryptogenic cirrhosis is a diagnosis of exhaustion. The history will be negative for alcohol use, and the autoimmune and viral workup will be negative. In a small number of these ambiguous patients, one will stumble onto nonalcoholic fatty liver disease as the cause of cryptogenic cirrhosis.[33] Nevertheless, liver transplant is the best therapy for liver failure despite the absence of a clear-cut etiology for the failure.

FULMINANT HEPATIC FAILURE

Fulminant hepatic failure (FHF) refers to a syndrome of clinical symptoms and physiologic responses associated with the rapid arrest of liver function. The syndrome is defined by the presence of hepatic encephalopathy occurring as the consequence of severe liver damage in patients without previous, clinically overt liver disease.[34] Fulminant hepatic failure progresses rapidly to death in 2–3 weeks without transplantation. Also known as acute hepatic necrosis, fulminant failure can occur most commonly due to viral etiologies (Hepatitis A, B, C, Delta), or chemical or drug toxicity (acetaminophen).[34] Less commonly, fulminant hepatic failure may be due to other etiologies like Wilson's disease, Budd-Chiari, veno-occlusive disease, acute fatty liver of pregnancy, and cryptogenic causes. These patients present acutely and are generally in critical condition. They require transplantation within one week of their presentation if they are to survive. Patients who do not make it to transplantation generally succumb to lethal herniation or sepsis.

INDICATIONS FOR LIVER TRANSPLANT

The most common indicatons for liver transplantation in the United States are HCV infecton (30–40%), alcoholic liver disease (10–12%), cryptogenic cirrhosis (9–10%), and other less common indications are HBV (5%), primary biliary cirrhosis (5%), primary sclerosing cholangitis (5%), metabolic diseases (5%), HCC, and fulminant liver failure. The major indications for liver transplantation in children are biliary atresia, cholestatic liver disease, metabolic disorders, malignancies including hepatoblastoma, and fulminant hepatic failure. Biliary atresia is the most common indication for liver transplantation in children and accounts for 41% of cases.[35]

Hepatitis C virus (HCV) infects about 1.8% or 3–5 million people in the United States.[36,37] Up to 20% of HCV-infected patients progress to cirrhosis after 20 years of infection.[38] Among patients with HCV-induced cirrhosis, 4% per year decompensate and 1–4% per year develop HCC.[39–41] The risk of HCC is increasing among HCV-infected patients.[42] Five-year survival is only about 50% once hepatic failure has developed, so this is the trigger point for referring patients for transplantation.[40,41] It has been projected that the number of HCV-infected patients with hepatic decompensation or HCC will continue to increase over the next decade.[37] Indeed, complications resulting from chronic HCV infection account for 40% of liver transplants in the United States.

Patients with hepatitis B cirrhosis and high viremia were not eligible for transplantation in the past because of the high risk of recurrence after transplantation with consequent rapid graft loss. Since the availability of antiviral medication, high viremia is treatable and transplantation has become a more realistic option with excellent graft and patient survival that is even superior to that of many other indications.[43] After transplantation, antiviral treatment, often including hepatitis B immune globulin, is continued to prevent recurrent infection.[44] HCC is a well-recognized indication for transplantation when the patients have Child B and C liver cirrhosis at the same time and there are no metastases. Generally, only patients who meet the Milan criteria of a single tumor up to 5 cm or up to three tumors, all less than 3 cm in diameter, and no major vascular invasion such as portal and hepatic vein, as determined by imaging studies,[45] are approved by the transplant organizations in most countries. Survival rates for these patients are comparable to those for cirrhosis leading to transplant without a complicating HCC recurrence. Discussions at present focus on expansion of these strict criteria.[46] Yao et al. have shown that patients who have single tumor 6.5 cm in diameter or smaller or three or fewer tumors with largest being 4.5 cm or less in diameter and a total tumor burden of 8.0 cm or less (the so-called "UCSF criteria") achieved results that were not different from those of patients meeting the Milan criteria. Vascular invasion would preclude transplantation.[47] Lee et al. proposed Asan Medical Center (AMC) criteria from the results of live donor liver transplant (LDLT) for HCC, based on explant pathology, that were largest tumor diameter ≤5 cm, number ≤6, and no gross vascular invasion. It had similar prognostic power but highest discriminatory power than Milan and UCSF criteria.[48] Radiofrequency ablation and chemoembolization have become bridging therapies to transplantation while patient is waiting on the liver transplant list.[49,50]

For alcoholic liver disease, the prerequisites for transplantation in most centers are alcohol abstinence for at least 6 months and active treatment for alcohol dependency before transplantation.[51,52]

Acute Liver Failure (ALF), also called "fulminant hepatic failure", and the more indolent variant, subfulminant hepatic failure, are characterized by the development of liver failure manifested by coagulopathy, jaundice, and encephalopathy leading to coma in the absence of chronic liver disease.[53] ALF accounts for 5–6% of all liver transplants.[54] Acetaminophen hepatotoxicity is the leading cause of ALF, whereas idiosyncratic drug-induced liver injury is the major cause of subfulminant hepatic failure.[53] Patients who have ALF can recover spontaneously, but those with subfulminant hepatic failure are expected to have 100% mortality without transplantation.[53,55] Transplantation indications for ALF are usually based on King's College criteria,[56] and/or Clichy criteria.[57] However, it is often recommended that patients with ALF who fail to meet King's College criteria still be considered for liver transplantation, because spontaneous recovery is not guaranteed.[1] Timely referral and liver transplantation is of paramount importance, because death from sepsis and cerebral edema may occur within days of onset of stage 3 or 4 hepatic encephalopathy.[1,53,55] Lee et al.[58] described that the timely LDLT using appropriate graft type sufficing at least more than 40% of patient's standard liver volume with minimal steatosis resulted in remarkably improved survival rate for adult ALF patients in this region where deceased organ donation is very scarce.

Graft failure with the need for retransplantation accounts for an increasing number of transplants. Shortly after transplantation, the main reason for re-transplantation is primary nonfunction of liver grafts and hepatic artery thrombosis. Late causes for re-transplantation include biliary complications and recurrent hepatitis C.[46] In general, the past few years have been characterized by an increasingly shorter list of absolute contraindications and a growing list of indications for liver transplantation.

The liver is, in essence, a dynamic protein factory with a tremendous reserve. Failure occurs when greater than 80% of hepatic function is compromised. Individuals with liver disease, regardless of etiology, often have a significant reserve and live at a high level of function until their functional demand out paces their reserve. Well-compensated cirrhotics have exceptional 5 year survivals upwards of 90%. However, once patients begin to experience complications of end-stage liver disease, liver transplantation offers the only effective alternative.

Complications of end stage liver disease fall into two broad categories: (1) complications secondary to portal hypertension, and (2) complications due to reduced liver mass. Complications that result from portal hypertension include intestinal tract bleeding from gastroesophageal varices or portal gastropathy. Fluid retention that results from portal hypertension is manifest as ascites and/or hydrothorax (hepato-hydrothorax). Portosystemic encephalopathy is a central nervous system manifestation of shunting blood around the liver which occurs with portal hypertension. Complications secondary to a reduced hepatic cell mass include coagulopathy, jaundice, and impaired drug metabolism. Hepatic encephalopathy is also believed to occur due to a reduced cell mass.

Hepatorenal syndrome (HRS) is the result of a complex cascade of events which commence with liver failure and portal hypertension eventually leading to renal failure. The diagnosis of HRS is made with the following criteria: oliguria with a urine to plasma osmolality >0.1; progressive azotemia; and rising creatinine in the presence of a urine sodium concentration <10 mEq/L. Treatment is supportive in nature including repletion of the intravascular volume by driving the central venous pressures, preferably with colloid. Two types of HRS have been described.[59,60] Acute onset or type I is a severe form associated with poor outcomes and type II develops gradually over time and is associated with better outcomes. Liver transplantation is the therapy of choice and results in resolution of HRS in the vast majority of patients. Those patients who do not recover renal function undergo a kidney transplant following recovery

Table 2. Model for end-stage liver disease score.

Criteria
   Bilirubin (mg/dL)
   International normalized ratio (INR) for prothrombin time
   Creatinine (mg/dL)

Formula*
MELD Score = 11.2 log(INR) + 3.78 log(Bilirubin) + 9.57 log(Creatinine)

Prognosis in hospitalized patients[†]:

Meld score	Three-month mortality
<9	4%
10–19	27%
20–29	76%
30–39	83%
>40	100%

*Malinchoc M, Kamath PS, Gordon FD, Peine CJ, Rank J, TerBorg PL. A model to predict poor survival in patients undergoing transjugular intrahepatic portosystemic shunts. Hepatology 2000;31:864–871
[†]Kamath *et. al* A model to predict survival in patients with end-stage liver disease. Hepatology 2001; 33:464–470.

from the liver transplant while on dialysis. When there is little hope of recovery, a combined liver and kidney transplant can be performed with good outcomes.[61]

MODEL FOR END-STAGE LIVER DISEASE

Since it has been exceedingly difficult to predict who will need to be transplanted given their current state of disease, the MELD system was devised. Once a patient has been diagnosed with ESLD, the timing of transplantation is dependent on the severity of liver disease. Livers are currently allocated according to the model for end-stage liver disease (MELD)[62] with hope to improve the allocation of grafts. MELD makes livers available to patients who have been deemed appropriate candidates for transplantation based on medical urgency. The model relies on three objective and reproducible parameters (Table 2). The ability of MELD to predict the 3-month mortality of patients with ESLD was validated in a study at the

Mayo clinic.[63] Moreover, MELD was shown to be as good as the CTP classification in terms of its ability to predict survival in patients with ESLD of diverse etiologies.

RECIPIENT OUTCOMES

The survival rates after DDLT are expected to be greater than 85% and 75% at 1 and 5-years post-transplantation, respectively.[64] Initially, the survival rate following LDLT was much lower than DDLT. However, LDLT has evolved to be a valuable strategy in reducing wait list mortality for pediatric patients and adult patients with chronic liver disease, ALF and HCC.

SUMMARY

Patients should be considered for liver transplantation if they have evidence of fulminant hepatic failure, a life-threatening systemic complication of liver disease or a liver-based metabolic defect, or, more commonly, cirrhosis with complications such as hepatic encephalopathy, ascites, HCC, hepatorenal syndrome, or bleeding caused by portal hypertension. Quality of life studies have shown that most patients have an excellent quality of life following transplantation, with 5-year patient survival at 75%. *De novo* malignancies and recurrence of native disease, however, remain significant challenges. Although living donor transplants are being performed more frequently, the most significant hurdle currently is the organ shortage.

REFERENCES

1. Ahmed A, Keeffe EB. Current indications and contraindications for liver transplantation. *Clin Liver Dis* 2007;11:227–247.
2. Murray KR, Carithers RL Jr. AASLD practice guidelines:evaluation of the patient for liver transplantation. *Hepatology* 2005;41:1407–1432.
3. Consensus Conference: indications for liver transplantation, January 19 and 20, 2005, Lyon-Palais Des Conges:text of recommendations (long version). *Liver Transpl* 2006;12:998–1011.
4. National Institutes Of Health Consensus Development Conference Statement: liver transplantation. June 20–23, 1983. *Hepatology* 1984: 4:107S–110S.
5. Jain A, Reyes J, Kashyap R, *et al.* Long-term survival after liver transplantation in 4000 consecutive patients at a single center. *Ann Surg* 2000;232:490–500.

6. Gordon RD, Fung J, Tzakis AG, et al. Liver transplantation at the University of Pittsburgh, 1984 to 1990. *Clin Transpl* 1001;105–117.
7. Abbasoglu O, Levy MF, Brkic BB, et al. Ten years of liver transplantation: an evolving understanding of late graft loss. *Transplantation* 1997;64–1801–1807.
8. Asfar S, Metracos P, Fryer J, et al. An analysis of late deaths after liver transplantation. *Transplantation* 1996;61:1377–1381.
9. Martin A, Hepatitis A. In: ER Schiff, MF Sorrell, WC Maddrey (eds). *Schiff's Disease of the Liver.* 9th edition, Lippincott Williams & Wilkins. 2003.
10. Davis GL, Hepatitis C. In: ER Schiff, MF Sorrell, WC Maddrey, (eds). *Schiff's Disease of the Liver.* 9th edition, Lippincott Williams & Wilkins. 2003.
11. Rizzetto M, Smedile A, Hepatitis D. In: In: ER Schiff, MF Sorrell, WC Maddrey, (eds). *Schiff's Disease of the Liver.* 9th edition, Lippincott Williams & Wilkins. 2003.
12. Vogel A, Wedemeyer H, manns M, Strassburg CP. Autoimmune hepatitis and overlap syndromes. *J Gastroenterol Hepatol.* 2002 Dec;17 Suppl 3: S389-S398.
13. McFarlane IG. Definition and classification of autoimmune hepatitis. *Semin Liver Dis* 2002;22(4):317–324.
14. Subramanian I, Vanek ZF, Bronstein JM. Diagnosis and treatment of Wilson' disease. *Curr Neurol Neurosci Rep* 2002;2(4):317–323.
15. Wolfsdorf JI, Weinstein DA.Glycogen storage diseases. *Rev Endocr Metab Disord* 2003;4(1):95–102.
16. Liu PP, de Villa VH, Chen YS, et al. Outcome of living donor liver transplantation for glycogen storage disease. *Transplant Proc* 2003;35(1):366–368.
17. Lee PJ. Glycogen storage disease type I: pathophysiology of liver adenomas. *Eur J Pediatr* 2002;161 (Suppl 1):S46–49.
18. Russo PA, Mitchell GA, Tanguay RM Tyrosinemia: a review. *Pediatr Dev Pathol* 2001;4(3):212–221.
19. Ganschow R, Grabhorn E, Helmke K, et al. Liver transplantation in children with Alagille syndrome. *Transplant Proc* 2001;33(7–8):3608–3609.
20. Lewis WD. Liver transplant and familial amyloidotic polyneuropathy. *Liver Transpl* 2002;8(11):1085–7.
21. Fidler HM, Hadziyannis SJ, Dhillon AP, et al. Recurrent hepatic sarcoidosis following liver transplantation. *Transplant Proc* 1997;29(5):2509–2510.
22. Hunt J, Gordon FD, Jenkins RL, et al. Sarcoidosis with selective involvement of a second liver allograft: report of a case and review of the literature. *Mod Pathol* 1999;12(3):325–328.
23. Pescovitz MD, Jones HM, Cummings OW, et al. Diffuse retroperitoneal lymphadenopathy following liver transplantation — a case of recurrent sarcoidosis. *Transplantation* 1995;60(4):393–396.

24. Shibolet O, Kalish Y, Wolf D, *et al.* Ilan Y Exacerbation of pulmonary sarcoidosis after liver transplantation. *J Clin Gastroenterol* 2002;35(4):356–358.
25. Marchesini G, Bugianesi E, Forlani G, *et al.* Non-alcoholic fatty liver, steatohepatitis, and the metabolic syndrome. *Hepatology* 2003;37(4):917–23.
26. Tankurt E, Biberoglu S, Ellidokuz E, *et al.* Hyperinsulinemia and insulin resistance in non-alcoholic steatohepatitis. *J Hepatol* 1999;31(5):963.
27. Alba LM, Lindor K. Review article: non-alcoholic fatty liver disease. *Aliment Pharmacol Ther* 2003;17(8):977–86.
28. Pelage JP, Denys A, Valla D, *et al.* Budd-Chiari syndrome due to prothrombotic disorder: mid-term patency and efficacy of endovascular stents. *Eur Radiol* 2003 Feb;13(2):286–93. Epub 2002 Jun 12.
29. Slakey DP, Klein AS, Venbrux AC, *et al.* Budd-Chiari syndrome: current management options. *Ann Surg* 2001;233(4):522–7.
30. Richardson P, Guinan E. Hepatic veno-occlusive disease following hematopoietic stem cell transplantation. *Acta Haematol* 2001;106(1–2):57–68.
31. Gottesman L, Turnbull AD, O'Reilly RJ. Surgical implications of hepatic venocclusive disease following bone marrow transplantation. *J Surg Oncol* 1988;37(2): 113–5.
32. Bischof M, Zierhut D, Gutwein S, *et al.* Veno-occlusive liver disease after total infradiaphragmatic lymphoid irradiation. A rare complication. *Strahlenther Onkol.* 2001;177(6):296–301.
33. Clark JM, Diehl AM. Non-alcoholic fatty liver disease: an underrecognized cause of cryptogenic cirrhosis. *JAMA.* 2003;289(22):3000–4.
34. Williams R, Riordan SM. Fulminant Hepatic Failure In: ER Schiff, MF Sorrell, WC Maddrey (eds). *Schiff's Diseases of the Liver.* 9th edition, Lippincott Williams & Wilkins, 2003.
35. Leary JG, Lepe R, Davis G. Indications for liver transplantation. *Gastroenterology* 2008;134:1764–1776.
36. Alter MJ, Kruszon-Moran D, Nainan OV, *et al.* The prevalence of hepatitis C virus infection in the United States, 1988 through 1994. *N Engl J Med* 1999;341: 556–562.
37. Davis GL, Albright JE, Cook SF, *et al.* Projecting the future healthcare burden from hepatitis C in the United States. *Liver Transpl* 2003;9:331–338.
38. Freeman AJ, Dore GJ, Law MG, *et al.* Estimating progression to cirrhosis in chronic hepatitis C virus infection. *Hepatology* 2001;34:809–816.
39. Serfaty L, Aumaitre H, Chazouilleres O, *et al.* Determinants of outcome of compensated hepatitis C virus-related cirrhosis. *Hepatology* 1998;27: 1435–1440.
40. Fattovich G, Giustina G, Degos F, *et al.* Morbidity and mortality in compensated cirrhosis type C: a retrospective follow-up study of 384 patients. *Gastroenterology* 1997;112:463–472.

41. El-Serag HB. Hepatocellular carcinoma: recent trends in the United States. *Gastroenterology* 2004;127 (Suppl 1):S27-S34.
42. Sangiovanni A, Prati GM, Fasani P, *et al.* The natural history of compensated cirrhosis due to hepatitis C virus: a 17-year cohort study of 214 patients. *Hepatology* 2006;43:1303–1310.
43. Kim WR, Poterucha JJ, Kremers WK, Ishitani MB, Dickson ER. Outcome of liver transplantation for hepatitis B in the United States. *Liver Transpl* 2004;10:968–974
44. Hwang, S, Lee SG, Ahn CS, *et al.* Prevention of hepatitis B recurrence after living donor liver transplantation: primary high-dose hepatitis B immunoglobulin monotherapy and rescue antiviral therapy. *Liver Transpl* 2008;14:770–778.
45. Mazzaferro V, Regalia E, Doci R, *et al.* Liver transplantation for the treatment of small hepatocellular carcinoma in patients with cirrhosis. *N Engl J Med* 1996;334:693–699.
46. Verdonk RC, van den Berg AP, Sloof MJ, Porte RJ, Haagsma EB. Liver transplantation: an update. *Neth J Med* 2007;65:372–380.
47. Yao FY, Ferrell L, Bass NM, *et al.* Liver transplantation for hepatocellular carcinoma: expansion of the tumor size limits does not adversely impact survival. *Hepatology* 2001: 33:1394–1403.
48. Lee SG, Hwang S, Moon DB, *et al.* Expanded indication criteria of living donor liver transplantation for hepatocellular at one large-volume centre. *Liver Transpl* 2008;14:935–945.
49. Befeler AS, Hayashi PH, Di Bisceglie AM. Liver transplantation for hepatocellular carcinoma. *Gastroenterology* 2005;128:1752–1764.
50. Freeman RB Jr. Transplantation for hepatocellular carcinoma: the Milan criteria and beyond. *Liver Transpl* 2006;12:S8-S13.
51. Lim JK, Keeffe EB. Liver transplantation for alcoholic liver disease: current concepts and length of sobriety. *Liver Transpl* 2004;10:S31-S38.
52. diMartini A, Day N, Dew MA, *et al.* Alcohol consumption patterns and predictors of use following liver transplantation for alcoholic liver disease. *Liver Transpl* 2006;12:813–820.
53. Lee WM. Acute liver failure. *N Engl J Med* 1993;329:1862–1872.
54. United Network for Organ Sharing (UNOS). United Network for Organ Sharing: Organ donation and transplantation (Internet). Richmond (VA). UNOS; 1995 (cited 2006 Feb 12). Available from: http://www.unos.org.
55. Yu AS, Keefe EB. Liver transplantation. In: D Zakim, TB Boyer (eds). *Hepatology: A Textbook of Liver Disease.* 4th edition, Philadelphia, Saunders, pp. 1617–1656. 2003.

56. o'Grady JG, Alexander GJ, Hayllar KM, Williams R. Early indicators of prognosis in fulminant hepatic failure. *Gastroenterology* 1989;97:439–445.
57. Bernuau J, Samuel , Durand F, *et al.* Criteria for emergency liver transplantation in patients with acute viral hepatitis and factor V (FV) below 50% of normal: a prospective study. *Hepatology* 1991;14:49A.
58. Lee SG, Ahn CS, Kim KH. Which types of graft to use in patients with acute liver failure? (A) Auxiliary liver transplant (B) Living donor liver transplantation (C) The whole liver. (B) I prefer living donor liver transplantation. *J Hepatol* 2007;46:574–578.
59. Wong F, Blendis L. New challenge of hepatorenal syndrome: *prevention* and treatment. *Hepatology* 2001;34(6):1242–51.
60. Kramer L, Horl WH. Hepatorenal syndrome. *Semin Nephrol* 2002;22(4): 290–301.
61. Margreiter R, Konigsrainer A, Spechtenhauser B, *et al.* Our experience with combined liver-kidney transplantation: an update. *Transplant Proc.* 2002;34(6): 2491–2.
62. Wiesner RH, McDiarmid SV, Kamath PS, *et al.* MELD and PELD: Application of Survival Models to Liver Allocation. *Liver Transplantation*, Vol. 7, No 7, 2001: PP567–580
63. Kamath PS, Wiesner RH, Malinchoc M, *et al.* A model to predict survival in patients with end-stage liver disease. *Hepatology* 2001;33:464–470.
64. Roberts MS, Angus DC, Bryce CL, *et al.* The survival after liver transplantation in the United States: a disease-specific analysis of the UNOS database. *Liver Transpl* 2004;10:886–897.

EMBOLIZATION OF LIVER TUMORS　　13

Leo Villegas* and Paul V. Suhocki[†]

INTRODUCTION

Surgery is the only potential cure for liver tumors. This chapter will describe basic concepts of alternative procedures that HPB surgeons must be familiar with in order to treat patients with liver tumors. To provide patients with the best multidisciplinary approach to their disease, surgeons should partner with radiologists and oncologists.

PORTAL VEIN EMBOLIZATION

Liver failure is the principal cause of death post-major hepatectomy. Portal vein embolization (PVE) has been used for over a decade as a preoperative strategy for borderline resectable liver tumors while planning for a major liver resection. This technique expands patients' eligibility for liver resections and decreases postoperative complications.

Kinoshita used PVE to prevent portal extension of HCC and observed contralateral hypertrophy.[1] In patients with gross liver disease and little spare normal liver parenchyma, this technique involves occluding the portal vein on the tumor-involved hemi-liver to stimulate the growth of the future liver remnant (selective hypertrophy). CT-generated volumetric data are used to

---

*Sacred Heart Health System, Pensacola, FL, USA
†Duke University Medical Center, Durham, NC 27710 USA

calculate volumes of the total liver (TLV) and the functional liver remnant (FLR). PVE is usually indicated when the FLR is below 20% of the TLV on a patient with otherwise normal liver function or less than 30% of chemo-induced steatohepatitis or less than 40% if cirrhotic.

Controversy still exists regarding the need for embolization of segment IV of the liver before a planned extended right hepatectomy. This could contribute to better hypertrophy of the segments I, II, III, but could also increase the risk of portal occlusion of the normal liver and induce liver failure.

PVE is performed via a percutaneous transhepatic approach utilizing ultrasound and fluoroscopy.[2] An ipsilateral approach (access through the portion of the liver to be resected) is recommended so as not to injure the FLR. The most frequent indication for PVE is the right PVE while planning a right trisegmentectomy. After inserting a 22-gauge Chiba needle into the right portal vein, a flush portography is performed with an angiographic 5-F pigtail catheter. Embolization is performed with polyvinyl alcohol particles and microcoils until hemostasis is achieved.

A CT scan is usually performed 4 weeks after PVE to evaluate the degree of FLR hypertrophy and the possibility of resectability. A technical success rate of PVE was recently reported to be nearly 99%, with less than 1% fatal liver failure after hepatectomy.[3] In a recent meta-analsysis, 85% of the patients underwent planned hepatectomy following PVE. PVE is safe, with a reported morbidity of 2.2% and no mortality.[4]

Tumor size post-PVE and LFT's pre-PVE were found to be predictors of resectability. PVE patients who underwent resection had a survival benefit compared to unresected (MS of 7 months), with 45% of patients remaining disease-free at 2 year follow-up.[5]

For patients with multifocal or bilobar liver colorectal metastases, a two-stage hepatectomy combined with PVE has been reported to allow curative resection for initially unresectable tumors. The tumors in the FLR are removed in the first surgery followed by PVE and a second extended hepatectomy. This technique resulted in a survival benefit (54% at 3 years) for initially unresectable patients.[6]

PVE still has some unresolved issues; some publications have reported a concern of PVE stimulating the growth of hepatic tumors. Kokudo was able to demonstrate in patients with colorectal liver metastasis a proliferative activity of the metastasis in the embolized liver.[7] The blood supply of intrahepatic metastasis may depend mostly on the hepatic artery flow. After PVE, it has been shown that the blood flow of the embolized segment is compensated by an increase in hepatic arterial flow.

ARTERIAL EMBOLIZATION: TAE, TACE, DRUG-ELUTING BEADS (HEPASPHERE®)

There has been an increasing incidence of hepatocellular carcinoma (HCC) in the U.S. Surgical resection (single tumor) and transplantation (Milan criteria) are traditionally considered the only curative options for these patients. The use of radiofrequency ablation has gained popularity for lesions </= 3.0 – 3.5 cm in diameter. Transplantation has been associated with a 70% 5-year survival, but a small fraction of patients are candidates and donor supply is limited.[8] Surgical resection, limited by cirrhosis, has a 40% 5-year survival, but recurrences are nearly 80%. Less than 25% of patients with HCC are candidates for curative treatments because most of them present with advanced disease. Today, transcatheter embolization is the preferred treatment for palliation in unresectable HCC. It can be used before or after radiofrequency ablation (RFA) and as a bridge for liver transplantation.

Trans catheter arterial bland embolization (TAE) and transarterial chemoembolization (TACE) have gained popularity in the treatment of inoperable or recurrent hepatocellular carcinoma or cholangiocarcinoma. The former induces tumor ischemia and necrosis while the latter technique combines exposure of the tumor to a chemotherapeutic agent with tumor ischemia and necrosis. TACE was introduced in 1977 by Yamada, while he first explored HCC blood supply from the hepatic artery to deliver chemotherapy.

In TAE, gelfoam particles, polyvinyl alcohol particles or trisacryl gelatin microspheres are used with/without lipiodol to occlude the tumor-feeding vessels. Chemoembolization (TACE) involves the addition of doxorubicin (most common), cisplatin, epirubicin or mitomycin C to the particles for embolization. Currently, there is no good evidence of which chemotherapeutic agent is most effective. Lipiodol is an iodinated ester that is selectively taken up and retained in HCC (up to a year) used in primary HCC and hepatic metastasis of colonic and neuroendocrine tumors.

Prior to embolization, hepatic angiography is performed from a common femoral approach with a 5-French catheter. The lesion is identified and the portal vein is assessed for patency. Patients are typically admitted overnight for observation of pain, nausea vomiting, fever, post-TACE syndrome, and leukocytosis. Bacteremia, liver abscess, or vascular complications (dissection) requiring re-intervention (stent) are closely monitored. After discharge, most will evaluate patients with a CT scan after 4–6 weeks.

Llovet and the Barcelona group published in 2002 a randomized clinical trial of TACE, TAE and symptomatic treatment for unresectable HCC.[9] The survival rates for 2 years were 63% for TACE, 50% for TAE, and 27% for the conservative arm. The trial was stopped when TACE showed survival benefit to conservative treatment (p = 0.025). No significant survival advantage was seen on TACE vs. TAE. Lo *et al.* performed another randomized clinical trial in Asia, evaluating the value of TACE with cisplatin and Lipiodol compared to a control group.[10] They demonstrated a 26% survival at 3 years compared to 3% in the control group (p = 0.002).

The Memorial Sloan-Kettering Cancer Center group published in 2006 the results of more than 800 embolization procedures. For patients with recurrent HCC following hepatectomy who underwent TAE (n = 45), they reported a 47% overall survival at 5 years, with an overall median survival of 46 months.[11]

In 2008, the Memorial Sloan-Kettering Cancer Center group reported 322 patients with unresectable HCC treated with TAE. The median survival was 21 months, with a 1-, 2- and 3-year overall survival rate of 66%, 46% and 33% respectively.[12] They hypothesized that TAE may be the critical component of catheter-directed embolotherapy.

Drug-eluting beads (DEB) are 100–900-micron diameter spheres that are loaded with chemotherapy (doxorubicin, cisplatin or irinotecan) and delivered to the liver by transcatheter technique. The beads slowly release the chemotherapeutic agent into the adjacent tumor, minimizing the systemic effects of the drug. At least a partial response to DEB was seen in almost half of the patients and with less doxorubicin-related side effects than compared with TACE alone. Potential survival benefits are still unproven.

New biological target agents for cancer have recently been combined with TACE for HCC. These include monoclonal antibodies that bind VEGF receptors (Bevacizumab (Avastin®)) and a multikinase inhibitor (Sorafenib (Nexavar®)).

RADIOEMBOLIZATION MICROSPHERES (THERASPHERE® & SIR-SPHERE®)

Conventional external-beam radiotherapy (EBR) for unresectable liver cancer is limited by the limited tolerance of the liver to radiation. This motivated an investigation of safer ways to deliver radiotherapy to liver tumors.

Radioembolization delivers radiotherapy via transcatheter embolization of radioactive microspheres. This allows for a high radiation dose to be delivered to the tumor cells, with relative sparing of the adjacent normal liver tissue. It is also associated with less arterial occlusion and a lower incidence of postembolization syndrome when compared with TACE.

Yttrium-90 (^{90}Y)–labeled microspheres are used for palliative treatment of primary and metastatic liver cancer. This technique was initially described in the 1960s, but there has been a resurgence of interest in the United States since 2000. TheraSpheres® (Canada) are glass microspheres and SIR-Spheres® (USA) are resin microspheres, each loaded with ^{90}Y. The emitted electrons from the spheres have a tissue penetration average of 2.5 mm with a maximum of 1 cm. Radioembolization can be performed as an outpatient. It can deliver up to 130–150 Gy to the tumor cells. With a 59-hour half-life, there is no measurable activity 10 days after embolization. SIR-Spheres have a lower activity per sphere and therefore have a greater embolic effect than Theraspheres. Theraspheres can be used in patients with portal vein thrombosis. ^{90}Y radioembolization was reported as a bridge for transplantation, with a complete necrosis of the tumor noted in 66% by pathologic examination.

In 2010, Salem *et al.* published a long-term outcome study after arterial radioembolization in a single-center, prospective, longitudinal cohort study of 291 patients with HCC.[13] Side effects included fatigue (57%), pain (23%), nausea/vomiting (20%), and bilirubin toxicity (19%). The response rate was 42–57% (WHO or EASL criteria). Survival differed between patients with Child-Pugh A and B (17 vs. 7 months).

Many patients with unresectable HCC develop portal vein thrombosis (1/3). TAE or TACE could increase the risk of liver failure if done while portal vein thrombosis coexists due to the lack of flow compensation. For this reason, TAE or TACE has been considered a contraindication when the patient has a portal vein thrombosis. Radioembolization has been described in patients with portal vein thrombosis; in 2008, the Northwestern University group published a study on 108 patients treated with Theraspheres for HCC with or without portal vein thrombosis.[14] They reported a partial response (decrease of at least 50% of the tumor size) of 42% using the World Health Organization (WHO) or 70% using the European association for the study of liver (EASL) criteria, a modification of the WHO that includes necrosis.

Studies in 2010 have compared TACE with TheraSphere for unresectable HCC, showing equivalent or better survival, a shorter treatment session and less toxicity in the TheraSphere group.

Iodine-131 (^{131}I)–labeled Lipiodol, Lipiocis® (France), has been used as an embolic agent, but its long half-life limits its use, requiring that patients be kept in isolation after the initial injection. With no survival difference, it seems that ^{131}I-lipiodol is much better tolerated (fewer side-effects) than chemoembolization, with the advantage of no particle embolization or concern with portal vein thrombosis. In 2008, Boucher et al. published a retrospective study evaluating patients with HCC post-hepatectomy treated with ^{131}I-lipiodol and matched them with a group of patients with resection alone. The mean time for recurrence was 26 vs. 21 (control group) months and disease-free survival better (p = 0.09) for the ^{131}I-lipiodol group (no difference in overall survival).

SUMMARY

Patients with liver tumors are challenging to treat. Many tumors are unresectable and long-term outcomes can be disappointing. Although there is growing data to support the benefit of different transarterial therapies, a combination of these therapies with new systemic chemotherapies, biological target agents or ablative procedures may be the future for unresectable patients. These are tools that the hepatobiliary surgeon must be familiar with while treating patients with liver cancer that are initially unresectable.

REFERENCES

1. Kinoshita H, Sakai K, Hirohashi K, et al. Preoperative portal vein embolization for hepatocellular carcinoma. World J Surg 1986, 10(5): 803–808.
2. Abdalla EK, Hicks ME, Vauthey JN. Portal vein Embolization: rationale, technique and future prospect. Br J Surg 2001, 88(2): 165–175.
3. Ribero D, Abdalla EK, Madoff DC, et al. Portal vein embolization before major hepatectomy and its effects on regeneration, resectability and outcomes. Br J Surg 2007, 94(11): 1386–1394.
4. Abulkhi. Preoperative portal vein embolization for major liver resections: a meta-analysis. Ann Surg 2008; 247: 49–57.
5. Mailey. Surgical resection of primary and metastatic hepatic malignancies following portal vein embolization. J Surg Onc 2009; 100: 184–190.
6. Jaeck. A two-stage hepatectomy procedure combined with portal vein embolization to achive curative resection for initially unresected multiple and bilobar colorectal liver metastasis. Ann Surg 2004; 240: 1037–49.

7. Kokudo. Proliferative activity of intrahepatic colorectal metastases after preoperative hemihepatic portal vein embolization. *Hepatology* 2001; 34: 267–72.
8. Llovet JM. Resection and liver transplantation for hepatocellular carcinoma. *Semin Liver Dis* 2005; 25: 181–200.
9. Llovet JM. Arterial embolization or chemoembolization versus symptomatic treatment in patients with unresectable hepatocellular carcinoma: a randomized controlled trial. *Lancet* 2002; 359: 1734–1739.
10. Lo CM. Randomized Controlled Trial of Transarterial Lipiodol Chemoembolization for unresectable hepatocellular carcinoma. *Hepatology* 2002; 35: 1164–1171.
11. Covey A. Particle embolization of recurrent hepatocellular carcinoma after hepatectomy. *Cancer* 2006; 106: 2181–9.
12. Maluccio MA. Transcatheter arterial embolization with only particles for the treatment of unresectable hepatocellular carcinoma. *J Vasc Interv Radiol* 2008; 19: 862–9.
13. Salem R. Radioembolization for hepatocellular carcinoma using yttrium-90 microsphere: a comprehensive report of long-term outcomes. *Gastroenterology* 2010; 138: 52–64.
14. Kulik LM. Safety and efficacy of 90Y radiotherapy for hepatocellular carcinoma with or without portal vein thrombosis. *Hepatology* 2008; 47 (1): 71–81.

RADIOFREQUENCY ABLATION 14

Syamal Bhattacharya*
and Carlos E. Marroquin[†]

NATURAL HISTORY OF HCC AND UNTREATED HCC

Hepatocellular carcinoma (HCC) is the 5th most common malignancy worldwide with 500,000 new cases annually. HCC is also increasing rapidly in the US. This is due to a variety of factors including the hepatitis C epidemic, immigration of populations with a high prevalence of chronic hepatitis B, and the obesity epidemic with increasing incidence of non-alcoholic fatty liver disease (NAFLD).[1] Among worldwide cancer-related deaths, it is the 3rd most common cause of mortality. While not exhaustive, common causes of HCC include: viral hepatitis (hepatitis B and C), heavy metal intoxication (Wilson's disease, hemachromotosis), alcohol consumption, obesity, and NAFLD. The common denominator among the causes of HCC is that they are all risk factors for the evolution of cirrhosis. In the western world, HCC develops in the setting of underlying cirrhosis in 80–95% of cases with hepatitis C being the main etiology. Therefore, cirrhosis is the strongest predisposing factor for

---

*Duke University Medical Center, Durham, NC 27710 USA
[†]University of Rochester, Rochester, New York, USA

HCC as repeated rounds of necrosis and regeneration are necessary to initiate the carcinogenic process. Moreover, HCC is the leading cause of death in cirrhotic patients.[2] In patients with untreated HCC, the median survival is dismal ranging from 0.7 months to 8.3 months.[3] Prognostic indicators of poor outcome in patients with HCC are multiple tumors, bilobar involvement, size >5cm, vascular invasion, and positive margin from previous resection.

USUAL THERAPEUTIC MODALITIES AND INDICATIONS

HCC surveillance has become a standard practice in patients with chronic liver disease. While therapy for hepatitis B and C significantly reduces the risk of HCC, the occurrence of HCC is not arrested. In patients with known cirrhosis, The AASLD recommendations are ultrasound surveillance every 6 months. As such, HCC surveillance is still recommended for patients with successfully treated viral hepatitis. Another group of patients that require periodic surveillance are transplant candidates. It is crucial to identify small tumors that may require therapy, either resection or local ablation, before transplantation.

After the diagnosis of HCC has been made, one needs to assess the patient's ability to tolerate therapy. Patients with HCC generally have two problems. In addition to their tumor burden, these patients also have underlying liver disease. Accurate evaluation of the underlying liver disease is critical as it directly influences the therapeutic modality selected and affects outcomes. While there are several tools to evaluate the extent of the underlying liver disease, one straightforward approach is the Child-Pugh classification which includes two clinical parameters (ascites and encephalopathy) and three biochemical parameters (bilirubin, albumin, and INR).[4] Because the Child-Pugh classification is imperfect, one should also scrutinize the degree of portal hypertension as evidenced by splenomegaly, varices, and thrombocytopenia (<100). Patients with underlying liver disease also have other medical comorbidities (cardiac, pulmonary, and renal) which should be taken into consideration prior to going forward with therapy. In general, Child's A cirrhotics are candidates for a nonanatomic resections as one objective is to spare as many functioning hepatocytes as possible. When patients have multiple lesions or are poorly compensated, other treatment considerations include orthotopic liver transplantation, hepatic artery chemoembolization, cryoablation, microwave coagulation therapy, percutaneous ethanol injection, and radiofrequency ablation (RFA).

INDICATIONS FOR RFA

Traditional surgical approaches to HCC are not possible in the majority of patients with HCC because of their underlying liver disease. These patients have decreased synthetic function with reduced reserve. While resections should only be performed in well-compensated Child's A cirrhotics, regional therapies such as RFA allow us to treat patients that are less well-compensated. As such, current indications for RFA for patients with known HCC include poor resection candidates secondary to patient deconditioning, poor transplant candidates, and inability to resect secondary to tumor location, portal vein thrombosis, tumor size, or multiple lesions. A common utilization of RFA is to bridge patients to transplantation. The rationale for pretransplant ablation is to control tumor growth and intrahepatic metastasis during the waiting period. In fact, the response to RFA may serve as a marker of favorable tumor biology that may also translate into improved outcomes after transplantation. Lastly, pretransplant ablation theoretically eliminates the risk of tumor cell dissemination that could occur with manipulation during the hepatectomy at the time of transplantation. While RFA is typically utilized in the treatment of HCC, it is also a useful tool in the management of colorectal and noncolorectal metastatic disease to the liver. RFA can be utilized in addition to resection to render patients NED Smaller lesions in the contralateral lobe that are not amenable to a non-anatomic resection may be ablated in conjunction with a resection of the opposite lobe. RFA should only be used in this adjunctive fashion when one believes, with reasonable certainty, that complete tumor clearance will result. Finally, the combination of resection and RFA should not risk decompensation in cases of inadequate liver reserve from small residual volumes or excessive steatosis.

HOW RFA WORKS

The RFA probe is introduced into the liver parenchyma either percutaneously, laparoscopically, or via an open technique. The electrode delivers energy spherically; a low level of electrical energy coalesces to yield an area of coagulation and subsequent necrosis. The diameter of energy spread is determined by the probe selection. One should select a probe that will ablate a sufficient region based on the tumor size without destroying healthy hepatocytes. Factors that play into the amount of energy required include maximal tumor diameter and tissue resistance. For example in the case of a 2-cm lesion, one might choose a 3-cm field to yield complete ablation of the tumor load while providing a 0.5–1-cm margin. Limitations of RFA include potential for tissue charring, uneven coagulation, and heat sink effect caused by the hepatic vasculature. In the case of charring, this is combated using water-cooled probes. The heat sink effect can be overcome by using multiple RFA probes or microwave ablation technology. While RFA continues to gain popularity, there are other complications attributed to this modality: damage to nearby structures, bleeding from the tumor bed, and potential for tumor seeding of the peritoneal cavity. A similar technique to RFA involves microwave ablation. The electrodes are, instead, attached to a microwave generator. Microwave energy is then delivered to destroy areas of the tumor. Multiple pulses of microwave energy can be delivered during one session, and multiple needle electrodes can be utilized to treat larger lesions. Selection of any particular system is dependent on user friendliness and service and requires a trial period to develop a comfort level.

INDICATIONS FOR PERCUTANEOUS VERSUS OPERATIVE APPROACHES

Deciding on a percutaneous versus operative approach can be relatively straightforward. While some centers will not perform a percutaneous ablation in a patient with ascites, others have not encountered any additional morbidity after ablating these patients following a pre-ablation paracentesis. Therefore, the presence of ascites is only a relative contraindication to percutaneous ablation. The percutaneous approach is ideal in that it can be performed with local anesthesia and conscious sedation. Avoiding general anesthesia is attractive in patients with HCC and known cirrhosis as general anesthesia can result in rapid decompensation in patients with underlying liver disease. Other considerations include patient BMI, previous abdominal operations, and adjacent structures. Tumors near the diaphragm or other vital structures are often better managed operatively, whether laparoscopically or open, than percutaneously.

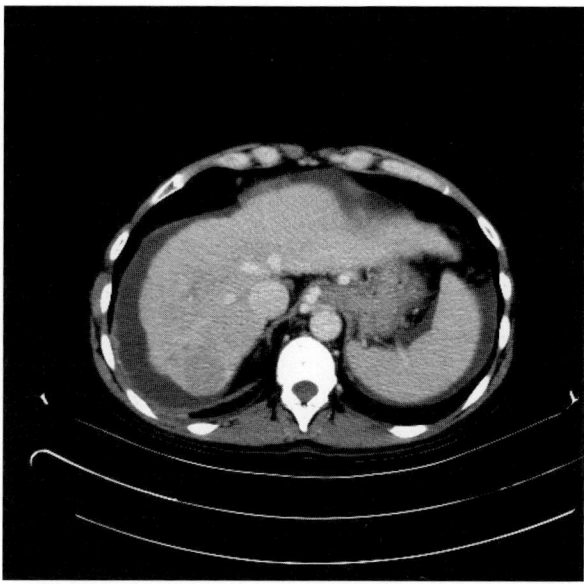

Figure 1. Lesion in the posterior sector of the liver with classic arterial enhancement and washout during the delayed phase. Posterior sectoral locations are ideal for a laparoscopic approach. The patient should be positioned in the left lateral decubitus position and trocars placed in sequence at the mid-clavicular line at about T-8, the anterior axillary line about T-10, and the posterior axillary line about T-10. The colon is mobilized away from the liver and the right triangular ligament is divided. This will expose these lesions and allow facile ultrasound localization and ablation.

Approaching a lesion near the diaphragm can be done laparoscopically with the patient in the left lateral decubitus position. While the patient is lying laterally, dividing the triangular ligament and mobilizing the right hemiliver facilitates laparoscopic localization and ablation. The best approach to a lesion located in the posterior sector, is an operative one as this allows mobilization of the colon away from the liver for the subsequent ablation (Figure 1). Similarly, lesions adjacent to the gallbladder fossa are best managed surgically as it may be necessary to perform a concomitant cholecystectomy to prevent subsequent gallbladder necrosis or hemobilia with cholecystitis. Multiple lesions are best handled operatively as visualization and access is facilitated by intraoperative ultrasound in our opinion.

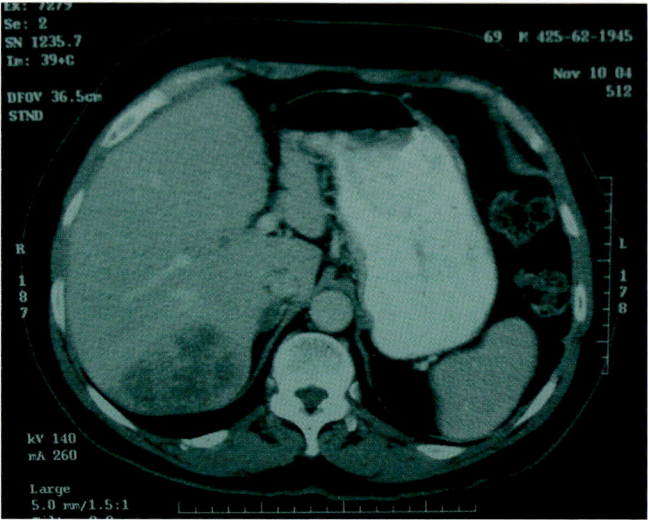

Figure 2. Lesions at or near the dome of the liver should be approached operatively. A percutaneous approach has a higher risk of pneumothorax and other thoracic injuries. These lesions are ideal for a laparoscopic approach with the patient in the left lateral decubitus position. The right triangular ligament is divided exposing these lesions. The right lobe can be medialized while using a rigid ultrasound probe to identify and ablate the lesion.

POSITIONING AND EQUIPMENT

Operative planning and patient positioning are critical for this procedure. Tumors that are located in the right anterior sector or left hemiliver can be approached laparoscopically or open with the patient supine. While lesions in the right posterior sector or high on the dome might be accessible in the supine position when a laparotomy is performed, they are best approached with the patient in the left lateral decubitus position during a laparoscopic approach (Figure 2). Intraoperative ultrasound is a must as it assists localizing the tumor and allows visualization of the probe placement and subsequent "ice ball" formation during the ablation. Ultrasound probes require a 10-mm port which should be positioned such that the index lesion and remaining liver can be interrogated for multifocal disease. Ideally, the intraoperative ultrasound utilized during a laparoscopic ablation should be a rigid probe. The nodules in a cirrhotic liver often provide the "illusion" of a tumor. Rigid probes optimize interface with the hepatic surface area allowing localization and characterization of difficult to localize lesions. During laparoscopic procedures, 5- and 10-mm, angled scopes are crucial to allow visualization through differing port sites and at different angles. Large or difficult to reach tumors may require a more complex approach necessitating the use of a gelport for hand assistance.

POSTOPERATIVE CARE

The postoperative care after a laparoscopic or open ablation is critical. The hematocrit should be measured serially to assess for bleeding. Moreover, because both hepatic failure and tumor lysis syndrome can result, basic chemistries (potassium, calcium, phosphate, creatinine), and hepatic synthetic function (INR, conjugated and unconjugated bilirubin) should be evaluated. AST/ALT derangements are not uncommon after an ablation. However, the development of an altered mental status, and acidosis with rising bilirubin and INR are of concern and should be closely monitored as these may be indicative of evolving liver failure. Once decompensation is suspected, imaging via CT or ultrasound should be performed to evaluate the possibility of compromised blood flow. Supportive care and preventing a secondary insults (hypotension, hypoxia) is the critical to successful outcomes. Treatment of tumor lysis syndrome is also supportive. Tumor lysis syndrome is a potentially fatal metabolic complication that results from rapid destruction of tumor cells. Cellular lysis results in hyperkalemia, hyperphosphatemia, hypocalcemia, hyperuricemia and potentially renal failure. Therefore, vigilant monitoring of fluids and electrolytes is important to prevent the onset of renal insufficiency, seizures and cardiac arrhythmias. Other less serious morbidities that are encountered with greater frequency include fever, nausea, abdominal discomfort and should be treated with antipyretics, antiemetics and expectantly. Pleural effusions can develop and should only be treated if symptomatic. Hemobilia is also encountered and may resolve without intervention but is often amenable to arterial embolization. Liver abscesses are known complications following an ablation. When a hepatic abscess results, it is often found during the outpatient follow-up and should be treated with percutaneous drainage and appropriate antimicrobial therapy. Finally, while the risk of needle track seeding is increased by lesions with a subcapsular location and poor tumor differentiation, the incidence is less than 1%.[5]

FOLLOW-UP

Follow-up should be scheduled with the surgeon hepatologist, and medical oncologist, preferably in a multi-disciplinary clinic. Alfa-feto protein (AFP) may be useful if it was elevated before treatment and it is critical to realize that AFP is often normal in HCC and commonly elevated in cirrhosis. Consequently, AFP has a low sensitivity and specificity and should not be used as a single source of surveillance. However, AFP does have a very high positive predictive value for the presence of HCC when it is persistently elevated above 200 ng/ml.[6–8] As such, AFP should be checked at 1, and 4 weeks post ablation and at the time of surveillance imaging studies with either CT scan or MRI. Imaging is recommended at 1 month post-operation, and then every 3 months for the subsequent 2 years. The interval can then be lengthened to every 6 months for the ensuing 2 years. Annual imaging can be obtained at the 4-year mark. When recurrence is detected, the option remains to repeat the therapy if the patient has hepatic functional reserve. Careful examination of the patient and review of function status and liver synthetic function must be carefully weighed. Critical judgment should be exercised in cases that may leave the patient with insurmountable liver failure.

RESULTS

When one considers that the median survival for someone with untreated HCC is on the order of months and potential surgical therapies are often limited by the patient's underlying liver disease, ablative techniques are emerging as viable therapies that truly provide a survival advantage in patients with no previous options. Studies have demonstrated a substantial survival advantage, for both RF and microwave ablation, that exceeds what can be expected from the natural history of untreated HCC.[9]

Total hepatectomy and transplantation may be the best treatment for patients with HCC in a cirrhotic liver. However, the current organ shortage leads to excessive waiting times for patients with tumors which increases the likelihood of "falling out" of criteria while waiting for a transplant. Regional therapy with ablative techniques may prevent "falling out" and provides a practical bridge to transplantation for these patients. While patients with multifocal or large unresectable tumors do not have a transplant option and traditionally had no real therapeutic options, ablative techniques offer the compensated cirrhotic treatment that potentially extends their life by arresting their tumor progression.

REFERENCES

1. Howe HL, Wingo PA, Thun MJ, *et al.* Annual report to the nation on the status of cancer (1973 through 1998), featuring cancers with recent increasing trends. *J Natl Cancer Inst* 2001; 93:(11), 824–842.
2. Llovet JM, Burroughs A, Bruix J. (2003) Hepatocellular carcinoma. *Lancet* 2003; (9399) 362:1907–1917.
3. Okuda K, Ohtsuki T, Obata H, *et al.* Natural history of hepatocellular carcinoma and prognosis in relation to treatment. Study of 850 patients. *Cancer* 1985; 56(4):918–928.
4. Schroeder RA, Marroquin CE, Bute BP, *et al.* Predictive indices of morbidity and mortality after liver resection. *Ann Surg* 2006; 243(3): 373–379.
5. Cedrone A, Rapaccini GL, Pompili M, *et al.* Neoplastic seeding complicating percutaneous ethanol injection for treatment of hepatocellular carcinoma. *Radiology* 1992;(3)183, 787–788.
6. Bruix J. Sherman M. Management of hepatocellular carcinoma. *Hepatology* 2005; 412(5): 1208–1236.
7. Trevisani F, D'Intino PE, Morselli-Labate AM, *et al.* Serum alpha-fetoprotein for diagnosis of hepatocellular carcinoma in patients with chronic liver disease: influence of HBsAg and anti-HCV status. *J Hepatol* 2001; 34(4): 570–575.
8. Oka H, Tamori A, Kuroki T, *et al.* Prospective study of alpha-fetoprotein in cirrhotic patients monitored for development of hepatocellular carcinoma. *Hepatology* 1994; 19(1): 61–66.
9. Omata M, Tateishi R, Yoshida H *et al.* Treatment of hepatocellular carcinoma by percutaneous tumor ablation methods: ethanol injection therapy and radiofrequency ablation. *Gastroenterology* 2004; 127(5 suppl 1): S159–S166.

REGIONAL THERAPIES FOR HEPATIC MALIGNANCY 15

Lindsay Talbot* and Dan G. Blazer III*

INTRODUCTION

Patients with isolated unresectable hepatic malignancies pose a significant challenge. Though systemic therapies have improved markedly in the past decade, long-term disease control is rare. Techniques for regional delivery of high-dose chemotherapeutics to the liver remain an area of active interest and have demonstrated some promise in delaying tumor progression and/or palliating symptomatology from hormonally active metastases. As opposed to local ablation strategies such as radiofrequency ablation (RFA), regional chemotherapy to the liver treats the entire organ, allowing for the destruction of micrometastatic disease. This chapter will briefly focus on three modalities for regional delivery of high dose chemotherapeutics to the liver: hepatic arterial infusion therapy (HAI), isolated hepatic perfusion (IHP), and percutaneous hepatic perfusion (PHP).

The liver is an attractive organ for the application of regional chemotherapy given its unique blood supply. It is dually perfused via the portal and hepatic arterial systems. The portal venous system provides approximately 75% of the blood flow to normal liver parenchyma, and the hepatic arterial system provides the remaining 25%. However, many hepatic tumors, primary or metastatic, are preferentially perfused via the hepatic arterial system, providing a natural segregation between normal

---

*Duke University Medical Center 3247, Durham, NC 27710 USA

and diseased tissue perfusion that can be exploited by administering agents via the hepatic arterial system. In addition, a number of chemotherapeutic agents demonstrate high first-pass extraction, allowing delivery of higher dose chemotherapy to the liver while minimizing systemic toxicity. Each of the regional therapy strategies covered in this chapter utilizes these anatomic and metabolic assets in order to maximize drug delivery to tumor-bearing tissue while minimizing systemic toxicity.

HEPATIC ARTERIAL INFUSION THERAPY

The development of an entirely implantable device that could deliver continuous infusion of chemotherapy through a catheter into the hepatic artery was developed in the 1970s.[1] Though surgical technique and the implantable HAI pumps themselves have evolved, the basic strategy has remained unchanged.

Formal laparotomy is required for placement of the HAI pump. Patients with portal vein thrombosis or insufficient hepatic or renal function are excluded as candidates. Patients with aberrant vascular anatomy must be identified preoperatively and may require alternative surgical approaches. In those patients with classic anatomy, the basic technique is to isolate the gastroduodenal artery (which branches off the hepatic artery in this setting) and insert the HAI catheter into the GDA rather than employing direct placement into the hepatic artery. Side branches are ligated to avoid chemotherapy perfusion into the stomach, duodenum, or pancreas, which can cause significant toxicity. Cholecystectomy is now routinely performed to avoid chemical cholecystitis. The pump reservoir is then implanted subcutaneously into the abdominal wall.

Delivery of HAI chemotherapy relies exclusively on first-pass metabolism of the chemotherapeutic agent to minimize systemic toxicity. Floxuridine (FUDR), an analog of 5-FU, is the most utilized chemotherapeutic agent. It concentrates preferentially in tumorous tissue and because of its high hepatic extraction enables delivery of very high concentrations of chemotherapy into the liver. Oxaliplatin, irinotecan, mitomycin C, and cisplatin have also been used. Unlike IHP and PHP, HAI therapy allows continuous infusion of chemotherapy over time rather than solely intraoperatively.

Complications associated with HAI therapy can be significant. Most important is the issue of biliary sclerosis. The addition of dexamethasone has been added to the regimen to ameliorate this important side effect. However, this toxicity remains a significant problem; patients must be monitored closely with serial bilirubin levels and dose reduction may be necessary. Other important complications include hepatic artery thrombosis, mechanical pump failure, and extrahepatic perfusion.

The majority of data demonstrating promise of HAI in the treatment of liver metastases has been in the management of colorectal liver metastases. Initial studies focused on patients with unresectable colorectal liver metastases, comparing HAI therapy with systemic chemotherapy versus systemic chemotherapy alone. Though studies showed initial promise with response rates in the HAI groups of 29–88% and improved survival against historical controls, more recent randomized clinical trials have not consistently demonstrated any survival benefit with HAI therapy, even when compared against older, less effective systemic chemotherapy regimens.[1] A recent meta-analysis of 10 randomized trials did not reach statistical significance for improved median overall survival.[2]

Studies have also looked at the potential utility of HAI therapy in the adjuvant setting after resection of colorectal liver metastases. In a study by Kemeny *et al.*, patients randomized after hepatic resection to HAI therapy with floxuridine plus systemic chemotherapy versus systemic chemotherapy alone demonstrated improved 2-year survival and time to progression of hepatic disease.[3] This early enthusiasm has been tempered by subsequent follow-up demonstrating no difference in survival.[4]

Though limited, studies have examined HAI therapy in noncolorectal liver disease, including primary hepatic tumors, neuroendocrine metastases, and other noncolorectal, non-neuroendocrine metastases such as breast, gastric, sarcoma and melanoma. For example, one recent study looking at HAI therapy for primary liver cancers again showed favorable response rates (47%) and 2-year survival of 67%.[5] Additional studies are required to establish the utility of HAI therapy in the management of the noncolorectal malignancies.

In summary, despite favorable response rates with HAI therapy and improved toxicity profile and given the significant advances in systemic chemotherapy for colorectal liver metastases, the role for HAI in colorectal and noncolorectal liver metastases remains controversial and currently is practiced in only a few select centers in the United States.

ISOLATED HEPATIC PERFUSION

Though the first clinical IHP was reported in 1961, the modern era of IHP emerged in the early 1990s with the clinical availability of TNF.[6] Unlike HAI therapy, which relies exclusively on agents with high first–pass metabolism for reduction of systemic toxicity, IHP is a technique which allows administration of high-dose chemotherapy to the liver by surgically attaining complete vascular isolation of the liver. Rather than choosing agents with high first-pass metabolism, agents such as melphalan and TNF have been widely utilized due to their low first-pass extraction and ability to remain confined within the perfusion circuit. In addition, the technique of IHP allows for the use of hyperthermia. Hyperthermia increases capillary endothelial permeability in tumor-associated vasculature and, for certain chemotherapeutic agents, appears to promote increased delivery of the cytotoxic agent to the tumor interstitium, thus enhancing tumor cell kill.

IHP requires formal laparotomy.[6] The right hemiliver and the suprahepatic IVC are mobilized. The infrahepatic IVC is mobilized above the renal veins. The right adrenal vein, retroperitoneal tributaries, and phrenic veins are ligated. The porta hepatis is dissected, cholecystectomy performed, and the hepatic artery and portal vein are isolated. The patient is then anticoagulated. The IHP circuit is established by clamping the IVC below the liver (above the renal veins). The outflow cannula is inserted above and directed such that the tip is positioned just below the hepatic veins. The inflow catheter is inserted via the GDA to perfuse the right and left hepatic arteries equally. The suprahepatic IVC, proximal common hepatic artery, and portal vein are all then occluded. During perfusion, systemic circulation is maintained by cutdown on the saphenous and axillary veins and institution of venovenous bypass. Simpler techniques have also more recently been described.[7]

Typical perfusion parameters include 60-minute perfusion at 40°C. Flow rates are generally around 1000 ml/minute. Melphalan has been the chemotherapeutic agent of choice for the past several years due to the lack of availability of TNF in the United States. Other agents such as 5-FU, mitomycin C, and oxaliplatin have also been utilized.

IHP has primarily been applied to those patients with unresectable colorectal, ocular melanoma, and neuroendocrine (NET) liver metastases. No randomized controlled trial data exist to this point. For unresectable colorectal liver metastases, phase I and II trials have shown response rates in the 60–70% range, even in patients who have progressed on modern systemic chemotherapy agents.[6] Unfortunately, duration of response has been limited (less than a year) and meaningful survival data are lacking. For ocular melanoma, similar response rates (62%) and duration of response have been achieved. Limited data exist describing utilization IHP for patients with NETs.

In conclusion, because of the complexity of the technique and significant potential morbidity, the technique of IHP has not been widely adopted. However, the technique has achieved impressive radiographic response rates and mortality rates for this procedure are less than 5% in centers with the appropriate expertise. Whether these responses translate to meaningful improvement in survival remains unanswered. Thus, IHP continues to hold promise as a potentially useful technique in patients with very limited options.

PERCUTANEOUS HEPATIC PERFUSION

Because of the complexity of IHP, significant potential morbidity, and the limitation to one treatment per patient, PHP has been investigated as an alternative. Similar to IHP, PHP relies on isolation of the liver circulation to deliver high dose hyperthermic chemotherapy. However, in the case of PHP, percutaneously placed balloon catheters are utilized, making formal laparotomy unnecessary.

In brief, a percutaneously inserted double balloon catheter system in the IVC (Delcath Systems, New York, NY) is used to isolate the hepatic circulation.[8] The catheter system is positioned in the retrohepatic IVC to isolate and collect hepatic venous outflow. The cephalad balloon blocks the IVC superior to the hepatic veins whereas the caudal balloon obstructs the IVC inferior to the hepatic veins. Contrast medium is injected to confirm proper placement of the balloons and lack of leakage in the circuit. Once the circuit is established, high dose chemotherapy is administered via the proper hepatic artery for 30 minutes. The effluent is collected between the balloons and then passes through a extracorporeal filtration system (two activated charcoal filtration cartridges in parallel) using a centrifugal pump which then returns the effluent to the systemic circulation via the internal jugular vein. Thus, rather than relying on high first pass effect (HAI therapy) or true isolation of hepatic circulation (IHP), the PHP technique uses an extracorporeal filtration system to limit systemic toxicity from the high dose chemotherapy. Filtration efficiency is 80–90%.

The feasibility of this technique was first published in 1994 by two separate groups.[9,10] More recently, a phase I dose escalation trial using melphalan was published by Pingpank et al.[11] In this study, 28 patients with a variety of unresectable hepatic tumors (majority of tumors were metastasis from ocular melanoma) underwent 74 treatments. Overall, radiographic response rate was 30%. In those patients with ocular melanoma, response rate was 50%. Given these encouraging results and manageable toxicity profile, a phase II trial is ongoing for patients with hepatocellular carcinoma, metastatic adenocarcinomas and neuroendocrine tumors in the liver and metastatic ocular and cutaneous melanoma (ClinicalTrials.gov Identifier NCT00096083). In addition, a phase III trial for patients with metastatic melanoma to the liver recently completed accrual (ClinicalTrials.gov Identifier NCT00324727) and results are pending.

CONCLUSIONS

Regional therapies for unresectable hepatic malignancies hold great promise in their ability to offer high dose chemotherapy to the liver that cannot be achieved by systemic administration. Though excellent response rates in the liver have been achieved with all three modalities — HAI, IHP, and PHP — durable response and convincing survival benefits have yet to be demonstrated. As newer, more effective agents are developed, these techniques remain attractive strategies for targeted delivery to the liver.

REFERENCES

1. Callahan MK, Kemeny NE. Implanted hepatic arterial infusion pumps. *Cancer J* 2010; 16(2):142–149.
2. Mocellin S, Pilati P, Lise M, *et al.*, Meta-analysis of hepatic arterial infusion for unresectable liver metastases from colorectal cancer: the end of an era? *J Clin Oncol*, 2007; 25(35):5649–5654.
3. Kemeny N., *et al.*, Hepatic arterial infusion of chemotherapy after resection of hepatic metastases from colorectal cancer. N Engl J Med, 1999; 341(27): 2039–2048.
4. Kemeny NE, Gonen M. Hepatic arterial infusion after liver resection. *N Engl J Med*, 2005; 352(7):734–735.
5. Jarnagin WR, *et al.*, Regional chemotherapy for unresectable primary liver cancer: results of a phase II clinical trial and assessment of DCE-MRI as a biomarker of survival. *Ann Oncol*, 2009; 20(9):1589–1995.

6. Jones A, and Alexander HR. Jr., Development of isolated hepatic perfusion for patients who have unresectable hepatic malignancies. *Surg Oncol Clin N Am*, 2008; 17(4):857–876, x.
7. Verzaro R, Zeh H, and Bartlett D, A safe and fast technique for isolated hepatic perfusion. *J Surg Oncol*, 2008; 98(5):393–396.
8. Alexander HR., Jr., and Butler CC., Development of isolated hepatic perfusion via the operative and percutaneous techniques for patients with isolated and unresectable liver metastases. *Cancer J.* 16(2):132–141.
9. Curley SA, *et al.*, Complete hepatic venous isolation and extracorporeal chemofiltration as treatment for human hepatocellular carcinoma: a phase I study. *Ann Surg Oncol*, 1994; 1(5):389–399.
10. Ravikumar TS., *et al.*, Percutaneous hepatic vein isolation and high-dose hepatic arterial infusion chemotherapy for unresectable liver tumors. *J Clin Oncol*, 1994; 12(12):2723–2736.
11. Pingpank, JF., *et al.*, Phase I study of hepatic arterial melphalan infusion and hepatic venous hemofiltration using percutaneously placed catheters in patients with unresectable hepatic malignancies. *J Clin Oncol*, 2005; 23(15): 3465–3474.

HEPATIC RESECTION 16

Michael E. Barfield* and Bryan M. Clary*

HISTORY OF OPEN LIVER SURGERY

The first open hepatic resection in a human is credited to Berta in 1716. A mentally ill patient presented with a self-inflicted knife wound, which resulted in a protruding portion of liver. This was amputated, and the patient recovered without complications.[1] Elective liver surgery, however, was regarded as extraordinarily dangerous throughout much of the 1800s and early 1900s.[1,2] Most surgeries were for traumatic injuries, and many patients met their ultimate demise as a result of inability to adequately control hemorrhage. In 1908, J. Hogarth Pringle published a major work in which he described compression of the portal vessels to control hemorrhage during laparotomy.[3] Thereafter, control of the hepatic blood flow was to be essential in facilitating liver surgery.

Glisson first described the anatomy of the hepatic vasculature based on external landmarks in 1654, and this guided liver surgeons' resection attempts throughout the late 1800s and the early 1900s.[4] The excessive mortality associated with hepatic resections during this time highlighted the need for more thorough understanding of intrahepatic vascular and biliary structures to facilitate safer surgical interventions. Many efforts were made at refining these descriptions, and the modern and more complete understanding of liver anatomy was facilitated by the work of two groups, Couinaud and Goldsmith and Woodburne.[5] These newer descriptions emphasized a functional anatomy that relied not on external landmarks

---

*Duke University Medical Center, Durham, NC 27710 USA

to guide surgeons but on the course of vascular structures within the liver. Even with the improvements in anatomical understanding, hepatic resections remained controversial throughout the 1950–1980 era, a position supported by mortality rates as high as 20%.[2] Over the past 20–30 years, liver surgery has been refined, and through advances in patient selection, preoperative management, resection techniques, and postoperative care, hepatic resections can be completed in experienced hands with mortality rates as low as 5%.

EPIDEMIOLOGY

Open hepatic resections are undertaken more commonly today than in the past for both malignant and benign lesions. Significant improvements in imaging modalities over the past 2 decades have enhanced surgeons' abilities to select patients who will successfully tolerate and potentially benefit from resection of malignant hepatic lesions. Patients with cirrhotic liver disease due to viral hepatitis have approximately 100-fold increased risk of developing hepatocellular carcinoma (HCC). Colon cancer may present with liver metastases in up to 15% of patients at their initial presentation. These patients go through the same workup described below to determine whether they are operative candidates. Additionally, it is important to fully evaluate these patients for sites of other metastatic disease, and this will be discussed further in the section "Preoperative and Adjunct Therapeutic Management Options".

WORKUP

The workup for all patients being seen for diagnosis and treatment of a liver lesion should be directed at determining the etiology of the lesion, the extent of oncologic burden (for patients with malignancies), the preoperative functional status of the liver and volume of the future liver remnant following (FLR) resection, and overall fitness for surgical resection.

A clinical history and physical examination is critical in ascertaining the etiology of the liver mass as well as in judging overall fitness and the health of the liver. Specific physical findings that reflect underlying liver disease include jaundice and external manifestions of portal hypertension (ascites, caput medusa, splenomegaly, liver firmness, etc.). Physical manifestations of advanced malignancy should also be sought including distant lymphadenopathy, umbilical fullness, and palpable abdominal masses.

Table 1. Child–Pugh cirrhosis classification.

Points assigned	Albumin (g/dL)	Bilirubin (mg/dL)	INR	Ascites	Encephalopathy
1	>3.5	<2	<1.7	None	None
2	2.8–3.5	2–3	1.7–2.3	Slight	1–2
3	<2.8	>3	>2.3	Moderate	3–4
Child–Pugh classification					
A	5–6 pts				
B	7–9 pts				
C	10–15 pts				

Baseline bloodwork including serum albumin, bilirubin, alkaline phosphatase, aspartate aminotransferase (AST), alanine aminotransferase (ALT), a coagulation profile, and a platelet count are routinely obtained. For patients with newly appreciated intrinsic liver disease, a hepatitis panel may help to clarify the underlying cause. Serum tumor markers including alpha-fetoprotein (AFP), CA19-9, CEA, and 5-hydroxyindoleacetic acid (5-HIAA) may also be required depending on the suspected pathology of the lesion. Patients will also require high quality imaging to determine respectability as well as which preoperative therapeutic modalities should be employed (discussed in the next section).

A large number of the patients presenting for resection of HCC lesions have cirrhosis at baseline, and the leading cause of mortality in this population is postoperative liver failure. Although healthy individuals may successfully undergo resection of up to 75% of healthy liver tissue, patients with underlying liver dysfunction at baseline require special attention in determining what constitutes an adequate FLR; therefore, the importance of determining preoperative hepatic function and hepatic reserve cannot be overemphasized. The Child–Pugh Classification (Table 1) is often utilized in this setting. Patients are assigned one, two, or three points for each parameter in the table. The results are summed, and the patient is then classified as A (5–6 points), B (7–9 points), or C (10–15 points). Hepatic resection for a class A patient can be undertaken with relative safety as these patients have hepatic reserve substantial enough to tolerate resection of up to 50% with peroperative mortality of 5% or lower. Class B patients have less reserve and can therefore, only tolerate limited resections (generally 25% or less) such as wedge excisions of exophytic masses to assure a sufficient

FLR. As indicated by the points assigned, these patients are generally less medically fit at baseline, and resection for a class B patient is still associated with mortality rates ranging as high as 10–15%. Patients with class C cirrhosis undergoing hepatic resection have experienced mortality rates far in excess of 25% and are therefore only considered for transplantation as a curative therapy. A number of centers incorporate additional and/or alternative preoperative assessments including the MELD criteria, preoperative portal vein:systemic venous pressure gradients, thrombocytopenia, and indocyanine green (ICG) clearance. It is clear that Child's–Pugh A patients with underlying renal dysfunction (identified in the MELD) and portal hypertension need to be carefully selected as most cannot tolerate moderately large volume hepatectomies although wedge excisions may still be feasible.

Additional steps in the workup for an open hepatic resection are much akin to those for other major abdominal procedures. Patients with a history significant cardiac or pulmonary disease or concerning symptoms must undergo a full evaluation. Patients of advanced age were previously considered poor surgical candidates; however with proper preoperative assessment and risk stratification, these patients can now safely undergo hepatic resections with reasonable recovery expectations.

IMAGING

The goals of imaging in patients undergoing partial hepatectomy are to define the extent of disease/tumor burden and to identify the anatomical considerations and feasibility of resection. The latter involves attention to inflow (portal triad) and outflow (hepatic, IVC), as well as the specific segments of the liver that are involved with tumor. Although details of specific imaging modalities are covered elsewhere in this book, a brief discussion of imaging as it relates to operative planning is as follows: For most tumor conditions, a CT of the abdomen and pelvis (chest included for malignant diagnoses) or an MRI of the abdomen and pelvis (complemented by a CXR or chest CT) are comparable in defining the inflow, outflow, parenchymal, and extrahepatic disease issues. It is critical when possible that intravenous contrast be utilized. In addition to identifying tumor location and vascular issues, the future liver remnant volumes can be estimated via CT scans with straightforward image manipulation by radiology. Although generally unnecessary for most hepatic resections, extended right hepatectomies and major resections in cirrhotics present important situations where estimating the FLR is helpful as preoperative portal vein embolization may decrease postoperative morbidity. Although new contrast reagents have facilitated the availability of CT cholangiography, most patients with suspect involvement of the central ducts (where reconstruction may be required intraoperatively) are evaluated with an MRCP prior to surgery.

Additional studies are tailored to the patient's specific histology and or symptoms. Bony pain and or new-onset headaches/neurologic symptoms may prompt plain films and or CT of the brain respectively. ^{18}F-fluoro-deoxyglucose positron emission tomography (^{18}FDG-PET) is approved for several metastatic histologies including colorectal and melanoma, but appears less helpful (and often not reimbursed) for primary hepatic malignancies. Reasonable data exist to suggest that patients with metastatic colorectal cancer are better selected for hepatectomy through the use of FDG-PET scanning, but false positives including activity in the pelvis following surgery and XRT are quite common, and care should be taken in excluding patients for mild levels of activity in these and other locations. In addition, many small lesions, mucinous lesions, and lesions recently treated with systemic therapy also lead to false-negative studies. The advent of combined CT/PET scanning has likely increased the incorporation of PET as a screening tool for hepatectomy, but the lack of IV CT-contrast (except when specifically requested) presents difficulties in appreciating inflow and outflow issues. The author utilizes PET selectively in colorectal cancer patients.

PATHOLOGY

The extent of the desired margin is dependent upon the histology and technical considerations. Many benign lesions including hemangiomas, FNH, cysts, and some adenomas are reasonably approached with minimal margin and in some instances enucleated when technically preferable. Although a margin of approximately 1 cm has been long adhered to in the treatment of malignancies, the inability to achieve such a wide margin should not necessarily preclude attempts at resection. For patients with colorectal metastases, the width of a negative margin (i.e. 1 mm versus. 10 mm) appears to have modest if any bearing on overall outcome. Although many advocate anatomic resections in HCC given the intrahepatic portal vein dissemination pattern, the parenchymal loss in these patients with intrinsic liver disease may trump margin considerations.

PREOPERATIVE AND ADJUNCT THERAPEUTIC MANAGEMENT OPTIONS

Generally, patients with primary hepatic tumors that are deemed to be anatomically resectable and have an adequate FLR may proceed to surgery after ruling out metastatic disease. In those patients with Child's A liver status and in whom an inadequate liver remnant is a concern, portal vein embolization of the ipsilateral side (the portion of the liver to be resected) can facilitate preoperative FLR hypertrophy and as a result, possibly minimize the risks of liver dysfunction postoperatively. This is predominantly an issue with right hepatectomy and extended hepatectomies (right or left) in patients with intrinsic liver disease. Also included in this category are jaundiced patients without prior liver disease whose tumors have caused central obstruction, such as Klatskin tumors. In these patients, preoperative biliary drainage and consideration of ipsilateral portal vein embolization are critical in preparing the FLR.

Patients presenting with liver metastases from colorectal cancer present special considerations to the surgeon. In most western centers, metastatic colon cancer is the most frequent indication for partial hepatectomy. The appropriate inclusion and timing of systemic therapy and the management of the primary tumor in patients with synchronous disease represent areas of complexity that require a full multidisciplinary approach. At present, there is no compelling data to argue for or against pre-hepatectomy systemic therapy when the hepatic disease is clearly resectable. Although the selection of patients may be modestly improved with short courses of prehepatectomy systemic therapy, there are some potential disadvantages including hepatotoxicity, a modest increase in perioperative morbidity, and the possibility of rendering small, deep lesions occult at the time of surgery. For patients with extensive intrahepatic tumor burdens precluding a single setting extirpation of their disease, a staged approach to resection may be feasible. In this approach, a partial hepatectomy is performed intentionally leaving residual disease behind with the intent of performing a completion resection at a later date. The most common scenario involves wedge excisions of the left liver and right hepatectomy (possibly preceeded by right portal vein embolization). A full discussion of the optimal management of synchronous patients is beyond the scope of this chapter, but is important to contemplate how best to prepare patients for hepatectomy in the context of their disease.

SURGERY

General Surgical Strategy

The primary goals of hepatectomy include tumor clearance while avoiding catastrophic hemodynamic complications and minimizing injury to the future liver remnant. The latter occurs in the setting of prolonged general hypotension (typically with significant bleeding or overenthusiastic low-CVP anesthesia), prolonged hepatic ischemia (Pringle), injury to the major support structures serving the FLR, and/or decisions to remove an excessive volume of parenchyma.

The basic steps of hepatectomy include the following:

(1) Exploration and exposure: The initial steps of any hepatectomy include an assessment of tumor burden, both within the liver (palpation, visual inspection, and intraoperative ultrasound) and outside of the liver (for suspected malignancies). Many hepatic surgeons prefer staging laparoscopy as the initial maneuver at the time of planned hepatectomy. The likelihood of identifying disease precluding resection varies according to the histology and quality of the preoperative imaging, but is generally less than 15–20%. It is possible to preclude favorable risk patients from laparoscopy such as metachronous patients with small, solitary colorectal metastases who have an even lower yield on laparoscopy. Once the final incisional plan (open versus. laparoscopic) is decided upon, a through inspection of the peritoneal cavity, regional and accessible nodes, and liver are mandated. Adequate exposure and mobilization of the liver is achieved to facilitate this assessment and prepare for the hepatectomy. When performing right hepatectomy, the left liver is not typically mobilized so as to minimize the possibility of torsion of the FLR. Similarly, the right liver is not mobilized during most left-sided hepatectomies.

(2) Control of inflow: Three basic strategies exist in taking the inflow (portal triad) serving the region of the liver to be removed.

   (a) Extrahepatic dissection: For many anatomic resections (hemihepatectomy and extended hemihepatectomy), a standard extrahepatic dissection can be performed with relative ease to selectively isolate the triad structures to be taken. These are discussed below with each specific procedure. The main drawback is the time required and the risk of injuring aberrant hilar structures that serve the FLR.

(b) Intrahepatic portal pedicle isolation and division: In an effort to minimize the time required by extrahepatic dissections and the risks to central structures, the pedicles can often be isolated by making a hepatotomy adjacent to the pedicle and passing a blunt instrument or one's finger around it. This is relatively easy for left hepatectomies while a bit more difficult for right hepatectomies and right posterior sectionectomies. The major downside of this maneuver is the relative unfamiliarity of many surgeons and the difficulty in patients with tumor abutting the hilum/major pedicles. A discussion of this strategy is outside the scope of this book and well covered in more exhaustive textbooks and atlases.
(c) Intrahepatic division during parenchymal transection: The third option is that of taking the pedicle once it is identified during the parenchymal transection. Although seemingly appropriate for just wedge excisions and left lateral sectionectomies, this can be utilized in some patients undergoing hemihepatectomies especially if a rapid method of parenchymal transection is incorporated.
(d) Pringle maneuver: The placement of a tourniquet around the duodenal hepatic ligament (Pringle maneuver) is often utilized to augment the above strategies. Newer parenchymal division strategies that minimize blood loss have led to a selective approach to the Pringle maneuver. When necessary, an intermittent approach to clamping is generally best and as practiced involves clamping for periods of 5–15 minutes followed by 5–10 minutes with the tourniquet released. Although the total duration of inflow occlusion can be extended through this intermittent approach to approximately 100 minutes in patients with normal liver and modest volume resections, it is rare for the Pringle occlusion to exceed beyond 30–40 minutes. Continuous inflow occlusion (either alone or in conjunction with clamping of the IVC) should not exceed approximately 30 minutes as the risk of liver dysfunction greatly increases with the need for longer durations.

(3) Control of outflow: For most hepatic resections, the hepatic veins are taken intrahepatically during the course of the parenchymal transection. Exceptions to this include situations where the tumor is immediately adjacent to the major hepatic veins near their junction with the IVC. In addition, many hepatic surgeons routinely take the right hepatic vein outside of the liver prior to right hepatectomy given its

relative accessibility. The increased mobility of the liver that occurs once the right hepatic vein is divided is also helpful especially in deep individuals with lesions in the dome of the right liver. The common trunk of the left and middle hepatic veins is less accessible and its dissection is associated with greater difficulty and risk. In uncommon circumstances for large lesions abutting the IVC, an approach of total vascular exclusion can be employed whereby the IVC is isolated above and below the liver.

(a) Right hepatic vein: In order to isolate the right hepatic vein, the falciform is divided superiorly with the dissection extending onto the right coronary ligament. Often, a notch or cleft is palpable at the site of the right hepatic vein that may be appreciated before the RHV is clearly seen. The right liver is completely mobilized by dividing the entirety of the right coronary ligament anteriorly and posteriorly. Small tributaries extending directly to the inferior cava from the posterior aspect of the right liver and caudate are ligated and divided. Superiorly a sling of fibrous tissue (hepatocaval ligament) encircles the IVC just below its junction with the hepatic veins. This "ligament" is often thin with just fibrous tissue, but on occasion can possess a significant amount of hepatic tissue and appear quite plump. The right hepatic vein: IVC junction lies immediately medial to this ligament. The ligament is divided with a stapler for ease and in the event that a portion of the IVC is drawn into the ligament by retraction. Once the hepatocaval ligament is divided, the lateral aspect of the RHV is exposed. A tunnel between the RHV and MHV is carefully created with a blunt instrumentthus isolating the RHV trunk for division (once the inflow has been divided).

(b) Left and middle hepatic veins: In most patients, it is possible to selectively isolate the common trunk of the left and middle hepatic veins outside of the liver. The left coronary ligament and falciform ligaments are divided thus mobilizing the left hemiliver. Underneath the left lateral section of the liver, the gastrohepatic ligament is incised and the peritoneum overlying the region of the left hepatic vein is incised. The ligamentum venosum can be seen traversing in the most medial aspect of the gastrohepatic ligament anterior to the caudate leading from the left portal vein to the left hepatic vein. This cordlike structure can be divided approximately 1 cm prior to its entry into the left hepatic vein and by doing so, a plane posterior to the common trunk of the MHV/LHV becomes apparent. Anteriorly, a plane is established between the RHV and MHV to complete a passage around the common MHV/LHV trunk.

(c) Total vascular exclusion: For some patients with tumors involving the major hepatic veins near their entry into the IVC, selective exclusion of the RHV or MHV/LHV trunk may not be feasible. For these patients, the option of IVC clamping may be reasonable. In performing total vascular exclusion, the IVC is isolated above the liver and just below the liver near the caudate process. The latter is quite straightforward although care need be taken to minimize risk to the left renal vein, right adrenal vein, and posterior lumbar branches. Isolation of the suprahepatic IVC is also generally straightforward — involving the division of the peritoneum overlying the anterior surface and alongside the crura. When the time comes to apply TVE, the inflow is occluded with a Pringle (and prior anatomic dissection of the inflow structures to be removed) followed by clamping of the supra- and infrahepatic IVC with vascular clamps. The anesthetic management is entirely different when applying TVE; specifically, patients often require volume loading as opposed to low-CVP approaches. In addition, the time available for parenchymal division is often limited as TVE is most commonly performed in a continuous manner. Application of the Pringle for a brief period (10 minutes) prior to application of TVE may provide a protective effect on the FLR and minimize postoperative liver dysfunction issues (preconditioning). In this approach, the Pringle is followed by a 10-minute period of revascularization prior to applying TVE.

(4) Parenchymal division: Parenchymal division can be accomplished through a variety of strategies and technologies. Historically, the parenchyma was crushed between the fingers (finger fracture technique) thus identifying structures to be clamped, clipped, or sutured. Intuitively, this was a very bloody process and was subsequently replaced with a more refined approach utilizing either a clamp (tonsil or Kelley) instead of the fingers or an ultrasonic dissection device (CUSA®) to isolate structures requiring ligation prior to division (both approaches under general inflow occlusion Pringle). Energy devices including standard electrocautery are generally sufficient for

peripheral and superficial limited transections. The standard electrocautery is limited by the eschar that forms with respect to the depth of coagulation and by the fact that the eschar commonly pulls away resulting in ongoing bleeding. Newer devices that flow saline across the catery tip minimize the eschar while allowing for deeper levels of coagulation. These precoagulation devices may be especially useful in cirrhotic patients where the stiffness of the liver limits strategies the require crushing of the parenchmya. Other energy devices which seal vascular structures (i.e. Harmonic Scalpel®, Ligasure®, Enseal®, etc.) have also been utilized to divide the parenchyma while minimizing the need for inflow occlusion. Care needs to be exercised in utilizing the precoagulation devices adjacent to important remnant structures (i.e. near the hilum). The marked improvement in surgical stapling devices has led many to perform the parenchymal division with multiple applications of the stapling device. Akin to the crush clamp technique, the thin anvil of the stapler is insinuated into the parenchyma (often with pretunneling by a Kelley clamp to provide direction) with the jaws brought together (crushing the tissue) and subsequently divided (staples preceeding division by the knife within the stapling cartridge). This is a very rapid method to divide the liver and has easy application to the minimally invasive setting. Nonetheless, stapling is expensive and not always applicable such as in circular wedge excisions, cirrhotic livers, and in regions of the liver where the margin will be very close. Ultimately, the liver surgeon needs to understand the advantages and limitations of the different parenchymal division strategies as one approach is not best for every possible scenario.

Anesthetic Considerations

The anesthetic management of patients undergoing partial hepatectomy cannot be underestimated with respect to their impact upon the perioperative outomes. In most patients (i.e. those where TVE is not incorporated), excessive volume administration and/or underlying patient cardiovascular considerations are associated with high central venous pressures and as a result, significant hepatic venous bleeding during the parenchymal transection or upon inadvertent entry into hepatic venous tributaries. For most complicated large volume hepatectomies or complex wedge excisions in precarious locations, a low-CVP approach is critical to minimize bleeding during the parenchymal division stage of the procedure. The anesthesiologist can affect the CVP through a variety of ventilator, pharmacologic (IV nitroglycerin, diuretic), and fluid administration (minimization) strategies. Monitoring of the CVP through the use of a central venous catheter aiming for CVP's in the 0–5 mmHg range preferable. It is equally important to avoid systemic hypotension in an effort to achieve a low-CVP and in some patients this necessitates concurrent low-level inotropic support (dopamine) until mild volume resuscitation and cessation of intravenous NTG can occur. It is equally important to communicate in advance when the prospects of significant blood loss present themselves. While transfusion of blood products can be life saving in the setting of significant hemorrhage, it is important to avoid unnecessary transfusions as they may lead to higher perioperative morbidity rates and possibly worse long-term oncologic outcomes. Most patients can tolerate hematocrits in the low-mid 20s when active hemorrhage is not present. It has been our observation that intraoperative hematocrit levels are errantly low, possible from fluid shift issues. Transfusion decisions based largely upon these readings may lead to excessive transfusions if taken in isolation. Although our practice is against the use of epidurals in hepatic surgery, many centers routinely employ epidurals for intraoperative and postoperative management. This decision should be routinely discussed with the anesthesia team. The disadvantages that have steered our hepatic surgery group away from epidurals include frequent hypotension postoperatively with attendant fluid boluses, prolonged urinary catheterization, the confusion that can result from multiple teams managing the patients postoperative pain, the requirement of some teams for FFP prior to epidural removal when the prothrombin time is elevated (not infrequent after large-volume hepatectomies), and the fact that many patients are well-managed with intravenous narcotics. However, we recognize it is an open question as there are potential advantages as well.

Choice of Incisions

For many patients, the procedure is started with a laparoscopic exploration. Utilizing either a Veress technique or open trocar placement approach, the abdomen is inspected laparoscopically for tumor burdens that preclude resection. Although this is identified in a minority of patients, that minority is exceptionally grateful for the lack of a large open incision and the process requires only a few additional minutes.

The general choice of incisions (open versus. laparoscopic, where to place the port or open incisions) should be considered before the beginning of the operation. The goal of the incision(s) is to allow for proper visualization and access of necessary instrumentation such that a safe and appropriate procedure can be carried out.

For procedures performed with traditional open incisions, a variety of incisional strategies can be employed including right subcostal, bilateral subcostal, right hockey-stick ("J"), upper midline, full midline, and trifurcated (upper abdominal transvers with midline extension) incisions. Except for patients with very large left-sided tumors, a hockey-stick incision is applicable to most tumor location/body habitus scenarios. This incision involves an upper midline component (extending from xiphoid to a point halfway between the umbilicus and xiphoid) and subcostal component extending from the bottom of the midline component laterally to approximately the anterior axillary line. The transition point from midline to transverse may need to be modified based upon body habitus to allow for adequate visualization and retractor blade depth issues. A bilateral subcostal incision also provides great exposure for most hepatectomies, especially in very obese patients where the costal angle is very broad and in patients with large left liver masses where the leftward extent provides better exposure than the hockey stick incision. A trifurcated incision is rarely necessary except in massive central or left liver tumors that are adjacent to the hepatic veins. Modest left liver wedge excisions and resections of the left lateral section of the liver are easily approached with an upper midline incision alone. For thin patients undergoing concomitant colon surgery, a full midline can provide enough exposure even for right posterior liver lesions. Ultimately, each surgeon has an incisional preference that works best for them in the context of their retractor systems, help, lighting, etc.

The fundamental aspects of liver surgery when performed with minimally invasive approaches are generally unchanged (adequate exposure and consideration of inflow/outflow/parenchymal issues) although the technical aspects are quite different. In general, patients selected for minimally invasive approaches (laparoscopic or hand-assisted) have modest-sized lesions and straightforward tumor locations without complex inflow/outflow considerations. Large lesions requiring substantial abdominal wall extraction site incisions and/or lesions in complex locations (adjacent to hilum and/or hepatic veins) are not well-served with MIS based approaches. The details of specific laparoscopic procedures are outside the scope of this condensed textbook but generally follow the strategies outlined below for the specific open hepatectomies.

Specific procedures

Described below are the most commonly performed anatomic resections. Nonanatomic wedge excisions generally require appropriate mobilization without inflow/outflow isolation prior to parenchymal transection. Although seemingly straightforward, wedge excisions can be quite challenging and complex. Aside from lesser degrees of control over the outflow/inflow structures, the appreciation for the depth of the transection is sometimes subtle and often in proximity to important structures. When possible, large wedge excisions should be set up so that a relatively linear path through the liver can be followed. Large circular-shaped wedge excisions are difficult and should be guided by tactile and ultrasound appreciation.

(1) *Left lateral sectionectomy*

Resection of segments 2 and 3 involves the removal of the liver residing to the left of the falciform (errantly termed the left lateral segment). This is one of the most common hepatic resection procedures and can be accomplished quite quickly. After visual inspection of the abdomen, the falciform is divided back to the region of the hepatic veins. The left coronary ligament is then divided. Unless the lesion is immediately abutting the left hepatic vein, no attempt is made to isolate the hepatic veins prior to parenchymal division. When the lesion in segment 2 or 3 is adjacent to the umbilical fissure, the pedicles to segment 2 or 3 are dissected within the umbilical fissure. When the tumor(s) is not in proximity to the umbilical fissure, dissection of the pedicles within the umbilical fissure is unwarranted and may risk injury to structures serving segment 4. In the latter situation, a parenchymal division is initiated (commonly with a Pringle maneuver applied) staying to the patients left of the falciform. The pedicles to segments 2 and 3 are divided (stapler or suture ligature) when encountered during the parenchymal transection. Near the superior aspect of the liver, the line of parenchymal division takes a sharp turn to the left taking the left hepatic vein intrahepatically with a vascular stapler or clamp. Larger tumors that abut the LHV near its junction with the IVC are typically best approached by a formal left hepatectomy taking the common MHV/LHV trunk outside of the liver.

(2) Left hepatectomy

Following initial exposure, an appropriate incision is then made. For most patients, a hockey stick or bilateral subcostal incision is generally sufficient. For thin patients, an upper midline incision may also provide adequate exposure and access. The left liver is mobilized by division of the falciform and left coronary ligaments. The standard approach to the inflow (left portal pedicle) involves an extrahepatic dissection at the base of the umbilical fissure. Care is taken to limit the dissection to the base of the umbilical fissure which is generally 2–3 cm away from the bifurcation of left and right portal structures and as such may minimize possible injury to right liver support structures. The left hepatic artery(ies) is encountered first, test occluded and divided. This then exposes the underlying left portal vein. When the caudate is to be preserved, the portal vein is isolated above the takeoff of the branch leading to the Spigellian lobe of the caudate. The isolated left portal vein is test occluded to ensure demarcation along Cantlie's Line and then divided with a stapler or between ties/suture ligation. Once the left portal vein is divided, the remaining tissue includes the left hepatic duct(s) and fibrous hilar plate. We typically leave division of the left hepatic duct until late in the parenchymal transection phase of the procedure. Attention is then turned to the hepatic venous outflow. If the tumor(s) is abutting the MHV/LHV, the common trunk is isolated and divided extrahepatically with a vascular stapler. It is also our practice to oversew this staple line with a running 3–0 proline suture to minimize the possibility of a rare, but catastrophic staple line disruption during later portions of the procedure. If the tumor is away from MHV/LHV:IVC junction, division of MHV branches and the LHV are reserved for later during the parenchymal transection when encountered. At this point, the parenchyma is scored just to the left of Cantlie's line and a parenchymal division initiated. The gallbladder is removed in a standard manner if not previously removed. Near the superior aspect of the liver (segment 4A), the line of transection takes a sharp left turn leaving a modest amount of left liver tissue adjacent to the MHV/LHV. These structures are taken intrahepatically when encountered.

(3) *Right hepatectomy*

Adequate mobilization of the right liver requires division of the falciform and right coronary ligament. This exposes the retrohepatic IVC which is then cleared of small tributaries with clips and/or ties. The RHV is then isolated and encircled with a vessel loop for later division. In the traditional approach to a right hepatectomy, the right portal pedicle structures are taken individually at the very base of the right liver. Care is taken to limit this dissection to the patient's right of the very bottom of the gallbladder fossa and is initiated with removal of the gallbladder. It is a common mistake to approach the right hepatic artery and/or right portal vein by dissecting on the left side of the common hepatic duct. This is unnecessary and increases the risk of injury to the left liver's support structures. The peritoneum at the base of the right liver is incised to expose the right hepatic artery(ies). Commonly at the base of the right liver, the right hepatic artery has already bifurcated into anterior and posterior divisions. These strutures are test-occluded (feeling for a retained left hepatic artery pulse at the base of the umbilical fissure) and then ligated and divided. This then exposes the portal vein. It is critical to understand the branching pattern of the portal vein from the preoperative imaging and intraoperative ultrasound. Many patients do not have a formal right portal vein, but instead have a trifurcation of the LPV, R anterior PV, and R posterior PV. Another common aberrancy is for an early takeoff of the R posterior PV leaving a common trunk for the R anterior PV and LPV, which then bifurcates. Both of these aberrancies necessitate isolating and dividing the R posterior PV and R anterior PV individually. Once isolated, these are test-occluded prior to division. It is also imperative when performing this extrahepatic dissection to visually see the LPV/main PV junction to ensure preservation of left liver inflow. The previously isolated RHV is then divided with a vascular stapler and the staple line oversewn with a running proline suture. The parenchyma is then scored to the right of Cantlie's line and the parenchymal division initiated.

(4) *Extended right hepatectomy (right trisectionectomy)*

The basic steps of an extended right hepatectomy parallel the steps of a right hepatectomy (control of the right liver inflow and right hepatic vein).

The principal difference lies in the plane of transection which involves all or part of segment 4 (that portion of the liver between midplane of the liver and the line of the falciform). In extending the parenchymal transection into segment 4, the inflow to this region of the liver and the middle hepatic vein will need to be addressed. Except for tumors within segment 4 that are immediately abutting the umbilical fissure, the strategy for taking the small portal pedicles serving segment 4 are taking during the course of dividing the parenchyma when the are encountered. Simliarly, the middle hepatic vein is typically taken intrahepatically when encountered during the parenchymal transection. Aside from control of the middle hepatic vein, the principal danger in performing an extended right hepatectomy is in avoiding injury to the inflow structures of the future liver remnant (left lateral section). Although avoiding injury to the left hepatic artery and left portal vein is generally straightforward, the confluence of the common hepatic duct and left hepatic duct is variable and in many patients may occur high and near the base of the gallbladder fossa. Lowering the hilar plate by incising the peritoneum at the base of segment 4B is a helpful maneuver in avoiding this inadvertent injury. If concern exists, a cholangiogram can be done to ensure that the ductal structures to the liver remnant are intact.

(5) *Extended left hepatectomy (left trisectionectomy)*

A formal extended left hepatectomy is among the most difficult resections given the relative lack of external landmarks on the surface of the liver that define the line of parenchymal transection. An extended left hepatectomy involves extension of the parenchymal transection plane into the right anterior section (either all or part). In an extended left hepatectomy, the left hepatic portal structures are taken as described above for the left hepatectomy. When the entirety of the anterior section must be removed (large tumors or those abutting the anterior section pedicles), the vasculobiliary strutures to this section can be selectively isolated and ligated. Although the vascular component of this is relatively straightforward, the biliary component is not and significant risk to injuring the right posterior section's duct exists. It is important to understand the branching pattern of the intrahepatic ducts prior to embarking upon an extended left. This information is available form preoperative MRI or an intraoperative cholangiogram.

(6) *"Wedge" excision*

Non-anatomic wedge excisions can easy or sometimes quite difficult. When performing wedge resections, selective control of the inflow and outflow are generally not obtained, but instead these structures are taken during the course of the parenchymal transection. Small lesions at the peripheral edge of the liver are easily resected often with the standard electrocautery without a Pringle and with minimal blood loss. Larger wedge excisions and/or those in more difficult locations often require a strategy for minimization of blood loss such as application of a Pringle during the resection or with a precoagulation device (saline-enhanced electrocautery, electrothermal bipolar tissue sealing systems, ultrasonic vibration shears). It is most advantageous if the plane of resection can be lined up as a linear pass as opposed to a curvilinear path. The depth of the transection is monitored by palpation and/or the intraoperative ultrasound.

Hemostasis

Following the parenchymal transection, hemostasis and a lack of biliary leakage must be ensured. In addition to the conduct of the parenchymal transection, a variety of strategies exist to achieve hemostasis. First and foremost is direct pressure. It is rare to not be able to temporarily stop bleeding from the parenchymal surface through the application of manual pressure. Larger bleeding sites in the parenchymal edge are often easily addressed by *en mass* compression of the surrounding parenchyma utilizing figure-of-eight sutures (0-silk or 1-chromic sutures). More diffuse oozing is managed with application of electrothermal energy. The most widely utilized device for this is the Argon Beam coagulator which is excellent at surface hemostasis. Small bleeders can be stopped with the standard electrocautery and/or the saline-enhanced electrocautery devices available from parenchymal transection. Topical hemostatic agents are also often useful including cellulose, bovine collagen, and human thrombin. Following control of hemostasis, careful inspection of the parenchyma must occur to identify bile leaks. A fresh white sponge placed against the parenchymal edge is an easy way to identify. Injection of the cystic duct stump with air or methylene blue dye is an alternative.

Postoperative Care

Patient management in the first day after surgery revolves around identifying and responding to bleeding and cardiopulmonary issues. It is our practice to check the hematocrit immediately after surgery, late in the evening, and early on the day following surgery. In this manner, three time points are available by the following morning to make decisions on DVT prophylaxis as well as the possibility of identifying early bleeding issues that might be clinically occult. Fluid management needs to be judicious especially in older patients, those with underlying heart disease and in those who had very large volume resections where fluid retention issues are quite common. Our practice is to accept hematocrit levels in the low mid 20s unless clinical circumstances suggest end-organ issues or the patient is too fatigued/lightheaded to mobilize. We do not, as a general rule, transfuse FFP even when the postoperative INR is quite high unless there is evidence of clinical bleeding. Equally, we do not administer vitamin K as these patients, despite the INR, are still hypercoagulable and at risk for thrombotic events. Pharmacologic DVT prophylaxis is started on postoperative day one if the hematocrit is relatively stable and no other contraindications exist. Patients without concomitant biliary/enteric procedures are left without nasogastric tubes upon leaving the operating room. A significant minority of patients will have gastric distension though requiring placement of a nasogastric tube postoperatively. Gastric dilatation should be actively sought in patients describing symptoms of or with signs of upper abdominal distension as failure to decompress a significant dilatation can be catastrophic. Urinary catheters are removed on postoperative day one except when oliguria is a concern. Our general strategy for pain control is patient-controlled intravenous administration of narcotics complemented by intravenous non-steroidal anti-inflammatory drugs (in patients without renal insufficiency). Although many groups utilize epidurals, our group as a general rule has been less than enthusiastic given the frequent hypotension, urinary retention, and other issues associated with their use. Patients are begun on clear liquids when they are without nausea and/or signs of an ileus.

OUTCOMES

In the current era of liver surgery, the expected mortality of partial hepatectomy should be generally very low and is largely predicted (negatively) by the presence of intrinsic liver disease, an inadequate volume of the future liver remnant, the performance of concomitant complex procedures, and profound underlying comorbidities. In general for patients undergoing partial hepatectomy for metastatic disease, the expected mortality rate should be 1–3%. Patients with metastatic disease who require extended hepatectomies still have mortality risk estimates of 5–10% even in high volume centers. Patients undergoing partial hepatectomy in the context of underlying disease have mortality risks that are approximately double those reported in the metastatic resection population. Overall and severe morbidity rates are still 30–50% and 15–30%, respectively. Among the more frequent severe morbidities are bile leak, postoperative liver dysfunction, cardiopulmonary issues (atrial fibrillation, symptomatic pleural effusions), oozing requiring postoperative transfusions, and prolonged ileus. For large hepatectomies, some degree of hyperbilirubinemia is to be expected. When the bilirubin levels exceed 5 mg/dl, the risks of death secondary to hepatic failure begin to greatly increase such that one-third of patients who reach this threshold die in the postoperative period. The time for full recovery in patients is generally expected to be 2–3 moths and patients should be counseled regarding this expectation.

REFERENCES

1. Dagradi A, Brearley R. The surgery of hepatic tumours. *Postgrad Med J* 1962; 38:670–687.
2. Foster JH, Berman MM. *Solid Liver Tumors*. Philadelphia, Saunders. 1977.
3. Pringle JH. V. Notes on the arrest of hepatic hemorrhage due to trauma. *Ann Surg* 1908; 48(4):541–549.
4. Townsend CM, Sabiston DC. *Sabiston Textbook of Surgery: The Biological Basis of Modern Surgical Practice*. Philadelphia, Saunders. 2004.
5. Fischer JE, Bland KI. *Mastery of Surgery*. 5th edition, Philadelphia, Wolters Kluwer Health/Lippincott Williams & Wilkins. 2007.

SURGICAL TECHNIQUES: LIVER PROCUREMENT AND TRANSPLANTATION

17

Deepak Vikraman* and Carlos E. Marroquin[†]

ORGAN RECOVERY

The cadaveric organ recovery proceeds in two distinct phases: the first is the warm dissection and the second is the cold dissection and extraction of the organs from the peritoneal cavity.

Adequate exposure is critical during the conduct of an abdominal organ recovery. The peritoneal cavity is entered through a midline laparotomy extending from the subxyphoid area to the pubic symphyses. Once the liver is visualized and a decision has been made to proceed with recovery, a median sternotomy is performed to enhance exposure and facilitate the subsequent recovery and allow exploration of the thoracic cavity to rule out thoracic malignancies. If an adequate retractor is not available, a cruciate incision should be fashioned to obtain better exposure. The cruciate incision is made 2–3 finger breaths below the costal margins extending from the midline laterally to the anterior axillary line and secured at four quadrants with heavy nonabsorbable suture like number 1 prolene or nylon (Figure 1). Examine the abdominal organs for any abnormality prior to proceeding with the recovery.

---

*Department of Surgery, Duke University, Durham, North Carolina
[†]Department of Surgery, University of Rochester, Rochester, New York

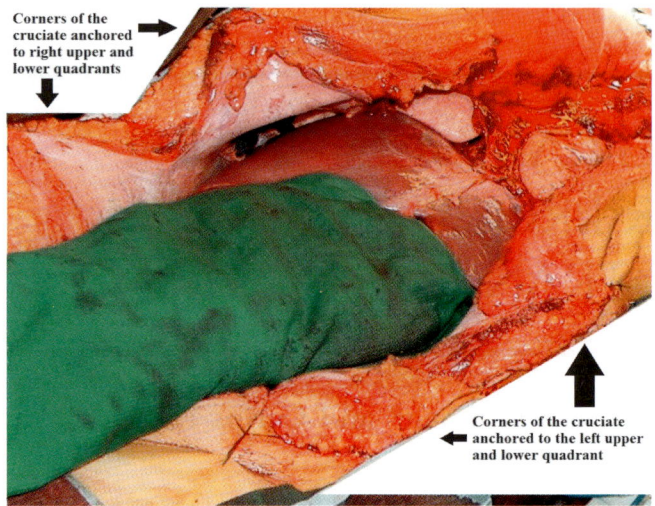

Figure 1. Optimal exposure has been created with a bilateral subcostal cruciate. Once a complete medial evisceration has been performed, wrapping the intestines facilitates control of small bowel during exposure of the great vessels.

The recovery process requires both supraceliac and infrarenal control of the abdominal aorta. Whether one starts with supraceliac or infrarenal exposure is not critical. However, prior to obtaining control, one needs to inspect the abdomen specifically looking for and abdominal aortic aneurysm (AAA). The presence of an AAA is not necessarily a contraindication to recovery, but will necessitate greater thoracic exposure of the aorta to allow perfusion of the liver through the thoracic aorta. If an AAA does exist, one will need to make a critical evaluation of the hepatic arteries as they may be substantially atherosclerotic.

Supraceliac aortic control is obtained after the left triangular ligament is divided. The gastrohepatic ligament is opened next. Careful inspection of the gastrohepatic ligament is performed looking for an accessory or replaced left hepatic artery which usually arises from the left Gastric artery.[1] If present, the accessory vessel is traced back to it origin by ligating and dividing its branches. This can be performed during the warm recovery or after reperfusion during the cold recovery. Supra celiac aorta is exposed through the crura of the diaphragm — dividing the crura provides the best exposure. The aorta is controlled with a single umbilical tape (Figure 2).

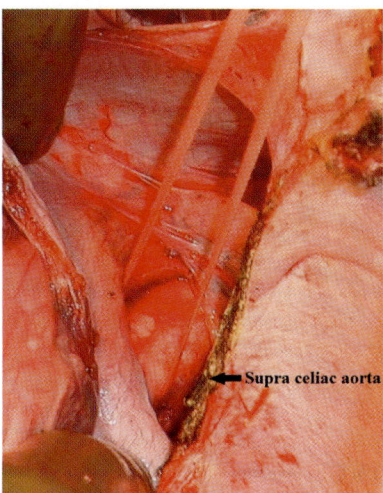

Figure 2. Control of the supra-celiac aorta is accomplished by incising the diaphragmatic fibers overlying the aorta as it leaves the chest. Dividing the left crus of the diaphragm will place one over the aorta; do not enter the esophagus. Alternatively, one can find the supra-celiac aorta through the left chest after taking down the left diaphragm. Once it has been skeletonized, pass a single umbilical tape around the aorta for supra-celiac control. The supra-celiac aorta will be cross clamped at this level at the time of perfusion.

Exposure of infrarenal aorta and inferior vena cava (IVC) is performed with a medial evisceration of the abdominal intestines. The white line of Toldt is incised, and the right colon is medialized; the duodenum is kocherized and the root of the mesentery is divided all the way to the ligament of Treitz. This exposes the abdominal aorta and IVC from their bifurcation to the level of the superior mesenteric artery (SMA) and left renal vein (Figure 3). During the course of performing the Kocher maneuver and exposing the SMA, one should inspect for a replaced or accessory right hepatic artery. The SMA is located just above the left renal vein. Traction of the duodenum and small bowel mesentery in a cephalad direction helps identify the artery. The peri arteriolar nerve plexus is incised longitudinally to expose the proximal 3–4 cm of SMA. This is the usual location where an accessory or replaced artery originates from the SMA in about 10–15% of deceased donors,[3] and takes a course posterior to the common bile duct. The aorta is controlled with an umbilical tape at the level of the bifurcation for cannulation of the Systemic circulation. The Inferior mesenteric artery

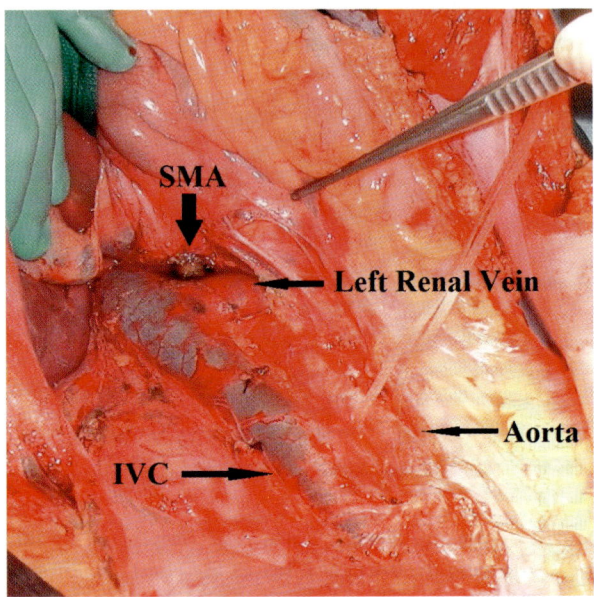

Figure 3. A medial visceral rotation is performed from the patient's right side exposing the abdominal aorta, and IVC. Once the aorta and vena cava are exposed, use a right angle clamp to get around the aorta just above the bifurcation and pass 2 umbilical tapes. Care must be taken to see behind the aorta prior to passing the clamp in an attempt to avoid the paired lumbar arteries. The vena cava is then surrounded with a large silk tie. At this point, the anterior wall of the aorta is dissected free of adventitial tissue and the left renal vein is exposed. At the superior border of the left renal vein, the SMA pulse can be appreciated at the base of the small bowel mesentery. Expose the base of the SMA as this will facilitate recovery of the pancreas and will facilitate the identification of a replaced right hepatic artery. Usually, a replaced right artery will arise from the SMA (~10%) for the first 2–3 cm. Skeletonizing the base of the SMA facilitates identification of a replaced right hepatic artery.

may be ligated and divided. The inferior mesenteric vein is identified to the left of the ligament of Treitz. The vein is skeletonized and controlled with 2–0 silk ties and prepared for splanchnic venous cannulation.[2]

The hilar dissection of the liver is initiated by excising the lymph node at the junction of the pancreas and the porta hepatis. This node is referred to by many in transplantation as "The Starzalian Node" as it establishes the location from which we initiate the dissection of the portal structures for a liver recovery that will subsequently be transplanted (Figure 4). The

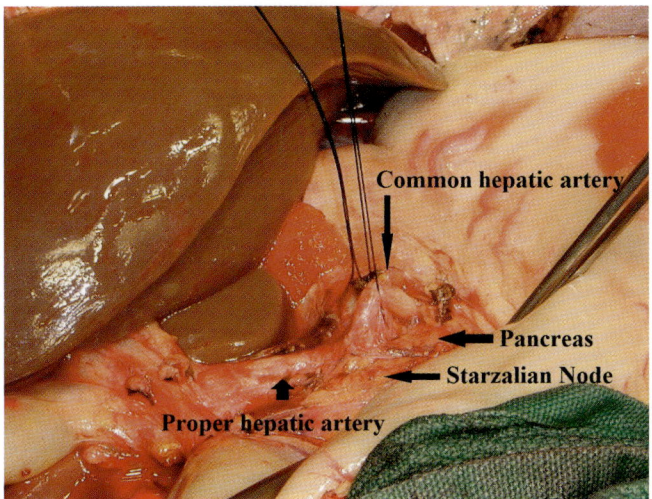

Figure 4. The dissection of the porta-hepatis is initiated at the level of the Starzalian Node. This dissection should proceed away from the hilum towards the celiac axis. The objective is to stay on top of the common hepatic artery working towards the celiac axis while avoiding the pancreatic parenchyma.

common hepatic artery runs along the superior edge of the pancreas under this lymph node. The artery is traced distally until the branching point of the gastro duodenal artery (GDA). The GDA is doubly ligated and divided. The common hepatic artery is then traced proximally towards the celiac axis to identify the splenic artery take off and the origin of the left gastric artery (Figure 5). The common bile duct is ligated close to the head of the pancreas and divided. The gall bladder is incised, bile is drained, and the biliary tree is flushed out with cold saline prior to cross clamp. The portal vein is skeletonized to the level of the head of the pancreas.

The donor is given a large doze of intravenous heparin (40,000 units or 300 IU/Kg) prior to cross clamp. Once heparin has circulated for three minutes, the distal aorta is tied off and the abdominal aorta is cannulated with a 20–24 French catheter for systemic flushing. Similarly, the Inferior or superior mesenteric vein is also cannulated with a 10 or 12 French catheter. The supraceliac aorta is cross clamped and the systemic and portal flush is begun through the inferior mesenteric vein or superior mesenteric vein and abdominal aorta (Figures 6a–6b). The infusion volumes average

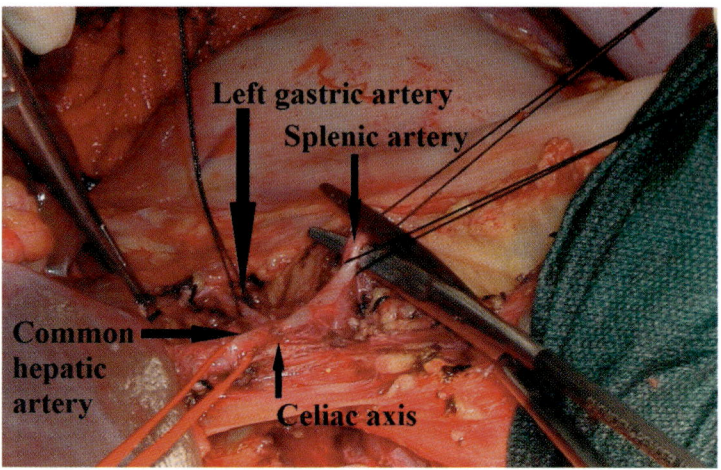

Figure 5. It is easier and more straight forward to isolate the vascular anatomy prior to cross-clamping; pulsatile flow facilitates identification of each vessel. These structures are all divided once the perfusion is complete.

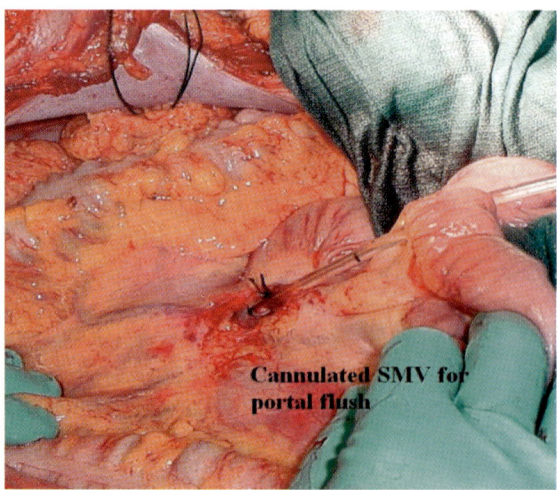

Figure 6a. Organ perfusion requires arterial and portal flow. The portal flow may be obtained by cannulating the SMV or IMV.

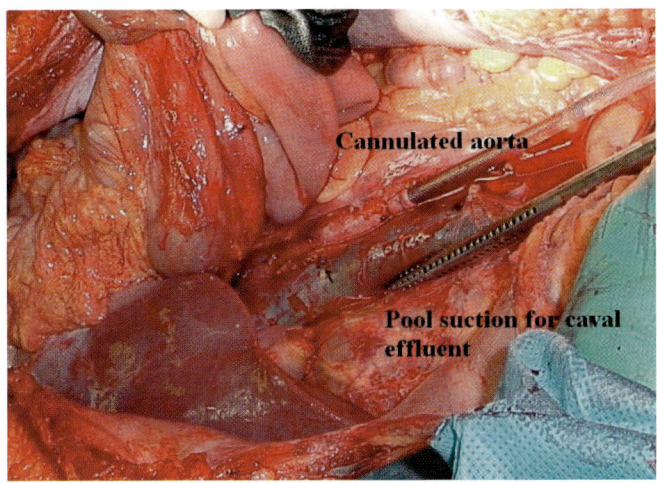

Figure 6b. One of the main objectives of the recovery procedure is to expose the infra renal aorta and vena cava with a complete medial evisceration. Here the cannula is in the aorta ready for perfusion and the cava will be opened to allow drainage of the perfusate into the pool suction that is inserted into the vena cava.

30–60 mL/Kg or approximately 3000 ml through the aortic cannula and 1000–2000 mL through the portal venous cannula for adults.[4] The commonly used solution for organ preservation is UW solution. A venotomy is made to drain the blood volume either in the thoracic IVC or infrarenal IVC. Ice is then applied on the organs to achieve topical cooling at the same time.

Once the flush is complete, the cold recovery is begun. The suprahepatic IVC is excised with a cuff of diaphragm. The infra hepatic IVC is divided just above the point in the cava where the left renal vein joins the IVC. The portal vein is divided at the level of the coronary vein. The left gastric and splenic arteries are divided distal to there origin from the celiac axis. The SMA is disconnected with a cuff of aorta. The aorta is then transected just superior to the renal arteries. At this point, all the vascular attachments of the liver have been disconnected and the liver is sharply excised by sharp dissection away from the retroperitoneum (Figure 7) and placed in cold preservative solution. It is important to recover the common iliac arteries and veins to the level of the distal external iliac arteries and veins as they may be needed to create an arterial or venous conduit during the conduct of the transplantation.

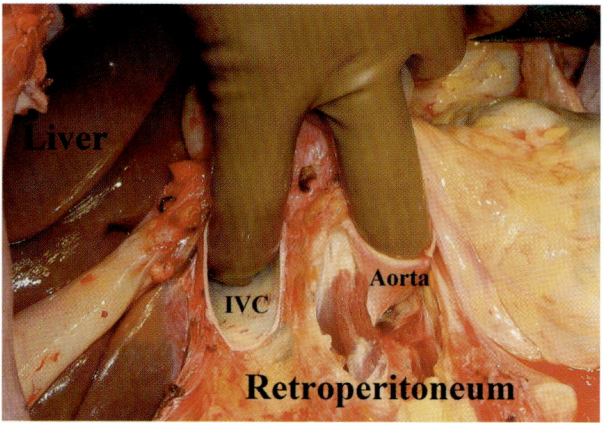

Figure 7. The final step involves cutting the liver away from the diaphragmatic and retroperitoneal attachments. Once the diaphragm is divided, the liver can be lifted out of the retroperitoneum as if grasping a bowling ball by the caval and aortic orifices while cutting the retroperitoneal muscles.

DONATION AFTER CARDIAC DEATH

Use of liver allografts from donation after cardiac death (DCD) donors has continued to increase steadily and now accounts for 5% of all liver-only transplants, compared to 0.9% of transplants performed in 2000. The number of centers utilizing DCD allografts has also increased quite markedly from 11 centers in 2000 to 62 in 2007(www.UNOS.org). Major factor contributing to this rise is the continued critical shortage of available organs for transplantation.

Specific protocols are in place to ensure that a patient is pronounced dead by a physician who is not involved with the recovery of donor organs. There is increased risk of ischemic injury to the organs and therefore usually young donors are accepted as DCD donors who are pronounced within 30 minutes of extubation.

From a technical standpoint, the difference from a standard donor is that, the vasculature is rapidly isolated using the same maneuvers and the preservation solution is flushed to rapidly cool the organs. The dissection of the organs is then done in the cold when there is no blood flow to the organs. So a sound knowledge of the anatomy and the anatomical variations is critical when when performing a DCD donor.

RECIPIENT PROCEDURE

The recipient hepatectomy is the most technically challenging part of the liver transplant as the development of portal hypertension will alter the anatomy with formation of vascularized adhesions and engorged varices. An experienced anesthesia team is crucial in a transplant procedure as they have to manage the excessive blood loss, fluid shifts, electrolyte imbalances and hemodynamic changes that occur during the process of the recipient hepatectomy and occlusion of the portal vein and inferior vena cava.

A generous bilateral subcostal incision will provide adequate exposure to the abdominal cavity. We rarely require a midline extension which was popular during the inception of liver transplantation. The liver is mobilized by dividing the falciform ligament, the left triangular ligament, the right triangular ligament and the gastrohepatic ligament. The hilar structures are subsequently skeletonized. The common hepatic duct, the branches of the proper hepatic artery, the portal vein and the accessory right hepatic artery if present are ligated and divided distally at the hilum of the liver. The portal vein is not ligated until the liver is ready to be explanted. One can occasionally encounter a substantial amount of back bleeding from the liver during the course of the hepatectomy. When this occurs, the portal vein may be divided earlier than usual to limit the blood loss.

The dissection of the inferior vena cava can be carried out depending on the technique utilized to implant the donor liver. In the standard procedure with caval replacement (Figure 8), after complete mobilization of the right and left lobes of the liver, the IVC is completely skeletonized by dividing the peritoneal lining from the diaphragm to above the insertion of the left renal vein. The right adrenal vein should be ligated and divided during this procedure. Once one is prepared to cross-clamp, a test clamp should be provided for anesthesia. This allows anesthesia to determine how to support the recipient during the implantation. At this point, the portal vein is clamped at the most distal site in the hilum and divided. The liver is explanted after placing vascular clamps on the supra hepatic IVC and infra hepatic IVC and excising the cava between the clamps along with the liver. If the test clamp were not tolerated, then one would have to consider implanting the liver using a piggyback technique or placing the patient on an extracorporeal bypass circuit.[5]

In the caval preservation technique or "piggy back" technique (Figure 9), the caudate lobe of the liver is dissected off the IVC and the

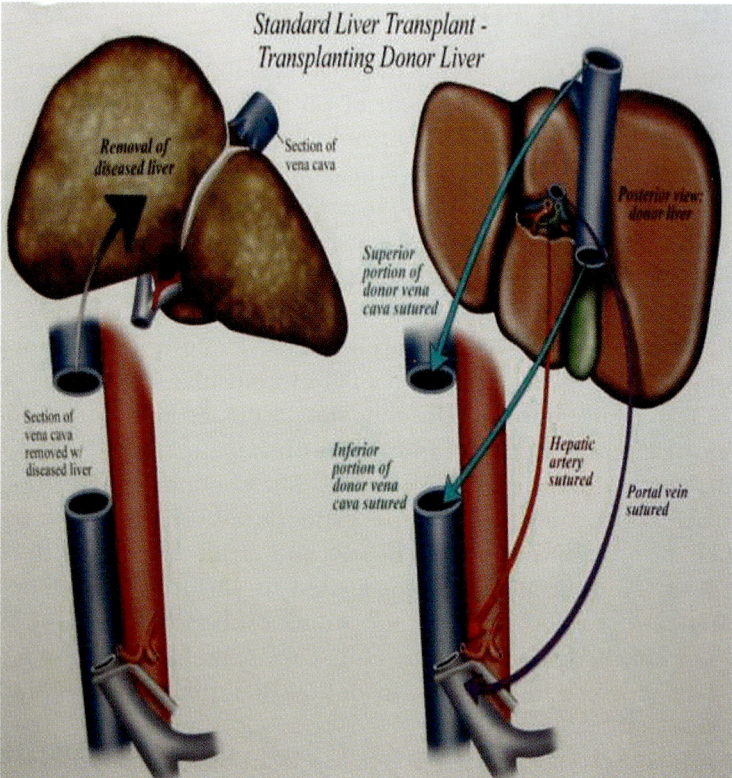

Figure 8. In the standard or end-to-end implantation technique, after complete mobilization of the right and left lobes of the liver, and complete mobilization of the IVC from the level of the diaphragm to the level of the renal veins, the IVC and liver are excised *en-bloc*. The liver is then brought up to the operative field. The suprahepatic caval anastamoses is performed in an end-to-end fashion and the liver is flushed of preservative solution. Following the hepatic flush, the infrahepatic caval anastamoses is completed and the portal vein anastamoses is performed and the liver is reperfused. Once the liver is reperfused and there is no obvious bleeding, the hepatic arterial anastomosis is performed followed by the biliary anastomosis.

short hepatic veins from the right lobe and the caudate lobe are ligated and divided, thereby completely mobilizing the liver off the IVC except for its attachment by the right, middle and left hepatic veins.[6] Once the liver has been mobilized off of the IVC, a test clamp is provided and the

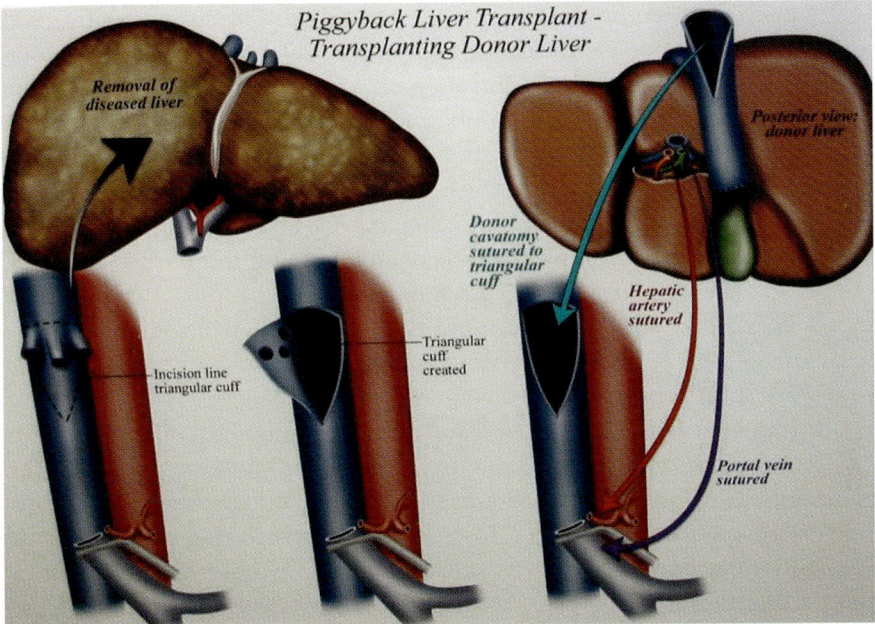

Figure 9. In the "piggy-back" technique, the right and left lobes of the liver are mobilized. The liver is subsequently completely mobilized off of the IVC. The liver is then brought up to the operative field and the suprahepatic caval anastomoses is performed in an end-to-end fashion to a cloacae fashioned between the hepatic veins or directly to a caval cuff created by excising the hepatic veins. The liver is flushed of preservative solution and the infra-hepatic cava is ligated or stapled. The portal vein anastomoses is performed in and end-to-end fashion and the liver is reperfused. Once the liver is reperfused and there is no obvious bleeding, the hepatic arterial anastamosis is performed followed by the biliary anastamosis.

portal vein is subsequently clamped high in the hilum and divided. The right hepatic vein is usually divided and a clamp is placed on the confluence of the middle and left hepatic veins. The liver is excised above the the confluence and past off of the field to pathology. Prior to the clamping the IVC and the portal circulation a test clamp is performed to assess the hemodynamic stability of the patient. If a test clamp were not tolerated in an effort to perform a "piggy back" technique, one would have to consider implanting the liver using an extracorporeal bypass circuit.

The liver is then brought to the operative field. The suprahepatic caval anastamoses is carried out in an end-to-end fashion utilizing 3–0 prolene sutures. This is followed by the infrahepatic caval anastamoses also utilizing 3–0 prolene sutures. Prior to completing the infrahepatic anastamoses, the liver is flushed with one liter of either cold albumin or lactated ringers solution through the portal vein to flush the high potassium load in the preservation solution through the infrahepatic cava. Following the hepatic flush, the infrahepatic anastamoses is completed and the portal vein anastamoses is performed with 5–0 prolene sutures. The portal vein anastamoses is carried out keeping in mind that the portal vein usually enlarges in diameter after reperfusion. As such, a "growth factor" is incorporated in to the last knot by purposefully tying an air knot.

Upon completion of the caval and portal venous anastamoses the liver is reperfused by removing the clamps in the following sequence. First, the suprahepatic clamp is removed and the suprahepatic anastamoses is carefully inspected for hemostasis. This is followed by restoring complete caval flow and the portal vein clamp is released last, providing complete restoration of blood flow to the liver. Meticulous hemostasis is then achieved.

If the liver is being implanted using the "piggy back" technique, the only difference in the procedure is that the suprahepatic vena cava of the donor liver is anastamosed to the confluence created between the middle and left hepatic veins or directly to the cava in a triangular cuff created by excising the hepatic veins (Figure 9). The infrahepatic caval orifice is ligated after flushing the preservation solution through the liver. Once the liver has been flushed, the portal venous anastomosis is created in an end-to-end fashion with great care to eliminate any redundancy. The hepatic arterial anastamoses is then carried out by anastamosing the proper hepatic artery of the recipient to the celiac trunk of the donor liver. Usually the recipient's gastroduodenal artery is ligated and divided.

This is followed by the biliary anastamoses, which could either be a choledochodochostomy between the donor and recipient ducts or a hepaticojejunostony with a roux limb. The biliary anastamoses is carried out using an absorbable suture; usually 5–0 or 6–0 PDS. Traditionally, transplant surgeons used T-tubes or Turcotte tubes to stent the biliary anastamoses. It is not our practice to stent our choledochodochostomies.

The abdomen is then closed in layers with either a single drain near the biliary anastamoses or multiple drains with additional drains behind the right and left lobes.

There are variations to the construction to the arterial and portal venous anastamoses, which are beyond the scope of this chapter.

REFERENCES

1. Todo S, Makowka L, Tzakis A, et al. Hepatic artery in liver transplantation. *Transplant Proc* 1987; 19:2406–2411.
2. Broelsch C. Removal of cadaver donor liver for adult recipient. In: T Buck (ed). *Atlas of Liver Surgery.* 1993. Churchill Livingstone. pp. 144–155.
3. Hiatt J, Busuttil RW. Surgical anatomy of the hepatic artery in 1000 cases. *Ann Surg* 1994; 220:50–52.
4. Renz JR, Yersiz H. The donor operation. In: R Busuttil, G Klintmalm (eds). *Transplantation of Liver.* 2005. Philadelphia, WB Saunders. pp. 545–559.
5. Marroquin CE, Kuo PC. Adult cadaveric liver transplantation. In: PC Kuo, RD Davis (ed). *Comprehensive Atlas of Transplantation.* 2005. Philadelphia, Lippincott W&W, pp. 99–114.
6. A Tzakis, S Todo, TE Starzl, et al. Orthotopic liver transplantation with preservation of the inferior vena cava. *Ann Surg* 1989; 210(5):649–652.

Section 2: Biliary Disease

BILIARY ANATOMY   18

Asvin Ganapathi* and Sandhya A. Lagoo-Deenadayalan*

INTRODUCTION

Anatomy is one of the basic tenets of surgery, as one must have sound anatomical knowledge to safely perform surgery. Surgeons are taught normal anatomy and some common variants. However, to be able to perform both simple and complex operations skillfully and safely, one must also possess a strong fund of knowledge about the anatomical variants that can potentially present during a procedure. One organ system that has many potential anatomic variants with regards to functional structures as well as vasculature and lymphatics is the biliary system.

The purpose of this chapter is to first briefly establish what is considered normal anatomy starting at the cellular level of the liver all the way through the biliary system into the duodenum. We will then explore the many different anatomic variants of the biliary system focusing primarily on the biliary system, while also trying to provide clinical adjuncts of the importance of these variants.

NORMAL

Liver

The formation and origination of secreted bile begins in the liver at the level of the hepatocytes. These cells form bile and secrete bile into

*Duke University Medical Center, Durham, NC 27710 USA

canaliculi, which surround the cells on all, but one side. The canaliculi empty into the hepatic cords, which drain into hepatic ductules that further empty into ducts. It is at this point that the anatomy becomes more clear based on the idea that there are anatomic segments of the liver, each with an associated bile duct.[1] Three main systems must be considered in understanding hepatic anatomy: the left, right, and caudate systems of the liver.

Left Hepatic System

Anatomically the left hepatic system is comprised of the drainage system of the left part of the liver consisting of segments 2, 3, and 4. Most commonly, the bile ducts of segments 2 and 3 merge with one or more ducts from segment 4 to form the confluence of the left hepatic system, creating the left hepatic duct (LHD) (Figure 1a). The LHD, normally 2–5 cm in length, runs in an extrahepatic fashion from left to right in the hilum, above and behind the left portal branch. This configuration is normally observed in approximately 82% of patients.[2,3]

Right Hepatic System

Similar to the left system, the right hepatic system drains the right side of the liver consisting of segments 5, 6, 7, and 8. This is accomplished through drainage from the anterior (segments 5 and 8) and posterior (segments 6

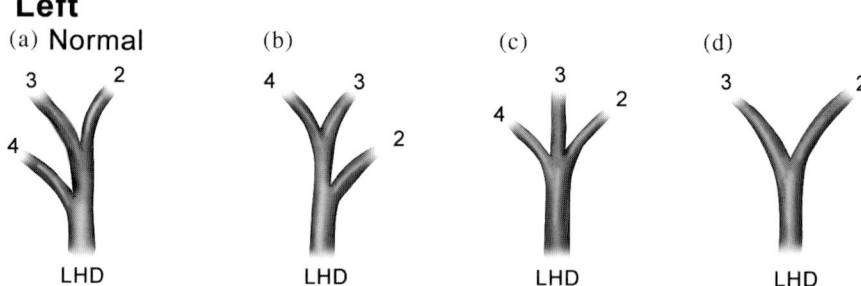

Figure 1. (a) Normal, most common biliary configuration of left hepatic system; (b) Anatomical variant with drainage of segments 2 merging with the combined drainage for segments 3 and 4; (c) Anatomic variation with confluence of segments 2, 3, and 4; (d) Drainage of segments 2 and 3 with absence of segment 4 drainage.

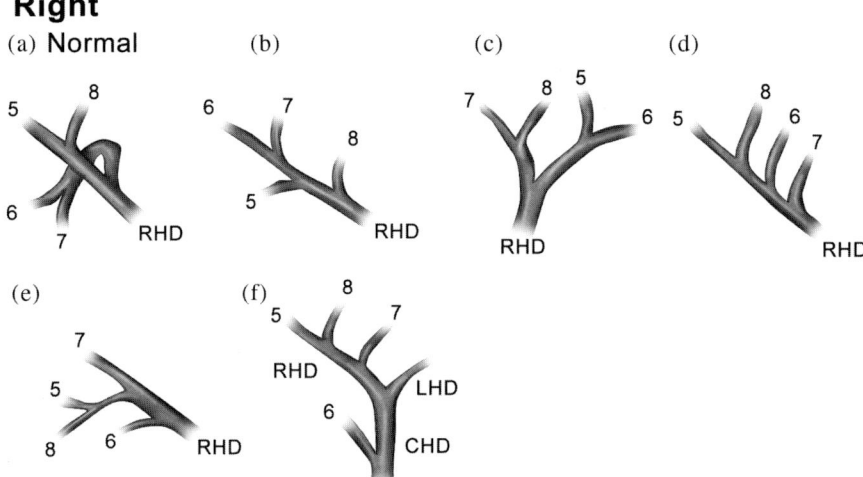

Figure 2. (a) Normal biliary drainage of right hepatic system; (b) Variant with segment 5 joining combined drainage of segments 5 and 6, with segment 8 joining last; (c) Anatomic variant with the merger of branch draining segments 5 and 6 and branch draining segments 7 and 8; (d) Drainage of segment 5 sequentially drained by drainage of segments 8, 6, and 7, in that order; (e) Drainage of segments 5 and 8 merging with the segment 7 and subsequent merger of segment 6; (f) Right hepatic duct comprised of segments 5, 7, and 8, and with drainage of segment 6 into CHD.

and 7) ducts. The anterior duct normally lies vertically to the left of the anterior branch of the portal vein, while the posterior duct is primarily horizontal, superior to the anterior branch of the portal vein. These two ducts then usually converge in a confluence above the right portal branch in an extrahepatic fashion to form the right hepatic duct (RHD) (Figure 2a).[3–5] Typically the RHD is approximately 1 cm in length and runs vertically.

Caudate System

The caudate lobe is unique in that this lobe has its own drainage system. Drainage occurs through 1 to 6 branches (on average 3).[4,6] These ducts will drain into both the right and left hepatic ducts with the right duct receiving one duct from the caudate lobe and the left duct receiving one to two from the caudate lobe. About 85% of the right part of the caudate lobe drains into the RHD, while approximately 93% of the left part of the caudate lobe drains into the LHD. Approximately 80% of the caudate drainage goes to both ducts, and 15% is drained only to the LHD and 5% only to the RHD. In general, these ducts are found posterior and above the portal branches.

Confluence/Common Hepatic Duct (CHD)/ Common Bile Duct (CBD)

The confluence is formed by the connection of the right and left hepatic ducts. This merger usually occurs anterior to the portal vein in the hilar plate and this particular pattern occurs in 40–80% of people.[4,5,7] The confluence leads to the formation of the common hepatic duct, which courses downward, anterior to the portal vein. Usually, the hepatic artery is found to the left of the CHD and the right hepatic artery crosses the CHD posteriorly. Following the merger of the cystic duct and CHD, the common bile duct is formed. The common bile duct travels anterior to the portal vein, caudad behind the first part of the duodenum, then obliquely on the dorsal aspect of the pancreas in the pancreatic groove. The CBD then joins the pancreatic duct and enters the second portion of the duodenum posteromedially at the ampulla of Vater.

Cystic Duct/Gallbladder

The gallbladder, which normally lies on the inferoposterior aspect of the right lobe of the liver, drains into the cystic duct. This structure then courses inferior and to the left of the gallbladder neck and then joins the CHD, on the right lateral edge of the CHD. This merger often occurs approximately 2 cm inferior to the confluence of the RHD and LHD.[8] Another aspect of the gallbladder that should be considered is the connection to the liver through the small ducts of Luschka, allowing bile to reach the gallbladder, without having to travel through the normal path of the biliary tree.

VARIANTS

The variations of the previously described structures are presented below. It should be noted that only variations that have been observed and described in the literature are discussed with theoretical variations presented in the literature not being included.

Left Hepatic System

As described earlier, normally the ducts draining segments 2 and 3 merge and then are joined by the drainage of segment 4 to create the LHD and this occurs in 59.3–82.4% of people. The most common variation described occurs when the drainage from segment 4 feeds into the duct from segment 3 and this structure then merges with the duct of segment 2 and the reported occurrence varies from 11.8% to 29.6% (Figure 1b). Another observed variant is where segments 2, 3, and 4 all merge together creating a "triconfluence", with the incidence ranging from 2–11.1% (Figure 1c).[2,3,9] Finally, a confluence of only segments 2 and 3 without any contribution from segment 4 has been described in 4% of patients in one series (Figure 1d).[3] Another rare occurrence is where segment 4 will directly drain into the CHD. Additionally, variations of segment 4 where there is a superior and inferior duct has been described and in this scenario these two ducts can merge in separate locations with the drainage from segments 2 and 3.[7]

Right Hepatic System

Normal configuration of the right hepatic system is the formation of a right anterior (RA), by segments 5 and 8, and right posterior (RP), by segments 6 and 7, duct that join to form the RHD and this occurs in 65.7–78.4% of subjects.[3,4,7] One common variation, occurring in approximately 20% of studied subjects in one study, is when a complete RP merges with an incomplete RA with two smaller segmental branches from the components of the right anterior liver, named as a "right triple" configuration by Hribernik et al.[3] Examples include the segment 8 branch joining the RP system first and then this common duct being joined by the segment 5 branch or having the segment 5 branch merge with the RP first, followed later by a separate branch from segment 8 (Figure 2b).[4] Hribernik et al. also described other less common arrangements such as the RP merging with three smaller segmental branches from the right anterior liver forming a "right quadruple" configuration or having segments 5 and 6 form one duct and segments 7 and 8 form another, with these two ducts joining to create the RHD[3] (Figure 2c). Healey and Schroy also described rare variations such as: (a) segment 6 draining into the RA with segment 7 joining later (Figure 2d), (b) segment 7 draining into the RA with segment 6 joining later (Figure 2e), and (c) segment 7 draining into the RA creating the RHD and having segment 6 drain into the CHD (Figure 2f).[4] Another variation described in the literature describes having segment 5 draining into the CBD.[7]

These variations of the biliary drainage of the left and right ductal systems become particularly important for patients undergoing partial hepatectomies and in the procurement and implantation of split liver transplantation. In these cases, surgeons not expecting anatomic variants can find themselves in an unanticipated situation where there is biliary leakage from an unexpected source. Additionally, in the case of liver transplantation, it can lead to a loss of a potential organ if one is not careful about the process of dividing the organ.

Caudate System

Because of the proximity of the caudate lobe to the rest of the liver, the drainage is usually split between the RHD and LHD. However, it should be noted that the caudate can have exclusive RHD or LHD drainage, or drain into the confluence of the RHD and LHD. When looking at the drainage of the caudate lobe, usually there are three systems that are described: (1) caudate process (CP), (2) right caudate (RC), and (3) left caudate (LC). In 44% of subjects each of these systems has a single duct that feeds into the biliary drainage of the remainder of the liver (Figure 3a). There are many variations of this arrangement, with the most common being the CP duct draining into the RC duct, with the LC duct being separate (26%) (Figure 3b). Another relatively common variation is where the RC duct and LC duct merge to form a common duct with the CP duct being separate (13%) (Figure 3c). Less commonly the RC can have two separate ducts along with a separate LC and CP duct (4%) (Figure 3d) or in another scenario with a separate LC duct, with the CP duct draining into one of the two RC ducts (6%) (Figure 3e). Likewise, the LC can be split into two isolated ducts with a separate RC and CP duct (2%) (Figure 3f). Finally, the CP, RC, and LC ducts can merge to form one common duct that provides common drainage for the entire caudate lobe (5%) (Figure 3g).[4]

In 85% of cases the CP drains into the RHD system, with the other 15% of cases being drainage into the LHD system. As would be expected in 93% of cases the LC drains into the LHD system, with only 7% of cases being

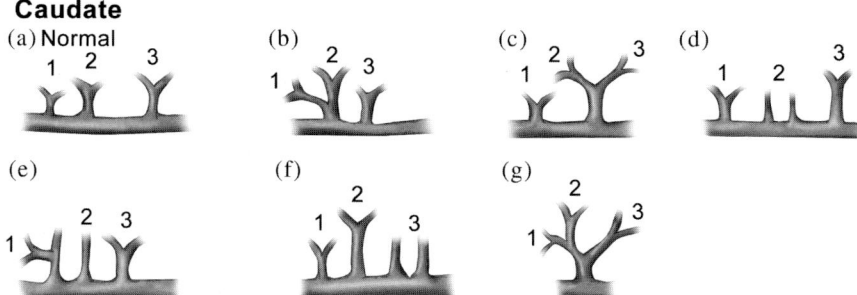

Figure 3. (a) Normal biliary drainage of caudate lobe with separate drainage of CP (1), RC (2), and LC (3); (b) Variant with combined drainage of CP (1) and RC (2) and separate LC (3) drainage; (c) Variant with independent CP (1) drainage and combined RC (2) and LC (3) drainage; (d) Variant with independent drainage of CP (1), RC (2), and LC (3), but with two separate drainage ducts for RC (2); (e) Drainage of CP (1) into one of 2 ducts drainage RC (2); (f) Independent drainage of CP (1) and RC (2), with 2 separate drainage ducts of LC (3); (g) Confluence of CP (1), RC (2), and LC (3) into a single drainage duct.

RHD system drainage. However, for the RC 52% of cases have the RHD system receiving the bile, while 48% of the time the LHD received the feed from the RC.[4]

Confluence/Common Hepatic Duct/Common Bile Duct

A complete RHD joins with a complete LHD to form the CHD in 40–80% of the population. However there are many variations (Figure 4a). One common configuration is the formation of a "triple confluence", where the LHD joins simultaneously with the RA and RP ducts (without a true RHD), occurring in 3–21.2% of subjects (Figure 4b). Another common variation is where the RP and RA join different parts of the biliary tree (8.9–31.2%). One example is the RP feeding into the LHD and this combination of these ducts merging with the RA duct (Figure 4c). An alternate configuration is where the RA merges with the LHD and the RP later feeds into the CHD.[3,10]

As mentioned earlier, the CHD helps form the CBD, which normally feeds into the duodenum, however variations can exist even here. Some of the commonly described variations include having accessory bile ducts,

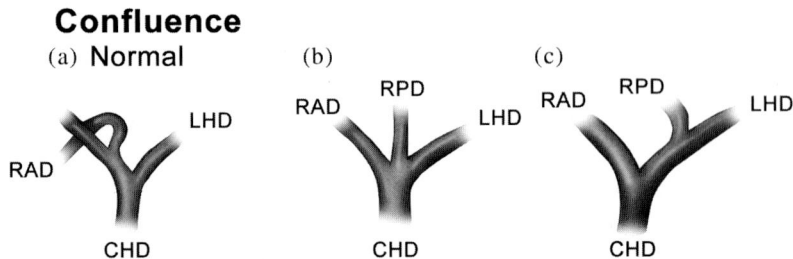

Figure 4. (a) Normal confluence with merger of complete RHD and complete LHD; (b) Variant with simultaneous confluence of RAD, RPD, and LHD; (c) Drainage of RPD into LHD with subsequent confluence with RAD.

which feed into various sections of the biliary tree, having the CHD enter the gallbladder and then be drained directly into the duodenum by the cystic duct, or having the RHD or LHD draining separately into the cystic duct.[12]

The anatomical variants of the confluence are again important in situations of partial hepatectomies (particularly in a left or right hepatectomy) or in split liver transplantation for reasons outlined above. The significance of variations in the CHD/CBD, while rare, should not be underestimated as they can lead to biliary leaks following cholecystectomies if the surgeon is not careful in identifying the anatomy.

Cystic Duct/Gallbladder

The cystic duct and gallbladder can also have variations. One abnormality is that of cystic duct agenesis, which likely occurs during the process of embryogenesis. Another cystic duct abnormality is more relative, as it refers to the length of the cystic duct. The cystic duct can sometimes be rather short, obscuring the anatomy normally expected during a cholecystectomy and this can lead to inadvertent clipping of the CBD. Another variation that exists is that of diverticulum that can be present along the cystic duct. In terms of a structural difference, a "double cystic duct" can be present. In this case, there are a few different configurations possible. One is a "Y" configuration where two cystic ducts originate from the gallbladder, which then join to form a common duct that helps form the CBD. An "H" configuration is where there is one cystic duct leaving from the gallbladder, and this then splits to form two separate ducts that separately help to make the CBD. The cystic duct can also have alternative points of entry into the biliary system, and in some cases can enter the duodenum separately from the rest of the biliary drainage leading to multiple sources of biliary drainage into the duodenum.[12] These variants are important to consider when one is performing a cholecystectomy, so that when one is clipping the presumed cystic duct, the patient's anatomy is considered such that there is no residual bile leak.

The gallbladder also has various anomalies that range from agenesis (can be present with or without a cystic duct) to multiple gallbladders. In the case of multiple gallbladders, up to three gallbladders has been described. In these cases, each gallbladder can have its own drainage via separate cystic ducts, or there can be a merger of initial cystic ducts to form one common duct. The gallbladder can also have septations creating multiple channels for drainage of bile. There can also be a deformity known as a Phyrigian cap, where the fundus of the gallbladder is folded. This is a non-pathologic condition, but can appear as a hepatic mass on imaging. Finally, the gallbladder can arise in ectopic locations with locations such as suprahepatically, retrorenally, in the anterior abdominal wall, the falciform ligament, and the left side of the lower abdomen being reported in the literature.[12] With regards to variations in the number and/or location of gallbladders, the clinical significance lies primarily in the clinical presentation of patients who present with gallbladder disease. For example, a patient with a retrorenal gallbladder would not necessarily present with the same symptoms as someone with a normally located gallbladder.

SUMMARY

As has been outlined above there are many variants to the biliary system that can present in a patient. While almost all of these variants are non-pathologic, surgeons should have knowledge of the variations so that inadvertent injury to the biliary tree can be avoided during hepatobiliary surgery.

REFERENCES

1. Hjortsjo CH. The topography of the intrahepatic duct systems. *Acta Anat (Basel)* 1951; 11: 599–615.
2. Castaing D. Surgical anatomy of the biliary tract. *HPB (Oxford)* 2008; 10: 72–76.

3. Hribernik M, Gadzijev EM, Mlakar B, *et al.* Variations of intrahepatic and proximal extrahepatic bile ducts. *Hepatogastroenterology* 2003; 50: 342–348.
4. Healey JE, Jr., Schroy PC. Anatomy of the biliary ducts within the human liver; analysis of the prevailing pattern of branchings and the major variations of the biliary ducts. *AMA Arch Surg* 1953; 66: 599–616.
5. Couinaud C, Le Foie. *Etudes anatomiques et chirurgicales.* Paris: Masson; 1957.
6. Kogure K, Kuwano H, Fujimaki N, *et al.* Relation among portal segmentation, proper hepatic vein, and external notch of the caudate lobe in the human liver. *Ann Surg* 2000; 231: 223–228.
7. Vakili K, Pomfret EA. Biliary anatomy and embryology. *Surg Clin North Am* 2008; 88: 1159–1174, vii.
8. Moosman DA, Collier FA. Prevention of traumatic injury to the bile ducts; a study of the structures of the cystohepatic angle encountered in cholecystectomy and supraduodenal choledochostomy. *Am J Surg* 1951; 82: 132–143.
9. Kitami M, Takase K, Murakami G, *et al.* Types and frequencies of biliary tract variations associated with a major portal venous anomaly: analysis with multi-detector row CT cholangiography. *Radiology* 2006; 238: 156–166.
10. Cucchetti A, Peri E, Cescon M, *et al.* Anatomic variations of intrahepatic bile ducts in a European series and meta-analysis of the literature. *J Gastrointest Surg* 2011; 15: 623–130.
11. Smadja C, Blumgart L. The biliary tract and the anatomy of biliary exposure. In: LH Blumgart (ed). *Surgery of the Liver and Biliary Tract.* New York, Churchill Livingstone, pp. 11–24. 1994.
12. Lamah M, Karanjia ND, Dickson GH. Anatomical variations of the extrahepatic biliary tree: review of the world literature. *Clin Anat* 2001; 14: 167–172.

IMAGING OF THE BILIARY TREE   19

Asad A. Shah* and Theodore N. Pappas*

INTRODUCTION

Advances in radiologic technology have given physicians many new and varied imaging modalities to use in diagnosing and treating patients with biliary disease. Basic imaging modalities such as ultrasound (US) and hepatobiliary iminodiacetic acid (HIDA) scan are still effective and continue to be used frequently. Magnetic resonance cholangiopancreaticography (MRCP) with or without contrast is a newer technique that provides excellent anatomic detail of the biliary system. Additionally, endoscopic retrograde choangiopancreatography (ERCP) and percutaneous transhepatic cholangiography (PTC) provide such detail as well as the ability to perform therapeutic interventions.

After developing a differential diagnosis based on history, physical examination, and laboratory workup, radiologic imaging is typically the next step in diagnosing suspected biliary disease. The suspected diagnosis or diagnoses will determine the imaging modality to be used. With typical biliary symptoms such as right upper quadrant pain, jaundice, nausea, or vomiting, ultrasound is the preferred initial diagnostic study. It can typically initially characterize or diagnose many biliary pathologies including gallstones (cholelithiasis), gallbladder inflammation (cholecystitis), biliary ductal dilatation, and gallbladder masses. If there is any uncertainty or the

---

*Duke University Medical Center, Durham, NC 27710 USA

need to further characterize other anatomic regions (i.e. distal common bile duct for stones, peritoneum for metastases etc.), other techniques can be employed including HIDA scan, MRCP, PTC, or ERCP.

Cost, accessibility, radiation exposure, and individual patient characteristics must all be taken into account before proceeding with a radiologic study. For example, a patient who has previously undergone a Roux-en-Y reconstruction may be unable to have an ERCP due to difficulty of advancing an endoscope through the aberrant anatomy. MRCP, ERCP, and PTC may be unavailable in some centers, particularly at off hours or on weekends.

This chapter describes the radiologic techniques typically used to image the biliary tree. It describes the methods of the studies, indications, advantages, disadvantages, and effectiveness of these imaging modalities with the goal of assisting physicians confronted with biliary pathology in diagnosing and treating biliary disease.

ULTRASOUND

Ultrasound, or sonography, is an inexpensive, non-invasive way to image most biliary tract disorders. It involves placing a round ultrasound probe (transducer) over the skin of the abdomen. This probe then emits high frequency sound waves which bounce back off the body's tissues and get transmitted into pictures of the body's internal structures. Ultrasound does not use radiation and can provide real-time imaging of the movement of structures or fluid within the body cavity.

The procedure should be performed after the patient has been fasting, if possible, to promote filling of the gallbladder with bile and thus easier visualization. Because of its non-invasive nature, availability, low cost, and overall excellent diagnostic accuracy, ultrasound is typically used as the first radiologic test in imaging the biliary tree. It is the most accurate method of identifying gallstones, with a sensitivity of greater than 95%.[1] Gallstones appear on ultrasound as echogenic foci producing acoustic windows (Figure 1). When false negatives do occur, they are typically in obese patients with small stones. Ultrasound can also identify intra- and extrahepatic biliary ductal dilatation.

Situations where the gallbladder may not be visualized include prior cholecystectomy, dramatic cholelithiasis filling the entire gallbladder, emphysematous cholecystitis, or the gallbladder being in an abnormal location. Disadvantages of ultrasound include limitations due to the individual

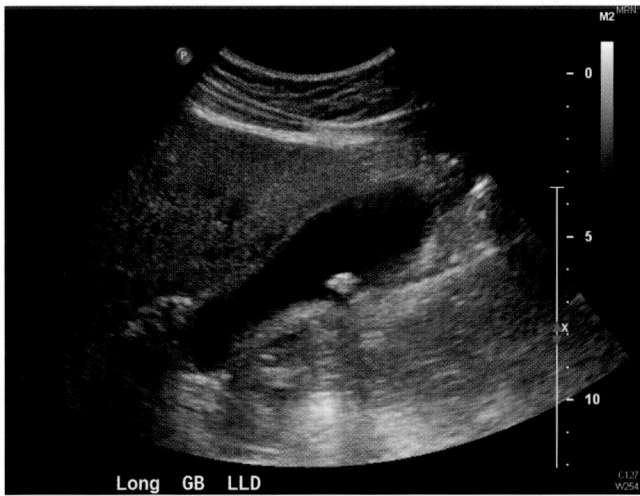

Figure 1. Ultrasound demonstrating a gallstone appearing as an echogenic foci.

examiner's skill and unfavorable anatomy, including bowel gas between the bile ducts and transducer preventing a suitable acoustic window.

Ultrasound is the best initial imaging test for acute cholecystitis. The positive predictive values of stones combined with either tenderness localized to the gallbladder (positive sonographic Murphy's sign), or the presence of a gallbladder wall thickness of >3 mm, are 92% and 95%, respectively. The negative predictive value of the absence of gallbladder stones and a negative sonographic Murphy's sign is 95%. However, gallbladder wall thickening may result from causes other than cholecystitis. These include nonfasting, generalized edematous states, hepatitis, pancreatitis, gallbladder wall varices, adenomyomatosis, and carcinoma (although the latter two usually cause focal rather than diffuse thickening).

Gallstone(s) may be impacted in the neck of the gallbladder and this region must be carefully examined. Other US signs of cholecystitis are gallbladder distension (diameter >5 cm), pericholecystic fluid, gallbladder wall striations and, occasionally, obvious wall hyperemia on doppler examination. Fine echoes seen within the gallbladder may be seen due to sludge or pus (gallbladder empyema). Sludge appears as nonshadowing, fine dependent echoes. Sludge is often seen in patients who are in chronically fasting states, on TPN, critically ill, on ceftriaxone, or pregnant. If liver function tests suggest duct obstruction, a careful evaluation of the common

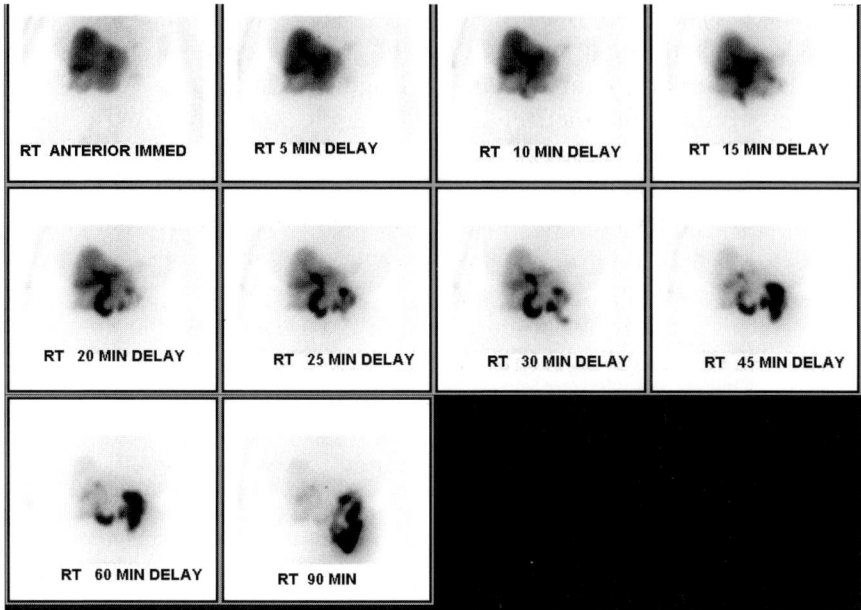

Figure 2. HIDA scan demonstrating acute cholecystitis. There is prompt excretion of radiotracer into the common bile duct and small bowel, but no activity within the gallbladder.

bile duct should be made for choledocholithiasis. The common bile duct should not be more than 10 mm in diameter.

HIDA

In a HIDA scan, 99m Tc iminodiacetic acid derivates injected intravenously, taken up by hepatocytes in the liver, and excreted into the biliary tree. The gallbladder is normally seen within 30 minutes of injection and the small intestine is seen within 60 minutes. The most common reason HIDA scans are performed is to evaluate for acute cholecystitis. In patients with acute cholecystitis, the cystic duct is usually obstructed and the gallbladder does not fill with contrast (Figure 2). If the gallbladder fills in between 1 and 4 hours, chronic cholecystitis is commonly present. However, nonfilling of the gallbladder alone is a nonspecific finding, as it can also be caused by eating, prolonged fasting, chronic cholecystitis, and severe liver disease.[2] HIDA is 86–100% sensitive and 94–100% specific for diagnosing acute cholecystitis.[3]

HIDA scans can also be used to evaluate for bile leaks. In patients who have a bile leak, the contrast accumulated in an abnormal location. HIDA can assess the leak is continuing and the magnitude of the leak, but it is not useful in locating the exact site of the biliary leak. HIDA can also show acute complete or near complete CBD obstruction, as there will be little or no activity in the small bowel, even on delayed images. HIDA is used to measure gallbladder ejection fraction to diagnose biliary dyskinesia and chronic cholecystitis. In infants, it can distinguish between biliary atresia from neonatal hepatitis, and can also identify choledochal cysts.

Negatives of the HIDA scan are that it takes longer, is more expensive, and does not evaluate adjacent organs, as compared to US. It is helpful when there is diagnostic uncertainty after ultrasound.

ERCP

ERCP is an invasive, yet atraumatic, method of imaging the biliary tree. It can be both diagnostic and therapeutic. ERCP is typically performed in an endoscopy suite. The patient is required to fast overnight. Any coagulopathies should be corrected before the procedure. Patients are sedated, typically with benzodiazepenes, and topical anesthetic is applied to the posterior pharyngeal wall. A duodenoscope is used to enter the duodenum and then a cannula is passed through the duodenoscope into the ampulla. Contrast material is then injected and the biliary and pancreatic ducts can typically be visualized.

The sensitivity of ERCP for detecting common bile ducts stones is 90–95%. For patients in whom there is a high suspicion of common bile duct stones, ERCP should be performed before cholecystectomy. Sphincterotomy can be readily performed and stones can be removed with a basket or stone retrieval balloon. The common bile duct can be cleared from stones in about 90% of cases. Stents are typically left in place when all stones can not be removed, the patient cannot tolerate a lengthy procedure, or if the papilla is edematous.

Advantages include being able to visualize the mucosa of the stomach, duodenum, and ampulla of Vater and perform biopsies as needed. Therapeutic procedures that can be performed include sphicterotomy, stone extraction, and placement of stents. Disadvantages include the inability to perform the procedure after some upper gastrointestinal tract reconstructions, when there is an obstructing ampullary lesion, and nonfilling of the ducts above an obstruction. Unless performed for surgical planning or drainage, ERCP should be avoided in patients with pancreatic pseudocysts, as infection and abscess formation can occur.

Risks of ERCP include those from the procedure itself and those from the anesthesia required for the procedure. Clinical pancreatitis is the most common complication and occurs in approximately 3% of patients after diagnostic ERCP and 7% after therapeutic ERCP. Up to 25% of patients have post procedure rise in serum amylase not accompanied by symptoms.[2] Cholangitis occurs in 0.6–0.8% of patients, typically in those with poor biliary drainage.[4] Whenever obstruction is present, patients should be placed on antibiotics for prophylaxis. When endoscopic sphincterotomy is performed, hemorrhage can occur in up to 5% of patients. This is usually seen during the procedure and can be controlled. Late bleeding may occur as well, usually 2–3 days after the procedure, but this generally stops on its own. When endoscopic stents are placed, the above mentioned complications may occur as well as perforation, stent occlusion, cholecystitis, duodenal stenosis, duodenal erosion, or stent migration. Oversedation and aspiration can also occur due to anesthesia.

ERCP is useful when postoperative bile leak is suspected because it can both identify and treat a leak. Stents can be placed across the leak with or without sphincterotomy. The stents are left in for many months. ERCP is also helpful in managing biliary strictures. Benign strictures typically occur postoperatively and cholangiography usually demonstrates a short smooth stricture. Malignant strictures often appear irregular, although imaging is not reliable in differentiating between benign and malignant processes. Guidewires can be placed across strictures followed by dilatation with serial plastic dilators or balloons. Brushing can be taken as well, although the yield of accurate tissue diagnosis is only 40–60%. Plastic or metal stents may be placed. Plastic stents are temporary and typically occlude by after 3 months. Metallic stents have a larger diameter and thus longer patency compared to plastic stents. They are typically used for palliation in the setting of malignant biliary strictures.

PTC

PTC has mostly been replaced by ERCP and MRCP due to a higher rate of complications with PTC, but it still has certain scenarios where it is particularly useful. Antibiotics are given prophylactically and the procedure is done under conscious sedation. Any coagulopathy should be corrected beforehand. The procedure involves placing a thin, flexible 22 or 23 gauze needle (i.e. Chiba) into the right or left intrahepatic ducts from the right flank or via the epigastrum under fluoroscopy. The right side is usually chosen due to its larger volume (typically) and easier accessibility. Ultrasound can also be used for puncture guidance. The stylet is removed from the needle and contrast is injected providing visualization of the bile ducts.

PTC can be used to visualize the biliary tree, place stents across obstructions, dilate obstructions, and remove stones. One indication for the procedure is situations when endoscopic cannulation is impossible. Examples of this include patients with previous surgery where the endoscope cannot reach the ampulla, when the ampulla is obstructed (i.e. large ampullay cancers), and when there are contraindications to ERCP. Another indication is for external drainage, particularly when endoscopic drainage is not possible. This frequently occurs when obstruction occurs at the liver hilum. Lastly, PTC is indicated when ERCP fails to visualize the entire biliary tree when complete visualization is needed.

Catheters can be placed across malignant strictures to provide internal and external drainage in 80–90% of cases. A simple drain may be placed to drain externally or a drain may be placed through the obstruction to allow internal or external drainage. Internal drainage has the advantage for patients in that they are not required to take care of the catheter and drainage system daily. However, they often become occluded within 3–6 months. Plastic or self-expandable metallic stents may be placed. Metallic stents result in improved biliary drainage due to their large diameter and smaller surface area. Percutaneous biliary drainage is preferred for perihilar obstructions. Infected bile can be drained and samples can be taken for microbiology and cytology. Success approaches 100% if the ducts are significantly dilated and about 75% if the ducts are slightly dilated or nondilated.

Complications occur in about 4–15% of patients and include hemobilia, bacteremia, and bile leak. Aspiration of some bile during the procedure reduces the risk of bile leak and endotoxemia by reducing intraductal pressure. Puncture of other organs can occur, particularly the lung, resulting in pneumothorax.

MRCP

MRCP is a relatively newer technique that can provide excellent imaging of the biliary tree. It is based on heavily T2-weighted images that portray static or slow moving fluids, such as bile, as high signal intensity images and surrounding tissues as low signal intensity images. Technological advances in MRCP such as three-dimensional images with fast advanced spin echo (FASE), maximum intensity projection (MIP), relaxation enhancement (RARE), and half-Fourier acquisition single-shot turbo spin-echo (HASTE) allow excellent visualization of the biliary tree with minimal breath-holding and no artifact. Ferric ammonium citrate solution can be given to the patient prior to the procedure to provide a negative contrast material for the T2-weighted images and remove signals from other abdominal fluids.

MRCP has numerous advantages as compared to ERCP. It is non-invasive, has no known complications, is not operator dependent, can provide imaging of the bile ducts both proximal and distal to any obstructions, and does not require any preparation or contrast administration. It is particularly helpful in patients who have undergone prior surgical reconstruction of the upper gastrointestinal tract resulting in anatomy that would not allow passage of an endoscope. It is also of use in patients who have proximal gastrointestinal stenoses, pancreatitis, cholangitis, or who are unable to undergo upper endoscopy for another reason. The advantages of MRCP can be limited by ascites or other fluid collections in the upper abdomen that will limit visualization of the bile ducts.

Patients should fast 4–6 hours before the procedure to promote gallbladder filling and gastric emptying. The gallbladder is visualized in

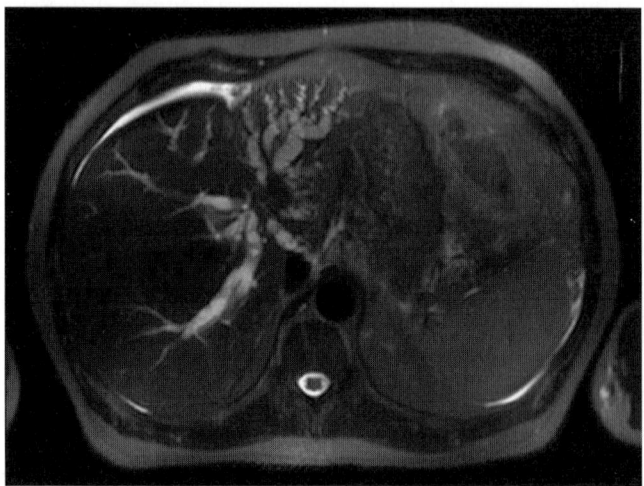

Figure 3. Cholangiocarcinoma.

approximately 90% of patients, while the cystic duct and hepatic duct bifurcation are visualized in 70–80% of cases. Biliary tract anatomic variants are frequently identified as well. Cholelithiasis is accurately identified in 80% of patients, while choledocolithiasis is accurately identified in 90–100% of cases. Small stones less than 2–3 mm can result in false negatives. Stones are seen as low signal intensities which are surrounded by hyperintense bile. However, air, artifact, blood clot, or neoplasm may have a similar appearance to stones. MRCP can accurately identify bile duct obstruction in nearly 100% of cases. This can be seen as ductal dilatation, a hypointense filling void surrounded by the hyperintense signaling of bile, or irregular borders of the biliary tree. MRCP can identify the level of obstruction and characterize the bile duct proximal and distal to the obstruction. It can detect the location and extent of cholangiocarcinomas (Figure 3). The sensitivity of MRCP in detecting pancreaticobiliary malignancies is 60–94%, while the specificity is 85–100%,[5] which is equivalent to that of ERCP. MRCP can also detect bile leaks rather easily, but cannot detect whether or not a leak is active.

REFERENCES

1. Ariyama J. Cholecystitis and Mirizzi syndrome. In: Okunda K, Mitchell DG, Itai Y, Ariyam J (eds). *Hepatobiliary Diseases: Pathophysiology and Imaging.* Oxford, Blackwell Science, 2001. pp.682–695.
2. Wald C, Scholz FJ, Pinkus E, *et al.* An update on biliary imaging. *Surg Clin North Am.* 2008;88(6):1195–220,viii.
3. Alobaidi M, Gupta R, Jafri SZ, *et al.* Current trends in imaging evaluation of acute cholecystitis. *Emerg Radiol* 2004;10(5):256–258.
4. Schoeman MK, Huibregtse K, Reeders J. Endoscopic cholangiography and pancreatography. In: DJ van Leeuwen, J Reeders, J Ariyama (eds). *Imaging in Hepatobiliary and Pancreatic Disease.* WB Saunders, 2000; pp. 309–332.
5. Hekimoglu K, Ustundag Y, Dusak A, *et al.* MRCP vs. ERCP in the evaluation of biliary pathologies: review of current literature. *J Dig Dis* 2008;9(3): pp. 162–169.

BENIGN GALLBLADDER DISEASE: CHOLELITHIASIS, POLYPS, GALLSTONE ILEUS   20

Kelley Hutcheson* and Dan G. Blazer III[†]

INTRODUCTION

The gallbladder is a pear-shaped organ located on the inferior surface of the liver. Its purpose is to collect, concentrate and store bile between meals. After eating, bile is ejected from the gallbladder, primarily in response to the release of cholecystokinin (CCK), where it travels through the common bile duct into the duodenum. Passage into the duodenum is also enhanced by relaxation of the sphincter of Oddi. Disruption in normal bile physiology can result in gallstone formation (cholelithiasis).

GALLSTONES

Cholelithiasis is common. Approximately 10–15% of the adult population, or more than 20 million people in the United States, have gallstones. It is estimated that there are about 1 million newly diagnosed patients annually. As a cause of hospitalization, gallstones are the most common and most costly digestive disease, with an annual estimated overall cost of more than $5 billion.

---

*Washington University School of Medicine, St Louis, Missouri, USA
[†]Duke University Medical Center, Durham, NC 27710 USA

Gallstones can be classified as cholesterol and pigment types. Cholesterol stones are at least 70% cholesterol and represent the vast majority (>85%) of stones in Western countries. Pigment stones may be black or brown and result secondary to the presence of calcium bilirubinate. They contain less than 20% cholesterol. Black stones typically form in the gallbladder and represent 10–15% of stones in Western industrialized countries, though they make up a higher percentage in Asian countries. They are also more commonly associated with hemolytic disorders, cirrhosis, and hyperalimentation. Brown stones are more commonly found in the bile ducts and are associated with bacterial contamination of the biliary tract. Though they represent a small minority in Western countries, they are much more common in Asian populations, in part due to the endemic nature of certain biliary parasites.

Gallstone formation is multifactorial but essentially results when the ability of the hepatobiliary system to maintain cholesterol or calcium salts in solution is overwhelmed. Bile is a complex aqueous solution which includes the biliary lipids — cholesterol, phospholipids, and bile salts. These lipids are typically maintained in an equilibrium that enables them to remain in solution. Factors affecting gallbladder motility or bile composition can disrupt this equilibrium and stone formation results. A more detailed description of gallstone pathophysiology is beyond the scope of this short review. Though a complete understanding of why certain people form gallstones remains to be elucidated, several risk factors for gallstone formation are well understood (Table 1).

Table 1. Known risks associated with developing cholelithiasis.

- Pregnancy
- Female sex
- Family history of gallstones
- Obesity (BMI >30kg/m^2)
- Ileal disease, resection or bypass
- Age >40 years
- Drugs: oral contraceptives, estrogen replacement therapy
- Diabetes mellitus
- Rapid weight loss
- Ethnicity: native American, Scandinavian
- TPN
- Hemolytic disease: heredity spherocytosis, thalassemia, sickle cell disease
- Hepatic cirrhosis

ASYMPTOMATIC CHOLELITHIASIS

Interestingly, despite the widespread prevalence of cholelithiasis, not all patients develop symptoms. Existing data indicate that 10% of patients will develop symptoms in the first 5 years after diagnosis and approximately 20% by 20 years. Thus, it is often said that patients develop symptoms at a rate of about 1–2% per year. Almost all patients will experience symptoms for some period of time before they develop a complication. Therefore, with few exceptions, prophylactic treatment of asymptomatic patients is not indicated. Diabetic patients should be treated promptly when symptoms first appear because of higher morbidity and mortality rates with emergency operations in this subset of patients. Incidental cholecystectomy during nonbiliary abdominal surgery in asymptomatic individuals is also not warranted. Though gallstones are associated with gallbladder cancer, risk of gallbladder malignancy, except in the case of a porcelain gallbladder, is also not a reasonable justification for prophylactic treatment as its incidence is so low (1 per 1000 patients per year).

SYMPTOMATIC CHOLELITHIASIS

The primary symptom related to cholelithiasis is biliary colic, which results when the gallbladder contracts against an obstructing stone. Attacks of biliary colic are discrete but severe enough that most patients can recall them when carefully questioned. The pain usually occurs in the epigastrium or right upper quadrant, is severe, and typically resolves after a few hours. It is commonly associated with ingestion of foods high in fat content. It can also be accompanied by other symptoms including nausea and vomiting, belching and bloating. Pain persisting longer than 1 day or accompanied by fever or jaundice usually reflects more serious illnesses including acute cholecystitis or choledocholithiasis and requires more urgent intervention. Patients with gallstones but an atypical clinical presentation should have other causes of right upper quadrant pain thoroughly evaluated, including peptic ulcer disease, pneumonia, renal calculi, liver disease, hernia, reflux, or angina prior to surgical intervention for gallstones.

When clinical suspicion for symptomatic cholelithiasis arises, right upper quadrant ultrasound is the diagnostic imaging modality of choice. In the workup of other clinical issues, incidental note may be made of the presence of gallstones on other imaging modalities, including computed tomography scans and MRI scans. For further details on the diagnosis of cholelithiasis, see Chapter 19.

When the presence of gallstones is established by imaging and the clinical picture suggests symptomatic cholelithiasis, surgical intervention is warranted. Once gallstone symptoms appear, they recur in the majority of patients. In addition, more severe complications of gallstone disease such as cholecystitis or cholangitis may occur.

Laparoscopic cholecystectomy is the procedure of choice for symptomatic cholelithiasis. For a full discussion of the technique of cholecystecomy, refer to Chapter 31. Almost 90% of patients with typical biliary colic become symptom-free after cholecystectomy and it remains the gold standard for management. Cholecystectomy is one of the top 10 procedures performed annually in U.S. hospitals. Annually, approximately 600,000 patients undergo cholecystectomy.

GALLBLADDER DYSKINESIA

There is a small group of patients without gallstones and no other identifiable abnormality of the gallbladder who have typical biliary pain. Biliary colic-type pain attributable to gallbladder dyskinesia is a diagnosis of exclusion. Other functional and organic disorders should be evaluated and excluded. These patients may have abnormal gallbladder emptying, usually defined as a gallbladder ejection fraction less than 35–40% with cholescintigraphy after injection of cholecystokinin. Pain may be relieved after gallbladder removal in some of these patients, with successs rates greater than 90% in appropriately selected patients.

GALLBLADDER POLYPS

Gallbladder polyps are outgrowths of the gallbladder mucosa wall that are usually found incidentally by ultrasonography or in pathologic specimens after cholecystectomy. Gallbladder polyps have been observed in 0.004–13.8% of resected gallbladders[4] and up to 4.5% of gallbladders assessed by ultrasonography.[5] Unlike gallstones, no association has been observed between the presence of polyps and certain risk factors including patient age, sex, weight, number of pregnancies, or use of exogenous female hormones. Several types of gallbladder polyps exist: cholesterol polyps (cholesterolosis), adenomas, adenomyomatosis, inflammatory polyps, and other rare benign lesions (leiomyomas, lipomas, hemangiomas).

Cholesterol polyps account for about half of all polypoid lesions of the gallbladder. Cholesterolosis results from epithelium-covered, cholesterol-laden macrophages in the lamina propria. The pathologic appearance of yellow deposits on a hyperemic mucosal background is the classically described "strawberry gallbladder." No particular risk factors have been identified. These lesions have no malignant potential.

Adenomatous polyps of the gallbladder are rare. Although the true incidence is unknown, the reported literature cites an incidence of less than 0.5%. Adenomas arise from the epithelial layer of the gallbladder and may be tubular or papillary. More than 90% of adenomas are solitary lesions. These lesions are considered premalignant. Though malignant transformation is rare, size appears to be an important risk factor for transformation. A size greater than 1 cm is associated with foci of carcinoma and resection is indicated. For a complete discussion of gallbladder andenocarcinoma, see Chapter 25.

Adenomyomatosis of the gallbladder is a rare condition characterized by localized or diffuse hyperplastic extension of the mucosa into a thickened muscular layer. These changes can result in focal thickening of the gallbladder and may resemble gallbladder carcinoma on imaging studies. However, these lesions are not considered premalignant.

Inflammatory polyps are the least common of the benign polyps. They are either sessile or pedunculated and are composed of granulation and fibrous tissue with plasma cells and lymphocytes. Polyps usually range from 5 to 10 mm in diameter, although they rarely grow larger than 1 cm. When large, these polyps can be confused with gallbladder carcinoma. They are associated with chronic cholecystitis.

Though gallbladder polyps may present with symptoms similar to biliary colic, the majority of these lesions are discovered incidentally by ultrasound or other imaging study during workup for other abdominal conditions. When gallbladder polyps are identified incidentally, the issue arises as to their management. No imaging study can reliably differentiate benign from premalignant polypoid lesions.

Given this uncertainty, most agree that patients with symptoms attributable to polypoid lesions should undergo cholecystectomy. In addition, large polyps (greater than 1 cm) are considered to have the greatest potential for malignant transformation and these patients should undergo cholecystectomy. Polyps of 1–2 cm size carry a greater than 40% likelihood of at least *in situ* carcinoma. Polyps larger than 2 cm are nearly always malignant with advanced cancer present in many cases. For patients, with lesions smaller than 1 cm, ultrasonographic surveillance may be implemented.

One group recommends follow-ups in 3 months, 6 months, and then yearly.[17] An increase in polyp size is an absolute indication for surgery.

Patients who have gallbladder polyps along with gallstones should undergo cholecystectomy regardless of polyp size or symptoms since gallstones are a risk factor for gallbladder cancer in patients with gallbladder polyps.[4,14] Gallbladder polyps in the setting of primary sclerosing cholangitis are frequently malignant and require cholecystectomy.[15]

GALLSTONE ILEUS

Gallstone ileus occurs in less than 0.5% of patients with cholelithiasis making it an unusual complication. Despite its overall rarity, it is responsible for 1–4% of all cases of mechanical small bowel obstruction and, in patients over 65 years of age, gallstone ileus may account for 25% of nonstrangulated small bowel obstruction.[19] There is a 5:1 female/male predominance. Thus, gallstone ileus is an important entity to consider in the differential diagnosis of an elderly female patient with symptoms of intestinal obstruction.

Gallstones most commonly enter the bowel lumen through a biliary enteric fistula, although rare cases have been reported after endoscopic sphincterotomy. Biliary enteric fistula complicates approximately 1–3% of patients with acute cholecystitis. Fistulae are formed with the duodenum in roughly two-thirds of cases, with colonic and gastric fistulas also described.

The specific mechanism which results in gallstone ileus involves three steps: fistula formation, stone passage, and stone impaction at a narrowing in the bowel. The mechanism of fistula formation begins with pericholecystic inflammation after cholecystitis leading to the development of adhesions between the biliary and enteric systems. The inciting gallstone then presses on the biliary wall causing pressure necrosis which causes erosion and fistula formation. Once gallstones have passed into the small bowel, they increase in diameter as they pass distally due to sedimentation of bowel contents. More than 90% of obstructing stones are longer than 2 cm in diameter, with the majority measuring over 2.5 cm.[21] The most common site of impaction for up to 70% of gallstones is the ileum, the narrowest segment of the intestine. The jejunum and stomach are the sites that are next most frequently affected.[20] Colonic obstruction is less frequent as the normal colonic diameter is sufficient to allow for stone passage. If colonic obstruction does occur, it tends to occur at sites of pre-existing pathology, such as a diverticular stricture. Appendiceal obstruction by a gallstone is reported but rare. It is also important to remember that multiple gallstones may be found along the obstructed bowel so all of the bowel should be examined at the time of surgical intervention.

Gallstone ileus classically presents as episodic subacute bowel obstruction in an elderly female. Transient gallstone impaction produces abdominal distention, pain, and vomiting, which subside as the gallstone becomes disimpacted. Symptoms intermittently recur as the progressively larger stone lodges in the more distal bowel lumen. As a result, vague intermittent symptoms are commonly present for days prior to evaluation or diagnosis. The mean symptom duration before hospital admission is roughly 5 days.[20] Hematemesis occasionally occurs due to hemorrhage at the site of the biliary enteric fistula. Gastric outlet obstruction secondary to gallstone impaction in the duodenum or pylorus is referred to as Bouveret's syndrome, whose presenting symptoms are epigastric pain, nausea, and vomiting.

On physical examination, the patient often appears dehydrated with vital signs reflecting this state: tachycardia, mild hypotension, even fever. Common abdominal signs include distension, tympany and hyper-resonant bowel sounds. Jaundice occurs in less than 15% of cases.[20] Due to the prevalence of gallstone ileus in elderly patients, many patients have serious comorbid medical conditions, including coronary artery disease, pulmonary disease, and diabetes mellitus which affect management decisions.

The most important factor affecting the diagnosis of this condition is clinical suspicion which must be maintained even in patients with no known history of biliary disease. Roughly one-half of patients found to have gallstone ileus have no prior history of biliary stone disease. Laboratory values are also nonspecific reflecting dehydration (electrolyte imbalances, leukocytosis, elevated aminotransferase levels). The diagnosis can be suggested by findings on a plain abdominal radiograph (pneumobilia, intestinal obstruction, direct or indirect visualization of a gallstone), although these findings may be present in only 30% of plain films. Computed tomography scanning offers better visualization of the impacted stone in most cases and has largely supplanted plain films in ascertaining the diagnosis, with successful diagnosis in up to three-quarters of cases.[19,22]

Prompt diagnosis of gallstone ileus and treatment are essential to relieve intestinal obstruction after adequate volume resuscitation. The main management controversy lies in the decision to perform concomitant biliary surgery at the time of operation. Surgical management options include enterolithotomy alone versus enterolithotomy and definitive biliary repair (cholecystectomy, repair of cholecystoenteric fistula), i.e. one-stage repair.

Most authors advocate enterolithotomy alone in the surgical management of gallstone ileus, given the commonly associated comorbidities in this typically frail elderly patient population. In Reisner's review of 1001 cases of gallstone ileus, postoperative mortality was higher in patients undergoing definitive one-stage repair versus enterolithotomy alone (17% versus. 11%). Enterolithotomy can be performed via laparoscopy or laparotomy. With either approach, a longitudinal enterotomy is made along the antimesenteric intestinal border proximal to the point of impaction. The stone is milked proximally and removed. The entire bowel must be examined to evacuate any additional stones, which occur in up to 16% of cases. The enterotomy is then closed in a transverse fashion to avoid narrowing of the bowel lumen. Manipulation of stones through the bowel must be done carefully to avoid transmural injury. The cecum is particularly vulnerable to undetected transmural injury and therefore milking of stones through it should not be performed routinely. Bowel resection using standard techniques is required where perforation, bowel ischemia, or unmoveable gallstones are identified.

Because persistent or recurrent symptoms related to biliary enteric fistula — recurrent gallstone ileus, cholecystitis, cholangitis — requiring reoperation may occur in up to 20% of patients, some authors advocate one-stage repair in fit, stable patients where the right upper quadrant is accessible for cholecystectomy and biliary tract inspection. In addition, interval elective laparoscopic cholecystectomy can be considered after enterolithotomy in patients with symptoms or residual cholelithiasis if nonbiliary disease does not pose an unacceptable risk for further surgery.

Nonsurgical treatments for gallstone ileus are desirable in high-risk patients too sick for conventional surgical treatment. Case reports of successful extracorporeal lithotripsy of obstructing stones in the jejunum, stomach, and colon have been reported[24,25,26] however, abdominal gas containing bowel loops may prevent visualization of the obstruction by ultrasonography, thereby precluding extracorporeal lithotripsy. Endoscopic removal of gallstones from the colon and duodenum has also been described.[27] Ultimately, however, surgery remains the gold standard therapy.

REFERENCES

1. SAGES. Society of American Gastrointestinal and Endoscopic Surgeons. http://www.sages.org/publication/id/PI11/.
2. Chari RS, Shah SA. Biliary system in townsend In: CM Townsend, RD Beauchamp, BM Evers, RL Mattox, (eds). *Sabiston Textbook of Surgery*. 18th edition, Philadelphia. Pennsylvania W.B. Saunders Publishing. 2007.
3. Gallstones and Laparoscopic Cholecystectomy, NIH Consens Statement 1992 Sep 14–16; 10(3):1–20. http://www.ncbi.nlm.nih.gov/bookshelf/br.fcgi?book=hsnihcdc&part=A11132.
4. Yang, HL, Sun, YG, Wang, Z. Polypoid lesions of the gallbladder: Diagnosis and indications for surgery. *Br J Surg* 1992; 79:227.
5. Jorgensen, T, Jensen, KH. Polyps in the gallbladder. A prevalence study. *Scand J Gastroenterol* 1990; 25:281.
6. Stringer, MD, Ceylan, H, Ward, K, Wyatt, JI. Gallbladder polyps in children — classification and management. *J Pediatr Surg* 2003; 38:1680.
7. Christensen, AH, Ishak, KG. Benign tumors and pseudotumors of the gall bladder. Report of 180 patients. *Arch Pathol* 1970; 90:423.
8. Feldman, M, Feldman, M Jr. Cholesterosis of the gallbladder; an autopsy study of 165 cases. *Gastroenterology* 1954; 27:641.
9. Shepard, VD, Walters, W, Dockerty, MB. Benign neoplasms of the gallbladder. *Arch Surg* 1942; 45:1.
10. Kubota, K, Bandai, Y, Noie, T, et al. How should polypoid lesions of the gallbladder be treated in the era of laparoscopic cholecystectomy?. *Surgery* 1995; 117:481.
11. Sugiyama, M, Xie, XY, Atomi, Y, Saito, M. Differential diagnosis of small polypoid lesions of the gallbladder: The value of endoscopic ultrasonography. *Ann Surg* 1999; 229:498.
12. Sugiyama, M, Atomi, Y, Yamato, T. Endoscopic ultrasonography for differential diagnosis of polypoid gall bladder lesions: Analysis in surgical and follow up series. *Gut* 2000; 46:250.
13. Gurusamy, KS, Abu-Amara, M, Farouk, M, Davidson, BR. Cholecystectomy for gallbladder polyp. *Cochrane Database Syst Rev* 2009; CD007052.
14. Terzi, C, Sokmen, S, Seckin, S, et al. Polypoid lesions of the gallbladder: Report of 100 cases with special reference to operative indications. *Surgery* 2000; 127:622.
15. Buckles, DC, Lindor, KD, Larusso, NF, et al. In primary sclerosing cholangitis, gallbladder polyps are frequently malignant. *Am J Gastroenterol* 2002; 97:1138.
16. Kmiot, WA, Perry, EP, Donovan, IA, et al. Cholesterolosis in patients with chronic acalculous biliary pain. *Br J Surg* 1994; 81:112.

17. Koga, A, Watanabe, K, Fukuyama, T, *et al.* Diagnosis and operative indications for polypoid lesions of the gallbladder. *Arch Surg* 1988; 123:26.
18. Up to Date: www.Uptodate.com.
19. Reisner, RM, Cohen, JR. Gallstone ileus: A review of 1001 reported cases. *Am Surg* 1994; 60:441.
20. Clavien, PA, Richon, J, Burgan, S, *et al.* Gallstone ileus. *Br J Surg* 1990; 77:737.
21. Deitz, DM, Standage, BA, Pinson, CW, *et al.* Improving the outcome in gallstone ileus. *Am J Surg* 1986; 151:572.
22. Ayantunde, AA, Agrawal, A. Gallstone ileus: diagnosis and management. *World J Surg* 2007; 31:1292.
23. Rodriguez-Sanjuan, JC, Casado, F, Fernandez, MJ, *et al.* Cholecystectomy and fistula closure versus enterolithotomy alone in gallstone ileus. *Br J Surg* 1997; 84:634.
24. Sackmann, M, Holl, J, Haerlin, M, *et al.* Gallstone ileus successfully treated by shock-wave lithotripsy. *Dig Dis Sci* 1991; 36:1794.
25. Bourke, MJ, Scheider DM, Haber, GB. Electrohydraulic lithotripsy of a gallstone causing gallstone ileus. *Gastrointest Endosc* 1997; 45:521.
26. Meyenberger, C, Michel, C, Metzger, U, Koelz, HR. Gallstone ileus treated by extracorporeal shockwave lithotripsy. *Gastrointest Endosc* 1996; 43:508.
27. Oakland, DJ, Denn, PG. Endoscopic diagnosis of gallstone ileus of the duodenum. *Dig Dis Sci* 1986; 31:98.
28. http://www.surgery.com/procedure/cholecystectomy/demographics.
29. Feldman's.

BENIGN GALLBLADDER DISEASE: CHOLECYSTITIS 21

Ryan Turley, Kelley Hutcheson and
Lisa Pickett*

ACUTE CALCULOUS CHOLECYSTITIS

Acute cholecystitis is clinically described by the triad of right upper quadrant pain, fever, and leukocytosis in conjuction with evidence of gallbladder inflammation. It is estimated that 25 million Americans have cholelitihiasis with 1–2% of these patients developing symptoms or complications per year. Based on these numbers, cholecystectomy is one of the most commonly performed surgeries in the United States, with 700,000 estimated to be performed annually.[1]

Pathogenesis

In the vast majority of cases, acute cholecystitis is a reactive inflammatory process resulting from cystic duct obstruction caused by gallstones. Cystic duct obstruction alone, however, is not sufficient to cause acute cholecystitis. Rather, the resultant biliary stasis or mucosal trauma seen in cystic duct obstruction causes the release of various inflammatory enzymes and mediators responsible for the development of acute cholelithiasis. One such enzyme is phospholipase A, which converts lecithin, a normal bile constituent, to lysolecithin. Studies have shown lysolecithin to be present in

---

*Duke University Hospital, Durham, NC 27710 USA

patients with acute cholecystitis and absent in normal individuals. In animal models, acute cholecystitis can be reproduced by ligating the cystic duct and installing lysolecithin into the biliary system.[2]

Inflammatory prostaglandins are also thought to be involved in the cascade leading to acute cholecystitis. Analysis of human tissue has demonstrated higher levels of prostaglandins in acute cholecystitis. Further supporting the role of prostaglandins in the development of the acute cholecystitis, a prospective, placebo-controlled study demonstrated diclofenac, a prostaglandin synthetase inhibitor, to prevent the development of acute cholecystitis in patients with pre-existing biliary colic.[3]

Although bacteria are not believed to precipitate acute cholecystitis, secondary biliary infection is common, with a frequency approaching up to 50%. Escherichia coli, Enterococcus, Klebsiella, and Enterobacter are the most common isolates. Infection of the gallbladder wall can lead to the formation of a cholecystic abcess or empyema. If gas-forming organisms are present, emphysematous cholecystitis can occur.[1]

Clinical Presentation

The hallmark triad of acute calculus cholecystitis includes right upper quadrant pain, fever, and leukocystosis. The typical abdominal pain is described in the right upper quadrant or epigastric area, and may radiate to the right shoulder or scapula. In constrast to biliary colic, the right upper quadrant pain associated with acute cholecystitis can be prolonged and steady. In fact, pain lasting more than 4–6 hours should raise the suspicion for acute cholecystitis. Many patients endorse nausea, bloating, vomiting and anorexia. Classically, there is a history of fatty food ingestion prior to onset of abdominal pain.

Physical Examination

Patients with acute cholecystitis are often in distress, febrile, and tachycardic. True acute cholecystitis leads to focal inflammation of local parietal peritoneum. Therefore, patients typically exhibit clinical symptoms of peritonitis. Patients generally lie still on the examining table to avoid pain associated with movement. Abdominal examination usually demonstrates voluntary and involuntary guarding.

The classic physical examination finding in acute cholecystitis is the "Murphy's sign". To elicit this sign, the examiner palpates just beneath the liver edge in the right upper quadrant of the abdomen. While palpating, the examiner asks the patient to inspire deeply, causing the gallbladder to descend toward the examiners hands. Patients with acute cholecystitis generally endorse worsening pain during inspiration or even have inspiratory arrest.

Diagnosis

The diagnosis of cholecystitis relies on a combination of clinical, radiological and, laboratory data. Acute cholecystitis should be suspected for any patient presenting with the clinical symptoms outlined above and with evidence of gallstones on an imaging study. Care should be noted, however, as radiographic evidence of cholelithiasis is in itself insufficient to diagnose acute cholecystitis.

A systematic review of 17 previously published studies examining the role of the history, physical examination and/or laboratory tests in adults with abdominal pain or suspected acute cholecystitis showed no single clinical or laboratory finding could accurately determine the diagnosis. However, the correct diagnosis was often made when the history, physical examination, laboratory, and radiologic findings were taken account together.[4]

Laboratory Evaluation

Laboratory workup in a patient with suspected acute cholecystitis includes a white blood cell count with differential, liver function tests including total bilirubin, alkaline phosphatase, and serum aminotransferases. Patients often have leukocytosis and increased band forms. In uncomplicated cholecystitis, serum total bilirubin and alkaline phosphatase are normal. Elevations of these values should prompt further investigation for possible complicating conditions including choledocholithiasis, cholangitis, and Mirizzi syndrome. However, mild elevations in serum aminotransferases and amylase can be seen in uncomplicated cholecystitis, hypothesized to occur from passage of small stones, sludge or infection.

Imaging studies

Patients presenting with clinical features suggestive of acute cholecystitis require further radiographic imaging tests to confirm the diagnosis. The two most common modalities include ultrasonography and nuclear cholescintigraphy

Ultrasonography

The first radiographic study for any patient with suspected acute cholecystitis should be a right upper quadrant ultrasound. Advantages of ultrasound include its portability, anatomic accuracy, and lack of ionizing radiation. It is most sensitive in a patient who has been fasting for at least 8 hours, as this leads to gallbladder distention and improved detection of echogenic objects such as stones. A systemic review of 30 previously published studies of ultrasound in detecting biliary disease approximated the sensitivity and specificity of ultrasonogarphy for detecting gallstones as 84% and 99%, respectively. For stones greater than 2 mm, the sensitivity of ultrasound is increased to greater than 95%.[5]

The mere presence of gallstones is insufficient to make the diagnosis of cholecystitis. However, ultrasound of the gallbladder can demonstrate other features supporting the diagnosis including pericholecystic fluid, gallbladder wall thickening greater than 4 mm, as well as the sonographic Murphy's sign. The sonographic Murphy's sign is elicited when the ultrasonographer elicits focal gallbladder tenderness directly under the ultrasound transducer. This clinical test is thought to be superior to the clinical Murphy's sign expressed on physical exam as the ultrasound transducer is more likely to be placed directly over the gallbladder.

Cholescintigraphy

If the diagnosis of acute cholecystitis remains uncertain after ultrasonagraphy, the next recommended radiographic study is cholescintigraphy or HIDA scan. During cholescintigraphy, technetium-labeled hepatic iminodiacetic acid (HIDA), is injected intravenously. HIDA is preferentially taken up by hepatocytes and excreted into bile. If the cystic duct is patent, this agent will enter the gallbladder, leading to its visualization without the need for concentration. The HIDA scan is also useful for demonstrating patency of the common bile duct and ampulla. Visualization of contrast within the common bile duct, gallbladder, and small bowel occurs within 30–60 minutes.

A positive HIDA scan is indicated by non-visualization of the gallbladder. The sensitivity and specificity of a HIDA scan for acute cholecystitis is approximately 97% and 90%, respectively.[5] Sources of false positives include cystic duct obstruction from a stone or tumor, severe liver disease, total parental nutrition, previous biliary sphincterotomy, and hyperbilirubinemia. False negative results are rare since most patients with acute cholecystitis have cystic duct obstruction.

Magnetic resonance cholangiography

Magnetic resonance cholangiopancreatography (MRCP) is a rapid, non-invasive technique for imaging bile and pancreatic ducts. Within the scope of cholecystitis, MRCP is reserved for ruling out choledocholithiasis in patients with a low to moderate pre-test probability in effort to avoid the more invasive endoscopic retrograde cholangiopancreatography (ERCP).

CT scan

Abdominal computed tomography (CT) is most useful for detecting complications of acute cholecystitis, such as gallbladder perforation or emphysematous cholecystitis. A diagnosis of cholecystitis by CT scan generally occurs during evaluation for other abdominal pathologies. Even though a CT scan can detect gallbladder wall thickening, pericholecystic fluid, and high-attenuation bile, it remains unnecessary for the diagnosis of acute cholecystitis due to the high sensivity, specificifity, and portability of ultrasound.

Management

Intravenous antibiotics with activity against gram-negative and anaerobic activity should be initiated at the time of diagnosis of acute cholecystitis and stopped after cholecystectomy.

The definitive treatment of acute cholecystitis is cholecystectomy. Historically, the timing of cholecystectomy has been controversial as many surgeons believed early surgery for acute cholecystitis resulted in more complications, longer operative time, and higher conversion rates from laparoscopic to open techniques. These surgeons would opt for 1 week of antibiotics with a delayed, elective surgery 6–8 weeks later However, meta-analysis of five randomized trials including 451 patients comparing early versus delayed laparoscopic cholecystectomy showed decreased length of stay and reduced costs in the laparoscopic group with no difference in morbidity, mortality or conversion rates.[6] Presently, early intervention within 2–3 days of presenting symptoms is recommended.

Cholecystectomy should be started laparoscopically and converted to open if safe dissection is prevented by inflammation obscuring important structures. Absolute contraindications to laparoscopy include intolerance to pneumoperitoneum or the presence of a severe coagulopathy. Predictors of conversion from laparoscopic to open cholecystectomy include increased patient age, male gender, elevated American Society of Anesthesiologists class, obesity, and thickened gallbladder wall (>4mm).[7]

Patients presenting with complications of acute cholecystitis (empyema, emphysema, or perforation) will need an emergent cholecystectomy. If this patient cannot tolerate general anesthesia, drainage via a percutaneous cholecystostomy is recommended. However, cholecystectomy is the preferred and optimal treatment in most cases. If inflammation precludes safe dissection of the cystic duct, a partial cholecystectomy and drainage is an acceptable alternative to avoid common bile duct injury.[1]

Percutaneous cholecystostomy

Percutaneous cholecystostomy is indicated in high-risk patients in whom a laparoscopic or open cholecystectomy imposes a significant high risk of morbidity or mortality. A percutaneous cholecystostomy can be placed at bedside under ultrasound guidance or by interventional radiology under a combination of ultrasonic and fluoroscopic guidance. Although temporizing in most cases, percutaneous cholecystostomy does not remove the gallbladder, which may be source of ongoing sepsis. After drainage and IV antibiotics, interval laparoscopic cholecystectomy can be performed 2–4 months later.

Complications

Untreated acute cholecystitis can lead to gangrene, empyema, biliary-enteric fistula formation, and even perforation with spillage of infected bile into the abdominal cavity. The latter can lead to peritonitis, sepsis, and eventual death. Complications from cholecystectomy include bleeding, wound infection, hernia, hematoma, abscess formation, and bile leaks. Most leaks result from iatrogenic transection of the small cholecystohepatic ducts commonly known as the "Ducts of Luschka". The majority of these leaks will resolve without further intervention. Cystic duct leaks occur in less than 1% of laparoscopic cholecystectomies and are generally diagnosed by ERCP, ultrasound, cholescintigraphy, or CT scan. Cystic duct leaks can be treated successfully via endoscopic stenting and sphincterotomy. Common bile duct injuries are reported to occur in 0.1–0.2% of cases.[7]

CHRONIC CALCULOUS CHOLECYSTITIS

Chronic calculus cholecystitis is defined as recurrent biliary colic or pain resulting from chronic cystic duct obstruction. Approximately 3% of cholecystectomies are performed for chronic inflammation of the gallbladder.[1]

Clinical Presentation

Chronic cholecystitis generally presents with recurrent right upper quandrant pain usually accompanied by nausea, vomiting, and intolerance of food. Most attacks last 1–5 hours but less than 24 hours. If the pain lasts more than 24 hours, acute cholecystitis should be considered. Approximately 30% of patients suffer an initial episode of pain consistent with classic biliary colic without having an additional episode over the next 24 months. After the initial episode of biliary pain, 6% of patients per year will develop sufficient symptoms to justify a cholecystectomy.[8]

The diagnosis of chronic cholecystitis requires radiographic evidence of gallstones and presenting symptoms consistent with recurrent biliary colic. These patients generally lack classic radiographic signs of acute cholecystitis such as pericholecystic fluid, gallbladder wall thickening, and a sonographic Murphy's sign. The physical examination for chronic cholecystitis is for the most part unremarkable, but patients can have slight tenderness in their right quandrant during an acute attack. Liver functions tests are usually normal for patients with chronic cholecystitis.

The standard imaging modality for patients with chronic cholecystitis is ultrasound. On occasion, a right upper quandrant ultrasound will fail to demonstrate stones or only sludge will be seen. If sludge presents on two more ultrasounds without signs of true gallstones, cholecystectomy is indicated if symptomatic.

Management

The standard management of chronic calculus cholecystitis is elective laparoscopic cholecystectomy. Cholecystectomy should be expedited for diabetic patients as they have a higher risk of developing acute cholecystitis or even gangrenous cholecystitis.[9] Cholecystectomy offers excellent long-term results for patients with symptomatic gallstones.

ACUTE ACALCULOUS CHOLECYSTITIS

Acute acalculus cholecystitis is defined as acute inflammation of the gallbladder in the absence of cholelithiasis. Acute acalculus cholecystitis accounts for approximately 2–15% of cases of acute cholecystitis and is associated with elderly age, critical illness, burns, trauma, major surgery, total parental nutrition, diabetes, immunosuppression, and childbirth. Acaclulus cholecystitis has been reported to occur in 0.2% of surgical intensive care admissions with a mortality approaching 40%.[10] Complications of cholecystitis such as gangrene, empyema, and perforation are more common in acalculus cholecystitis as compared to calculous cholecystitis.[1]

Pathogenesis

The underlying mechanism leading to acalculus cholecystitis remains poorly understood. In the end, patients with acute acalculus cholecystitis have developed sufficient biliary stasis or mucosal inflammation leading to the release of inflammatory enzymes and mediators responsible for acute cholecystitis. Common risk factors for developing acalculus cholecystitis are indeed associated with bile stasis. Also, the critically ill often require vasoconstrictors to raise their blood pressure leading to mucosal ischemia and initiation of the inflammatory cascade.

Diagnosis

The diagnosis of acute acalculus cholecystitis can be subtle, usually requiring a high index of suspicion in patients with known risk factors. Patient complaints include classic biliary colic with accompanying fevers or nonspecific symptoms of fatigue and nausea. In the critically ill, the diagnosis is made during workup for persistent fevers of unknown origin. Workup is similar to calculus cholecystitis. Ultrasound will show gallbladder wall thickening and pericholecystic fluid without stones. HIDA scan is useful in patients with localized ascites as the pericholecystic fluid and gallbladder wall edema may be difficult to interpret.

Treatment

Treatment of acalculus cholecystitis is similar to calculus cholecystitis. However, many patients, especially those in the ICU, will be unfit to undergo laparoscopic cholecystectomy. Thus, percutaneous cholecystectomy is often the treatment of choice, with 90% patients demonstrating clinical improvement.[11] Patients with acalculus cholecystitis are more likely to develop emphysematous cholecystitis (denoted by gas within the gallbladder or gallbladder wall emphysema). These patients are best treated with emergent cholecystectomy or cholecystostomy to prevent rapid deterioration.

MIRIZZI SYNDROME

Mirizzi syndrome (MS) is the partial obstruction of the common hepatic bile duct secondary to chronic inflammation and impaction of gallstones in the adjacent gallbladder. MS occurs in about 0.1–0.7% of patients with cholelithiasis and is associated with an increased risk of gallbladder cancer.[12]

Pathogenesis

MS occurs in patients whose anatomy places the cystic duct in parallel to the common hepatic duct. Impaction of a gallstone in the cystic duct or neck or inflammation directly resulting from an impacted stone leads to common hepatic obstruction. Patients subsequently have intermittent or constant jaundice which can lead to cholangitis or even biliary cirrhosis from longstanding obstruction.[13]

Diagnosis

Symptoms of MS are similar to those of cholecystitis or choledocholithiasis including biliary colic, jaundice, and abnormal liver function tests. Diagnosis generally starts with a right upper quandrant ultrasound. If the laboratory tests are abnormal most patients will need a ERCP which has been reported to be 100% accurate for diagnosing MS.[14]

Based on imaging, MS is further subtyped into the Csendes classification:

Type I: External compression of the common bile duct.
Type II: A cholecystobiliary fistula is present involving less than one third the circumference of the bile duct.
Type III: A fistula is present involving up to two-thirds the circumference of the bile duct.
Type IV: A fistula is present with complete destruction of the wall of the bile duct.[15]

Treatment

Surgical treatment for MS based on type can be challenging. Type I MS can generally be treated with cholecystectomy alone in a fundus-down technique. If inflammation prevents satisfactory dissection of the Calot's triangle, a partial cholecystectomy with stone extraction is sufficient. Given the high risk of gallbladder cancer in MS patients, a frozen section should be sent to pathology.

For type II MS or above, a biliary fistula takedown is necessary and usually requires more complex reconstructions. If remnant gallbladder tissue appears healthy, the fistula can be repaired with this tissue with concurrent placement of a T-tube distally in the common bile duct. If the tissue is compromised, a Roux-en-Y reconstruction is recommended. For these patients, serious consideration should be given to transferring to a tertiary care center where complex biliary reconstructions are more commonly performed.[12]

REFERENCES

1. Elwood DR. Cholecystitis. *Surg Clin North Am* 2008; 88(6):1241–1252, viii.
2. Roslyn JJ, DenBesten L, Thompson JE, Jr., Silverman BF. Roles of lithogenic bile and cystic duct occlusion in the pathogenesis of acute cholecystitis. *Am J Surg* 1980; 140(1):126–130.
3. Browning JD JS. Gallstone disease. In: M Feldman, ed. *Sleisenger & Fordtran's Gastrointestinal and Liver Disease.* 8th edition, Philadelphia, Saunders Elsevier, 2006; pp. 1387–1343.
4. Trowbridge RL, Rutkowski NK, Shojania KG. Does this patient have acute cholecystitis? *JAMA* 2003; 289(1):80–86.

5. Shea JA, Berlin JA, Escarce JJ, et al. Revised estimates of diagnostic test sensitivity and specificity in suspected biliary tract disease. *Arch Intern Med* 1994; 28; 154(22):2573-2581.
6. Gurusamy KS, Samraj K. Early versus delayed laparoscopic cholecystectomy for acute cholecystitis. *Cochrane Database Syst Rev* 2006; (4):CD005440.
7. Chari R, SA Shah. Biliary section. In: C Townsend (ed). *Sabiston Textbook of Surgery*. Philadelphia, 2007; pp. 1547-1587.
8. Friedman GD. Natural history of asymptomatic and symptomatic gallstones. *Am J Surg* 1993; 165(4):399-404.
9. Fagan SP AS, Rahwan K, et al. Prognostic factors for the development of gangrenous cholecystitis. *Am J Surg* 2003; 186:481.
10. Kalliafas S, Ziegler DW, Flancbaum L, et al. Acute acalculous cholecystitis: incidence, risk factors, diagnosis, and outcome. *Am Surg* 1998; 64(5):471-475.
11. Barie PS, Eachempati SR. Acute acalculous cholecystitis. *Curr Gastroenterol Rep* 2003; 5(4): 302-309.
12. Zaliekas J, Munson JL. Complications of gallstones: the Mirizzi syndrome, gallstone ileus, gallstone pancreatitis, complications of "lost" gallstones. *Surg Clin North Am* 2008; 88(6):1345-1368, x.
13. Johnson LW, Sehon JK, Lee WC, et al. Mirizzi's syndrome: experience from a multi-institutional review. *Am Surg* 2001; 67(1):11-14.
14. Yeh CN, Jan YY, Chen MF. Laparoscopic treatment for Mirizzi syndrome. *Surg Endosc* 2003; 17(10):1573-1578.
15. Csendes A, Diaz JC, Burdiles P, et al. Mirizzi syndrome and cholecystobiliary fistula: a unifying classification. *Br J Surg* 1989; 76(11):1139-1143.
16. Reisner RM, Cohen JR. Gallstone ileus: a review of 1001 reported cases. *Am Surg* 1994; 60(6):441-446.
17. Clavien PA, Richon J, Burgan S, et al. *Br J Surg* 1990; 77(7):737-742.
18. Deitz DM, Standage BA, Pinson CW, et al. Improving the outcome in gallstone ileus. *Am J Surg* 1986; 151(5):572-576.
19. Ayantunde AA, Agrawal A. Gallstone ileus: diagnosis and management. *World J Surg* 2007; 31(6):1292-1297.
20. Sackmann M, Holl J, Haerlin M, et al. Gallstone ileus successfully treated by shock-wave lithotripsy. *Dig Dis Sci* 1991; 36(12):1794-1795.
21. Bourke MJ, Schneider DM, Haber GB. Electrohydraulic lithotripsy of a gallstone causing gallstone ileus. *Gastrointest Endosc* 1997; 45(6):521-523.
22. Meyenberger C, Michel C, Metzger U, et al. Gallstone ileus treated by extracorporeal shockwave lithotripsy. *Gastrointest Endosc* 1996; 43(5):508-511.
23. Oakland DJ, Denn PG. Endoscopic diagnosis of gallstone ileus of the duodenum. *Dig Dis Sci* 1986; 31(1):98-99.

BENIGN GALLBLADDER DISEASE: BILE DUCT INJURIES

22

Dawn M. Elfenbein[*] and
Mark Shapiro[*]

EPIDEMIOLOGY

Injury to the common bile duct is a dreaded complication of cholecystectomy. Although rare in terms of absolute percentages (less than 1%), the high volume of this surgery makes it likely that a surgeon will encounter a patient with, or will cause, a major bile duct injury. Injuries to the bile duct may also occur as a result of abdominal trauma; both blunt and penetrating trauma may cause injury. Other abdominal surgeries where the surgeon is working in close proximity to the liver may also result in iatrogenic bile duct injury. However, over 750,000 laparoscopic cholecystectomies are performed each year in the United States, and the vast majority of duct injuries occur during this operation.

The introduction of laparoscopy has turned cholecystectomy into an outpatient procedure, with many benefits to patients including shorter recovery time, less pain and smaller scars. However, population-based studies suggest that the incidence of bile duct injury is approximately two times higher, although still less than 1%, when using the minimally

---

[*]Duke University School of Medicine, Department of Surgery, Durham, North Carolina, USA

invasive approach.[1] Prompt recognition of these injuries is essential to improving outcomes, and during a laparoscopic approach, in addition to having a higher rate of injury to a major bile duct, recognition of an injury is more challenging than in the open surgery.

Although surgeon inexperience has been identified as one risk factor for common duct injury, one-third of these injuries occur in surgeons who have performed more than 200 laparoscopic cholecystectomies.[2] Misidentification of the biliary anatomy can happen to even the most experienced laparoscopic surgeons, and is by far the most common reason for injury to a major duct. The results of several large surveys indicate that somewhere between one-third and one-half of all general surgeons have caused a major bile duct injury. Several techniques have been proposed to reduce the incidence of this preventable complication. Intraoperative cholangiogram is used by some surgeons routinely, and there is good evidence that it aids in the early identification of injuries, as well as reduces the incidence and severity of injury.[3] However, because this absolute reduction in risk is quite low (0.4% risk of injury with IOC versus 0.6% risk of injury without), and doing a cholangiogram adds significant time and expense to the operation, there is not yet consensus about routine versus selective use of this imaging. Fellowship training in minimally invasive procedures is a recent postresidency training option, but the vast majority of these operations are performed by general surgeons without formal postresidency training. Therefore, it falls upon every surgeon who operates in the upper quadrants of the abdomen to be able to recognize when an injury has occurred and to know the best management of these injuries.

Patients whose injuries are identified at the time of surgery and promptly repaired have the best outcomes, but 55–90% of injuries are not recognized at the time of surgery.[4] Initial symptoms may be non-specific, and often occur after a patient has been discharged from the hospital. The classic signs and symptoms of a biliary leak include jaundice, biloma, sepsis, biliary fistula and biliary peritonitis. A surgical clip placed on a major duct can cause obstructive jaundice and cholangitis without biloma. Suspicion for a bile duct injury should be high in any patient who does not seem to be recovering easily after laparoscopic cholecystectomy, or in any patient who remains unwell after 48 hours. A missed bile duct injury may result eventually in strictures, which can present months or years after the injury. Patients with strictures may present with recurrent cholangitis and secondary biliary cirrhosis.

Extrahepatic traumatic biliary injuries are rare, and represent much less than 1% of all traumatic injuries. Penetrating trauma to the upper abdomen or blunt injuries can both cause injury to a major bile duct. Recognition of these injuries can be a challenge, and often the first sign that an injury has occurred is in the formation of a biloma days after the injury.[5]

WORK UP AND IMAGING

Patients who remain unwell after cholecystecomy should undergo a thorough investigation for bile duct injury. Physical examination findings may include jaundice and scleral icterus, abdominal pain that may range from vague pain to frank peritonitis, palpable mass in the case of a large biloma, fever, or bilious drainage from surgical drains. Laboratory evaluation should start with liver function biochemistry. Postoperative increase in alanine aminotranferase may be seen in up to 34% of patients, and may be a normal finding, but increases in bilirubin or alkaline phosphatase occur in only 9% and 4% of patients, respectively.[6] Increases in these in the postoperative period suggest either bile duct injury or stones in the common duct.

The initial imaging study for such patients should be ultrasonography. Ultrasound can detect common duct dilatation, which can be seen either in an obstructing type injury (such as from a surgical clip) or when stones are in the distal common duct. A bile leak-type injury will not cause duct dilatation, but an ultrasound can determine if there are any intra-abdominal fluid collections.

Computed tomography plays an ever-increasing role in diagnosis, and it does have a role in biliary injury. In patients who present with signs of intra-abdominal sepsis to the emergency room, a computed tomography is often the study of choice, and can be useful in identifying intra-abdominal fluid collections. Computed tomography can also identify intrahepatic ductal dilatation, which is associated with distal obstruction. Neither computed tomography nor ultrasonography delineates the precise injury, however, and every patient must undergo cholangiography in order to plan the appropriate management. At this time in the work-up, however, if fluid collections are identified, it is advisable to aspirate or place percutaneous drains prior to proceeding to cholangiography.

Endoscopic retrograde cholangiography (ERC) is often available and is technically easy to perform. Magnetic resonance cholangiopancreatography (MRCP) is a non-invasive alternative, but is available in fewer institutions and does not have the added benefit of being therapeutic that ERC offers. If a bile duct is transected, however, ERC will only show the anatomy

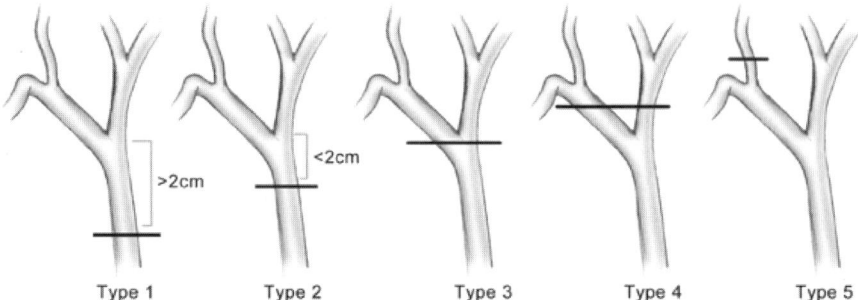

Figure 1. Percutaneous transhepatic cholangiogram showing a common bile duct injury.

up to the point of obstruction, and a percutaneous transhepatic cholangiography (PTC) is necessary to visualize the proximal anatomy and decompress the biliary tree. Often patients undergo more than one of these imaging techniques in order to fully visualize the injury (Figure 1).

MANAGEMENT OPTIONS

Once a patient with a bile duct injury is identified, the surgeon needs to understand that the mechanism of injury, location on the bile duct, timing of recognition, and potential involvement of nearby structures (i.e. vascular involvement) can all influence the most appropriate management. There are a variety of interventions currently available, ranging from endoscopic stent placement to image guided drainage to surgical reconstruction, and a thorough understanding of the pattern of injury is essential to determine the best treatment for an individual patient.

Bile leakage seen during any operation in the upper quadrants of the abdomen should prompt the surgeon to examine carefully for the source. Bile leaking from the gallbladder is usually thick and greenish, whereas bile from the common duct is much thinner and yellow. If a biliary injury is suspected, it is advisable to obtain an intraoperative cholangiogram to delineate the anatomy. If an injury is identified and the surgeon is a trained biliary surgeon or if one is immediately available, the procedure should be converted to an open operation and the injury should be repaired immediately (see Chapter 31: Bile Duct Injury Repair). If such expertise is unavailable, large bore drains should be placed and transfer of the patient should be considered. It is well documented that outcomes are improved when performed by an experienced hepatobiliary surgeon, and attempts at exploration by a less experienced surgeon may exacerbate the injury.

If an injury is not discovered intraoperatively, but suspected in the early postoperative period or in a trauma patient, a thorough work up with imaging as outlined above should commence. First and foremost, any bile collections must be drained. Undrained bile collections can become infected, are associated with postoperative complications, and may even be lethal. Always start by draining the bile, and then proceed to high quality imaging to delineate the anatomy of the injury. Several classification systems have been in use to describe the injury and to aid in management.

The Bismuth classification for biliary strictures is a simple and useful classification that can be quite helpful in determining the type of surgical repair the patient will require. Because surgical repair of bile duct injuries is often delayed for a period of weeks after the initial injury — long enough for strictures to form — this classification can be used quite successfully, and it is straightforward. The location of the stricture is paramount. Type I involve the common bile duct with a hepatic stump of >2 cm, Type II leaves a hepatic stump of <2 cm. Type III is a high injury that preserves the ductal confluence, and Type IV is a stricture that has destroyed the confluence. Type V is a tight sectoral duct stricture with or without common bile duct injury (Figure 2).

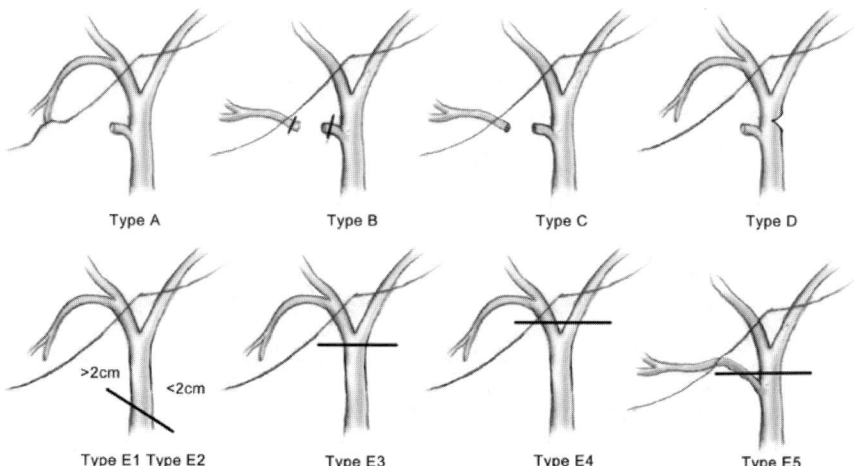

Figure 2. Bismuth classification.

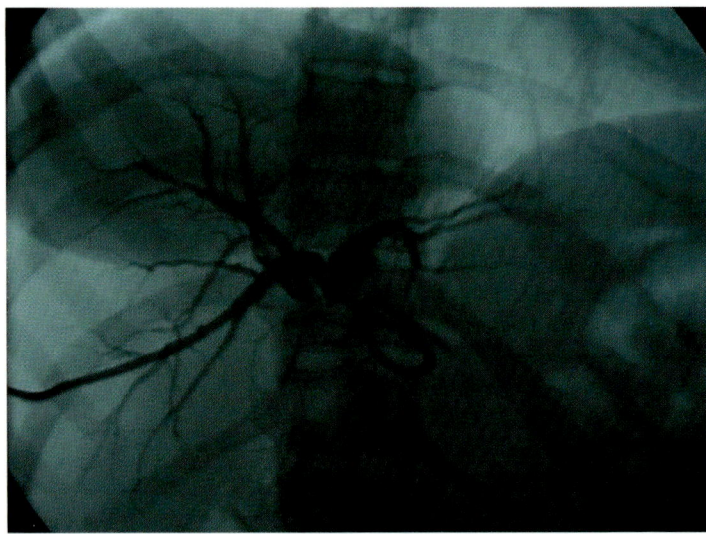

Figure 3. Strasberg scale.

The Bismuth classification does not take into account the severity of the initial bile duct injury, so the Strasberg scale was developed in 1995 as a modified version of the Bismuth classification of strictures. A type E injury on the Strasberg scale is a circumferential injury of the major bile ducts, and is further divided into five subtypes corresponding to the five locations of stricture on the Bismuth classification. Type A injuries are minor and result from injury to a minor duct at the cystic duct or liver bed. Type B injuries are ones that occlude (often from a surgical clip) part of the biliary tree that drains sections of the liver. The most common type B injury is injury to an aberrant right hepatic duct. Type C injuries are bile leaks from a duct not in communication with the common bile duct, and Type D injuries are bile leaks from ducts that are in communication with the common bile duct (Figure 3).

Several other classification schemes have been proposed that take into account other important aspects of the injury, and are useful in certain situations. The Mattox classification of extrahepatic biliary tree injuries focuses on the mechanism of injury and is useful in trauma. Type I injuries are contusions to the gallbladder or portal triad; Type II injuries are lacerations or perforations of the gallbladder; a type III injury is the complete avulsion of the gallbladder from the liver; Type IV injuries include partial (<50%) laceration of the common bile or hepatic duct; and Type V injuries are severe (>50%) transection of the common bile duct, intraduodenal or intrapancreatic ducts.

The Stewart–Way Laparoscopic Biliary Tract injury scale describes the types of injuries that can occur (incomplete transections, strictures, complete transection, or excision of right hepatic duct system), but is of little use for patient management. The Hannover classification has recently been proposed and includes additional discriminators for peripheral bile duct lesions and vascular injuries within the liver hilum, but with over 21 different patterns of injuries, may be somewhat cumbersome to use in everyday practice.

The use of nonoperative modalities for management of bile duct injuries is limited, as most injuries require definitive surgical repair. Patients who present with biliary sepsis, however, will need to have the sepsis controlled before repair. Possible modalities used in this situation include image-guided percutaneous drainage of fluid collections, percutaneous transhepatic decompression, and endoscopic decompression. For minor injuries, including cystic duct leak, endoscopic stent placement may be all that is required, but major injuries will eventually require repair once the patient is stabilized.

SURGERY

The goals for definitive operative repair of common bile duct injuries are to re-establish flow of bile into the gastrointestinal tract, prevent cholangitis and further strictures, and prevent progressive liver injury. The procedure of choice in almost all instances is a Roux-en-Y hepaticojejunostomy. In cases of complete division, primary end-to-end anastomosis of the cut ends of the duct over a T-tube is generally not recommended because of a high stricture rate, though some advocate this strategy in cases that are immediately recognized and there is not extensive tissue loss. In injuries detected at any time after the initial surgery, Roux-en-Y hepaticojejunostomy after drainage of collections and control of sepsis is the procedure of choice. Details about this procedure can be found in Chapter 31: Bile Duct Injury Repair.

OUTCOMES

The long-term results of bile duct injury repairs at the Johns Hopkins Hospital were reported in 2000.[7] A total of 156 patients underwent repair between 1990 and 2000; 75% of patients sustained injury during laparoscopic cholecystectomy, 22% during open cholecystectomy, and the rest during other surgery or trauma. The vast majority (93%) of injuries occurred outside the institution; one patient whose injury occurred at Hopkins underwent primary end-to-end anastamosis, but all other patients underwent Roux-en-Y hepaticojejunostomy. There were 13 failures (9.3%) after reconstruction, and 5 of those patients (38.5%) had undergone attempted repair prior to referral, again reinforcing the higher success rates in hands of experienced hepatobiliary surgeons and the strong recommendation to consider transfer once an injury has occurred.

In a recent study of 56 patients in Amsterdam who presented to a tertiary care center with complications after primary repair of the duct during the initial cholecystectomy, one-third of the patients required secondary surgical repair, while the majority of patients were managed using endoscopic or radiographic interventions alone.[8] This high rate of failure of primary anastomosis is unacceptable to some, while others interpret this study as one possible management strategy for injuries detected at the time of surgery where there is minimal tissue loss and no inflammation. Primary anastomosis is a simpler procedure than a hepaticojejunostomy, and two thirds of patients repaired this way did not require further operations. In the Hopkins study, of the 13 patients who failed reconstruction, only one patient underwent surgical revision, again demonstrating the success of endoscopic and radiographic interventions in managing strictures. Ideally, strictures should be avoided, not managed, and repair with Roux-en-Y hepaticojejunostomy in the hands of an experienced hepatobiliary surgeon has been demonstrated to be the procedure that leads to the greatest long-term success after bile duct injury.

REFERENCES

1. Jablonska B, Lampe P. Iatrogenic bile duct injuries: etiology, diagnosis and management. *World J Gastroenterol* 2009; 15(33):4097–4104.
2. Archer SB, Brown DW, Smith CD, Branum GD, Hunter JG. Bile duct injury during laparoscopic cholecystectomy: results of a national survey. *Ann Surg* 2001; 234(4):549–558; discussion 558–549.
3. Flum DR, Dellinger EP, Cheadle A, *et al.* Intraoperative cholangiography and risk of common bile duct injury during cholecystectomy. *JAMA* 2003; 289(13):1639–1644.
4. Connor S, Garden OJ. Bile duct injury in the era of laparoscopic cholecystectomy. *Br J Surg* 2006; 93(2):158–168.

5. Sawaya DE, Jr., Johnson LW, Sittig K, *et al.* Iatrogenic and noniatrogenic extrahepatic biliary tract injuries: a multi-institutional review. *Am Surg* 2001; 67(5):473–477.
6. Andrei VE, Schein M, Margolis M, *et al.* Liver enzymes are commonly elevated following laparoscopic cholecystectomy: is elevated intra-abdominal pressure the cause? *Dig Surg* 1998; 15(3):256–259.
7. Lillemoe KD, Melton GB, Cameron JL, *et al.* Postoperative bile duct strictures: management and outcome in the 1990s. *Ann Surg* 2000; 232:430–441.
8. de Reuver PR, Busch OR, Rauws EA, *et al.* Long-term results of a primary end-to-end anastomosis in a perioperative detected bile duct injury. *J Gastrointest Surg* 2007; 11:296–302.

BENIGN GALLBLADDER DISEASE: POSTCHOLECYSTECTOMY SYNDROME AND STRICTURE

23

Judson B. Williams[*] and
Sandhya A. Lagoo-Deenadayalan[*]

INTRODUCTION

Cholecystectomy results in resolution of symptoms in a majority of patients who have been accurately diagnosed with gallbladder disease, either secondary to cholelithiasis or biliary dyskinesia. Postcholecystectomy pain has been reported since the advent of the operation, predating the development of minimally invasive techniques. In the early postoperative period following cholecystectomy, bile duct injury, obstruction or leak may manifest as nonspecific abdominal pain, anorexia, fever, nausea, or vomiting. Intra-abdominal fluid collection should raise the suspicion of a bile leak and bile duct dilatation should raise the suspicion for obstruction. Intra-abdominal fluid collections may be due to bile, blood, or enteric contents from an unrecognized hollow viscus injury. Delays in treatment may increase morbidity and the surgeon should maintain a high index of suspicion for biliary injury or leak in the early postoperative period. Iatrogenic

---

[*]Duke University Medical Center, Durham, NC 27710 USA

biliary tract injuries commonly result in significant morbidity and will be specifically addressed in Chapter 31.

This chapter defines and considers late postcholecystectomy problems. In particular, we will consider postcholecystectomy syndrome and the common biliary causes including stricture. Postcholecystectomy syndrome refers to a heterogeneous group of symptoms and findings in patients who have undergone cholecystectomy. These may include both biliary and nonbiliary disorders, commonly encompassing abdominal pain, dyspepsia, flatulence, and bloating. The term postcholecystectomy syndrome is misleading in that the symptoms and findings it describes typically antedate the operation and are uncommonly referred to the operation itself. Postcholecystectomy syndrome may often be encountered in patents that had been offered a cholecystectomy without concrete evidence of gallbladder disease. Nonetheless, in patients with abdominal symptoms following cholecystectomy, for whom the pathophysiology of these symptoms remains unclear despite an extensive workup, the classification "postcholecystectomy syndrome" may be applied.

DIFFERENTIAL DIAGNOSIS

The differential diagnosis for symptoms following cholecystectomy includes every major organ system. The table below indicates the breadth of possibilities. The surgeon must be aware of potential nonbiliary causes of symptoms, some life-threatening, and evaluate such patients appropriately.

CYSTIC DUCT REMNANT

Postcholecystectomy symptoms have been attributed to disease of the cystic duct remnant, including fistulas, granulomas, and neuromas. Remnant gallbladder tissue is subject to these same complications. While there are no symptoms specific to cystic duct remnants, ERCP and MRCP are both useful modalities for defining the biliary anatomy in patients with possible cystic duct remnant disease. Treatment includes the excision of the cystic duct remnant. Completion cholecystectomy is advised for any diseased gallbladder remnant.

While also rare, stones in a cystic duct remnant are more commonly identified as a cause of postcholecystectomy syndrome than are granulomas or neuromas. Cystic duct remnant stones may be discovered with ERCP or

Table 1. Causes of abdominal symptoms following cholecystectomy.

Cardiovascular	Coronary artery disease, mesenteric ischemia, aortic aneurysm, aortic dissection
Pulmonary	Pneumonia, pleural effusions, malignancy
Biliary	Sphincter of Oddi dysfunction, stricture, cystic duct remnant, malignancy, choledochocele, common bile duct stone, transpapillary passage of crystals
Pancreatic	Pancreatitis, pancreatic pseudocyst, pancreas divisum, malignancy
Gastric	Peptic ulcer disease, gastroesophageal reflux, malignancy
Small bowel and Colon	Inflammatory bowel disease, constipation, irritable bowel syndrome, adhesions, internal hernia
Infectious	Wound infection, liver abscess, hepatitis, cholangitis, herpes simplex virus
Neurologic	Intercostal neuritis, wound neuroma
Musculoskeletal	Muscle strain, thoracolumbar disc disease, costochondritis
Psychiatric	Substance abuse, somatization disorder, major depressive disorder, general anxiety disorder, Munchausen syndrome
Other	Pharmaceutical reaction, malingering, renal disease

MRCP while evaluating for more common causes of postcholecystectomy syndrome. When ERCP is done to exclude common duct calculi, the surgeon should also consider the possibility of associated or isolated stones of a remnant cystic duct or remnant gallbladder. Selective cystic duct cannulation should be considered when no common duct stones are identified. Most surgeons prefer endoscopic removal at the time of ERCP for its ease and safety. Options for excision of the remnant include laparoscopic or open surgical approaches. When a remnant duct stone is difficult to remove, fragmentation techniques including shock wave lithotripsy may be employed in centers where this technology is available. Extracorporeal shockwave lithotripsy is especially useful when an operation is contraindicated.

CHOLEDOCHOLITHIASIS

Stones in the common bile duct are a potential late cause of postcholecystectomy symptoms. Stones found within 2 years of cholecystectomy are considered to be retained stones and were most likely present at the time of operation. This occurs in roughly 1–2% of patients undergoing a laparoscopic cholecystectomy without a cholangiogram. Less frequently, stones may form primarily in the biliary ductal system. Stones found more than 2 years after cholecystectomy are considered recurrent stones and are unlikely to have been present at the time of operation. Regardless of the etiology, choledocholithiasis can result in biliary pain, jaundice, cholangitis, and pancreatitis. Liver biochemical laboratory values, particularly alkaline phosphatase, may be elevated. Stones are extracted endoscopically following endoscopic papillotomy.

ERCP has been the criterion standard for diagnosing retained stones and offers the additional benefits of papilla visualization and therapeutic modalities. For initial diagnostic intent, MRCP is beginning to replace ERCP in many centers as evidence grows that ERCP can be avoided in upwards of 50% of patients at low to moderate risk for choledocholithiasis, as may be the case in patients with postcholecystectomy syndrome. MRCP is non-invasive, requires no contrast to be administered, and carries a sensitivity of 95–100% and specificity of 88–89% for detecting choledocholithiasis.

In the absence of stones by imaging, bile microlithiasis may be considered as a cause for postcholecystectomy pain. Patients with postcholecystectomy pain believed to be of biliary origin, but with normal-appearing MRCP or ERCP, may benefit from a microscopic examination of bile for crystals or microlithiasis. Ursodeoxycholic acid treatment is indicated in these patients if microlithiasis is identified.

SPHINCTER OF ODDI DYSFUNCTION

A number of patients with postcholecystectomy pain are diagnosed with an abnormality of the sphincter of Oddi. Sphincter of Oddi dysfunction can result in biliary-type pain, jaundice, and pancreatitis. Delayed drainage of contrast medium, greater than 45 minutes, may be seen at the time of ERCP.

Papillary stenosis, a fixed narrowing of the sphincter, may occur as a result of trauma from instrumentation, or the passage of gallstones or cholesterol crystals. Pancreatitis and infection are other causes of papillary inflammation. Patients suffering papillary stenosis may develop episodic, severe upper abdominal pain several years after cholecystectomy. Evaluation typically includes laboratory studies, ultrasound, ERCP, and CT scan to exclude other causes. Elevated LTFs, difficulty cannulating the ampulla, distal bile duct dilatation, or delayed drainage of contrast from the common bile duct may be seen. No study is diagnostic and only approximately one in five patients with presumed papillary stenosis will have elevated LFTs or lower bile duct anatomic abnormalities.

A functional disturbance at the sphincter of Oddi, referred to in the past as ampullary spasm or sphincter dyskinesia, is an idiopathic process. Biliary manometry demonstrates increased sphincter pressures from tonic or phasic smooth muscle contractions. An increased basal pressure, paradoxic response to cholecystokinin, retrograde propagation of phasic-wave contractions, or an increased frequency of phasic-wave contractions may contribute to abnormal sphincter pressures.

Treatment for sphincter of Oddi dysfunction is endoscopic sphincterotomy. Endoscopic sphincterotomy reduces bile duct and sphincter pressures with excellent results.

STRICTURE

Despite improvements in experience and technology, the incidence of bile duct injuries after cholecystectomy remains at 0.2% for open and 0.5% for laparoscopic procedures. Unfortunately, only 30% of injuries are recognized at the time of operation. Patients with a bile leak typically present early whereas patients with postoperative biliary strictures alone will present with jaundice or cholangitis months to years after the initial injury. The clinical signs of a bile duct injury include malaise, nausea, anorexia, right upper quadrant abdominal pain, ileus, fever, chills, jaundice, and sepsis. Biliary leaks can be diagnosed by ERCP, and the patient should undergo stent placement, with CT guided drainage of the biloma.

Cholangiography should be performed to establish the presence of ductal stricture and identify the level of the stricture. Delayed management of stricture can range from endoscopic intervention to bilioenteric bypass to liver transplantation. Direct operative bilioenteric bypass remains the gold standard for long-term treatment of biliary strictures. Chapters 32 and 34 discuss operative approaches in more detail, however, we will note here that successful repair hinges on the use of proximal bile duct with minimal inflammation, creation of a tension-free anastomosis with a Roux-en-Y jejunal limb, and direct mucosa-to-mucosa anastomosis. Recent reports have suggested that primary repair of the bile duct is associated with an up to 50% long-term failure rate. The use of a Roux-en-Y jejunal limb is also favored over a direct choledochoduodenostomy or choledochojejunostomy because it allows for the creation of an "access loop" of the proximal portion of the Roux-en-Y limb for future interventional radiologic access.

ERCP with stenting for major bile duct injuries has become more commonplace and has been shown to be associated with acceptably low morbidity and mortality. This approach is particularly attractive for the patient with multiple comorbidities at high risk with open operation. Long term results are still needed to assess durability. Strictures which are from long, lateral lacerations of the common bile duct and common hepatic duct (1.5–2 cm in length) often represent more recalcitrant injuries with high endoscopic failure rates.

REFERENCES

Lee VS, et al. Complications of laparoscopic cholecystectomy, *Am J Surg* 1993; 165:527.

Terhaar OA, et al. Imaging patients with "post-cholecystectomy syndrome": an algorithmic approach, *Clin Radiol* 2005; 60(1):78–84.

Zhou PH, et al. (2003) Endoscopic diagnosis and treatment of post-cholecystectomy syndrome, *Hepatobiliary Pancreat Dis Int* 2003; 2(1):117–20.

BENIGN GALLBLADDER DISEASE: CHOLEDOCHOLITHIASIS AND CHOLANGITIS

24

Loretta Erhunmwunsee* and
Aurora D. Pryor[†]

CHOLEDOCHOLITHIASIS

Epidemiology & Presentation

Choledocholithiasis typically arises from the gallbladder and is present in up to 10–15% of patients with symptomatic gallstone disease. Those ductal stones not arising from the gallbladder are considered primary, having formed in the intrahepatic or extrahepatic ducts. Primary stones are particularly seen in the elderly, people with Asian ancestry and those with chronic bile duct inflammation.[1] The risk factors associated with common bile duct (CBD) stones are the same as those seen with normal gallstone disease, i.e. being female, overweight, peripartum, middle aged or in association with a significant weight gain or loss. Patients who have infection of the common bile duct are also at increased risk for stone development. Patients with choledocholithiasis typically present with RUQ pain,

---

*Duke University Medical Center, Durham, NC 27710 USA
[†]Stony Brook Medicine, State University of New York at Stony Brook, USA

jaundice and/or fever. Choledocholithiasis can lead to gallstone pancreatitis, cholangitis, or obstructive jaundice and thus can cause significant morbidity and mortality if not diagnosed efficiently and treated effectively.

Work-up/Imaging

On work-up, abnormally elevated hepatobiliary biochemical values are frequently noted. A study of 1002 patients undergoing lap cholecystectomy revealed that having any abnormal elevation among the five liver function tests (LFTs) (GGT, AST, ALT, bilirubin or alkaline phosphatase) had a 87.5% sensitivity for diagnosing common bile duct stones. Total bilirubin had the highest specificity at 87.5% and highest accuracy at 98%. The negative predictive value for individual tests was highest for GGT at 97.9%.[2] Thus biochemical parameters are very helpful in diagnosing CBD stones.

Patients with RUQ pain, jaundice or elevated LFTs will usually undergo an ultrasound evaluation (US), which has a low sensitivity for detection of choledocholithiasis but a high specificity.[3] In many patients, an US is the only radiologic work-up necessary. A dilated common bile duct (>6mm) in the setting of gallstones with elevated bilirubin and alkaline phosphatase is enough to suspect choledocholithiasis. An abdominal CT scan may frequently be performed to rule out other causes of biliary obstruction and is useful for detecting choledocholithiasis with reported sensitivity of 88%, specificity of 97%, PPV 94% and NPV of 94%.[4] A HIDA scan can also give evidence of an obstructing common bile duct stone with nonfilling of the duodenum.

MRCP also belongs in the armamenterium of non-invasive tests used in detecting CBD stones. In one study, the sensitivity for detection of CBD stones by high-spatial resolution isotropic 3D T2-weighted MRCP was high for stones greater than 3mm at 94% to 100%. Specificity for detection of all stones was 97% to 99% using MRCP.[5] The negative predictive value ranges from 96–100%.[6] If an MRCP is interpreted as negative for CBD stones, to the performance of a diagnostic ERCP and its inherent complications can be avoided.

Studies have also been performed to determine the efficacy of endoscopic ultrasound (EUS) in detecting CBD stones. Studies have found EUS to have an accuracy comparable to that of ERCP for the diagnosis and exclusion of choledocholithiasis.[7] A meta-analysis of EUS-guided ERCP versus ERCP alone revealed that doing a preprocedure EUS reduced the need for ERCP by 67.1% when EUS did not detect choledocholithiasis. The complication rate was then significantly lowered by the use of EUS.[8] Studies are ongoing to determine the role for EUS in diagnosis and exclusion of bile duct stones.

ERCP should not be used solely as a diagnostic tool because of its invasive nature and inherent complication potential. ERCP is typically reserved for patients who will likely require therapeutic intervention for a persistent common bile duct stone that has been confirmed by one of the above imaging techniques. ERCP's role in management of choledocholithiasis will be discussed in more detail in the treatment section.

Treatment

In spite of the fact that a large percentage of common bile duct stones pass into the duodenum spontaneously, their presence warrants serious attention because their potential complications could be life-threatening. As such, the typical patient who is found to have choledocholithiasis should undergo cholecystectomy to prevent further episodes. But whether the common bile duct is explored before, during, or after the cholecystectomy is determined by the clinical situation and the surgeon's preference. Surgeons may choose to have their patient with evidence of choledocholithiasis undergo preoperative ERCP for clearance of the common bile duct, Other surgeons prefer to perform an intraoperative cholangiogram (IOC) to rule out a stone while performing their laparoscopic cholecystectomy, especially if LFTs have resolved. If a stone is present on IOC, the surgeon will decide whether to perform a common duct exploration versus requesting a postoperative ERCP for clearance of the stone. Many of these choices depend on the efficacy of ERCP at the local institution. Surgeons will more frequently choose ERCP if it is easy to access with lower risk and better efficacy.[9]

Ercp sphincterotomy

Most patients thought to have persistent CBD stones will undergo an ERCP, which has a greater than 90% success rate at removal of these stones. Sphincterotomy is the first line therapy performed during this procedure. Sphincterotomy includes the incision of the sphincter of Oddi and is typically followed by balloon or basket extraction of the stone. If the duct cannot be completely cleared, a stent is typically placed. For the difficult stone, mechanical, laser or electrohydrolic lithotripsy can also be used. ERCP sphincterotomy is highly effective at clearance of CBD stones but it was associated with a 9.8% complication rate in a large multicenter trial with over 2000 patients. They also noted a 5.4% risk of pancreatitis, 2% risk of bleeding and a 1% risk of procedure-related cholangitis.[10] For these reasons, it is best to reserve the procedure for patients with a conclusive diagnosis.

Although ERCP is highly effective at clearing the CBD, cholecystectomy is still standard of treatment for this disease as it treats the source of future stones. Patients who do not undergo prophylactic cholecystectomy after ERCP clearance of CBD stones have significantly higher rates of recurent biliary pain, jaundice, cholangtitis, repeat ERCP and death.[11]

Operative Techniques for Common Duct Clearance

Operative cholangiogram

Every surgeon who plans on performing laparoscopic cholecystectomy (LC) must master this technique. Many surgeons perform IOC routinely because there is evidence that it may lower the frequency of severe bile duct injuries. At the minimum, an IOC should be performed in patients with evidence of common bile duct stones, i.e. elevated LFTs, jaundice, gallstone pancreatitis, cholangitis, etc. who did not undergo preoperative ERCP. Once the cystic duct has been exposed, scissors are used to incise the duct less than 50% of the circumference close to the gallbladder. The cholangiogram catheter is then inserted via either a trocar or a small puncture made in the abdominal wall over the cystic duct, into the cystic duct opening. Sterile saline is then instilled to assure good flow. The catheter is kept in place with a hemoclip, clamp or balloon. Dilute contrast is then instilled through the catheter while films are obtained. Still films can be obtained, but real-time fluoroscopy is preferred. There should be visualization of the left and right hepatic ducts, the cystic and common bile duct and filling of the duodenum should be apparent. Maneuvers such as manipulating the bed into Trendelenberg position or tilting the table may aid in visualization of all structures. If common duct stones are detected, a common bile duct exploration can be performed. Biliary ultrasound is gaining some favor in determining the presence of common duct stones as well.

Laparoscopic common bile duct exploration

Once a stone is seen on IOC, some simple clearance maneuvers are usually performed prior to a formal CBD exploration. High volumes of saline may be injected to encourage flushing of the (small) stone. Glucagon injection may also help to relax the Sphincter of Oddi. If these maneuvers are not successful, one of two access techniques for laparoscopic CBD exploration can be performed. The transcystic approach accesses the cystic duct while the transductal approach accesses the common bile duct. The transcystic approach is easily used for small stones (<8 mm) and those stones located just below the cystic duct with great success. The transcystic approach is typically considered less morbid and patients typically have a shorter length of stay when compared to the transductal approach. Fortunately, most CBD stones can be cleared via the transcystic approach; although, the cystic duct may need to be dilated with balloon dilators up to 5–8 mm in order for smooth extraction of stones.

The transcystic approach may be more difficult, however, if the cystic duct is very tortuous, if the cystic and CBD have a very acute angle, or if there are many valves of Heister within the cystic duct. When stones are >10 mm, or proximal to the insertion of the cystic duct, the transductal approach is indicated. This approach is if the CBD is less than 10 mm, however, as rates of postoperative stricture will be higher. During the transductal approach an anterior, vertical choledochotomy is performed. This incision should not be larger than the diameter of the largest stone.

Once the accessing approach has been decided, i.e. transcystic vs. transductal, one must determine the extraction approach. In general if a stone is <2 mm, it will pass spontaneously. If they are visible on IOC, however, it is best to clear, these stones. Flushing the duct with normal saline, as mentioned above, using a red, rubber or balloon catheter while dilating the sphincter of Oddi with glucagon is frequently a successful strategy. For stones that can not be cleared simply by flushing, of a basket might be used to extract the stone. Biliary balloon catheters can also be used to help dilate the sphincter or push/pull a stone. Fluoroscopic guidance is usually helpful in these situations.

For larger stones that are associated with a dilated CBD (>6 mm), flushing and basket extraction may not be successful. A choledochoscope and its associated plastic introducer system is then frequently used either transcystically or via the CBD for a direct-vision basket maneuver. A 3-mm choledochoscope is frequently used and the basket typically advanced through the operating channel of the scope. In experienced hands, this technique is successful in 80–90% of patients.[12]

If there is impaction of stones, a number of different options are available. First, a T-tube can be placed in the CBD for drainage and an ERCP performed later. Secondly, an anterograde sphincterotomy can be performed. Usually this is done at the 10 o'clock position of the sphincter so as not to injure the pancreatic duct, which is usually at the 4 o'clock position. Electrohydraulic lithotripsy via a choledochoscope can also be performed, although this is rarely performed due to lack of experience and the risk of injury to the common bile duct. Lastly, conversion to open may be considered.

When the completion cholangiogram reveals clearance of the duct, the cystic duct that was accessed via a transcystic approach can be ligated with two clips or an endoloop. If a choledochotomy was performed, it may be closed primarily or a T-tube may be placed and the CBD closed with interrupted absorbable suture, such as Maxon.

A study comparing 122 patients with choledocholithiasis randomized to undergo either preoperative ERCP followed by LC or LC with laparoscopic common bile duct exploration revealed no difference in the efficacy of stone clearance between groups. They did show that the length of hospital stay was significantly longer for the preoperative ERCP group (55 hours vs. 98 hours p <0.001) but there was no difference between patient satisfaction or overall cost.[13] Thus, both options are viable depending on the surgeon's experience and the clinical scenerio.

Open common bile duct exploration

This procedure is typically performed in patients who are already undergoing open cholecystectomy or for whom laparoscopic surgery would be difficult. In those undergoing a laparoscopic procedure, conversion to open exploration may be considered when large or multiple stones are present in the CBD. Conversion is also appropriate for surgeons less experienced with advanced laparoscopic techniques. To start the procedure, the CBD is exposed in the lesser omentum and a vertical, anterior choledochotomy is performed just proximal to the duodenum. Stay sutures are placed on either side of the duct. The duct can then be flushed with sterile saline distally using a red rubber catheter with

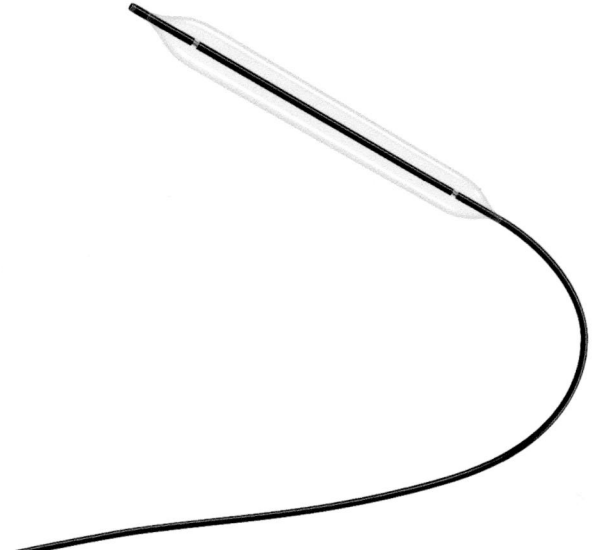

Figure 1. Fogarty Balloon Catheter for Bile Duct Manipulation.

removal of stones. If this is unsuccessful, then a fogarty balloon or dilatation catheter (Figure 1) can be used to bring up stones both distally and proximally. If the balloon or dilatation catheter does not work, a choledochoscope and its basket (Figure 2) may be used to directly visualize and extract stones. For impacted stones, a T-tube can be secured in the duct for extraction of stones from the tube at a later time after edema that is associated with the stones has settled. Choledochoenterostomy is a last resort when very large or difficult stones cannot be cleared by the above maneuvers. It involves mobilizinging the duodenum with a wide Kocher maneuver and closing the bile duct with the anastomosis. It is rarely performed today.

CHOLANGITIS

Epidemiology

Acute cholangitis is an infection of the biliary tree that typically occurs as a result of biliary tract obstruction. Bile duct stones are the number one

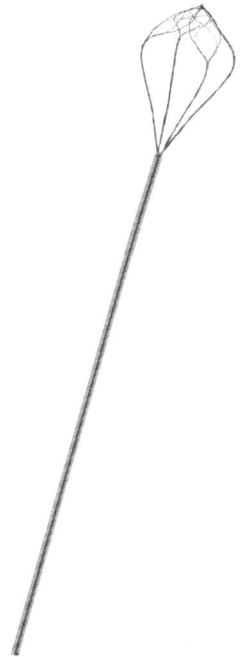

Figure 2. Endoscopic Basket for Stone Removal.

cause of the obstruction. Previous biliary therapy is the second most common cause of acute cholangitis. Bacteria typically arise from the duodenum causing bacterobilia in the setting of bile duct stones. Continued obstruction increases the intraductal pressure, which in the setting of bacterobilia leads to cholangitis. Charcot's triad of fever, right upper quadrant pain and jaundice occurs in up to 70% of patients. Reynold's pentad, which is characterized by the additional features of hypotension and altered consciousness, occurs in less than 10% of cases. Ninety percent of patients with acute cholangitis will have fever. A smaller percentage might have mild abdominal pain as well,[1] particularly in the setting of cholecystitis.

Work-Up/Imaging

Patients will likely have elevated WBC levels and invariably elevations in the liver function panel as well. Bile cultures are typically positive in patients with cholangitis. Blood cultures can also be positive. Gram-negative organisms, such as E. coli, Klebsiella and Enterococcus are typically isolated from bile. Patients with severe disease, the elderly, or those who have had biliary surgery are more likely to have a polymicrobial infection that includes anaerobes, MRSA, VRE or even fungi.

The same imaging options exist for diagnosing cholangitis as were discussed earlier for choledocholithiasis.

Management Options

Patients with mild disease should be treated with antbiotics. Those who respond should undergo biliary decompression within 24–48 hours. If the patient worsens or is without improvement, more urgent decompression should be performed. Eighty percent of patients will be effectively treated with supportive therapy and antibiotic treatment alone. Appropriate antibiotic use and early is necessary. Patients with severe disease should be closely monitored, rehydrated and started on antibiotics. These patients will likely require emergent/urgent ERCP decompression. Their instability may necessitate bedside performance in the ICU.

Antibiotics

Early broad-spectrum antibiotic use is paramount in treatment of patients with presumed acute cholangitis. Antibiotics should have strong gram-negative coverage with adequate biliary excretion. Patients who are sicker, older or who have had biliary surgery or manipulation may need even broader therapy. Antibiotics can be targeted once cultures come back. The Duration of therapy depends on the severity of disease.

Endoscopic Drainage

ERCP stone extraction with sphincterotomy is typically performed in stable patients. In patients with severe disease, however, the goal is to provide adequate drainage, which can even be via a nasobiliary tube, in as short a time as possible. Sphincterotomy or stent placement can be performed later once the patient is stable. Drainage via the percutaneous transhepatic route is also an option in patients who have altered anatomy or in whom endoscopic drainage is unsuccessful.

Surgical Drainage

Surgical drainage in patients with acute cholangitis is rarely performed now secondary to the success and decreased morbidity seen with endoscopic, and to a lesser extent percutaneous, treatment. A randomized trial from Hong Kong found 34% morbidity and 10% mortality rates in 41 patients with severe disease who underwent endoscopic decompression compared with 66% morbidity and 32% mortality rates in 41 patients who underwent primary surgical therapy.[14] The improved endoscopic outcomes are especially true in those with severe disease or older age. In most cases, surgical management is only considered if neither endoscopic nor percutaneous therapies are successful. If operative treatment is warranted, either laparoscopic or open common duct exploration could be performed. The details of both procedures are as discussed earlier.

CONCLUSION

Choledocholithiasis and cholangitis are potentially life-threatening diseases that must be diagnosed quickly and treated effectively. Laparoscopic common bile duct exploration, via the transcystic or transductal approach, may be utilized for clearance of CBD stones. Its use in the management of acute cholangitis is not first-line, however. Both disease states have seen the rise of endoscopic treatment over the last several years. In the case of CBD stones, ERCP can be performed before or after cholecystectomy for clearance of the CBD with good results. And in the case of cholangitis, urgent or even emergent ERCP drainage is the standard of care after resuscitation and broad-spectrum antibiotic initiation.

REFERENCES

1. Attasaranya S, Fogel EL, Lehman GA. Choledocholithiasis, ascending cholangtitis and gallstone pancreatitis. *Medical Clinics of North America* 2008; 92:925–960.
2. Yang MH, Chen TH, Wang SE, *et al.* Bicochemical predictors for absence of common bile duct stones in patients undergoing laparoscopic cholecystectomy. *Surg Endosc* 2008; 22:1620–1624.
3. Sugiyama M and Atomi Y. Endoscopic ultrasonography for diagnosing choledocholithiasis: a prospective comparative study with ultrasonography and computed tomography. *Gastrointest Endosc* 1997; 45:143-146.

4. Neitlich JD Topazian M, Smith RC, et al. Detection of choledocholithiasis: comparison of unenhanced helical CT and endoscopic retrograde cholangiopancreatography. *Radiology* 1997; 203:753–757.
5. Nandalur KR, Hussain HK, Weadock WJ, et al. Possible biliary disease: diagnositic performance of high-spatial-resolution isotropic 3D T2-weighted MRCP. *Radiology* 2008; 249:883–890.
6. Reinhold C, Taourel P, Bret PM, et al. Choledocholithiasis: evaluation of MR cholangiography for diagnosis. *Radiology* 1998; 209:435–442.
7. Prat F, Amouyal G, Amouyal P, et al. Prospective controlled study of endoscopic ultrasonography and endoscopic retrograde cholangiography in patients with suspected common bile duct lithiasis. *Lancet* 1996; 347:75–79.
8. Petrov MS and Savides TJ. Systematic review of endoscopic ultrasonography versus endoscopic retrograde cholangiopancreatography for suspected choledocholithiasis. *Br J Surg* 2009; 96:967–974.
9. Poulose BK, Arbogast PG and Holzman MD. National analysis of in-hospital resource utilization in choledocholithiasis management using propensity scores. *Surg Endosc* 2006; 20:186–190.
10. Freeman ML Nelson DB, Sherman S, et al. Complications of endoscopic biliary sphincterotomy. *N Engl J Med* 1996; 335:909–918.
11. McAlsiter V, Davenport E, Renouf E, et al. Cholecystectomy deferral in patients with endoscopic sphincterotomy. *Cochrane Database of Systematic Reviews*, 2007; Issue 4.
12. Topal B Aerts R, Penninckx F, et al. Laparoscopic common bile duct stone clearance with flexible choledochoscopy. *Surg Endosc* 2007; 21:2317–2321.
13. Rogers SJ, Cello JP, Horn JK, et al. Prospective randomized trial of LC+LCBDE vs. ERCP/S+LC for common bile duct stone disease. *Arch Surg* 2010; 145:28–33.
14. Lai EC, Mok FP, Tan ES, et al. Endoscopic biliary drainage for severe acute cholangitis. *N Engl J Med* 1992; 326:1582–1586.

GALLBLADDER CANCER 25

Asad A. Shah*, Srinevas K. Reddy[†], Dan G. Blazer III* and Bryan M. Clary*

EPIDEMIOLOGY, RISK FACTORS, PRESENTING SIGNS

Epidemiology

Gallbladder cancer (GBC) is a relatively rare but deadly form of cancer. There will be an estimated 9760 new cases of GBC in the United States in 2009, as well as an estimated 3370 deaths from it.[1] There is significant ethnic and geographic variability in the incidence of GBC. American Indian Alaska Natives and Asian Pacific Islanders have the highest age adjusted incidence of GBC, while white men have the lowest. Hispanics have more than double the rate of GBC compared to non-Hispanics. Higher incidences of GBC occur in South America, particularly Chile. The disease affects women two to six times more frequently than men, with this difference being greatest in regions with the highest rates of GBC. Overall, the incidence of GBC has been decreasing over the last decade.

Risk Factors

Numerous studies have demonstrated a relationship between GBC and gallstones, although there is no direct evidence proving causation. Gallstones can lead to gallbladder (GB) inflammation by directly irritating

---

*Duke University Medical Center, Durham, NC 27710 USA
[†]University of Maryland Medical Center, Baltimore, MD, USA

the mucosa or by altering GB function leading to delayed or incomplete emptying resulting in bile stasis and GB dilatation. This inflammation can then cause cellular dysfunction, ultimately resulting in dysplasia and carcinoma. Larger stones and a longer duration of cholelithiasis further increase the risk of developing GBC, possibly due to increased inflammation. Gallstones are present in 70–90% of patients with GBC, but only 0.5–3% of patients with cholelithiasis develop GBC.

GB polyps have also been linked to GBC, although there is no direct evidence showing that polyps are necessarily precursors to adenocarcinoma. Most GBCs contain dysplasia and carcinoma *in situ* adjacent to them. Patients with dysplasia and carcinoma *in situ* are younger than those with invasive carcinoma, which suggests a temporal and progressive sequence from polyps to carcinoma. Polyps suspicious for carcinoma include those that are sessile, solitary, greater than 1 cm in diameter, contrast enhancing on computed tomography (CT), or have visible blood supply on ultrasound (US).

Other risk factors for GBC include chronic biliary infection, congenital biliary cysts, and obesity.

Presenting Signs

Most GBCs are found incidentally after cholecystectomy. When symptomatic, the most common presenting symptoms include abdominal pain, biliary colic, and jaundice either from direct invasion of the bile ducts or nodal compression within the hepatoduodenal ligament.

WORK-UP

Physical examination is nonspecific in the workup of GBC. Jaundice, hepatomegaly, or an abdominal mass may be noted. Laboratory studies are also nonspecific, but may include elevated liver enzymes, carcinoembryonic antigen (CEA), and CA 19–9.

Imaging

Ultrasound (US) is an inexpensive and readily available means to image the GB. In patients with GBC, it will show a mass in about 90% of patients. GBC on US may be seen as a mass, diffuse or focal wall thickening, or loss of definition between the GB and liver. Echogenicity is variable. US cannot,

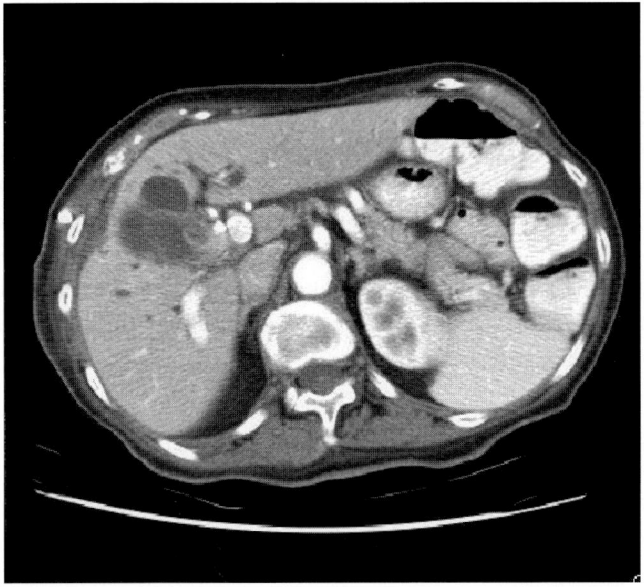

Figure 1. T3N1 GBCa invading through the gallbladder wall and into the liver.

however, differentiate a GBC from other GB lesions including cholesterol polyps or adenomatous polyps. Overall, US is a good initial screening test, but other imaging modalities are needed to further characterize any lesions and determine resectability.

Computerized tomography (CT) is very useful in the diagnosis and management of GBC. On CT, GBC can present as a low attenuation mass with variable enhancement, a polypoid mass (or masses) greater than 1 cm or as GB wall thickening (Figure 1). CT is also informative in regards to determining resectability. It can detect lymphatic spread, infiltration into the liver, bile ducts, and/or other neighboring organs, and metastases. CT is accurate in staging GBC, as it can differentiate the T stage of GBC in 70–100% of cases and determine resectability in 80–100% of patients.

Positron emission tomography (PET) is being used with increasing frequency in the staging of various malignancies. It is frequently used to detect metastatic, recurrent, or residual disease, as well as characterize the primary tumor. Overall, the limited studies done using PET for GBC have shown that it infrequently results in a change in operative management. As most GBCs are diagnosed after cholecystectomy, there is already local inflammation in the region of interest, that decreases the specificity of PET scanning.

Magnetic resonance imaging (MRI) is excellent for diagnosing and staging GBC. On MRI, GBC typically appears as hypointense on T1 images and hyperintense or heterogeneous on T2 images. MRI can accurately depict the local extent of the tumor, particularly into the liver. Cholangiography (MRC) or angiography (MRA) may be used with MRI as well to detect invasion into the peritoneum, bile ducts, vessels and duodenum, or to detect liver metastases or biliary obstruction. Combined preoperative MRI, MRA, and MRC have been shown to have sensitivities and specificities of 100% and 89% for bile duct invasion, 100% and 87% for vascular invasion, 67% and 89% for hepatic invasion, and 56% and 89% for lymph node metastasis, respectively.[2]

PATHOLOGY

GBC is an aggressive malignancy and about 75% of patients are deemed unresectable at initial presentation. Patients typically present with advanced locoregional disease or metastases. Greater than 80% of GBCs are adenocarcinomas which can be categorized into papillary, tubular, mucinous, and signet cell types (Figure 2). Other histologies such as squamous cell carcinoma, neuroendocrine tumors, and lymphoma are occasionally found.

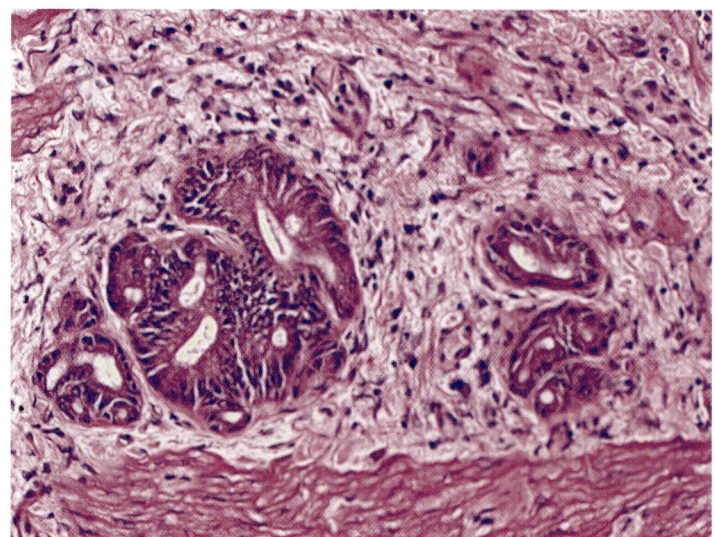

Figure 2. Invasive, well-differentiated adenocarcinoma of the gallbladder.

Spread occurs via the blood, lymphatics, nerves, and peritoneum. The tumor can invade the liver directly via short communicating veins draining the GB into the liver or via veins supplying the extrahepatic bile ducts. Invasion can also occur into the hilum along Glisson's sheath. Additionally, the tumor can spread transperitoneally into various local and distant structures including the common bile duct, colon, duodenum, and stomach. Peritoneal carcinomatosis may occur as well.

There are several different staging criteria for GBC. TNM staging established by the American Joint Committee on Cancer (AJCC) is most often used (Tables 1,2). Prognosis is strongly correlated with TNM staging and this system is most widely used in the United States. Other staging systems, including the modified Nevin system and the Japanese Biliary Surgical Society, are important historically but are less frequently utilized now.

SURGERY AND OTHER MANAGEMENT OPTIONS

Given the rarity of GBC and the perception of overall dismal prognosis by many physicians, there is marked heterogeneity in the management of GBC. Many patients are not offered the appropriate operation or the proper adjuvant therapy. Given this significant heterogeneity, studies describing long-term outcomes are difficult to evaluate and compare. However, tumor thickness, nodal disease, resection margin, and age have been found to be common variables associated with survival.

Incidental Disease

GBC is detected in GB specimens after cholecystectomy done for presumed benign disease in approximately 0.5–2% of cases. If GBC is found and a patient undergoes definitive surgical resection at a later point, studies have proven that a prior cholecystectomy does not affect survival. There is no difference in survival for patients diagnosed with GBC during versus after cholecystectomy, and there is no difference in survival or recurrence in patients who underwent laparoscopic versus open cholecystectomy.

Extended Cholecystectomy

Simple cholecystectomy is sufficient treatment for T_1 disease. However, extended cholecystectomy is necessary for long-term survival for T_2 and

Table 1. The American Joint Committee on Cancer (AJCC) TNM staging system for gallbladder cancer.

Primary tumor (T)	
TX	Primary tumor cannot be assessed
T0	No evidence of primary tumor
Tis	Carcinoma *in situ*
T1	Tumor invades lamina propria or muscle layer T1a: tumor invades lamina propria T1b: tumor invades muscle layer
T2	Tumor invades perimuscular connective tissue; no extension beyond serosa or into liver
T3	Tumor perforates the serosa (visceral peritoneum) and/or directly invades the liver and/or one other adjacent organ or structure such as the stomach, duodenum, colon, or pancreas, omentum, or extrahepatic ducts
T4	Tumor invades the main portal vein or hepatic artery or invades two or more extrahepatic organs or structures
Regional lymph nodes (N)	
NX	Regional lymph nodes cannot be assessed
N0	No regional lymph node metastases
N1	Metastases to nodes along the cystic duct, common bile duct, hepatic artery, and/or portal vein
N2	Metastases to periaortic, pericaval, superior mesenteric artery, and/or celiac artery lymph nodes
Distant metastases (M)	
M0	No distant metastases
M1	Distant metastases

Adapted from www.nccn.org. In: American Joint Committee on Cancer.: AJCC Cancer Staging Manual. 7th ed. New York, NY: Springer, 2010.

T_3 disease. Tumor thickness is associated with increased frequency of nodal disease and residual liver disease. Lymph node involvement occurs in 40–50% of patients with T2 or T3 disease and vascular, lymphatic, and perineural invasion is common. Additionally, patients with these tumors have

Table 2. AJCC stage groupings for gallbladder cancer.

Stage 0	TisN0M0
Stage I	T1N0M0
Stage II	T2N0M0
Stage IIIA	T3N0M0
Stage IIIB	T1–3, N1, M0
Stage IVA	T4, any N, M0
Stage IVB	Any T, N2, M0; Any T, Any N, M1

Adapted from www.nccn.org. In: American Joint Committee on Cancer.: AJCC Cancer Staging Manual. 7th ed. New York, NY: Springer, 2010, pp 139–44.

positive margins 25% of the time after cholecystectomy. Therefore, patients with T_2 or T_3 disease require at minimum an extended cholecystectomy for definitive surgical resection. This resection consists of wedge resection of segments IVb and V to at least 3 cm depth from the GB bed as well as regional lymphadenectomy including nodes around the cystic duct, liver hilum, portal vein, and hepatoduodenal ligament.

In an analysis of a large German registry of incidental gallbladder cancers, 200 of 439 cases were T2 tumors. Twenty-one percent of patients with T_2 tumors had positive nodal disease and subsequent radical resection improved 5-year survival from 35% to 55% (p = 0.04). Node negative disease was necessary to achieve long term survival, with a 5-year survival of 55% vs. 0% if there was node positive disease (p = 0.0078).[3] Other studies have also shown improved survival after extended cholecystectomy for T2 disease and many studies have shown this improvement for T3 disease as well.

Unfortunately, extended cholecystectomy is still performed infrequently for patients with thick GB cancers. The Surveillance Epidemiology and End Results (SEER) database demonstrated that only 6.7% of patients with T2 disease and 6.0% of patients with T3 disease had resection of three or more lymph nodes, the number indicated by the AJCC as adequate for a lymphadenectomy.[4] Additionally, when *en bloc* resection was performed, 45% of specimens contained no lymph nodes and 75% included two for fewer.[4] Thus, even patients undergoing aggressive resection are not receiving proper oncologic operations.

Bile Duct Resection

Survival for most patients with GBC is not improved with the resection of the extrahepatic bile ducts. CBD resection is typically performed when the cystic duct stump margins is positive for tumor after cholecystectomy. Although patients with a positive cystic duct stump margin are more likely to have disease in their CBD, this is not associated with decreased survival, as compared to the stage of disease and the presence of residual tumor in the liver bed. Additionally, the number of lymph nodes resected in portal lymphadenectomies seems to be independent of whether a CBD resection is performed or not.

Extended Hepatic Resection

The exact role of extended hepatic resection is yet to be determined. The rationale behind the more invasive procedure is that for tumors in the GB neck, Hartmann's pouch, or extending into the triangle of Calot, radical cholecystectomy will only provide a minimal margin. Additionally, as many GBC operations are performed after laparoscopic cholecystectomy, the Triangle of Calot is often scarred, making it difficult to differentiate tumor from postoperative inflammation. Extended hepatic resection can allow one to stay out of the plane of the prior surgery, thus theoretically promoting an improved oncologic resection. Studies are still needed to compare its efficacy and safety compared to extended cholecystectomy alone.

Adjuvant Therapy

Adjuvant radiotherapy has been proven beneficial (retrospectively) for GBC. One study demonstrated an overall survival improvement to 15 months compared to 8 months without radiation ($p < 0.0001$), with the benefit being mostly seen in patients with T2 or greater tumors and node positive disease.[5] Similarly, chemotherapy has shown benefit in GBC. One study comparing mitomycin C and 5-FU versus observation for patients with GBC showed a 5-year survival of 26% in the treatment group versus 14% in the control group ($p = 0.0367$).[6] These benefits are promising, but still need to be proven in high powered, prospectively randomized studies.

OUTCOMES

Overall, the outcome for GBC is poor. Survival statistics are variable given the numerous small series, various geographic locations of the studies, and evolving treatment trends in the disease. Many studies indicate an overall 5-year survival of 10–40%, though these outcomes can be improved up to 60% after margin negative resection. T1N0 lesions have survival rates of over 85%.

REFERENCES

1. National Cancer Institute. 2009. http://www.cancer.gov/cancertopics/types/gallbladder. Accessed July 30, 2009.
2. Kim JH, TK Kim, HW Eun, *et al.* Preoperative evaluation of gallbladder carcinoma: efficacy of combined use of MR imaging, MR cholangiography, and contrast-enhanced dual-phase three-dimensional MR angiography. *J Magn Reson Imaging* 2002; 16:676–684.
3. Goetze TO, V Paolucci. Benefits of reoperation of T2 and more advanced incidental gallbladder carcinoma. *Ann Surg* 2008; 247:104–108.
4. Coburn NG, SP Cleary, JCC Tan *et al.* Surgery for gallbladder cancer: a population-based analysis. *J Am Coll Surg* 2008; 207:371–382.
5. Wang SJ, D Fuller, JS Kim, *et al.* Prediction model for estimating the survival benefit of adjuvant radiotherapy for gallbladder cancer. *J Clin Oncol* 2008; 26:2112–2117.
6. Takada T, H Amano, H Yasuda. Is postoperative adjuvant chemotherapy useful for gallbladder carcinoma? *Cancer* 2002; 95:1685–1695.

CHOLEDOCHAL CYSTS   26

Brian R. Untch* and
Abigail E. Martin*

INTRODUCTION

Choledochal cysts are a rare, but challenging problem for pediatric and adult hepatobiliary surgeons. An understanding of the variety of anatomic variants and clinical presentations is necessary for optimal surgical treatment of these patients.

EPIDEMIOLOGY

The estimated incidence of choledochal cysts is 1:100,000 to 150,000 live births, and may be higher in some Asian countries. This increased incidence of choledochal cysts in Asian countries is poorly understood.[1] Females are affected at a preponderance of 3:1 or 4:1. While initially considered a childhood disease associated with jaundice, these cysts are now increasingly discovered in adults by way of CT imaging during the work up for abdominal pain.

CHOLEDOCHAL CYST CLASSIFICATION

As seen in Figure 1, there are multiple types of choledochal cysts. The currently accepted classification system is based on one initially proposed

---

*Duke University Medical Center, Durham, NC 27710 USA

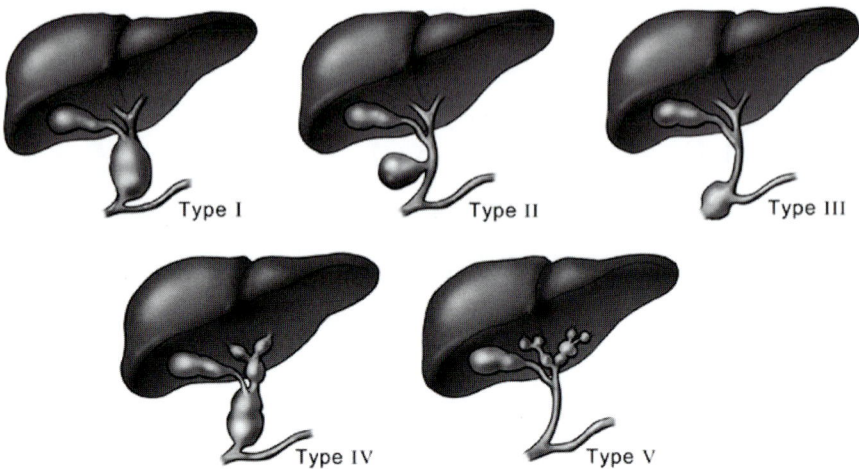

Figure 1. Type I cysts represent either cystic dilatation of the extrahepatic bile ducts (type Ia), focal dilatation of the extrahepatic bile duct (type Ib), or fusiform dilatation of the extrahepatic bile ducts (type Ic). Type II represents a diverticulum of the bile duct. Type III is often termed a choledochocele and is located within the duodenal wall. Type IV cysts are multiple cysts of the both the intra- and extrahepatic bile ducts (type IVa) or multiple cysts of the extrahepatic ducts (type IVb). Type V cysts, or Caroli's disease, is multiple areas of intrahepatic duct dilatation.

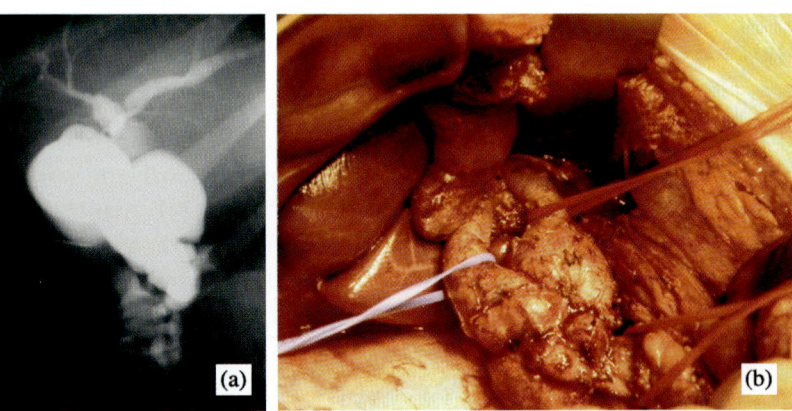

Figure 2. (a) Percutaneous cholangiogram of a type I choledochal cyst. (b) Intraoperative photograph of same choledochal cyst. The blue vessel loop is encircling the cyst duct, and the red vessel loop is encircling the common bile duct just superior to the cyst. Images used courtesy of Francois Luks, Division of Pediatric Surgery, Warren Alpert Medical School of Brown University.

by Alonso Lej *et al.*, including types I, II, and III cysts, and then expanded upon by Todani *et al.*, who added descriptions of types IV and V cysts.[2,3] The classification system is important since clinical presentation, risk of malignant degeneration, and surgical approaches are dictated by cyst morphology. Type 1 choledochal cysts, cystic or fusiform dilation of the entire extrahepatic biliary tree, are the most common cyst type accounting for >50% of patients. Type II cysts are simple diverticuli of the extrahepatic duct and are the most uncommon. Type III cysts, or choledochoceles, exist at the distal most portion of the duct inside the duodenal wall, and may have either biliary or GI mucosa. Type IV cysts are defined as multiple cysts throughout the biliary tract. Type IV cysts are further divided into IVa, which involve the intra- and extrahepatic ducts, and IVb, which affect only the extrahepatic ducts. Type V cysts are also known as Caroli's disease, and are defined as single or multiple cysts of the intrahepatic biliary tree.

PATHOGENSIS

Whether cholecochal cysts are congenital, acquired, or represent a continuum is unknown, however, several mechanisms of formation have been suggested in the literature. Pancreaticobiliary maljunction, or abnormal pancreaticobiliary junction (APBJ) has been observed in patients with choledochal cysts, although only two-thirds of patients with APBJ have choledochal cysts.[4] APBJ occurs when the bile duct and pancreatic duct merge outside the duodenal wall and at a distance from the sphincter of Oddi. Babbit hypothesized that choledochal cysts can form when a patient with APBJ has reflux of pancreatic enzymes resulting in inflammation and weakening of the bile duct wall. Evidence for this mechanism includes high amylase levels within the cysts of patients and canine animal models in which surgical creation of an APBJ leads to the development of choledochal cysts.[5] An extension of Babbit's theory is that APBJ with associated complete or partial obstruction results in elevated back pressure and subsequent acquired cyst formation.[6] The source of obstruction has been suggested to be accumulation of debris, congenital stenosis, or sphincter of Oddi dysfunction. In support of this hypothesis, when sphincteroplasty is performed in the above described canine model, there are less severe epithelial changes within the bile duct.[5]

Another proposed mechanism is that choledochal cysts develop due to ductal obstruction or distension during embryogenesis. Bile duct ligation in the neonatal sheep can produce choledocal cysts, interestingly, in adults — the only observed effect is distention of the gallbladder.[7] These observations suggest that neonatal biliary epithelium reacts to biliary obstruction differently than in the adult and produces, by an unknown mechanism, a choledochal cyst. Numerous developmental abnormalities have been observed with choledochal cysts, suggesting a common mechanism. Enteric atresias, pancreatic divisum and aplasia, and hepatobiliary malformations are either the result of a common developmental pathway abnormality or could represent secondary effects of the choledochal cyst itself. One potential genetic mutation that may be associated with choledochal cysts is the familial adenomatous polyposis coli gene. It has been suggested that the missing tumor suppressor gene could result in a weakening of the biliary epithelium and thus lead to cyst formation.[8]

The previously described mechanisms for the pathogenesis of choledochal cysts apply to the formation of type I and type IV cysts. It has been suggested that type II choledochal cysts may represent a simple duplication cyst, and this is supported by reports of type II cysts that do not communicate with the biliary tree.[9] Similarly, type III cysts have also theorized to represent duplication cysts since either duodenal or biliary epithelium may be present.[10] Because Caroli's disease is limited to the intrahepatic biliary tree, its pathogenesis is thought to be due to problems in the morphogenesis of the ductal plate of the hepatic hilum during gestation, and may be related to similar diseases of the ductal plate such as biliary atresia and congenital hepatic fibrosis.[1] Caroli's disease has also been linked to polycystic kidney disease and may be related to mutations in the PKHD1 gene.[11]

CANCER RISK

Patients who have undiagnosed or untreated choledochal cysts have a 20- to 30-fold increased risk of biliary tract cancer. The incidence of malignant degeneration of the cysts increases with age, and in adults diagnosed with choledochal cysts, up to 30% may already have evidence of malignancy.[12] In addition, these cancers develop 2 to 3 decades earlier than similar tumors in the general population. Choledochal cysts allow for chronic inflammation, bile stasis, and introduction of pancreatic enzymes to the biliary endothelium which may lead to the development of dysplasia leading to carcinoma. Adenocarcinoma accounts for a majority of the neoplasms arising from choledochal cysts, but other types including squamous cell carcinoma and anaplastic carcinoma have been reported. The risk of malignant degeneration is greatest for type I and IV cysts, with type II and III cysts having a low risk of malignancy.[13]

PRESENTATION

A majority of choledochal cysts present within the first decade of life. Patients who present in the first year of life often fail to thrive and have jaundice due to obstruction and this condition is often confused with biliary atresia. In children older than 1 year of age, the triad described by Alonso-Lej of abdominal pain, jaundice, and a right upper quadrant mass is only present in up to one-third of patients, although many children will have two of these symptoms.[14] Choledochal cyst should be considered in the differential diagnosis of patients who present with unexplained jaundice or pancreatitis. Adult patients have a more varied symptomatology. Abdominal masses are seen less often in adults, and more commonly these patients present with pancreatitis and intermittent cholangitis due to biliary stone formation. Chronic abdominal pain is nearly always present. If unrecognized and untreated, chronic cholestasis can lead to biliary cirrhosis and its sequellae.[15] In 1–12% of patients, the initial presentation occurs when the cyst spontaneously ruptures causing bile peritonitis and sepsis.[16] Choledochoceles are often asymptomatic but if large can present as either gastric outlet obstruction or intussusception.[16] Types IV and V choledochal cysts may also lead to the formation of intrahepatic abscesses due to persistent bacterial colonization or may present as portal hypertensive symptoms due to advanced biliary cirrhosis.

DIAGNOSIS

A high level of suspicion is needed to make the diagnosis when patients present with vague abdominal complaints. Laboratory values are usually nonspecific, although patients may show varying levels of conjugated hyperbilirubinemia due to obstruction. Ultrasound is often used as an initial test and is excellent at identifying types I, II, and IV cysts, but may be limited in identifying either types III and V cysts or the rare cases of cyst rupture. CT scanning can demonstrate both intra- and extrahepatic cysts, and is also useful in identifying thickening of cyst walls and associated masses that may represent cancer.[17] Patients without choledochal cysts but with chronic biliary obstruction from other causes can develop dilation of the biliary tract that may be difficult to distinguish from choledochal cysts. In these cases, the cause of biliary obstruction, such as choledocholithiasis, should be addressed and subsequent imaging performed. Other cystic lesions that may mimic choledochal cysts on imaging studies include echinococcal cysts, pancreatic pseudocysts, and biliary cystadenomas.[16]

The differential diagnosis for neonatal patients presenting with jaundice includes biliary atresia, and in these cases, HIDA scan should be performed. Biliary atresia is suggested on HIDA when no tracer is seen entering the bowel. HIDA scans are also effective in identifying extrahepatic choledochal cysts as the tracer can be seen filling the cyst and then entering the bowel. This imaging approach is less effective in identifying intrahepatic lesions.[18]

The gold standard for imaging choledochal cysts had been endoscopic retrograde cholangiopancreatography (ERCP) since this modality can definitively demonstrate the continuity of the cyst with the biliary tree. High rates of post-ERCP pancreatitis and cholangitis have been reported and have led to greater use of magnetic resonance cholangiopancreatography (MRCP). MRCP is as sensitive as ERCP for identifying cysts, however is less reliable for identifying APBJ and small biliary stones.[19] The lower costs and complications associated with MRCP make this the initial diagnostic procedure of choice for many practitioners. ERCP can also be combined with endoscopic ultrasound to diagnose type III lesions.

TREATMENT

The mainstay of treatment for choledochal cysts is surgical excision. The goals of treatment are to prevent malignant degeneration and prevent recurrent episodes of cholangitis, choledocholithiasis and pancreatitis. Historically, attempts at internal drainage of the cysts via either cystduodenostomy or cystjejunostomy have been complicated by unacceptably high rates of recurrent symptoms and the development of malignancy. For these reasons, excision of the cyst and reconstruction with hepaticojejunostomy is now the treatment of choice for types I and IVb cysts.[20] Pericystic inflammation can lead to difficulty in dissecting the cyst free from the portal vein posteriorally. In these cases, the wall of the cyst can be left *in situ*, although a mucosectomy should be performed to avoid future malignant degeneration and the patient should receive lifelong surveillance. Unfortunately, approximately 25% of patients undergoing hepaticojejunostomy will go on to develop stenosis of the anastomosis and be at risk for biliary obstruction complications.[21]

Types II and III cysts have lower malignant potential than the other categories. Thus, treatment of type II cysts involves a simple excision of the diverticulum. Type III choledochoceles can be addressed with endoscopic sphincterotomy or by unroofing the cyst via a transduodenal approach. Either method allows for free drainage of bile to avoid obstructive symptoms. Due to the intrahepatic biliary tree involvement in types IVa and V cysts, either partial hepatectomy for localized disease or liver transplantation for extensive disease is often required. In some cases of asymptomatic but diffuse Caroli's disease, transplantation can be avoided but regular surveillance for malignant disease is required.[20]

Despite cyst excision, approximately 5% of patients go on to develop biliary malignancy even after appropriate surgical therapy. This is likely related to cyst remant left at the time of operation or unknown cancer present prior to cyst excision. For this reason patients should be screened lifelong with imaging studies and liver function tests. Treatment of cholangiocarcinoma should proceed according to accepted oncologic protocols, including wide resection of the biliary tree and adjacent liver and regional lymph node dissection.

CONCLUSION

Choledochal cysts continue to present a diagnostic and therapeutic challenge to pediatric and adult hepatobiliary surgeons alike. As imaging modalities improve, the incidence of choledochal cysts may increase. In order to prevent recurrent episodes of cholangitis and the risk of malignant degeneration, complete surgical excision will remain the mainstay of treatment for these patients.

REFERENCES

1. Singham J, Yoshida E, Scudamore C. Choledochal cysts: part 1 of 3: classification and pathogenesis. *Can J Surg* 2009; 52:434–440.
2. Alonso-Lej F, Rever W, Pessango D. Congenital choledochal cyst, with a report of 2, and analysis of 94 cases. *Int Abstr Surg* 1959; 108:1–30.

3. Todani T, Watanabe Y, Narusue M, *et al.* Congenital bile duct cysts: classifcation, operative procedures, and review of thirty-seven cases including cancer arising from choledochal cyst. *Am J Surg* 1977; 134:263–269.
4. Sugiyama M, Atomi Y, Kuroda A. Pancreatic disorders associated with anomalous pancreaticobiliary junction. *Surgery* 1999; 126:492–497.
5. Han S, Han A, Kim M, *et al.* The role of sphincteroplasty in adverse effect of anomalous pancreaticobiliary duct union in an animal model. *Pediatr Surg Int* 2007; 23:225–231.
6. Miyano T, Suruga K, Chen S. A clinicopathologic study of choledochal cyst. *World J Surg* 1980; 4:231–238.
7. Spitz L. Experimental production of cystic dilatation of the common bile duct in neonatal lambs. *J Pediatr Surg* 1977; 12:39–42.
8. Behrns K, Shaheen J, Grimm I. Type I choledochal cyst in association with familial adenomatous polyposis. *Am J Gastroenterol* 1998; 93:1337–1339.
9. Jindal R, Harris N, McDaniel H, *et al.* Presentation of choledochal cysts without intrabiliary communication on endoscopic retrograde cholangiopancreatography. *Liver Transpl Surg* 1996; 2:468–471.
10. Kagiyama S, Okazaki K, Yamamoto Y, *et al.* Anatomic variants of choledochocele and manometric measurements of presure in the cele and the orifice zone. *Am J Gastroenterol* 1987; 82:641–649.
11. Sgro M, Rossetti S, Barozzino T, *et al.* Caroli's disease: prenatal diagnosis, postnatal outcome and genetic analysis. *Ultrasound Obstet Gynecol* 2004; 23:73–76.
12. Soreide K, Soreide J. Bile duct cyst as precursor to biliary tract cancer. *Ann Surg Onc* 2007; 14:1200–1211.
13. Todani T, Tabuchi K, Watanabe Y, *et al.* Carcinoma arising in the wall of congenital bile duct cysts. *Cancer* 1979; 44:1134–1141.
14. Lipsett P, Pitt H, Colombani P, *et al.* Choledochal cyst disease. A changing pattern of presentation. *Ann Surg* 1994; 220:644–652.
15. Rao K, Chowdhary S, Kumar D. Choledochal cyst associated with portal hypertension. *Pediatr Surg Int* 2003; 19:729–732.
16. Singham J, Yoshida E, Scudamore C. Choledochal cysts: part 2 of 3: Diagnosis. *Can J Surg* 2009; 52:506–511.
17. Han J, Choi G. Carcinoma in a choledochal cyst. *Adbom Imaging* 1996; 21:179–181.
18. Spottswood S, Jolles P, Haynes J, *et al.* Choledochal cyst with biliary atresia: scintigraphy and correlative imaging. *Clin Nuc Med* 2001; 26: 555–556.

19. Matos C, Nicaise N, Deviere J, *et al.* Choledochal cysts: comparison of findings at MR cholangiopancreatography and endoscopic retrograde cholangiopancreatography in eight patients. *Radiology* 1998; 209:443–448.
20. Singham J, Yoshida E, Scudamore C. Choledochal cysts: part 3 of 3: management. *Can J Surg* 2010; 53:51–56.
21. Rothlin M, Lopfe M, Schlumpf R, *et al.* Long-term results of hepaticojejunostomy for benign lesions of the bile ducts. *Am J Surg* 1998; 175:22–26.

PRIMARY BILIARY CIRRHOSIS AND PRIMARY SCLEROSING CHOLANGITIS 27

**Vanessa Teaberry* and
Alastair Smith[†]**

INTRODUCTION

The immune-mediated cholangiopathies, namely primary biliary cirrhosis (PBC) and primary sclerosing cholangitis (PSC) are uncommon but important disease entities. Surgical trainees might well ask what place a discourse such as this about two largely "nonsurgical" conditions such as PBC and PSC has in a surgical text. Conversely, the initial assessment and management of jaundice and to a lesser degree cholestatic liver test abnormalities remains very much in the realm of the general surgeon.

PRIMARY BILIARY CIRRHOSIS

PBC is a chronic, incurable and progressive cholestatic disease that is characterized by the presence of serum antimitochondrial antibody (AMA), inflammation and injury to biliary epithelial cells (cholangiocytes) and eventual loss of interlobular-sized bile ducts. The clinical course of PBC is very variable, but may culminate in intractable cholestasis, biliary cirrhosis

---

*Duke University Medical Center, Durham, NC 27708 USA
[†]Duke University Medical Center, Durham, NC 27710 USA

and complications of end-stage liver disease (ESLD), thereby requiring consideration of liver transplantation.

Epidemiology and Etiology

The incidence of PBC is 2.7 per 100,000 person years (4.5 for women, 0.7 for men) and has been increasing, probably as the result of a greater awareness of the disease and improved diagnostic capabilities. The female to male disease ratio is 9:1. The median age at diagnosis is 50 years although the range is wide. Patients are typically Caucasian.

Members of a family having a PBC patient are up to 100 times more likely to develop PBC than members of the general population. It appears that incidence may also vary by geographic region. These observations suggest that clustering observed within families may have less to do with genetics and more to do with similar environmental exposures.

Pathophysiology

Patients who develop PBC share both a genetic predisposition to the disease and exposure to certain environmental factors (triggers). The impact of the former is suggested by association with alleles from major histocompatibility complex loci, although these vary depending on the population studied, and the considerably increased prevalence of PBC reported among first-degree relatives. The triggers are believed to stimulate the immune system by a form of molecular mimicry. Examples of triggers include bacteria, e.g. *E. coli* especially as the cause of urinary tract infections, viruses such as the human β-retrovirus, and environmental toxins, e.g. nail polish and past cigarette smoking.

PBC is a T-cell–mediated phenomenon: large numbers of CD4+ and CD8+ cells may be observed in the portal triads of liver biopsy specimens. These lymphocytes are autoreactive against the pyruvate dehydrogenase subunit E2. Under normal circumstances, this subunit is found on the inner mitochondrial membrane only; however, among PBC patients, the E2 subunit is also expressed on the luminal surface of cholangiocytes. The mechanism by which this altered subunit expression occurs is not currently known but the result is that epithelial cells become the target for destruction by the patient's own CD8+ lymphocytes.

Presentation and Diagnosis

More than half of all PBC patients have no symptoms at diagnosis. However, asymptomatic patients will generally develop symptoms within 2–4 years of diagnosis. The most common symptom among PBC patients is fatigue, either with or without daytime somnolence. The presence or absence of this complaint does not correlate with disease severity. In some patients, fatigue is the primary manifestation of untreated hypothyroidism rather than PBC, and will improve with replacement therapy. Pruritus is the second most common symptom. Twenty-five to fifty percent of patients complain of hyperpigmentation: this is secondary to melanin deposition rather than hyperbilirubinemia. Other symptoms include a variety of musculoskeletal (joint and bone pain, stiffness) and cutaneous complaints (xanthelasmata), as well as features consistent with Sjogren's syndrome (dry mouth and eyes).

The diagnosis of PBC should be considered in any patient (symptomatic or not) with an elevated serum alkaline phosphatase concentration that is clearly of liver origin, i.e. increased gamma glutamyl transpeptidase. Assuming that intra- and extrahepatic bile duct dilatation does not exist, the presence of serum AMA should be sought (up to 95% of patients with PBC demonstrate this, and the antibody is 98% specific for PBC). If present in a titer of least 1:80, the diagnosis of PBC is secure. Liver biopsy is not required for diagnosis, although important information about hepatic fibrosis may be gained and thus help guide discussion about the anticipated clinical course. Conversely, liver biopsy is absolutely necessary in patients who lack serum AMA, in whom alternative explanations for cholestatic liver test abnormalities exist, e.g. drug reaction, and in whom the possibility of coexisting autoimmune hepatitis must be addressed. A detailed description of the variability of histologic abnormalities is beyond the scope of this chapter.

In most patients with PBC, serum concentrations of immunoglobulin M are elevated. Antinuclear antibodies are present in at least 50% of patients; their presence is believed to be associated with more rapid disease progression. Upwards of 50% of patients have hypercholesterolemia, invariably an increase in HDL concentration. Liver synthetic function is generally intact at diagnosis, and remains preserved until the late stages of the disease.

The mean survival for patients with early stage disease is 50–75% that of the general population, but only approximately 5–8 years from the onset of symptoms in the absence of treatment. Survival increases to 84% at 10 years and 66% at 20 years with treatment.

Treatment

Ursodeoxycholic acid (UDCA), administered in a daily dose of 13–15 mg/kg body weight, is the only US Food and Drug Administration-approved therapy for PBC. It is generally well tolerated, and should be continued indefinitely. Treatment with UDCA improves liver blood test results, delays histologic progression and enhances transplant-free survival among responders. UDCA also improves survival in symptomatic patients as previously mentioned.

Treatment of PBC complications, e.g. pruritus, metabolic bone disease and vitamin D deficiency, related conditions such as Sicca syndrome, as well as screening for primary liver cancer and gastroesophageal varices are fundamental to proper overall management of the patient with PBC.

Whereas PBC represented the leading indication for liver transplantation in the United States and Europe at its inception, this is no longer the case. Currently, PBC is the sixth commonest indication for liver transplantation (this is the only surgical intervention for patients with PBC). Priority is based upon satisfactory completion of transplant evaluation and the prevailing model for end-stage liver disease (MELD) score (see Chapter 12). Both short- and long-term outcomes of liver transplantation for PBC are superior to those for other indications. PBC does recur in the graft (at least 30% at 10 years) but graft loss secondary to recurrence is very low and does not change the overall long-term survival of the graft or the patient.

PRIMARY SCLEROSING CHOLANGITIS

PSC is an inflammatory cholangiopathy that follows a relapsing and remitting course. It is possible that PSC actually represents a spectrum of clinically similar diseases causing progressive inflammation, fibrosis and scarring of the intra- and extrahepatic bile ducts with different causes rather than one disease.

Epidemiology

A population-based study performed in Olmsted County, Minnesota found the incidence of PSC to be 1.25 per 100K person years for men and only

0.54 in females. This is in direct contrast to patients with PBC, who are almost always female. Men tend to be in the fourth or fifth decade of life at diagnosis (median age 40 years), whereas female PSC patients tend to be diagnosed later in life. No definite pattern of inheritance has been identified for PSC; however the prevalence of PSC among first-degree relatives of affected patients is nearly double that of the general population.

PSC may occur in conjunction with other autoimmune diseases, most notably chronic inflammatory bowel disease, specifically ulcerative colitis (UC), although PSC can occur in patients with Crohn's colitis, albeit with much less frequency. The incidence of UC in PSC patients has been reported to be as low as 25% and as high as 90% depending on the study (73% in Olmsted County) although only about 5% of UC patients will have PSC. PSC is more common in male UC patients and those with pancolitis. The reason for the large number of PSC patients also having UC is thought to be due to bile ductular cells expressing antigens that cross-react with those on colonic epithelium. Despite their occurrence in the same patient, the two diseases are often clinically distinct in their temporal manifestation. The most extreme example of this is UC occurring in a PSC patient after liver transplantation.

Like PBC, the PSC patient is very likely to be asymptomatic at the time of diagnosis, but rather than experiencing a slow progression to more severe disease, the PSC patient is more likely to have periods of relative disease severity interspersed with intervals during which the disease is more quiescent. The median survival for asymptomatic patients is 10–12 years from the time of diagnosis without liver transplant. Survival is somewhat lower for those patients who are symptomatic at diagnosis.

Pathophysiology

As above, PSC commonly occurs with other autoimmune syndromes, especially inflammatory bowel disease, and also less commonly autoimmune hepatitis. It is thought that the inflammation seen in PSC may also have an autoimmune cause. Further supporting this hypothesis, patients with PSC have elevated serum IgH levels (50%), antismooth muscle and antinuclear antibodies (75%), elevated P-ANCA (80% of patients with a 100% specificity for PSC over other liver diseases), and increased CD4+ T cells. These CD4+ T cells are believed to target the bile duct epithelial cells.

Despite suspicions that PSC may be an autoimmune disorder, the "trigger" has not been identified and therefore, the etiology of PSC remains largely unknown. However, several factors are believed to contribute to its development. Bacterial translocation into the portal circulation (especially in the setting of increased permeability across the inflamed colonic wall in UC) is thought to be causative by leading to chronic inflammation of the biliary tree. Another theory is that biliary epithelial injury may arise as the result of accumulation of toxic bile acids produced by colonic bacteria or chronic viral infection. Lastly, ischemia is thought to potentially play a role due to the fact that ischemic injury histologically resembles the lesions seen in PSC, although clinically no data exists to support this hypothesis.

Early stage disease may be characterized by ulceration of the ducts without stricture formation. However, the disease inevitably progresses to the loss of intra- and extrahepatic bile ducts and cholestatic cirrhosis. PSC patients also carry a lifetime risk of developing cholangiocarcinoma of about 10–15%. In patients with concomitant IBD, cirrhosis and variceal bleeding are independent factors associated with the highest risk of cholangiocarcinoma development. Unfortunately, cholangiocarcinoma is extremely difficult to diagnose and is found to be unexpectedly present in 10% of liver transplant recipient explants. This places the transplant recipient at high risk of recurrence in the transplanted organ and carries a poor prognosis.

Presentation and Diagnosis

PSC patients often have no symptoms at diagnosis, but cholestatic liver test abnormalities only, i.e. increased serum alkaline phosphatase and gamma GT concentrations, with or without elevation of total serum bilirubin, aspartate and alanine aminotransferase concentrations. If the patient is symptomatic at diagnosis the total serum bilirubin concentration may reflect the severity of an exacerbation of a disorder that is characterized by relapse and remission.

Although asymptomatic at presentation, the PSC patients will eventually develop some distinctive symptoms. Commonly, patients will complain of jaundice, RUQ pain, pruritus, weight loss, and fatigue. Additionally, they may experience episodes of fevers, rigors, and night sweats that may represent transient cholangitis. One-third will also develop choledocolithiasis with or without cholangitis throughout the course of their disease.

In contrast to PBC, imaging studies are essential when making a diagnosis of PSC. Endoscopic retrograde cholangiopancreatography is

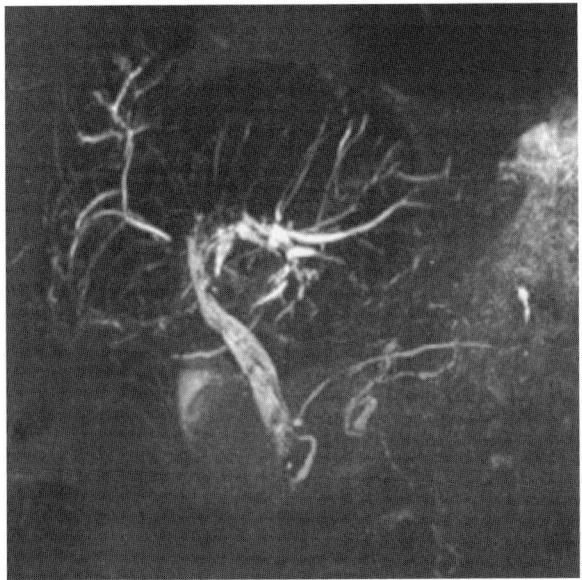

Figure 1.

preferable to percutaneous transhepatic cholangiography for imaging the biliary tree of a patient who is either known to or is suspected to have PSC; however, MRCP may be substituted should a non-invasive modality be desired. The obvious downside of MRCP is its lack of interventional capability. ERCP images may reveal diffuse multifocal strictures and focal dilations of the intra- and extrahepatic ducts in a characteristic appearance in 87% of patients (Figure 1). This structuring can involve the cystic duct and even the gallbladder. With respect to histology, liver biopsy is of limited utility in diagnosis but can be useful in staging. The findings of fibrous obliteration of small ducts and an onion skin pattern of fibrosis that starts in the portal triads and expands into the parenchyma are pathognomonic for PSC (Figure 2).

Treatment

Various therapies including Ursodiol and several immunomodulatory agents (including corticosteroids, cyclosporine, methotrexate, FK506, and Etanercept) have been studied for their efficacy in PSC, but none have

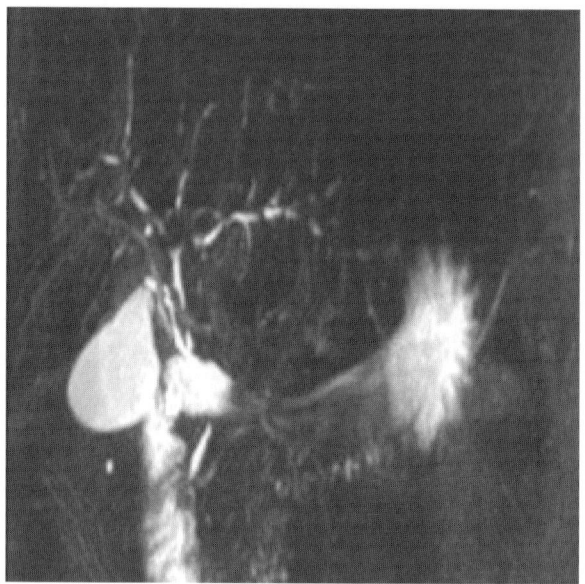

Figure 2.

been shown to alter the natural history of the disease. As a result of this, medical treatment is aimed at symptom relief, leaving intervention as the mainstay of management. Contemporary retrospective studies have shown that endoscopic therapy such as stenting or dilation of a dominant stricture may allow patients more years free of transplant than would have been predicted by the Mayo risk score. The caveat of endoscopic therapy for a dominant stricture is that it is difficult to differentiate a benign stricture from cholangiocarcinoma and therefore careful sampling of biliary epithelium with brushings and/or biopsies should be taken at the time of the procedure.

Liver transplantation represents the only definitive treatment option and is the primary surgical therapy for PSC; however, occasionally a patient with only extrahepatic disease and minimal liver dysfunction may be a candidate for a biliary reconstruction with biliary enteric drainage. This may be done with the caveat that such an operation carries risks of infection and acceleration of liver insufficiency and may make an eventual liver transplant more technically difficult. Regardless, the median survival from the time of diagnosis without transplant is 10–12 years in an asymptomatic patient and shorter for those that are symptomatic. As in PBC, the Mayo risk score may be used to determine timing of listing for transplant.

Table 1. Histologic grades

Stage 1:	Inflammation focused on the bile duct, but confined to the portal area.
Stage 2:	Inflammation focused on the bile duct, but extending beyond the limiting plate, i.e. interface hepatitis.
Stage 3:	The presence of fibrosis.
Stage 4:	Cirrhosis and regenerative nodule formation.

As with all indications for liver transplantation, organs are allocated using the MELD score. However, even in patients with a low MELD score and PSC, transplant is indicated in the setting of recurrent cholangitis, hilar cholangiocarcinoma and/or hepatocellular cancer. Post-transplantation survival rates are similar to those for other liver transplant indications although PSC patients have a higher incidence of nonanastomotic strictures. These strictures most likely represent disease recurrence as up to 20% of patients will experience return of their disease at 10-years post-transplant. About 1/3 of those patients with disease recurrence will progress to end-stage liver disease in their allograft. Risk factors for recurrence include age, sex mismatch, male recipient, concurrence with IBD especially if the colon is intact, CMV status, recurrent acute rejection especially if steroid resistant, OKT3 use, cholangiocarcinoma prior to transplant, extended criteria donors, and prolonged steroid usage. The goal when evaluating a PSC patient for liver transplant is for the patient to be transplanted prior to the development of cholangiocarcinoma.

REFERENCES

1. European Association for the Study of the Liver Clinical Practice Guidelines: Management of the cholestatic liver disease. *J Hepatol* 2009; 51:237–262.
2. Lindor KD, Gershwin ME, Poupon R, *et al.* Primary biliary cirrhosis. *Hepatology* 2009; 50:291–308.
3. Chapman R, Fevery J, Kalloo A, *et al.* Diagnosis and management of primary sclerosing cholangitis. *Hepatology* 2010; 51:660–678.
4. Mendes F, Lindor KD. Primary sclerosing cholangitis: overview and update. *Nature Reviews: Gastroenterology and Hepatology* 2010; 7:611–619.
5. Selmi C, Bowlus CL, Gershwin ME, *et al.* Primary biliary cirrhosis (review). *Lancet* 2011; 377:1600–1609.

BILE DUCT CANCER: PERIPHERAL AND HILAR CHOLANGIOCARCINOMA 28

Melissa Danko* and Dana Portenier[†]

INTRODUCTION

Cholangiocarcinoma (CC) is a bile duct tumor that can occur anywhere along the extra- or intrahepatic biliary system. These rare tumors are located most commonly at the hepatic duct bifurcation. Extrahepatic cholangiocarcinoma (ECC) arises within the hepatoduodenal ligament and is classified as hilar or distal tumors. Intrahepatic cholangiocarcinoma (ICC) originates in the liver. Over the past few decades, many advances have been made in the diagnosis, therapy, and palliation of this disease.

Epidemiology

In the United States, the incidence of cholangiocarcinoma is 1–2 cases per 100,000 population or about 5,000 new patients per year. The data from multiple cancer societies and registries are difficult to interpret as intrahepatic cholangiocarcinomas are often included with primary liver cancers and extrahepatic bile duct cancers are often grouped with gallbladder cancer. Over the past 2 decades, the incidence of ICC has been rising in

---

*Vanderbilt University School of Medicine, Nashville, TN, USA
[†]Duke University School of Medicine, Durham, NC, USA

Europe, North America, Asia, Australia, and Japan, while the rates of ECC are declining. In the United States, cholangiocarcinoma accounts for about 3% of all gastrointestinal tumors, while ICC accounts for 10–15% of all primary hepatic cancers.

Presentation and Risk Factors

Typically, cholangiocarcinoma presents between the 6th and 8th decade of life; the incidence of biliary tract cancers increases with age. It is slightly more common in men than women, and this might be reflective of the higher incidence of primary sclerosing cholangitis in men. In its early stage, cholangiocarcinoma may have no symptoms or can be associated with nonspecific symptoms. The majority of cholangiocarcinomas present with jaundice, specifically more than 90% of those with perihilar or distal tumors. Conversely, patients with intrahepatic cholangiocarcinoma do not develop jaundice until late in the course of their disease and are often only diagnosed with imaging studies. Other clinical features include pruritis, mild abdominal pain, fever, fatigue, weight loss, and anorexia.

Numerous diseases have been associated with cholangiocarcinoma including choledochal cysts, primary sclerosing cholangitis, and hepatolithiasis. These diseases all share certain characteristics such as biliary stasis, bile duct stones, and infection. Patients with cirrhosis have a 10-fold higher risk of developing CC. Hepatitis B and C are also recognized as risk factors in the development of intrahepatic cholangiocarcinoma. The inherited cancer syndrome Lynch syndrome II has been associated with an increased risk of bile duct cancer. An additional rare genetic disorder called multiple biliary papillomatosis is also linked to an increased risk of cholangiocarcinoma.

The future risk for cholangiocarcinoma may be increased by previous biliary enteric anastomosis. Other risk factors for cholangiocarcinoma include liver flukes, Thorotrast, asbestos, vinyl chloride, dietary nitrosamines, and medications, such as digoxin, isoniazid, and first-generation oral contraceptives.

WORKUP

Physical Exam and Laboratory Evaluation

Other than jaundice, the physical exam of patients with cholangiocarcinoma is usually normal. At the time of presentation, the total serum bilirubin of most patients with perihilar and distal biliary tumors is greater than 10 mg/dL. If there is obstruction of the two main hepatic ducts or the common bile duct, markers of biliary epithelial injury, including alkaline phosphatase and γ-glutamyltransferase, are also elevated. Serum CA 19–9 may be increased as well and seems to correlate with the stage of the disease, although this marker usually decreases once the biliary obstruction is relieved. CEA levels may also be elevated in cholangiocarcinoma.

Imaging

Radiological imaging is important for the diagnosis and treatment planning of cholangiocarcinoma. It is performed to determine the extent of the tumor, assessing the involvement of the bile ducts, liver, and hilar vessels as well as distant metastases. The initial radiographic study should be an abdominal ultrasound or triple-phase CT scan. While intrahepatic cholangiocarcinomas are easily visualized with these studies, perihilar and distal tumors are often difficult to evaluate. A hilar cholangiocarcinoma is suggested by a dilated intrahepatic biliary system with a normal or collapsed gallbladder and extrahepatic biliary tree. Distal cholangiocarcinomas cause dilation of the gallbladder and both the extra- and intrahepatic biliary trees. The overall accuracy of CT scan in predicting resectability of CC ranges from 60% to 85%. Duplex ultrasound with color Doppler has a 93% sensitivity and 99% specificity in assessing portal venous or hepatic artery invasion. CT cholangiography has recently been shown to be superior to conventional CT for the diagnosis of hilar CC.

MRI and magnetic resonance cholangiopancreatography (MRCP) create a three-dimensional reconstruction of the biliary tree and have been shown to have diagnostic accuracy comparable with endoscopic retrograde cholangiopancreatography (ERCP) or percutaneous transhepatic cholangiography (PTC). It is suggested that MRCP be performed prior to decompression of the biliary system. MRI can also be helpful in diagnosing lymph node metastases, portal venous invasion, and arterial invasion.

Once biliary dilation has been documented, biliary anatomy has traditionally been defined by cholangiography, which provides dynamic images of the biliary system. This can be performed by the percutaneous transhepatic route (PTC) or the endoscopic retrograde route (ERCP), both of which are invasive. The percutaneous route is favored in patients with perihilar tumors as it defines the proximal extent of the tumor most reliably, and this is the most important feature in determining resectability. ERCP is limited in the assessment of the proximal biliary tree, while PTC cannot assess the distal extension of the tumor if complete biliary obstruction is present.

Special ultrasound techniques have been developed and adopted for use over the years. Endoscopic ultrasound (EUS) can detect abnormalities that are not able to be easily identified using a percutaneous approach. EUS also has the advantage of being able to perform image-guided fine needle aspirations for cytology that assist in preoperative staging. Intraductal ultrasound can be performed by placing high-frequency US probes into the common bile duct using ERCP guidance, increasing the diagnostic accuracy of ERCP.

In 30% of patients with cholangiocarcinoma, PET will detect intrahepatic or distant metastases, having a higher rate of success for distant metastases (about 70%). PET scanning has a sensitivity of 85% for cholangiocarcinomas that measure at least 1 cm in size. A major limitation of PET is that patients with biliary inflammatory conditions, including cholangitis or PSC, may have false-positive results, while patients with mucinous cholangiocarcinoma have poor uptake of fluorodeoxygluose producing false-negative scans.

Optical coherence tomography (OCT) is a new technique that utilizes infrared light to produce cross-sectional images. Preliminary studies have suggested that OCT has the ability to produce high-quality images of the biliary tree that correlate with histological findings. Currently it is not widely available, and its diagnostic role in CC has not been well-established.

Differential Diagnosis

Cholangiocarcinoma should always be in the differential for a patient presenting with obstructive jaundice. Other hepatopancreatobiliary diseases that can present similarly include hepatocellular carcinoma, pancreatic adenocarcinoma, and gallbladder cancer.

PATHOLOGY AND CLASSIFICATION

The Bismuth classification is used to classify perihilar cholangiocarcinoma according to its anatomic location. Type I tumors are confined to the common hepatic duct. Type II tumors involve only the common hepatic duct bifurcation. Types IIIa and IIIb tumors extend into either the right or left secondary intrahepatic ducts, respectively. Type IV tumors involve the secondary intrahepatic ducts bilaterally or have multifocal distribution.

Cholangiocarcinoma can spread along the biliary tree, directly invade adjacent structures and lymph nodes, or seed distant metastasis. Papillary and nodular tumors are mostly associated with mucosal extension, while sclerosing tumors spread more via submucosal extension. About 45% of cholangiocarcinomas have lymph node metastasis. The regional hilar nodes are most commonly involved, but the para-aortic lymph node basins can also be the site of metastasis.

Important prognostic factors for cholangiocarcinoma include portal vein involvement and lobar atrophy.

Cholangiocarcinoma is staged by the TNM classification of the AJCC, with intrahepatic cholangiocarcinoma being classified as a primary liver malignancy (Tables 1, 2).[1] For hilar or Klatskin tumors, the Memorial Sloan–Kettering Cancer Center has created a staging system called the T-stage criteria. This staging system does not take into account the lymph node status or metastasis and only includes the location and extent of ductal involvement, presence or absence of hepatic lobar atrophy, and presence or absence of portal vein invasion.

Percutaneous fine-needle aspiration biopsy, brush and scrape biopsies, and cytologic examination of bile have all been utilized to confirm a tissue

Table 1. American joint committee on cancer staging of intrahepatic cholangiocarcinomas.

Stage	Tumor	Node	Metastasis
I	T1	N0	M0
II	T2	N0	M0
IIIA	T3	N0	M0
IIIB	T4	N0	M0
IIIC	Any T	N1	M0
IV	Any T	Any N	M1

T1, solitary tumor without vascular invasion; T2, solitary tumor with vascular invasion or multiple tumors none >5 cm; T3, multiple tumors >5 cm or tumor involving a major branch of the portal or hepatic vein(s); T4, tumor(s) with direct invasion of adjacent organs other than the gallbladder or with perforation of visceral peritoneum; No, no regional lymph node metastasis; Ni, regional lymph node metastasis; M0, no distant metastasis; M1, distant metastasis.

Table 2. American joint committee on cancer staging of extrahepatic cholangiocarcinomas.

Stage	Tumor	Node	Metastasis
0	Tis	N0	M0
IA	T1	N0	M0
IB	T2	N0	M0
IIA	T3	N0	M0
IIB	T1–T3	N1	M0
III	T4	Any N	M0
IV	Any T	Any N	M1

Tis, carcinoma *in situ*; T1, tumor confined to the bile duct histologically; T2, tumor invades beyond the wall of the bile duct; T3, tumor invades the liver, gallbladder, pancreas, or unilateral branches of the portal vein (right or left) or hepatic artery (right or left); T4, tumor invades any of the following: main portal vein or its branches bilaterally, common hepatic artery, or other adjacent structures such as the colon, stomach, duodenum, or abdominal wall; N0, no regional lymph node metastasis; N1, regional lymph node metastasis; M0, no distant metastasis; M1, distant metastasis.

diagnosis of cholangiocarcinoma. Unfortunately, the sensitivity of these methods in detecting a malignancy is low, and a benign result is not reliable. Ultimately, 7–15% of patients presenting with and having intraoperative findings consistent with a malignant biliary obstruction will have benign lesions of histological analysis of surgical specimens.

Over 90% of cholangiocarcinomas are well to moderately differentiated adenocarcinomas.

MANAGEMENT OPTIONS

When surgical resection is possible, it does provide an opportunity for long-term disease-free survival. Unfortunately, many patients diagnosed with cholangiocarcinoma are only candidates for palliative bypass or procedures performed to achieve biliary drainage to prevent the serious complications of cholangitis and liver failure.

Preoperative biliary drainage is controversial. Biliary drainage is considered if the total bilirubin is greater than 10 mg/dL. It is associated with an increased risk for cholangitis and a longer postoperative hospital stay in patients with obstructive jaundice who undergo resection. If drainage is not performed, cholestasis, biliary cirrhosis, and liver dysfunction may develop rapidly.

Radiographic criteria that suggests unresectablility of perihilar cholangiocarcinomas includes bilateral hepatic duct involvement up to secondary radicals, bilateral hepatic artery involvement, encasement or occlusion of the portal vein proximal to its bifurcation, atrophy of one hepatic lobe with contralateral portal vein encasement, atrophy of one hepatic lobe with contralateral biliary radical involvement, or distant metastases. The AJCC stages III and IV patients with distal ECC and intrahepatic CC are generally considered unresectable. Curative treatment is possible only with complete resection (R0).

Nonoperative palliation is offered to patients with unequivocal evidence of unresectable cholangiocarcinoma. This can be achieved either endoscopically or percutaneously. The endoscopic approach is usually favored in patients with distal cholangiocarcinoma, while percutaneous drainage is preferred in those with perihilar tumors. Metallic stents have become favored over plastic ones for their longer patency and fewer subsequent manipulations.

Medical interventions have not been proven to be very effective against cholangiocarcinoma. Radiation therapy has been suggested to improve survival in patients with unresectable cholangiocarcinoma, however there have been no randomized-control trials showing this. Adjuvant radiation therapy has been shown to have a benefit in patients with positive surgical margins. Chemotherapy has not been shown to improve survival in patients with unresectable or resectable disease. Only in ECC has combined adjuvant chemoradiation been shown to have a small survival advantage. Photodynamic therapy has been emerging as a potential palliative option for patients with unresectable cholangiocarcinoma.

SURGICAL MANAGEMENT

Procedure

Patients who have no evidence of metastasis or locally unresectable disease and are reasonable risk surgical candidates should undergo surgical exploration. Preoperative portal vein embolization is often utilized when a major liver resection is indicated. Recently, staging laparoscopy has been advocated to identify liver or peritoneal metastasis while avoiding a laparotomy.

Intraoperatively hepatic or peritoneal metastases or locally unresectable disease is found in more than half of these patients. Unfortunately, laparoscopy is limited in its ability to detect vascular or nodal involvement. In patients with metastatic disease, preoperative biliary stents should be left in place and a cholecystectomy should be performed. In patients with unresectable locally advanced perihilar disease, there are a number of palliative options including Roux-en-Y hepaticojejunostomy. For resectable patients, the anatomical classification of cholangiocarcinoma usually determines the treatment approach. Distal or extrahepatic cholangiocarcinoma is usually treated with pancreaticoduodenectomy. Intrahepatic biliary tumors are treated like hepatocellular carcinoma with hepatectomy as the gold standard when possible. Lymph node dissection is not recommended for ICC as it has not been shown to improve survival. Perihilar cholangiocarcinoma is managed by resection of the bile duct preferably with accompanying hepatic resection, cholecystectomy, and regional lymphadenectomy. For Bismuth type I and II lesions, the bile ducts and gallbladder are resected *en bloc* with 5–10 mm bile duct margins, regional lymphadenectomy, and Roux-en-Y hepaticojejunostomy. Type II lesions may need an accompanying hepatic lobectomy. Routine caudate lobectomy is often performed for type II and III tumors. When technically possible, gross surgical margins should be >2 cm for the papillary and nodular tumor types and >1 cm in the infiltrating type.

The use of liver transplantation for the treatment of cholangiocarcinoma is controversial. It is being investigated for patients with liver dysfunction that precludes resection and for patients requiring total hepatectomy for negative margins. More recent promising results have been achieved with neoadjuvant chemoradiation treatment followed by liver transplantation. Transplantation should be reserved for selected patients enrolled in research protocols and selected centers.

Surgical palliation is considered in patients who have unresectable disease at the time of surgical exploration, patients who cannot undergo repeated endoscopic or percutaneous interventions, or patients who have a long expected survival and who will tolerate an operation. Biliary-enteric anastomosis has superior patency compared to stents. It also eliminates the need for multiple stent exchanges.

Complications

Preoperative biliary drainage can introduce bacteria into the biliary tract via stent placement, causing more morbidity at the time of surgery.

Postoperatively, patients are at risk for episodes of cholangitis. Patients undergoing partial hepatectomy for CC are also at risk for postoperative liver failure.

OUTCOMES

Distal cholangiocarcinoma treated with a pylorus-preserving pancreaticoduodenectomy has a 5-year survival rate ranging from 15% to 25% but can be as high as 50% in certain patients who have a complete resection and node-negative disease. Positive surgical margins and lymph nodes are predictive of poor outcome. Outcomes for intrahepatic cholangiocarcinoma depend on disease stage, in particular the lymph node status, and margin status. Three-year survival rates for those patients undergoing complete resection vary from 22% to 66%. Positive resection margins, vascular and lymphatic invasion, and periductal infiltrating disease are predictors of poor outcome. For perihilar cholangiocarcinoma, curative resections are possible in less than half of cases and most resections do not provide long-term disease control. Despite this, some studies have reported 5-year survival rates above 50% when a more aggressive surgical approach is employed, which unfortunately is associated with increased surgical mortality rates.

REFERENCES

1. Greene FL, Page DL, Fleming ID, *et al.*, *American Joint Committee on Cancer Staging*. 6th edition, New York, Springer-Verlag. 2002.
2. Townsend CM, Beauchamp RD, Evers BM, *et al.*, *Sabiston Textbook of Surgery: The Biological Basis of Modern Surgical Practice*. 18th edition, Elsevier. 2008.
3. Aljiffry M, Abdulelah A, Walsh M, *et al.* Evidence-based approach to cholangiocarcinoma: A systematic review of the current literature. *J Am Coll Surg* 2009; 20(1):134–147.
4. Ustundag Y, Bayraktar Y. Cholangiocarcinoma: A compact review of the literature. *World J Gastroenterology* 2008; 14(42):6458–6466.

INTERVENTIONAL BILIARY TECHNIQUES 29

Nicholas D. Andersen[*] and
Paul V. Suhocki[†]

PERCUTANEOUS CHOLECYSTOSTOMY

Percutaneous cholecystostomy (PC) allows for nonoperative management of acute cholecystitis in patients where emergency surgery is contraindicated due to comorbidities or critical illness. The diagnosis of acute cholecystitis is usually made by a constellation of right upper quadrant pain, fever, leukocytosis, and imaging findings suggestive of gallbladder inflammation. Patients have typically failed 24 hours of antibiotics prior to proceeding to PC. In other circumstances, PC is used to rule out cholecystitis as a cause of sepsis in critically ill patients with imaging studies suggestive of gallbladder inflammation.

At our center, PC is performed under local anesthesia and conscious sedation using fluoroscopic and sonographic guidance. An 18-gauge needle is advanced transhepatically or transperitoneally into the gallbladder followed by a guidewire and serial dilators. An 8-F drainage catheter is then placed with the tip in the gallbladder. Contrast is injected to confirm appropriate placement of the catheter. Bile is aspirated for gram stain and culture and the catheter is anchored to the skin. Tubes are placed to bulb suction and flushed with 10-mL normal saline every 8 hours to maintain patency.

---

[*]Duke University Medical Center 3443, Durham, NC 27710 USA
[†]Department of Radiology, Room 1502 (MS3808), Durham, NC 27710 USA

Culture data is used to guide antibiotic treatment, with antibiotics continued for 7–14 days after resolution of symptoms when biliary pathogens or bacteremia are present. PC removal is considered after resolution of cholecystitis. Prior to PC removal, a cholangiogram is performed to assess for gallstones and patency of the cystic duct. If the cystic duct is patent and stones are not present, the PC can be safely removed. If gallstones are present or the cystic duct is occluded, the tube should remain until after the resolution of comorbid conditions when cholecystectomy is performed. If the patient's condition continues to preclude surgical cholecystectomy, the drainage cathether can be left indefinitely.

In our series published in 2003, PC was performed in 45 patients with presumed acute cholecystitis and contraindications to surgical cholecystectomy. The technical success rate was 100%. Ninety-one percent of patients had gallstones or sludge while 9% had neither. Twenty-two percent of patients were in the ICU, of which the majority had acalculous cholecystitis. Drainage tubes remained for an average of 54.3 days. Seventy-eight percent of the patients improved clinically within 5 days, while 20% died within 30 days. Complications included hemoperitoneum (2.2%), tube leakage (4.5%), tube blockage (9%), and tube dislodgement (2.2%). Of the 35 survivors, 31% remained asymptomatic after tube removal, while 42% were able to undergo surgery for cholecystectomy or cholecystoenterostomy. These data are consistent with other reports demonstrating the safety and utility of PC for the treatment of acute cholecystitis in high-risk surgical patients.

PERCUTANEOUS TRANSHEPATIC CHOLANGIOGRAPHY AND BILIARY DRAINAGE

Percutaneous transhepatic cholangiography (PTC) allows access to the biliary system for diagnostic cholangiography or interventional procedures. PTC is preferred over endoscopic transampullary biliary access primarily in the setting of biliary lesions proximal to the left and right main hepatic ducts, Roux-en-Y intestinal anatomy, need for external biliary drainage catheters, or failure of prior endoscopic attempts. PTC can be used to determine the etiology of cholangitis, biliary obstruction, bile leak, or primary biliary disease. Percutaneous biliary drainage (PBD) entails placement of a tube or stent for external or internal biliary drainage, and allows for relief of biliary obstruction due to benign or malignant causes

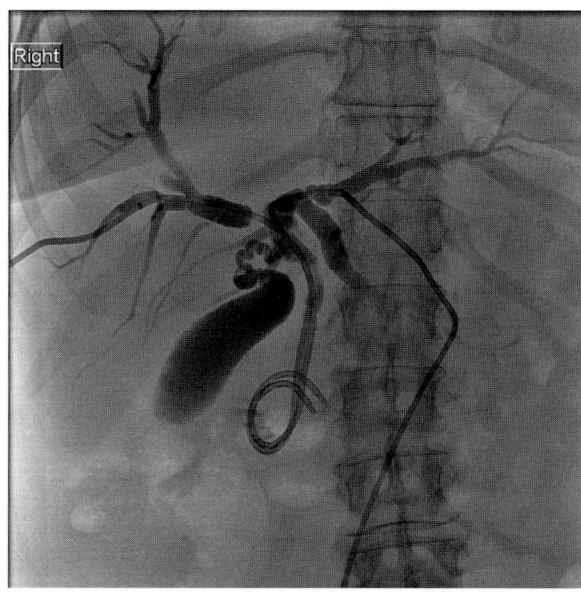

Figure 1. Klatskin tumor causing bilateral biliary obstruction treated with bilateral PBD placement.

(Figure 1). Benign causes of biliary obstruction most frequently include postoperative bile duct injuries or strictures from laparoscopic cholecystectomy or liver transplantation. Interventional manipulations can allow for dilation or stenting of biliary strictures, removal of bile duct stones, diversion of bile, or obtaining bile duct brushings or biopsies for pathology. Contraindications to PTC include coagulopathy, which should be corrected prior to the procedure, given that PTC entails blind percutaneous needle puncture through the liver parenchyma to access the biliary system.

Complications of PTC are reported in 0.5–9% of procedures and are higher in the setting of coagulopathy, cholangitis, stones, malignant obstruction, or proximal obstruction. Minor complications include transient hemobilia, rigors, ascites leakage, tube clogging, and tube dislodgement. Major complications include sepsis, bacteremia, cholangitis, bile leak, prolonged hemobilia, pancreatitis, pneumothorax, and hemothorax. Hemobilia is a feared complication owing to the blind nature of the technique. However, hemobilia can usually be treated by upsizing the drainage catheter to tamponade the site of bleeding, although occasionally embolization is required or an arteriobiliary fistula may develop. PTC was typically thought to have a higher complication rate than ERCP in the setting of nondilated bile ducts, which are more challenging to access percutaneously. Nondilated ducts are more typically seen in the setting of postoperative strictures. However, PTC/PBD has been shown to be successful in as many as 90% of patients with nondilated bile ducts with no increase in the number of complications.

At our center, PTC is performed under local anesthesia and conscious sedation using fluoroscopic and sonographic guidance. Coagulopathy is reversed and antibiotics are given before all procedures. A 22-gauge needle is advanced transhepatically to access the biliary system, with injection of contrast under fluoroscopy to confirm intrabiliary puncture. Once a peripheral bile duct is accessed, cholangiograophy can be performed and a microwire and serial dilators are used to position a drainage catheter. Pigtail drainage catheters can be locked in the duodenum if the obstructing lesion is able to be traversed, allowing for internalization of biliary drainge. If the lesion is unable to be traversed, a PBD may remain centrally at the level of obstruction, allowing only for external biliary drainage. Drainage catheters are sutured to the skin using 2–0 permanent suture. PBDs are replaced every 12 weeks to prevent occlusion.

BILIARY STENTS AND OTHER INTERVENTIONS

Biliary stents are typically used to relieve benign or malignant biliary obstruction and allow for internal drainage and removal of external biliary drains. Benign strictures can be stented as a bridge to definitive surgical repair or in concert with serial dilations. Malignant strictures can be stented to relieve obstruction prior to surgical resection, or as a palliative measure in the setting of unresectable disease.

Plastic stents were first developed, but have largely been supplanted by bare metal or polytetrafluoroethylene (PTFE) covered self-expandable metallic stents due to poor patency and need for frequent stent exchange (Figure 2). Compared to plastic stents, bare metallic stents offer a larger diameter, a lower incidence of infection, and a lower rate of migration given tissue or tumor ingrowth and incorporation into the bile duct wall. Re-occlusion rates as low as 9% have been reported with the use of bare metallic wall stents, compared to 35–45% for plastic stents. PTFE- covered stents allow the advantage of reduced tumor ingrowth and therefore

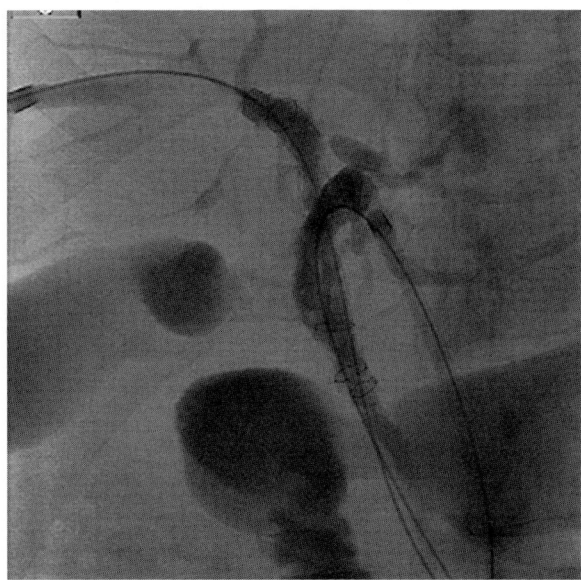

Figure 2. Bilateral covered biliary wall stents for cholangiocarcinoma with intrabiliary tumor thrombus causing obstruction.

longer patency compared to bare metallic stents (6–8 months for bare metallic stents vs. 12–18 months for covered stents). However, lack of tissue ingrowth leads to a higher rate of stent migration.

Other advanced interventional techniques reported by our center include percutaneous choledochocholedochostomy and percutaneous choledochojejunostomy. In the first case, an 80-year-old male developed hilar obstruction with an isolated biliary tree following a major liver resection. A percutaneous channel was created between the isolated obstructed biliary system to the contralateral biliary system draining via an internal PBD. This allowed for complete internalization of biliary drainage. In the second case, a 69-year-old male experienced a transected aberrant right hepatic duct following Roux-en-Y choledochojejunostomy. The leaking aberrant bile duct was in close proximity to the newly created Roux limb, allowing for creation of a percutaneous choledochojejunostomy by passing a needle from a transjugular liver access set through the aberrant hepatic duct and into the Roux limb of the jejunum. A PBD was placed through the newly formed percutaneous channel and locked in the jejunum, bringing the transected bile duct and the jejunum into juxtaposition. Six weeks later, cholangiogram confirmed a healed connection between the aberrant bile duct and the jejunum without evidence of leak, and the PBD was removed. These techniques and other advanced creative solutions may be attempted at centers of excellence under the guidance of a multidisciplinary team of surgeons, endoscopists, and interventionalists.

REFERENCES

1. Davis CA, Landercasper J, Gundersen LH, *et al.* Effective use of percutaneous cholecystostomy in high-risk surgical patients: techniques, tube management, and results. *Arch Surg* 1999; 134(7):727–731; discussion 731–722.
2. Byrne MF, Suhocki P, Mitchell RM, *et al.* Percutaneous cholecystostomy in patients with acute cholecystitis: experience of 45 patients at a US referral center. *J Am Coll Surg* 2003; 197(2):206–211.
3. Burke DR, Lewis CA, Cardella JF, *et al.* Quality improvement guidelines for percutaneous transhepatic cholangiography and biliary drainage. *J Vasc Interv Radiol* 2003; 14(9 Pt 2):S243–246.
4. Park JS, Kim MH, Lee SK, *et al.* Efficacy of endoscopic and percutaneous treatments for biliary complications after cadaveric and living donor liver transplantation. *Gastrointest Endosc.* 2003; 57(1):78–85.
5. Funaki B, Zaleski GX, Straus CA, *et al.* Percutaneous biliary drainage in patients with nondilated intrahepatic bile ducts. *AJR Am J Roentgenol.* 1999; 173(6):1541–1544.
6. Nicholson AA, Royston CM. Palliation of inoperable biliary obstruction with self-expanding metal endoprostheses: a review of 77 patients. *Clin Radiol.* 1993; 47(4):245–250.
7. Liapi E, Georgiades CS, Geschwind. Transhepatic interventions for obstructive jaundice. In: JL Cameron (ed). *Current Surgical Therapy.* 9th edition, Philadelphia, Mosby Inc. 2008.
8. Workman MJ, Suhocki PV, Meyers WC, *et al.* Percutaneous transhepatic choledochocholedochostomy in the management of the postoperative patient. *J Vasc Interv Radiol.* 1998; 9(2):359–362.
9. Suhocki PV, Clavien PA. Percutaneous transhepatic creation of a choledochojejunostomy between an excluded aberrant bile duct and a Roux-en-Y limb. *AJR Am J Roentgenol.* 1999; 172(3):655–657.

SURGICAL TECHNIQUES: LAP/OPEN CHOLECYSTECTOMY

30

Sean Lee* and
Aurora D. Pryor[†]

INTRODUCTION

Laparoscopic cholecystectomy (LC) is one of the most commonly performed surgical procedures with over 750,000 procedures annually in the United States.[1] The first laparoscopic cholecystectomy is credited to Phillipe Mouret in 1987, and this procedure represented the first major technical change in cholecystectomy since Langenbuch first performed an open cholecystectomy in 1882. Although early data on LC revealed significantly reduced postoperative pain, hospital length of stay, and improved patient satisfaction compared to open cholecystectomy, studies also revealed a concerning trend toward increased rates of biliary injury and mortality.[2,3] With modern training and techniques, the bile duct injury rate with LC has stabilized around 0.5%.[4] To minimize bile duct injury, Steven Strasberg described the "critical view of safety".[5] The critical view requires the dissection of all connective and fatty tissue from the triangle of Calot, leaving only the cystic duct, cystic artery, and liver bed, with clear visualization of these two structures entering the gallbladder. With this view, the

---

*Duke University Medical Center, Durham, NC 27710 USA
[†]State University of New York at Stony Brook, USA

cystic artery and duct are clearly and reliably identified. Other authors have advocated the routine use of intraoperative cholangiography (IOC) to visualize the biliary tree and confirm lack of injury.[6] Either of these techniques is appropriate for reproducible and safe LC.

INDICATIONS/PATIENT SELECTION

The most common indications for LC are symptomatic cholelithiasis, acute cholecystitis, gallstone pancreatitis, and biliary obstruction from gallstone disease. Please see Section 2 of this textbook for more detailed discussions of these indications. Relative contraindications to LC include significant previous abdominal surgery, pregnancy, cirrhosis, and neoplasms of the gallbladder.

SURGICAL TECHNIQUE

Patient Positioning

The patient is placed in a supine position, with arms out to the sides. The primary video monitor is placed over patient's right shoulder and second monitor over left shoulder, with the surgeon standing at the patient's left side and the assistant at the patient's right side. An orogastric tube should be placed and suction applied to decompress the stomach and permit better exposure of the hepatocystic triangle. Following port placement, a 30-degree Trendelenburg positioning of the operative table is used to help with exposure.

Accessing the Peritoneum

Initial access to the peritoneum may be gained by one of several techniques, including the open technique, Veress needle insertion, and transparent trocar use.

Accessory Trocar Placement

Once initial access to the peritoneum is obtained, remaining trocars are placed under direct visualization using a laparoscope placed through the first trocar. A 30-degree scope is recommended for optimal visualization during the procedure. There are many possible trocar configurations, and even the number of trocars used can range between one and four or more. A key tenet to maintain in any setup is appropriate triangulation of instruments to facilitate a clear view and the unobstructed use of the multiple necessary instruments.

The most common configuration utilizes four trocars. The first, usually a 10- or 12-mm trocar, is placed periumbilically. The second is placed just below the xiphoid process in the midline and can be a 5- or 10-mm trocar. The third, a 5-mm trocar, is placed two fingerbreadths inferior to the right costal margin in the midclavicular line. The fourth is another 5-mm trocar and is placed two to three fingerbreadths below the right costal margin in the anterior axillary line. The two most lateral ports are for the assistant. Through the most lateral port, a grasper is placed on the fundus of the gallbladder to retract it cephalad. Through the midclavicular line port, a grasper is placed to manipulate the gallbladder infundibulum, primarily retracting it inferolaterally toward the right anterior superior iliac spine. The above trocar positions should be modified based on each patient's anatomy, again with the goal of allowing appropriate reach, triangulation of instruments, and passage of necessary instruments.

A newer technique gaining in popularity is the single incision LC in which only one peritoneal access incision needed to perform LC. This incision is usually made in the periumbilical area, and may be larger than the standard periumbilical LC incision in order to accommodate special ports or multiple instruments. Two limitations to this procedure are the difficulty managing multiple instruments in one incision while holding pneumoperitoneum and obtaining enough triangulation of instruments to allow appropriate retraction and visualization. Devices have been developed to address these limitations, including various multiple port trocars, and articulating cameras and instruments, making the single incision technique more accessible to a wider variety of surgeons.

Exposure of the Cystic Duct and Artery

A 5-mm grasper is inserted through the lateral-most 5-mm trocar, placed on the fundus of the gallbladder, and used to retract the gallbladder cephalad. The liver is thereby lifted off the duodenum and hilar structures. It is frequently helpful to reposition this grasper closer to the infundibulum to accentuate this exposure. Trendelenburg position to 30 degrees also assists in visualization of the infundibulum of the gallbladder. Initially, the infundibulum is usually obscured by adherent fatty tissue. A second 5-mm grasper is thus inserted through midclavicular trocar, and used to stabilize the gallbladder lateral to the adherent fat. A Maryland dissector, or other similar instrument, is then inserted through the subxiphoid trocar, and used to bluntly dissect the adherent fat off the gallbladder. When dissecting, the adherent tissue is pulled down toward the base of the infundibulum, and care should be taken to ensure all movements are kept in the field of view to minimize the risk of inadvertent injuries. For densely adherent tissue, short bursts of electrocautery on the dissecting instrument may be helpful, but the operator must avoid thermal injury to the gallbladder and surrounding structures.

Once cleared of fat, the infundibulum is retracted inferiorly and laterally. This moves the gallbladder and cystic duct towards the right, moving the cystic duct away from and out of parallel alignment with the common bile duct, helping to prevent inadvertent common duct injury. Dissection of the peritoneum and fatty tissue from the infundibulum then proceeds starting posteriorly and moving anteriorly. Once the anterior side of the gallbladder has been freed, retraction is changed to superomedial on the infundibulum to expose the posterior surface for its dissection. Once both sides have been carefully dissected, the cystic duct and artery are usually visible. Often careful blunt dissection between the structures is required to distinguish one from the other. The cystic artery lies cephalad to the duct, and usually somewhat posterior. It is also typically posterior to the cystic duct node. Aberrant anatomy may be seen, so careful identification of all structures is mandatory.

Once the dissection is complete, the cystic duct should be clearly visualized as a tubular structure acting as the inferior continuation of the gallbladder infundibulum, and the cystic artery should be seen to be clearly separate from the cystic duct and also clearly running to the gallbladder. No other tubular or cystic structures should be seen within the hepatocystic triangle, and thus the liver should be clearly visible behind the cystic duct and artery. The infundibulum itself should also be clear of adherent tissue. The common duct and/or hepatic artery may be visible, but should not be intentionally exposed as this only adds to possible complications. A clear view from all directions of the cystic duct and artery running from the gallbladder toward the porta hepatis without other structures within the hepatocystic triangle between the cystic duct, artery, and liver represents a good critical view of safety.[5]

Division of the Cystic Duct and Artery

Once the cystic duct dissection is completed and the critical view obtained, a dissector is used to softly milk the duct towards the gallbladder in order to reduce any stones within it back into the gallbladder. A 5- or 10-mm laparoscopic clip applier is usually used through the subxiphoid incision. One clip is placed near the junction of the cystic duct and gallbladder, and two more slightly distal to the first. Endoshears are used to divide the duct. The cystic artery is then divided similarly.

Intraoperative Cholangiogram (IOC)

Following the application of the first clip on the cystic duct, an IOC may be obtained. Although some surgeons perform IOC with every LC, citing the relatively high rate of retained stones, others argue for selective IOC. Indications for IOC include: abnormal or unclear anatomy at time of surgery, suspected choledocholithiasis, and suspected biliary injury. Once the clip is placed on the cystic duct–gallbladder junction, the cystic duct is partially transected. A 4 or 5 French saline-flushed catheter is then placed in the abdomen either percutaneously through a large bore angiocatheter or with a specially designed laparoscopic instrument. The catheter is inserted into the cystic duct, and advanced several millimeters. It is secured either with a clip, a clamp on the instrument, or a balloon. A fluoroscope is then brought into position, and 10–15 mL of water-soluble contrast is injected under fluoroscopy. Contrast should freely enter the common duct, and the biliary tree should be visible from the second-degree branches of the right and left hepatic ducts to the duodenum. Plain films can alternatively be used, but are not preferred as they are static.

Removal of the Gallbladder from Liver and Abdomen

Once the cystic structures have been divided, attention is turned towards dissecting the gallbladder from its attachments to the liver. This is most commonly performed with cautery. A hook cautery device is placed through the subxiphoid trocar, and dissection begins in the areolar tissue at the inferior aspect of the gallbladder. Retraction in the cephalad direction facilitates the dissection by placing the areolar plane under tension. The surgeon must use care to remain within the proper plane. If a hole is made in the gallbladder, grasping its edges can control seepage, and any stones should be removed from the abdomen either immediately or after removal of the gall bladder. Once the gallbladder is nearly free, it is often useful to stop the dissection and inspect the gallbladder fossa for bleeding or bile leakage. Any bleeding is controlled with electrocautery. Any bile leakage should be carefully inspected, and the source identified and controlled. Irrigation of the gallbladder fossa facilitates a complete inspection. Once the inspection is completed, the last remaining areolar fibers are divided, and the gallbladder is removed. A retrieval bag may be used and is recommended if bile leakage has occurred. Often, repositioning the camera to an alternate port and insertion of the bag through the umbilical port simplifies the process of getting the gallbladder into the bag, and also removal of the gallbladder since the umbilical trocar site is usually the largest. If needed, the trocar is removed, and possibly the fascial incision is enlarged by stretching it with a Kelly forceps or even by incising further to facilitate gallbladder removal. Once the gallbladder is out of the abdomen, the gallbladder fossa is again irrigated as is the liver itself. The irrigant should be clear, without significant blood or bile, prior to completing the case. Once irrigation is complete, accessory ports are removed under direct visualization. The umbilical port site requires fascial closure if the port was placed by cutdown or if the fascial opening was enlarged. Placement of an operative drain in the gallbladder fossa is another option available to the surgeon. Drains can be inserted through 5-mm port sites, eliminating the need for another incision. Although usually unnecessary, in cases where severe inflammation or other circumstances lead to larger than expected blood loss or concern for bile leak, drainage may be appropriate.

Postoperative Management

Most patients are managed in an ambulatory setting, and are discharged either the same day or on postoperative day one. Antibiotics are not usually necessary, unless the clinical scenario was complicated by cholangitis or severe cholecystitis. Diet can usually be resumed within a few hours of surgery. Pain control should include injection of local anesthetic during the procedure in order to help minimize postoperative narcotics.

REFERENCES

1. Flum DR, Cheadle A, Prela C, *et al.* Bile duct injury during cholecystectomy and survival in medicare beneficiaries. *JAMA* 2003; 290:2168.
2. Richardson MC, Bell G, Fullarton GM, *et al.* Incidence and nature of bile duct injuries following laparoscopic cholecystectomy: an audit of 5913 cases. *Br J Surg* 1996; 83:1356.
3. Strasberg SM. Avoidance of biliary injury during laparoscopic cholecystectomy. *J Hepatobiliary Pancreat Surg* 2002; 9:543.
4. Rusell JC, Walsh SJ, Mattie AS, *et al.* Bile duct injuries, 1989–1993. A statewide experience. *Arch Surg* 1996; 131:382.
5. Strasberg SM, Hertl M, Soper NJ. An analysis of the problem of biliary injury during laparoscopic cholecystectomy. *J Am Coll Surg* 1995; 180:101.
6. Fletcher DR, Hobbs MS, Tan P, *et al.* Complications of cholecystectomy: risks of the laparoscopic approach and protective effects of operative cholangiography: a population-based study. *Ann Surg* 1999; 229:449.
7. Pappas TN, Harnisch M, Pryor AD. *Atlas of Laparoscopic Surgery.* Springer. 2007.
8. Soper NJ, Swanstrom LL, Eubanks WS. *Mastery of Endoscopic and Laparoscopic Surgery.* 3rd edition, Lippincott, Williams, and Wilkins. 2009.

SURGICAL TECHNIQUES: BILE DUCT INJURY REPAIR 31

Sapan Desai* and
Dan G. Blazer III*

INTRODUCTION

Despite over 20 years of experience with laparoscopic cholecystectomy, the risk of bile duct injury remains higher than its open counterpart and laparoscopic cholecystectomy remains the most common cause of bile duct injury. Current estimates place the risk of bile duct injury with laparoscopic cholecystectomy at 1 in 500 cases, compared to less than 1 in 1000 patients with open cholecystectomy. Other less common causes of bile duct injury include direct trauma to the biliary tree and iatrogenic injury from other hepatopancreaticobiliary procedures. A more thorough discussion of the etiology of bile duct injury is presented in Chapter 22. This chapter will focus on the surgical principles and techniques of repair.

CLASSIFICATION

Once bile duct injury is detected, precise characterization of the type of injury is critical. The Strasberg classification is commonly used (Chapter 22, Figure 2), which represents an expanded classification of the original Bismuth classification of biliary strictures.[4]

---

*Duke University Medical Center, Durham, NC 27710 USA

Class A injuries include leaks of the cystic duct stump or leaks from the gallbladder fossa. These injuries typically present with a bile leak and formation of a biloma. A class B injury represents occlusion of an aberrant right hepatic duct and may be silent initially. Long term, these injuries can result in atrophy of the involved liver. Class C injuries represent transection of aberrant right hepatic ducts, resulting in fistula and biloma formation. Class D injuries involve partial (<50%) transection injuries to major bile ducts and typically result in biloma.

Class E injuries are injuries to the main bile ducts. E1 injuries are injuries to the common hepatic/bile duct >2 cm distal to the confluence of the right and left hepatic ducts. E2 injuries occur <2 cm from the confluence. E3 injuries represent injury at the confluence. E4 injuries are even higher, involving the main left or right ducts or even more proximal injuries. E5 injuries represent simultaneous injury to the common hepatic duct and an aberrant right hepatic duct.

DIAGNOSIS

Patients with acute bile duct injury may present with abdominal pain, fevers, or jaundice. The presentation varies depending on the nature of the injury. In a patient with suspected bile duct injury, CT scan is commonly the initial study of choice. Acute bile duct injury can present with a bile leak leading to a biloma, readily identified with CT imaging. Infection of the biloma can form a subdiaphragmatic or infrahepatic abscess; bilomas need immediate percutaneous drainage to prevent septic complications.

Once acute fluid collections have been managed, characterization of the injury is necessary. HIDA scan can demonstrate the presence of a bile leak or duct occlusion but does not give precise anatomic information. Endoscopic retrograde cholangiopancreatography (ERCP) is typically the next best test. ERCP can demonstrate complete or partial obstruction of the biliary system and presence of a leak. In the setting of partial obstruction, ERCP may offer complete visualization of the entire biliary tree and complete characterization of the injury.

However, if there is complete obstruction of the biliary tree, ERCP will demonstrate a cutoff sign and no delineation of the proximal anatomy is possible. Here, percutaneous transhepatic cholangiography (PTC) is required for complete characterization. All intrahepatic ducts must be visualized and multiple duct cannulations may be necessary, depending on the nature of the injury. Importantly, ERCP and PTC are not only diagnostic but can be therapeutic and may obviate the need for surgical intervention.

TIMING

Bile duct injury can be recognized intraoperatively, in the immediate postoperative period, or after long-term degeneration has occurred in the liver and biliary tree. Intraoperative recognition of a major bile duct injury does not mandate immediate repair. In fact, unless the surgical team is experienced with exposure and reconstruction of these injuries, drainage and referral to an experienced hepatobiliary center is favored. Repair of the bile duct injury by the primary surgeon is associated with a lower success rate compared to repair by a specialist.[11] The best chance for long-term durability of repair is the initial reconstruction.

Once the patient has been referred to an experienced center, the timing of repair is controversial. Some centers favor immediate repair (less than 72 hours since time of injury) when possible whereas other centers favor delayed repair when acute inflammatory issues have resolved.[6] Regardless, no attempt at reconstruction should be made until all fluid collections have been managed and sepsis is controlled. An unstable patient is not a candidate for immediate repair.

MANAGEMENT PRINCIPLES

Not all patients require operative repair of bile duct injuries. Type A injuries do not require surgical reconstruction. These patients often present with biloma. After percutaneous drainage of the biloma, they are often managed with temporary biliary stenting until the leak resolves. Type B injuries are often silent, resulting only in long-term atrophy of the involved liver. Rarely is surgical repair indicated. Type C injuries, if involving minimal liver volume, may convert to a type B injury with long-term percutaneous drainage and may not need reconstruction. However, persistent biliary fistula mandates reconstruction.

Types D and E injuries represent injuries to the major bile ducts and require surgical repair. The principal goal in the management of these injuries is restoration of biliary-enteric drainage from all parts of the liver. In those patients requiring surgical repair, Roux-en-Y hepaticojejunostomy is the reconstruction technique of choice.

SURGICAL MANAGEMENT

Exposure

As described eloquently by Strasberg, surgical reconstruction involves two parts: appropriate exposure of the bile duct to be repaired and reconstruction with Roux-en-Y hepaticojejunostomy.[16] A generous right upper quadrant curvilinear incision with vertical midline extension or a Mercedes-Benz-type incision may be used in larger patients. Little inflammation or scar tissue is generally present in immediate repair, but significant adhesions may be encountered in patients who undergo delayed repair.

Immediate repair is typically reserved for those patients with E1 and E2 type injuries. The porta hepatis is exposed and the bile duct is cut back to healthy tissue. Sharp transection techniques are employed to avoid risk of devascularization. Some advocate anterior ductotomy to allow for a longer side-to-side anastomosis rather than the more typical end-to-side technique.

In those patients with more proximal/complex ductal injuries (E3 and E5), exposure and preparation of the bile ducts can be difficult. These techniques go beyond the scope of this short chapter and the reader is referred to other references that describe these principles of exposure for left and right hepatic ducts.[16,17]

Repair

Once the bile duct has been exposed and prepared for anastomosis, tension-free Roux-en-Y hepaticojejunostomy is utilized for reconstruction and establishment of biliary-enteric continuity. The jejunum is divided approximately 20–25 cm distal to the Ligament of Treitz. A 50–60 cm Roux limb is prepared in standard fashion. We favor a stapled side-to-side functional end-to-side enteroenterostomy. A mesenteric defect is created to the right of the mesenteric vessels. The Roux limb is then brought retrocolic for anastomosis. The limb must reach in tension-free fashion and must be well-vascularized.

The anastomosis is then fashioned in an end-to-side or side-to-side fashion. We use 4–0 or 5–0 absorbable monofilament sutures (depending on duct size) in interrupted fashion. Our technique is illustrated in Figure 1. We first load our anterior row sutures on the bile duct using double-armed sutures and place the suture on shodded clamps. A small

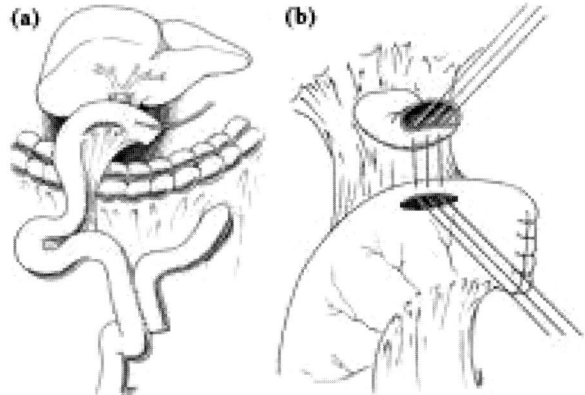

Figure 1. Hepaticojejunostomy. (a) Double-armed sutures are placed on the anterior row first, followed by the creation of an enterotomy within the Roux limb. Single-armed sutures are then used to take full thickness stitches through the jejunum and bile duct to create the posterior row. (b) Final appearance.

enterotomy is made in the Roux limb. Next, using single-armed sutures, we take full-thickness bites through the jejunum and bile duct for the posterior row. Knots on the posterior row are tied on the inside. We then complete our anterior row and these knots are tied on the outside. Meticulous technique is critical. We typically leave a drain, which is generally removed prior to discharge unless there is a leak.

OUTCOMES

In experienced centers, surgical mortality for bile duct reconstruction hovers at 1–2%.[12] About 10% of patients will eventually develop restenosis.[12] Of note, stricture formation is fivefold higher if a primary end-to-end reanastomosis is attempted, again underlining the importance of hepaticojejunostomy as the cornerstone of repair. The outcomes are slightly better for distal bile duct injuries compared to proximal bile duct damage.

The most significant predictor for postoperative complications is the existence of high-grade liver disease, such as biliary cirrhosis or portal hypertension. As a result, surgical interventions in patients who present months or years later after their injury are at 20–30% mortality, and nearly half of these patients will develop complications that require non-invasive management.[7]

In summary, satisfactory outcomes after bile duct injury hinges on early recognition of injury, immediate control/prevention of sepsis with drainage of bilomas/fluid collections, precise anatomic delineation of the type of injury, and surgical repair with a tension-free Roux-en-Y hepaticojejunostomy by an experienced hepatobiliary surgeon.

REFERENCES

1. Blumgart LH, Hann LE. Surgical and radiological anatomy of the liver and biliary tract. In: LH Blumgart, Y Fong (eds). *Surgery of the Liver and Biliary Tract.* New York, WB Saunders, pp. 13–14. 2000.
2. Branum G, Schmitt C, Baillie J, et al. Management of major biliary complications after laparoscopic cholecystectomy. *Ann Surg* 1993; 217:532–541.
3. Chapman WC, Halevy A, Blumgart LH, et al. Postcholecystectomy bile duct strictures: Management and outcome in 130 patients. *Arch Surg* 1995; 130:597–602.
4. Clavien PA, Sanabria JR, Strasberg SM. Proposed classification of complications of surgery with examples of utility in cholecystectomy. *Surgery* 1992; 111(5): 518–526.
5. Lee VS, Chari RS, Cucchiaro G: Complications of laparoscopic cholecystectomy. *Am J Surg* 1993; 165:527.
6. Lillemoe KD, Melton GB, Cameron JL, et al. Postoperative bile duct strictures: Management and outcome in the 1990s. *Ann Surg* 2000; 232:430–441.
7. Melton GB, Lillemoe KD, Cameron JL, et al. Major bile duct injuries associated with laparoscopic cholecystectomy: Effect of surgical repair on quality of life. *Ann Surg* 2002; 235:888–895.
8. Murr M, Gigot JF, Nagorney DM: Long-term results of biliary reconstruction after laparoscopic bile duct injuries. *Arch Surg* 1999; 134:604.
9. Pitt HA, Grace PA. Cancer of the pancreas. Pylorus-preserving resection of the pancreas. *Baillieres Clin Gastroenterol.* 1990; 4(4):917–930. Review.
10. Sicklick JK, Camp MS, Lillemoe KD, et al. Surgical management of bile duct injuries sustained during laparoscopic cholecystectomy: Perioperative results in 200 patients. *Ann Surg* 2005; 241:786–792.
11. Stewart L, Way LW: Bile duct injuries during laparoscopic cholecystectomy: Factors that influence the results of treatment. *Arch Surg* 1995; 130:1123–1128.
12. Walsh RM, Henderson JM, Vogt DP, et al. Long-term outcome of biliary reconstruction for bile duct injuries from laparoscopic cholecystectomies. *Surgery.* 2007; 142(4):450–6; discussion 456–457.

13. Way LW, Stewart L, Gantert W, *et al.* Causes and prevention of laparoscopic bile duct injuries: Analysis of 252 cases from a human factors and cognitive psychology perspective. *Ann Surg* 2003; 237:460–469.
14. Winslow ER, Fialkowski EA, Linehan DC, *et al.* "Sideways": results of repair of biliary injuries using a policy of side-to-side hepatico-jejunostomy. *Ann Surg.* 2009; 249(3):426–434.
15. Yan JQ, Peng CH, Ding JZ, *et al.* Surgical management in biliary restricture after Roux-en-Y hepaticojejunostomy for bile duct injury. *World J Gastroenterol.* 2007; 13(48):6598–6602.
16. Strasburg SM and Hawkins W. Reconstruction of the Bile Duct: *Anatomic Principles and Surgical Techniques in Mastery of Surgery.* 5th edition; 2007.
17. Hopp J. Hepaticojejenostomy using the left biliary trunk for iatrogenic biliary lesions: The French Connection, *World J. Surg.* 1985; 9:507.

SURGICAL TECHNIQUES: COMMON BILE DUCT EXPLORATION   32

Sebastian G. de la Fuente
Aurora D. Pryor* and
Theodore N. Pappas[†]

INTRODUCTION

The incidence of choledocholithiasis in patients undergoing elective cholecystectomy is approximately 5–15%. Treatment options in these patients include endoscopic retrograde cholangiopancreatography (ERCP) with sphincterotomy followed by cholecystectomy, cholecystectomy with intraoperative or postoperative ERCP, or cholecystectomy with intraoperative cholangiogram followed by common bile duct (CBD) exploration. Since the widespread introduction of ERCP, surgical exploration of the CBD in the United States has been limited to patients with failed ERCP attempts or when the resources are not available. In the current era, the classic open surgical approach is rarely performed and most surgeons familiar with the technique retrieve CBD stones laparoscopically. Laparoscopic CBD exploration can be accomplished either via the transcystic approach or through a

---

*Department of Surgery, Stony Brook Medicine, Stony Brook, NY 11794-8191, USA
[†]Department of Surgery, Duke University Medical Center, Durham, NC 27710 USA

choledochotomy. The anatomic characteristics of the biliary system, as well as the size and location of the stones, will dictate the route is indicated.

Since the introduction of laparoscopic cholecystectomy, the question of which therapeutic approach is superior has sparked some debate. A recent Cochrane Database Review assessed the management of choledocholithiasis by four different approaches: (1) ERCP versus open surgical CBD exploration, (2) preoperative ERCP versus laparoscopic bile duct exploration, (3) postoperative ERCP versus laparoscopic CBD clearance, and (4) ERCP versus laparoscopic bile duct clearance in patients with previous cholecystectomy. The study included 13 trials that randomized a total of 1352 patients. A significantly increased number of total procedures per patient was seen in the ERCP arms. ERCP was also found to be less successful than open surgery in CBD stone clearance with a tendency towards higher mortality rate. In addition, laparoscopic CBD exploration was as efficient as pre- and postoperative ERCP and with no significant difference in morbidity and mortality. In this review, the laparoscopic trials universally reported shorter hospital stays; however, insufficient data were reported for cost analysis.

OPEN COMMON BILE DUCT EXPLORATION

The most common indication for open CBD exploration is failure of other techniques. Most experts recommend avoiding surgical exploration when the CBD is found to be less than 3 mm in diameter. Clearance of the duct should always be confirmed either with choledoscopy of cholangiography.

The procedure can be performed via a right subcostal incision or an upper midline laparotomy. An extended Kocher maneuver is performed to facilitate palpation of the retroduodenal and intrapancreatic bile duct. Once the CBD has been identified, the duct is entered through a 1–1.5 cm longitudinal incision usually at the level of the cystic duct confluence. A transcystic approach can also be attempted. Stones that are easily identified can be milked up or down and extracted. For stones that are not easily accessible, administration of intravenous glucagon (1–2 mg) stimulates relaxation of the sphincter of Oddi and facilitates flushing the stone into the duodenum. Irrigation of the duct can be also performed upwards when intrahepatic stones are encountered. Some surgeons prefer using a biliary Fogarty balloon for stone extraction and to confirm ampullary patency.

Once patency of the biliary system has been confirmed, closure of the choledochotomy can be accomplished primarily with fine reabsorbable

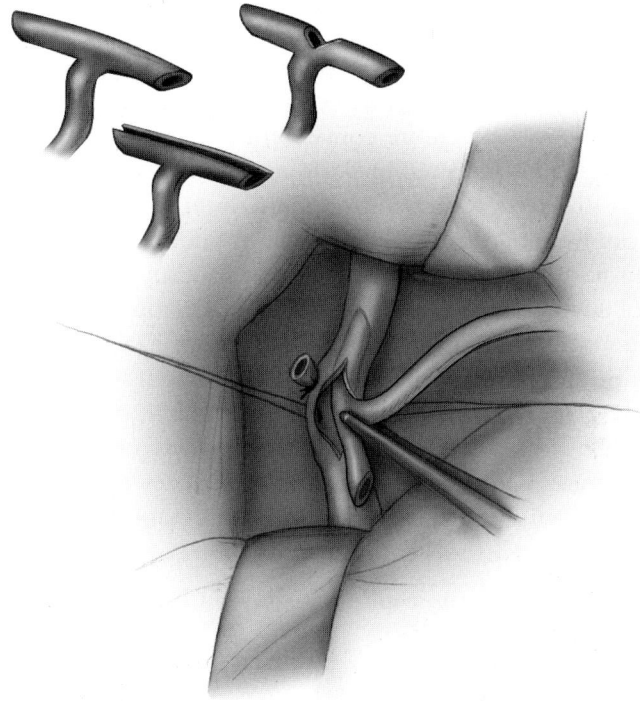

Figure 1. A T-tube is inserted in the common bile duct, and the choledochotomy incision is closed over it with fine absorbable sutures. Placement of a T-tube allows postoperative cholangiographic examination of the bile system.

sutures or over a T-tube fashioned to fit the CBD properly (Figure 1). When there is concern about ongoing obstruction or if a postoperative cholangiogram is needed, a T-tube is usually preferred. Revision of the literature shows five clinical trials investigating the use of T-tube versus primary closure following CBD exploration. These studies included a total of 165 patients randomized to primary closure and 159 patients randomized to T-tube closure. The primary closure patients show a significantly lower positive bile culture and wound infection rates. Even though bile peritonitis was higher in the T-tube patients (2.9%) compared to the primary closure group (1%), this was not statistically significant. In general, primary closure following CBD exploration seems to be as safe and effective as closure over a T-tube; however, long-term outcomes such as CBD postoperative stenosis rates is lacking. The T-tube is generally left in placed for approximately 2–3 weeks and removed after biliary patency is confirmed.

LAPAROSCOPIC APPROACH

Laparoscopic CBD exploration provides patients with choledocholitiasis undergoing laparoscopic cholecystectomy with the benefits of a single-stage procedure, which is more convenient and economical than a combine cholecystectomy followed by postoperative ERCP. A randomized trial published by Rhodes *et al.* of an intention-to treat model showed that duct clearance can be achieved in 100% of patients compared to 93% of those undergoing postoperative ERCP. Duration of treatment in this study was a median of 90 min (range 25–310) in the laparoscopic group as opposed to 105 min (range 60–255) in the postoperative ERCP group (p = 0.1, 95% CI for difference -5 to 40). The median hospital stay was 1 day in the laparoscopic group compared with 3.5 days (range in the ERCP group (p = 0.0001, 95% CI 1–2). Other more sophisticated techniques are also available but rarely performed in the United States (Table 1). Potential complications of this approach are described in Table 2.

Table 1. Laparoscopic techniques of CBD clearance.

- Transcystic approach:
  - Under fluoroscopic guidance
  - Using fiberoptic methods
  - Flushing techniques, baskets, Fogarty ballon
- Choledochotomy approach:
  - With internalized biliary stent
  - Without biliary stent (preferred)
- Laparoscopic antegrade sphincterotomy
- Laparoscopic bilioenteric anastomosis

Table 2. Potential complications of laparoscopic CBD exploration.

- Cystic duct stump postoperative leaks
- Bile duct perforation
- Creation of false lumen and dissection
- Hemobilia
- Pancreatitis
- Intestinal perforation

TRANSCYSTIC LAPAROSCOPIC CBD EXPLORATION

The trancystic approach is the preferred method by most surgeons performing laparoscopic CBD exploration. This is in part due to the lack of intracorporeal suturing needed as it is required when a choledochotomy is used. The position of the trocars for the laparoscopic cholecystectomy is the one used for transcystic CBD exploration. Once the cystic ductotomy for the cholangiogram is created, any visible stones are extracted with atraumatic graspers (Figures 2 and 3). If the cystic duct is found to be of inadequate size, a dilator can ease extraction of the stones. Gently irrigation with warm saline solution is then done to flush the stone down into the duodenum. As described above, flushing of larger stones can be facilitated by administration of intravenous glucagon.

If the flushing techniques are unsuccessful, the surgeon may opt for stone extraction under choledoscopic or fluoroscopic guidance. Available choledoscope sizes range from 3 to 10 Fr in diameter and can be utilized to push stones through the ampulla, should that be required.

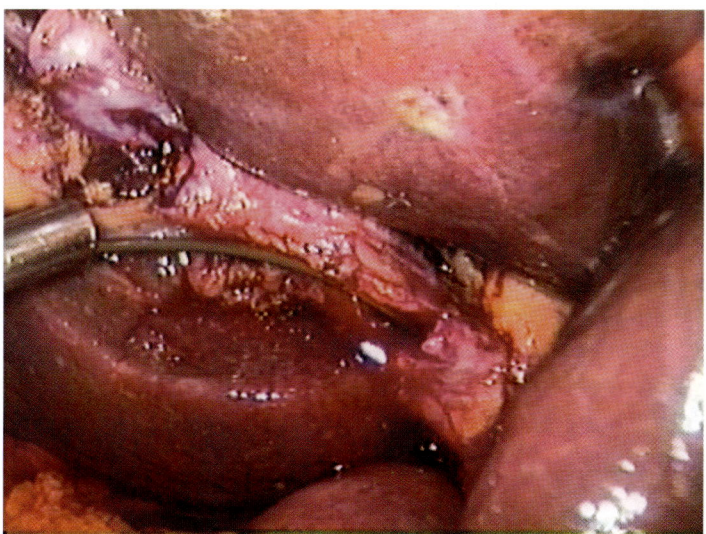

Figure 2. Cannulation of the cystic duct for cholangiography. The cholangiogram catheter is typically introduced through the subxiphoid 5-mm trocar. *Images courtesy of Juan Pekolj, MD and Rodrigo S. Claria, MD, Hospital Italiano, Buenos Aires, Argentina.*

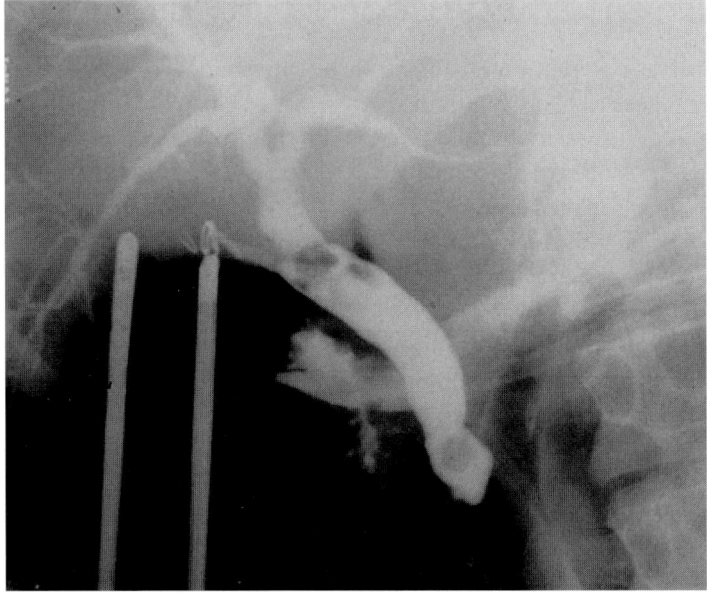

Figure 3. Cholangiogram demonstrating stones at the junction of the cystic duct and CBD and in the retroduodenal duct.

With the fluoroscopic technique, a guidewire is introduced and followed by either a Dormia basket or Fogarty biliary balloon (Figure 4). These can be passed through the 14-gauge catheter used for the cholangiogram. A completion cholangiogram then follows to assure biliary patency. Alternatively, confirmation of duct clearance can be obtained by passing the choledoscope down into the duodenum. Finally, the cystic duct stump is closed with clips or a standard Endoloop.

With this technique, the success rate of CBD exploration ranges from 71% to 98% in experience hands. Retained stones can occur in up to 5% of patients. Failure of the transcystic approach should lead to either conversion to an open approach, a choledochotomy, or postoperative ERCP.

LAPAROSCOPIC CBD EXPLORATION VIA THE CHOLEDOCHOTOMY ROUTE

The choledochotomy approach is indicated in situations when the trancystic approach is impossible, such as inability to cannulate the cystic duct

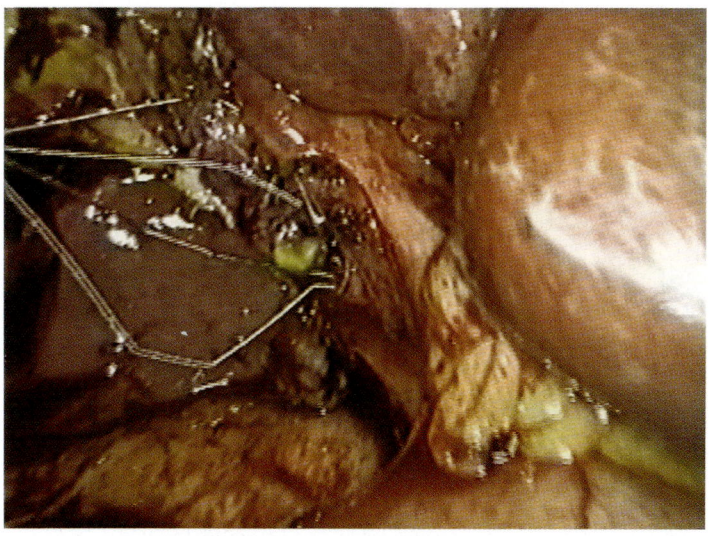

Figure 4. Extraction of CBD stones using the Dormia or helical basket. In this case, a choledochotomy was performed to allow extraction of large CBD stones. *Images courtesy of Juan Pekolj, MD and Rodrigo S. Claria, MD, Hospital Italiano, Buenos Aires, Argentina.*

or stones proximal to the CBD–cystic duct junction. Dissection starts in a routine fashion with the exposure of the Calot's triangle and ligation of the cystic duct. Once this has been accomplished, the CBD is exposed over a length of 1.5 cm. A choledochotomy is then made in the anterior surface of the duct with endoscissors or a laparoscopic blade. Stay sutures can be placed to allow retraction of the duct. The duct is then irrigated and confirmation of patency is carried out as described for the trancystic approach. If proximal stones are suspected, the choledoscope is passed cephalad and stones are removed with the Dormia basket or atraumatic forceps. As mentioned above, when the risk of postoperative CBD obstruction is low, a primary closure of the choledochotomy may be performed. This is done with fine 4–0 absorbable sutures in a running fashion (Figure 4). If there is concern about ongoing obstruction, the choledochotomy should be closed over a T-tube.

Overall, the success rate of CBD stones extraction through a choledochotomy ranges from 80% to 97% with complication rates below 15%. Long-term bile duct strictures have been described when primary closure is performed, but these can often be managed endoscopically.

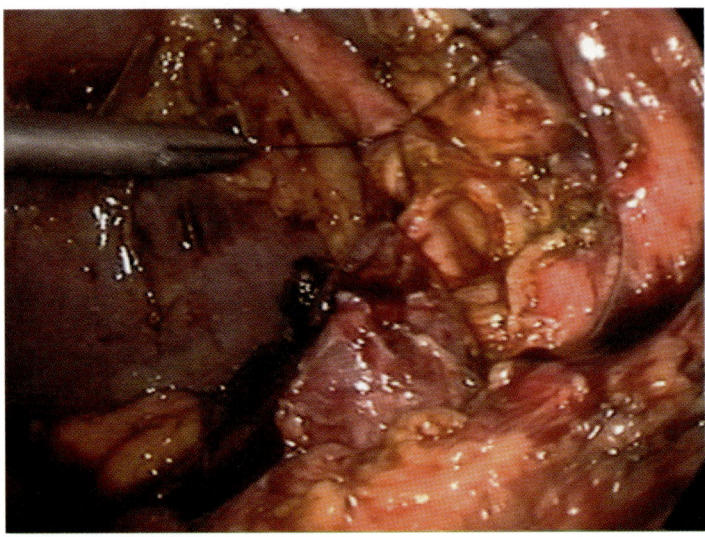

Figure 5. Primary closure of the choledochotomy is performed with fine absorbable sutures. This technique requires advance laparoscopic skills and can be performed with low postoperative complication rates in experience hands. *Images courtesy of Juan Pekolj, MD and Rodrigo S. Claria, MD, Hospital Italiano, Buenos Aires, Argentina.*

REFERENCES

1. Rhodes M, Sussman L, Cohen L, *et al.* Randomised trial of laparoscopic exploration of common bile duct versus postoperative endoscopic retrograde cholangiography for common bile duct stones. *Lancet* 1998; 17;351:159–161.
2. Nathanson LK, O'Rourke NA, Martin IJ, *et al.* Postoperative ERCP versus laparoscopic choledochotomy for clearance of selected bile duct calculi: a randomized trial. *Ann Surg* 2005; 242(2):188–192.
3. Pappas TN, Slimane TB, Brooks DC. 100 consecutive common duct explorations without mortality. *Ann Surg* 1990; 211(3):260–262.
4. Topal B, Aerts R, Penninckx F. Laparoscopic common bile duct stone clearance with flexible choledochoscopy. *Surg Endosc* 2007; 21(12):2317–2321.
5. Martin DJ, Vernon DR, Toouli J. Surgical versus endoscopic treatment of bile duct stones. *Cochrane Database Syst Rev.* 2006; 19(2):CD003327.
6. Gurusamy KS, Samraj K. Primary closure versus T-tube drainage after laparoscopic common bile duct stone exploration. *Cochrane Database Syst Rev.* 2007; 24(1): CD005641.

SURGICAL TECHNIQUES: BILE DUCT RESECTION/ RECONSTRUCTION

33

Sarah Evans* and
Carlos E. Marroquin[†]

PATHOPHYSIOLOGY OF BILIARY STRICTURES

Biliary strictures can be due to benign or malignant etiologies resulting in scarring and narrowing or external compression of the biliary tree. Malignant strictures are the most frequent cause and typically manifest with painless jaundice. Pancreatic head adenocarcinoma, cholangiocarcinoma, and ampullary tumors are the most common malignant causes of biliary stricture. The treatment of malignant biliary strictures depends upon the extent of disease, severity of symptoms, and overall health and life expectancy of the patient. There are multiple causes of benign biliary strictures with the most common resulting from iatrogenic surgical injuries, chronic choledocholithiasis, primary sclerosing cholangitis, and benign pancreatic disease; specifically, acute and chronic pancreatitis.

The etiology of iatrogenic surgical injuries and primary sclerosing cholangitis are discussed in detail in preceding chapters and will not be the focus in this section, though the surgical techniques described here can apply to the management of these two disease processes. However, it is

*Duke University, Durham, North Carolina, USA
[†]University of Rochester, Rochester, New York, USA

important to emphasize that while dominant extrahepatic strictures secondary to primary sclerosing cholangitis can be resected with the creation of a bilioenteric anastomosis, surgical management should be a last resort as dissection in the porta hepatis could lead to adhesions which may prohibit or make future liver transplantation exceedingly difficult. Benign pancreatic disease can produce transient or permanent biliary stricture or stenosis. Acute pancreatitis resulting in edema and narrowing of the intrapancreatic portion of the common bile duct can produce an obstructive jaundice that usually resolves on its own, whereas chronic pancreatitis can produce pancreatic fibrosis and consequently biliary cirrhosis, leading to permanent biliary stricture requiring surgical or endoscopic management.

The goal of treatment of biliary obstruction, regardless of cause, is to restore biliary flow and alleviate symptoms of obstructive jaundice such as cholangitis, pruritis and malabsorption. In some situations of either benign or malignant biliary stricture, stent placement without surgical intervention is the optimal treatment. In other situations, surgical intervention with a bilioenteric anastamosis, with or without bile duct resection, is advised. The type of bilioenteric anastamosis performed is dependent on the level of biliary obstruction. For all types of bilioenteric anastamoses, the goal is a mucosa-to-mucosa anastamosis between a segment of the gastrointestinal tract and a healthy, well perfused, non-diseased bile duct.

PREOPERATIVE IMAGING AND STENT PLACEMENT

Ultrasound and computed tomographic (CT) imaging are often the initial imaging modalities used to evaluate a patient with obstructive jaundice. Ultrasound can often identify ductal dilatation and suggest the level of obstruction, and a CT scan can provide greater detail on the size and location of a mass and the presence of metastases or vascular involvement. Magnetic resonance cholangiopancreatography (MRCP) can also be used and provides more detail than either CT or ultrasound. Regardless of the location of the lesion, direct cholangiography should then be used to clearly visualize the biliary tract and plan an operative approach. For lesions proximal to the bifurcation, this is best performed via percutaneous transhepatic cholangiography (PTC), whereas for a distal obstruction, endoscopic retrograde cholangiography (ERCP) is optimal. Moreover, while cholangiography is diagnostic allowing tissue biopsy for diagnosis, it is also therapeutic allowing drainage with internal stent placement or percutaneous drainage in cases of biliary obstruction.

It is important to note, however, that biliary decompression is not necessary nor recommended in all cases of biliary obstruction. Debate surrounds the routine use of preoperative biliary decompression, and studies indicate that decompression in the asymptomatic patient does not decrease postoperative morbidity or mortality.[1] Advocates of its use argue that decompression makes dissection easier by both decreasing swelling of the surrounding liver tissue, as well as facilitating the identification of the obstructed biliary ducts at the hilum. Others, however, contend that preoperative biliary decompression with stents or external drains should only be utilized in the setting of cholangitis because decompression can minimize bile duct dilation, making it more difficult to create a bilioenteric anastamosis of an adequate size to allow sufficient biliary drainage. We have tended to drain patients who present with cholangitis and those with significant cholestasis as it provides information into the degree of hepatic reserve. Patients who undergo an effective mechanical decompression with no appreciable correction of their cholestasis likely have poor hepatic reserve and may not tolerate an aggressive operative approach.

For patients who are not surgical candidates due to severe comorbidities, poor hepatic reserve, or a very short expected survival, placement of a biliary stent may be the treatment of choice. In some cases of obstruction due to benign causes such as chronic pancreatitis or iatrogenic injury, balloon dilation or plastic stent placement should be considered in patients who are a high surgical risk. Metallic stents, which have a lower occlusion rate than plastic stents,[2] should be reserved for palliation of patients with unresectable malignant obstructions, as their use precludes the possibility of a future surgical biliary bypass.

PREOPERATIVE EVALUATION AND PREPARATION

Biliary resection and reconstruction are performed to remove malignant tumors, if present, and to relieve and prevent symptoms of obstructive jaundice and cholangitis. While patients with benign biliary strictures may be young and free of other comorbidities, most patients with malignant biliary strictures are elderly with compromised cardiac or pulmonary function. In these patients, it is important to optimize cardiac and pulmonary function prior to surgery. Resections for gallbladder cancer and cholangiocarcinoma frequently require major liver resection as well, and it is therefore essential to evaluate for underlying liver diseases, such as cirrhosis, to ensure that the patient will not decompensate following resection.

In addition, severe coagulopathy that cannot be corrected is an indictor of poor hepatic reserve and often a contraindication to surgery.

Biliary obstruction can cause cholangitis, and this should be treated prior to surgery. In addition, all patients undergoing biliary tract surgery should receive perioperative antibiotics that cover common biliary tract organisms, such as *Escherichia coli* and *Klebsiella pneumoniae*. The use of perioperative antibiotics is especially important in patients who have had a preoperative indwelling stent placed or have biliary obstruction, as these two situations can increase the risk of infection. External biliary drainage via percutaneous catheters can also lead to fluid and electrolyte imbalances which should be corrected prior to surgery. Biliary obstruction can also lead to malabsorption, and it may be necessary to delay surgery to improve the nutritional status of a patient. In short, once the anatomic feasibility of any one procedure has been assessed, it is critically important to perform a global evaluation of the patient with particular focus on the hepatic reserve.

CONDUCT OF ABDOMINAL ACCESS AND EXPOSURE

A right subcostal incision generally allows adequate exposure for most biliary resections and bilioenteric anastomoses. However, extending this incision to a bilateral subcostal incision may be necessary. The ligamentum teres should be divided and the falciform ligament should be freed from the abdominal wall. Adhesions between the colon and the liver should be carefully divided. The Kocher maneuver is then used to mobilize the duodenum and expose the distal bile duct. When the biliary resection is being performed for malignancy, laparoscopy should be performed with careful inspection of the peritoneum for evidence of metastatic implants prior to proceeding with a laparotomy.

BILE DUCT RESECTION

Resection of Hilar Bile Duct Tumors

For potentially resectable hilar bile duct tumors, bilateral transhepatic biliary stents transversing the tumor should be placed preoperatively. This will allow easier identification of the main right and left hepatic ducts. The bile duct is divided distal to the tumor and the stents are passed out through the proximal end. The distal bile duct is then oversewn and the proximal bile duct, tumor, and gallbladder are dissected free from surrounding structures. The hepatic ducts are dissected proximally to reach healthy, nonfibrotic ducts and a resection margin is sent to pathology for frozen section verification of an adequate margin which will subsequently be incorporated into a bilioenteric anastamosis. The hepatic ducts are divided and the specimen is removed en bloc. Bilioenteric continuity is then restored with an end-to-side retrocolic Roux-en-Y hepaticojejunostomy as described below. Resection of a benign proximal biliary obstruction can be performed in a similar fashion.

End-to-side Roux-en-Y Hepaticojejunostomy for Proximal Obstructions

An end-to-side Roux-en-Y bilioenteric anastomosis can be used to restore continuity after resection of a proximal bile duct malignancy or benign stricture or to provide durable, long-term bypass of a proximal benign stricture. The jejunum is divided with a GIA stapler 40 cm distal to the ligament of Treitz and an entero-enterostomy is created in either a side-to-side or end-to-side fashion in two layers (Figure 1). Our preference is to

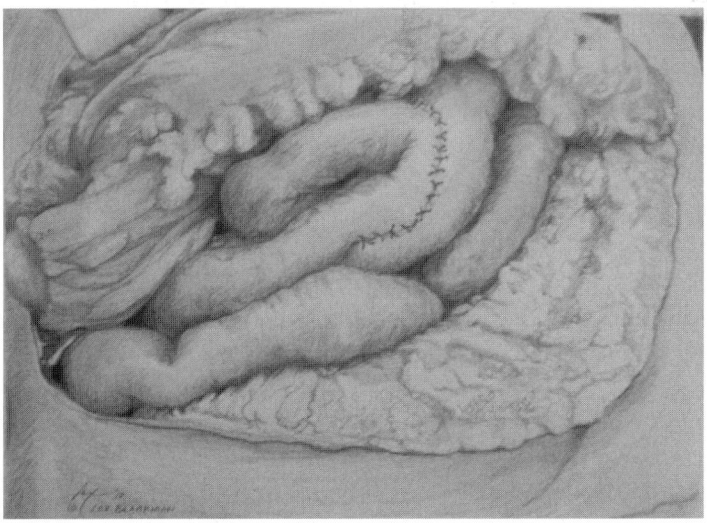

Figure 1. Enteroenterostomy.

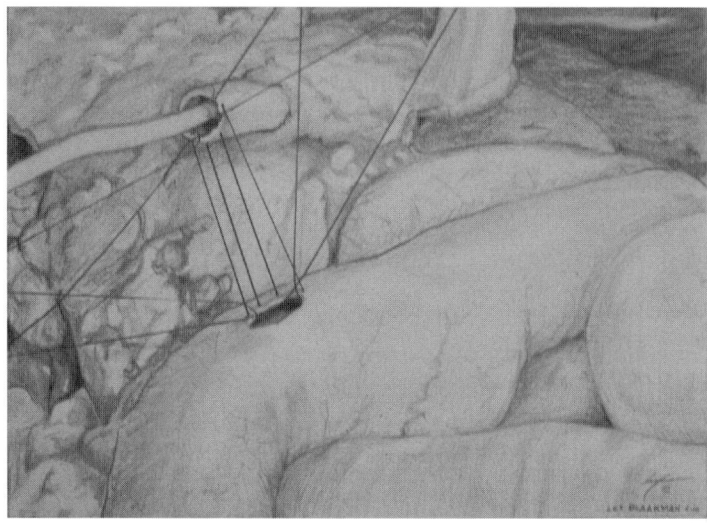

Figure 2. Posterior row anastomosis.

perform the anastamosis in a hand sewn manner utilizing interrupted 3–0 silk sutures on the outer layer and a running 3–0 PDS on the inner layer. The distal end of the jejunum is brought up in a retrocolic fashion through the transverse mesocolon to lie next to the undersurface of the liver adjacent to the bile duct. This position allows for the creation of a tension-free anastomosis. Absorbable 5–0 or 6–0 PDS sutures should be used to complete the bilioenteric anastomosis. The incision made in the jejunum should be slightly smaller than the orifice of the bile duct as the jejunal defect tends to stretch.

The posterior row sutures are placed first (Figure 2). Double-armed sutures should be placed sequentially working from left to right along the posterior row. The sutures are passed through the jejunum from inside to outside and subsequently through the bile duct from outside to inside. The knots will ultimately be on the inside of the anastomosis once secured. As they are placed, the sutures should be clamped and kept in order. After the entire posterior row of sutures is placed, the posterior row of sutures should be tied while the jejunum is pushed into the bile duct to remove tension and facilitate apposition between the bile duct and jejunal mucosa. The anterior row of sutures is then placed, again from left to right, outside to inside of the jejunal limb then inside to outside of the anterior wall of

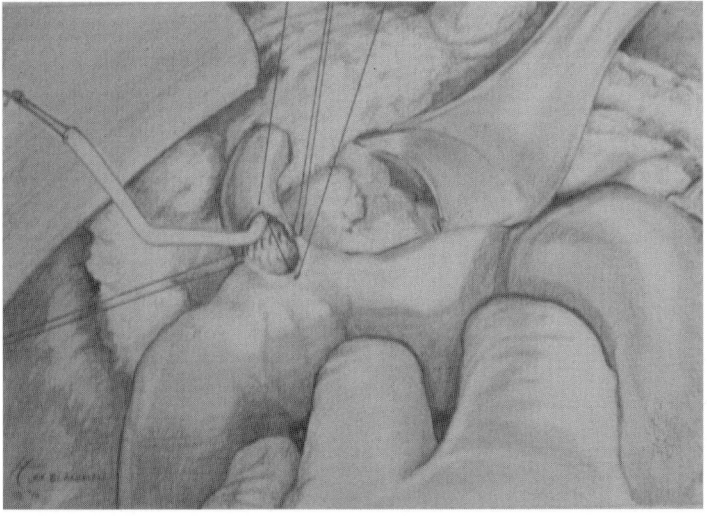

Figure 3. Anterior row anastomosis.

the bile duct (Figure 3). The needles should be cut and the sutures clamped as they are placed. The anterior row is completed by tying the sutures with the knots located on the outside of the anastamosis (Figure 4). In situations where multiple, separate bilioenteric anastamoses are needed, when possible, the surgeon should attempt to approximate adjacent bile ducts with simple interrupted sutures, creating a cloacae, so that they may be treated as a single duct for the enteric anastamosis.

Alternatively, the jejunojenunal anastomosis can be stapled. The side of the proximal end of the proximal jejunum is secured in opposition to the jejunum with 3–0 silk sutures. A small enterotomy is then made in each segment of jejunum, and a GIA stapler is used to create an anastamosis. The two small enterotomies can be closed with a TA-55 stapler or hand-sewn. To avoid an internal hernia, the mesenteric defect is closed with an interrupted 3–0 silk suture.

Side-to-Side Roux-en-Y Intrahepatic Hepaticojejunostomy for Biliary Decompression

In cases of nonresectable intrahepatic biliary cancer including cholangio-carcinoma and gallbladder cancer, palliative biliary decompression can

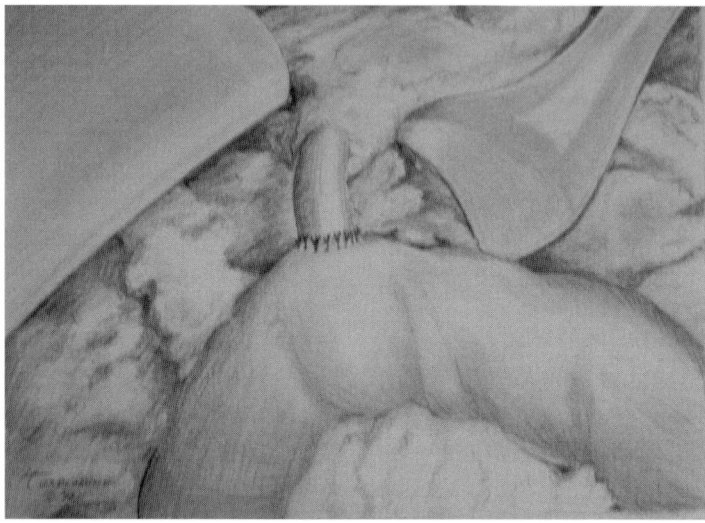

Figure 4. Completed anastomosis.

often be accomplished using the segment III ducts or right anterior sectoral duct. Upon exposure of the right or left hepatic ducts, a 40-cm jejunal roux-limb is created. Once the jejunal limb is placed in the appropriate position adjacent to the bile duct, a 2–3-cm incision is made longitudinally in the bile duct and a slightly shorter incision is made longitudinally in the adjacent jejunum. A side-to-side bilioenteric anastamosis is then created in the same fashion as for an end-to-side hepaticojejunostomy. This anastomosis may be performed in a running fashion with a 5–0 PDS. In patients with malignancy and isolated ductal systems, the drainage of only one side of the liver is acceptable as long as the other side is not contaminated.

DISTAL OBSTRUCTION

A distal bile duct obstruction can be bypassed by creating an anastamosis between the common hepatic duct, common bile duct or gallbladder, and the duodenum or jejunum. The choice of which procedure to perform for a particular patient depends on whether the obstruction is from a malignant or benign etiology, whether the patient has had a prior cholecystectomy and/or a patent cystic duct, on the overall operative risk of the patient, and the life expectancy of the patient.

End-to-Side Roux-en-Y Choledochojejunostomy or Extrahepatic Hepaticojejunostomy

Following dissection of the hepatic duct or common bile duct proximal to the tumor, the bile duct is divided and the distal end is sutured closed. The proximal bile duct is then sutured to the jejunum in a similar technique as that described for an intrahepatic hepaticojejunostomy. A 40-cm jejunal limb is created and the mesenteric defect is closed as previously described.

Side-to-Side Roux-en-Y Hepaticojejunostomy or Choledochojejunostomy

Following exposure of the common hepatic duct and common bile duct, a 40-cm roux limb is created. An approximately 2-cm incision is made longitudinally in the duct and a slightly shorter incision is made in the distal jejunal limb. The first suture should be placed in the apex of the jejunal incision and midpoint of the bile duct incision. The remaining sutures are then placed and clamped so that all knots are on the outside. The sutures are then tied in the order that they were placed. Alternatively, a single, double armed 5–0 or 6–0 absorbable suture can be used in a continuous running technique. After the creation of the bilioenteric anastamosis, the jejunojejunostomy is created as previously described.

Cholecystojejunostomy

In patients who have not had a prior cholecystectomy and in whom the cystic duct joins the hepatic duct sufficiently proximal to the tumor, a cholecystojejunostomy may be performed. However, this reconstruction should not be performed in patients who have the risk of developing malignant obstruction of the cystic duct due to the proximity of the tumor to the hepatocystic junction, as a patent cystic duct is essential for decompression. This reconstruction has inferior long-term function as compared to a choledochojejunostomy, but can be performed more rapidly, and therefore may be the ideal operation for a high-risk patient with limited life expectancy.

    A loop of proximal jejunum is placed in opposition to the fundus of the gallbladder. A 2–3-cm incision is made in both the gallbladder and the jejunum. To ensure the reconstruction provides adequate biliary drainage, incising the gallbladder should cause the collapse of the common hepatic duct. To complete the anastamosis, a continuous running 5–0 or 6–0 absorbable suture starting on the posterior side can be used. If preferred, interrupted 5–0 or 6–0 absorbable sutures could also be used, first placing an apex suture, followed by the posterior then anterior row of sutures. A clamp should be placed on the sutures as they are placed, and all sutures should be tied at the end in the order in which they were placed with the knots on the outside.

Side-to-Side Choledochoduodenostomy

A choledochoduodenostomy is most frequently used to bypass benign biliary strictures and after common bile duct exploration for a retained gallstone. For a successful reconstruction, the common bile duct must be dilated to a diameter of at least 1.5 cm to allow for effective biliary drainage.

After the common bile duct is exposed, if not already performed, a cholecystectomy is performed. A 2.0-cm longitudinal incision is then made in the distal common bile duct just proximal to where the duodenum crosses over the common bile duct. Seven to eight centimeters from the pylorus, a longitudinal duodenal incision is made. This incision should be slightly shorter than the incision in the bile duct as the tissue of the duodenum is more compliant and will stretch slightly. A single-layer interrupted anastamosis with a 5–0 or 6–0 absorbable suture is created by placing an apical suture through the inferior apex of the bile duct incision and posterior midpoint of duodenal incision. This suture, and all subsequent sutures, are placed so that the knot is on the inside. The entire posterior row of sutures is then placed and tagged. All sutures are tied in the order in which they were placed. This is repeated for the anterior row with the knots on the outside.

Laparoscopic Bilioenteric Bypass

While the breadth of surgeries that can be routinely performed laparoscopically has increased greatly over the past few years, laparoscopic bilioenteric bypass procedures remain relatively uncommon. Dissection of the portahepatis and the creation of a small bilioenteric anastamosis require a great deal of technical skill and training. Of the various anatomic reconstructions, a cholecystojejunostomy is technically the easiest to perform, and this procedure has been shown to be as safe as the open procedure.[3] Recently, studies have also shown laparoscopic choledochoduodenostomy to be a safe alternative to the open approach.[4]

We would like to acknowledge Alexander Blaakman for providing the illustrations for this chapter.

REFERENCES

1. Wang Q, Gurusamy KS, Lin H, et al. Preoperative biliary drainage for obstructive jaundice. *Cochrane Database of Systematic Reviews* 2008; 3:CD005444.
2. Perdue DG, Freeman ML, DiSario JA, et al. Plastic versus self-expanding metallic stents for malignant hilar biliary obstruction: a prospective multicenter observational cohort study. *J Clin Gastroenterol* 2008; 42(9):1040–1046.
3. Casaccia M, Diviacco P, Molinello P, et al. Laparoscopic palliation of unresectable pancreatic cancers: preliminary results. *Eur J Surg* 1999; 165:556–559.
4. Khalid K, Shafi M, Dar H, et al. Choledochoduodenostomy: reappraisal in the laparoscopic era. *ANZ J Surg* 2008; 78:495–500.

FURTHER READING

Blumgard LH, D'Angelica M, Jarnagin WR. *Surgery of the Liver, Biliary Tract, and Pancreas.* 4th edition Philadelphia, PA, Saunders Elsevier, pp. 455–474. 2007.

Selzner M Clavien PA. Surgery of the biliary system. In: PA Clavien J Baillie (eds). *Diseases of the Gallbladder and Bile Ducts: Diagnosis and Treatment.* Malden, MA, Blackwell Science pp. 140–148. 2001.

Bailen LS Libby ED. The management of benign and malignant biliary strictures. In: NH Afdhal M Dekker (eds). *Gallbladder and Biliary Tract Diseases,* New York, NY, Informa Healthcare pp. 843–867. 2000.

SURGICAL TECHNIQUES: TRANSDUODENAL TECHNIQUES 34

Sean Lee* and
Katia Papalezova[†]

INTRODUCTION

Over the last several years, serial advances in endoscopic technology and techniques have permitted endoscopic therapies to supplant surgery as the treatment of choice for benign diseases of the ampulla of Vater. Periampullary malignancies are traditionally treated with pancreaticoduodenectomy; and for all but the smallest and least-aggressive tumors, this remains the treatment of choice. Indications for transduodenal ampullectomy are therefore limited, and depend largely on the clinical experience of the surgeon to apply appropriately. Benign or small premalignant tumors that have an acceptably low risk of recurrence or progression after local resection and that are not amenable to or have already failed endoscopic resection may be appropriately pursued by a transduodenal approach, especially in patients who may be at high risk for more invasive procedures or when palliation is the primary goal of the resection.[1] Adenomas of the papilla with high-grade dysplasia and villous

---

[†]Montefiore Medical Center, The University Hospital for Albert Einstein College of Medicine, Green Medical Arts Pavillion, 3400 Bainbridge Avenue, Bronx, New York 10467 USA

or tubullovillus adenomas >2 cm in size may be appropriate for transduodenal excision or pancreaticoduodenectomy, whereas while tubular adenomas of the papilla may also be excised transduodenally, endoscopic excision is also effective.[2] Local lymph node dissection may also be of benefit, especially when operating for early stage (Tis or T1) neoplasms.[3] A clear idea of the nature of a tumor preoperatively is thus essential, and although these tumors are often discovered on CT or upper endoscopy, a subsequent ERCP or EUS should be considered to provide a clearer picture of the size and extent of the tumor.[4,5] Even with complete preoperative workup, intraoperative frozen sectioning has been shown to accurately detect the presence of malignancy, and should be utilized during local resections of periampullary tumors to ensure aggressive disease is not missed.[6] If the surgeon screens patients appropriately, is technically meticulous, and follows appropriate oncologic principles, transduodenal excision can be achieved with low morbidity, extremely low mortality, and acceptable long-term outcomes.

Obstructive ampullary diseases are now almost exclusively addressed endoscopically. Transduodenal sphincteroplasty is currently utilized for patients who have failed endoscopic treatment and those whose anatomy precludes endoscopic access to the ampulla (e.g. patients who have undergone procedures utilizing Roux-en-y gastric reconstruction).[7,8] Although these procedures have become less common with the rise of endoscopic techniques, transduodenal procedures continue to have specific applications and remain useful tools in the surgeon's armamentarium.

TRANSDUODENAL AMPULLECTOMY

The patient is positioned supine on the operating room table. Either an upper midline or extended right subcostal incision may be used depending on patient's body habitus and their history of previous surgeries. A complete examination of the abdomen should be undertaken, especially in the case of suspected malignancy, in order to evaluate for metastatic or loco-regional spread of disease. An abdominal retractor, such as a Bookwalter, is then placed to facilitate exposure. The right colon and hepatic flexure are mobilized, and a complete Kocher maneuver is performed to medialize the duodenum and expose its posterior surface.

Once the duodenum is mobilized, palpation of the ampulla is performed. A 4-cm longitudinal duodenotomy is made in the lateral (antimesenteric) wall of the second portion of the duodenum over the ampulla. Multiple stay sutures are placed on the sides of the duodenotomy to further facilitate exposure. Some authors[9] suggest that the operation is facilitated by the dilation of the biliary and pancreatic ducts, and therefore recommend delaying biliary decompression until postoperatively. A figure-of-eight stay suture is placed through the tumor. A fine-tipped electrocautery is then used to excise the mass at its base starting at the 11 o'clock position. Retraction of the mass inferiorly allows careful incision of the posterior duodenal tissues toward the common bile duct (CBD). Once the duct is entered, 4–0 or 5–0 absorbable sutures are placed through the duct, starting inside the lumen, and through the medial duodenal wall exiting through the duodenal lumen. The excision is continued in a clockwise direction, with sutures placed as the excision progresses. This helps to prevent retraction of the CBD, facilitating ease of the anastomosis. As dissection continues near the 2 o'clock position, the pancreatic duct (PD) is encountered, marked by the expression of clear pancreatic fluid when it is opened. The PD is anastomosed to the medial wall of the duodenum in a similar fashion to the CBD. Continued opposing retraction is maintained through the remainder of the excision to optimize the margins of the resection. Once the tumor is excised, it is oriented using marking sutures, and sent to pathology for frozen section. If clear margins are reported, we proceed with the reconstruction. The common walls of the PD and CBD are closed to each other with interrupted 4–0 or 5–0 absorbable sutures to form a common septum. The resulting common channel has then been completely closed as it was anastomosed to the medial duodenal wall as dissection was carried out. Inspection of the anastomosis is carried out carefully, and further interrupted sutures are placed where needed. It is crucial to ensure the patency of both ducts after all sutures are placed, and before proceeding with closure of the duodenotomy. Once ductal patency has been confirmed, the duodenotomy is closed in a transverse direction to avoid narrowing using one or two layers of 3–0 suture. A closed suction drain is unnecessary following an uncomplicated procedure, but may be left after a difficult procedure at the discretion of the surgeon. The abdomen is irrigated, and fascial and skin closures are preformed in the standard fashion.

LAPAROSCOPIC TRANSDUODENAL AMPULLECTOMY

A few authors[10,11] have advocated the application of laparoscopy to transduodenal ampullectomy for nonmalignant or minimally invasive periampullary tumors with a size or extent beyond the indications for endoscopic papillectomy. Port placement includes a 12-mm port at the umbilicus, a 10-mm port in the mid-right upper quadrant, and two 5-mm ports, one near the right costal margin in the anterior axillary line and one in the left mid abdomen. Similar exposure is gained via mobilization of the right colon and Kocherization of the duodenum. A flexible laparoscope aids in the procedure. Once exposure is gained to the second portion of the duodenum, ultrasonography is used to identify the location of the tumor. This guides the placement of a longitudinal 4-cm duodenotomy opposite to the site of the tumor. The ampullectomy is performed using electrocautery or ultrasonic shears. Given the orientation of the camera, dissection is started inferiorly and progresses counterclockwise superiorly. The pancreatic and CBD are transected and the excision is completed. The specimen is placed into a specimen bag, removed from the abdomen, and sent for frozen sectioning. The apposing edges of the CBD and PD are joined together with interrupted intracorporeal sutures. The conjoined CBD and PD lumen is then anastomosed to the duodenum using interrupted intracorporeal sutures. The duodenotomy is then closed transversely.

TRANSDUODENAL SPHINCTEROPLASTY

The technique for transduodenal sphincteroplasty is the same as that for transduodenal ampullectomy until access is gained to the ampulla. After mobilization of the colon and Kocherization, a transverse duodenotomy is made at the junction of the second and third portions of the duodenum over the ampulla. Two Allis clamps are placed, one on either side of the papilla. A probe is inserted into the papilla and a needle electrocautery is used to open the tissue overlying the probe for a length of 1–1.5 cm. A 3–0 absorbable suture is placed at the apex of the incision securing the wall of the common bile duct to the duodenal mucosa. A second stitch is placed at the lateral-most position of the incision. A third stitch is placed at the 2 o'clock position overlying the main pancreatic duct after a probe is placed into the duct to protect it from injury. Several more interrupted 3–0 sutures are placed circumferentially to complete the sphincteroplasty. Closure is completed as described above.

REFERENCES

1. Branum GD, Pappas TN, Meyers WC. The management of tumors of the ampulla of Vater by local resection. *Ann Surg* 1996; 224(5):621–627.
2. Paramythiotis D, Kleeff J, Wirtz M, et al. Still any role for transduodenal local excision in tumors of the papilla of Vater? *J Hepatobiliary Pancreat Surg* 2004; 11(4):239–244.
3. Beger HG, Treitschke F, Gansauge F, et al. Tumor of the ampulla of Vater: experience with local or radical resection in 171 consecutively treated patients. *Arch Surg* 1999; 134(5):526–532.
4. Posner S, Colletti L, Knol J, et al. Safety and long-term efficacy of transduodenal excision for tumors of the ampulla of Vater. *Surgery* 2000; 128(4):694–701.
5. Martin JA, Haber GB. Ampullary adenoma: clinical manifestations, diagnosis, and treatment. *Gastrointest Endosc Clin N Am* 2003; 13(4):649–669.
6. Clary BM, Tyler DS, Dematos P, et al. Local ampullary resection with careful intraoperative frozen section evaluation for presumed benign ampullary neoplasms. *Surgery* 2000; 127(6):628–633.
7. Morgan KA, Romagnuolo J, Adams DB. Transduodenal sphincteroplasty in the management of sphincter of Oddi dysfunction and pancreas divisum in the modern era. *J Am Coll Surg* 2008; 206(5):908–914; Discussion 914–907.
8. Miccini M, Amore Bonapasta S, Gregori M, et al. Indications and results for transduodenal sphincteroplasty in the era of endoscopic sphincterotomy. *Am J Surg* 2010; 200(2):247–251.
9. Maithel SK, Fong Y. Technical aspects of performing transduodenal ampullectomy. *J Gastrointest Surg* 2008; 12(9):1582–1585.
10. Rosen M, Zuccaro G, Brody F. Laparoscopic resection of a periampullary villous adenoma. *Surg Endosc* 2003; 17(8):1322–1323.
11. Ahn KS, Han HS, Yoon YS, et al. Laparoscopic transduodenal ampullectomy for benign ampullary tumors. *J Laparoendosc Adv Surg Tech A* 2010; 20(1):59–63.

Section 3:
Diseases of the Pancreas

PANCREAS ANATOMY AND ANATOMIC VARIANTS 35

Mani A Daneshmand* and Eugene P. Ceppa[†]

GROSS ANATOMY

The pancreas is an abdominal organ in the retroperitoneal space at the level of the second lumbar vertebrae. It is posterior to the stomach and bounded by the duodenum and spleen. The pancreas is divided into five segments: the head, the uncinate process, the neck, the body, and the tail. The uncinate process is a portion of the head that extends posterior to the superior mesenteric vessels. The main portion of the head extends anteriorly and medially along the curvature of the duodenal c-loop. It abuts the inferior vena cava, right renal artery, right renal vein, and the left renal vein posteriorly. Superiorly, the common bile duct traverses the head of the pancreas as it travels to the duodenum. Continuing laterally to the left, the neck of the pancreas passes anterior to the superior mesenteric vessels into the body of the pancreas and the organ terminates in the tail at the splenic hilum. The tail of the pancreas exists between the layers of the splenorenal ligament along with the main splenic vessels.

---

*Duke University School of Medicine, Durham, North Carolina, USA
[†]Indiana University School of Medicine, Department of Surgery Indianapolis, Indiana, USA

DUCTAL ANATOMY

The main pancreatic duct, also known as the duct of Wirsung, runs along the entire course of the pancreas. It originates at the tail of the pancreas, courses through the substance of the gland and joins the common bile duct at the head of the pancreas forming the hepaticopancreatic ampulla (Ampulla of Vater) which opens into the duodenum at the major duodenal papilla. The uncinate process is drained by an accessory pancreatic duct, also known as the duct of Santorini. Commonly, this duct drains into the main pancreatic duct but in less than 10% of people, it is a separate duct that drains into the duodenum at the minor duodenal papilla.

BLOOD SUPPLY

The pancreas has a rich and redundant blood supply from the celiac and superior mesenteric axes. The anterior and posterior superior pancreaticoduodenal arteries, which are branches off of the gastroduodenal artery of the celiac axis, perfuse the head and neck of the pancreas. The uncinate, head, and neck are also perfused by the anterior and posterior interior pancreaticoduodenal arteries which are branches off of the superior mesenteric artery. Finally, the body and the tail of the pancreas are supplied by direct vessels off of the splenic artery. This extensive network of arterial blood supply is instrumental in maintaining pancreatic viability after partial resections of this gland. Similarly, the venous drainage of the gland is quite robust. In general, the pancreatic veins run in parallel to the arterial blood supply. While a majority of the venous drainage originates from the body and tail via the splenic vein, there is extensive pancreatic drainage to the superior mesenteric and portal venous systems as well. Specifically, the superior pancreaticoduodenal veins drain directly into the portal vein; meanwhile the inferior pancreaticoduodenal veins unite to form the Henle trunk just proximal to the superior mesenteric vein. The confluence of the superior mesenteric and splenic vein forms the portal vein.

LYMPHATIC ANATOMY OF THE PANCREAS

There is no standard nomenclature for the description of the lymphatic drainage of the pancreas, yet abdominal lymph node stations have been described in the past with a particular focus around the pancreas. A majority of the peripancreatic lymphatic channels parallel the blood supply of the gland and terminate in nodal basins surrounding the gland. These pancreatic nodal basins can be divided into five main groups (superior and inferior head of the pancreas, superior border, inferior border, and splenic hilum). The superior nodes drain the anterior (level 17a) and posterior (level 13a) superior head of the pancreas and reside primarily on along the pancreaticoduodenal vessels. Similarly, the inferior drainage of lymph from the head of the pancreas is collected by the anterior (level 17b) and posterior inferior (level 13b) lymph nodes. The superior border nodal basin drains the anterior portion of the gland to lymph nodes in both the region inferior to the pylorus (level 6) and the common hepatic artery (level 8). The inferior border lymph nodes follow along the cephalad border of the gland (level 18) and drain into basins at the common bile duct (level 12), at the origin of the superior mesenteric artery (level 14A), and the right para-aortic lymph nodes (level 16). Finally, the splenic lymphatics start at the tail of the pancreas and drain predominantly into the hilum of the spleen (level 10).

NERVOUS ANATOMY

The pancreas is innervated by the autonomic nervous system. Sympathetic innervation arises from divisions of the splanchnic nerves from T5 through T11 with the predominant focus of nerves between T8 and T10. Parasympathetic innervation arises from divisions of the vagus nerve. They provide motor fibers to the blood vessels, pancreatic ducts, and pancreatic acini. Both also provide afferent visceral pain fibers to the gland.

ANATOMIC VARIANTS

In 60% of patients, the main and accessory pancreatic ducts drain independently into the duodenum (in the major and minor papillae, respectively). In a majority of these cases, there is intraglandular communication between the two ducts. Thirty percent of patients have an atretic accessory duct and their only pancreatic drainage is through the main pancreatic duct and the major duodenal papilla, while 10% of patients have either no accessory duct or the accessory duct does not communicate with the main pancreatic duct. In a majority of instances, the main pancreatic duct is larger than the accessory duct; rarely, the accessory duct may in fact be larger than the main duct. More rare variations include duplications of the accessory duct, a loop in the main duct, anomalous course of the accessory duct, and triple pancreatic ducts.

During organogenesis, the dorsal and ventral pancreatic ducts join to form the adult pancreas. Failure of this fusion (either complete or partial) results in pancreas divisum. In cases of pancreas divisum, the dorsal pancreas drains into the duct of Santorini and into the duodenum through the minor papilla. The ventral pancreas (primarily the head and uncinate process) alternatively drain into the duodenum through the major papilla.

Other anatomic variants of the pancreas include ectopic and accessory pancreas, annular pancreas, and pancreatic cysts. Ectopic pancreas occurs more commonly in the stomach, duodenum, ileum, or umbilicus. This ectopic pancreas tissue, however, can also be found in the colon, appendix, gall bladder, omentum, or mesentery. Annular pancreas is a normal pancreas tissue that encircles the duodenum at its second portion. This tissue is usually in continuity with the head of the pancreas. Often times, annular pancreas presents as duodenal obstruction in children.

REFERENCES

1. Skandalakis LJ, Rowe Jr JS, Gray SW, *et al.* Surgical embryology and anatomy of the pancreas. *Surg Clin North Am* 1993; 73:661–697.
2. Steer ML. Pancreas divisum and pancreatitis: Implications and rationale for treatment. In: HG Beger, M Buchler, H Ditschuneit, P Malfertheiner, (eds). *Chronic Pancreatitis.* New York, Springer-Verlag, 1990; 245–252.
3. Sugiyama M, Baba M, Atomi Y, *et al.* Diagnosis of anomalous pancreaticobiliary junction: value of magnetic resonance cholangiopancreatography. *Surgery* 1998; 123:391.
4. Avisse C, Flament JB, Delattre JF. Ampulla of Vater: anatomic, embryologic, and surgical aspects. *Surg Clin North Am* 2000; 80:201.
5. Koshi T, Govil S, Koshi R. Problems in diagnostic imaging: pancreaticoduodenal arcade insplanchnic arterial stenosis. *Clin Anat* 1998; 11:206.

IMAGING OF THE PANCREAS 36

Kristy Rialon[*], Courtney Coursey[†]
and Rendon C. Nelson[‡]

NORMAL CT ANATOMY

Understanding anatomy of the pancreas at CT is essential as this is the imaging modality of choice at many institutions. The splenic vein serves as a useful landmark for identification of the pancreas at CT since the pancreas sits directly anterior to the splenic vein. The splenic vein has a straight course from the splenic hilum to its junction with the superior mesenteric vein. The uncinate process, pancreatic head, and pancreatic neck are located posterior to the superior mesenteric vein, along the medial margin of the duodenal C loop, and anterior to the superior mesenteric vein, respectively. The pancreatic body is located between the left margin of the superior mesenteric vein and the medial margin of the left kidney. The pancreatic tail is located anterior to the left kidney. The gland itself is approximately 12–15 cm in length and decreases in size with age.

---

[*]Duke University Medical Center, Durham, NC 27710 USA
[†]Emory University School of Medicine, Atlanta, GA 30322 USA
[‡]Duke University Medical Center, Durham, NC 27710 USA

The celiac trunk, gastroduodenal artery, and superior mesenteric artery are readily identifiable at routine CT (Figure 1a). With modern CT technology including thin sections (e.g. 0.625 mm and 1.25 mm), arterial phase imaging, volume rendering and maximum intensity projection techniques, smaller pancreatic arteries including the anterior and posterior arcades can be seen at CT (Figure 1b). The splenic vein and superior

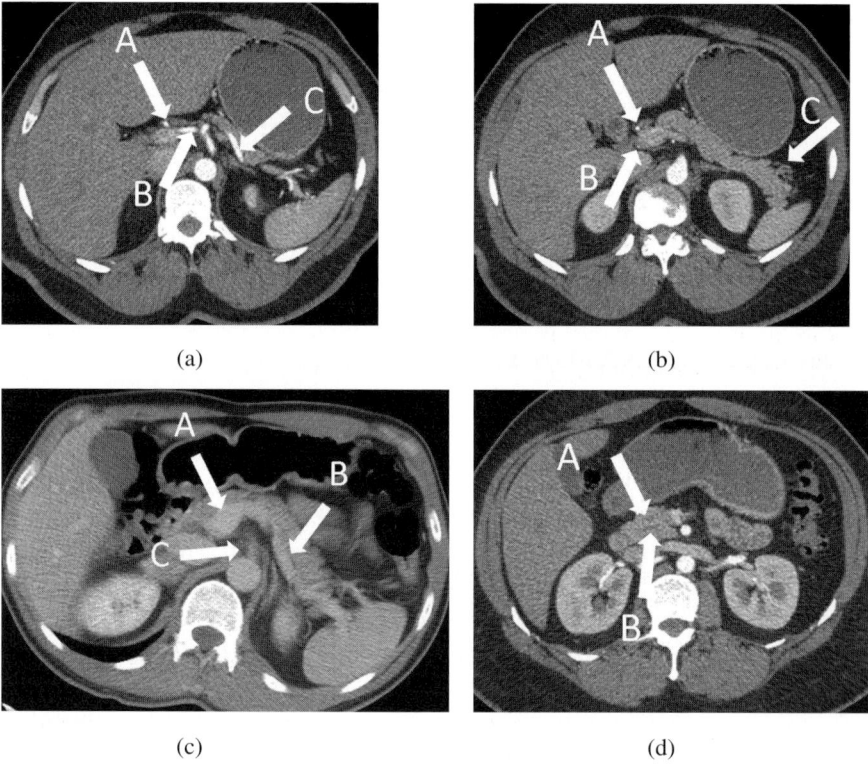

Figure 1. Arterial and venous anatomy. Axial CT images obtained after administration of intravenous contrast material. [A] Arterial phase image obtained at the level of the gastroduodenal artery. (b) Common hepatic artery and (c) splenic artery are also readily visible. [B] Arterial phase image obtained slightly more inferiorly than [A] demonstrates the (a) anterior and (b) posterior superior pancreaticoduodenal arteries. (c) The great pancreatic artery is also visible. [C] Delayed phase image with (a) the superior mesenteric vein, (b) splenic vein and (c) celiac artery labeled. [D] Normal, nondilated (a) dorsal and (b) ventral pancreatic ducts are faintly visible in this portal venous phase image.

mesenteric vein (the major pathways of pancreatic venous drainage) are readily identifiable at routine CT (Figure 1c). The superior mesenteric vein courses cranially to the right of the superior mesenteric artery until it joins the splenic vein to form the portal vein. The nondilated dorsal and ventral pancreatic ducts are also frequently visible at routine IV contrast-enhanced CT (Figure 1d). The duct normally measures a maximum of 3–4 mm in diameter in the head and tapers smoothly to the tail.

Lymphatic drainage of the pancreas is via paraceliac lymph nodes, superior mesenteric lymph nodes, splenic lymph nodes, and retroperitoneal lymph nodes. These lymph nodes are generally below the resolution of CT unless they are pathologically enlarged.

MDCT PROTOCOLS FOR EVALUATION OF THE PANCREAS

Multidetector CT (MDCT) is the imaging method of choice for evaluation of the pancreas at many institutions. With MDCT (as compared to older, single-detector scanners), one can obtain thinner slices (e.g. 0.625 mm) with improved spatial resolution. Images of the entire abdomen and pelvis can be obtained in as few as 5–10 seconds with 64-slice MDCT scanners. The two MDCT protocols used to evaluate the pancreas at our institution are given in Table 1 along with the advantages and disadvantages of each protocol.

Single phase imaging with images acquired in the portal venous phase of enhancement (images acquired approximately 60 seconds after intravenous contrast administration) is the workhorse protocol for evaluation of suspected pancreatitis and its complications. Although findings of pancreatitis such as peripancreatic inflammation ("fat stranding") are visible at CT without the use of intravenous contrast material, intravenous contrast material is mandatory for the assessment of possible pancreatic necrosis as pancreatic enhancement is evaluated in the determination of possible pancreatic necrosis.

Multiphase imaging with images acquired in the arterial (approximately 30 seconds postcontrast) and pancreatic (approximately 40–70 seconds postcontrast) phases of enhancement should be reserved for the evaluation and staging of known and suspected pancreatic malignancies. The arterial phase images in a dual phase protocol are helpful in the evaluation of arterial involvement of pancreatic adenocarcinomas and also in the evaluation of

Table 1

	Unenhanced CT abdomen and pelvis protocol	Enhanced CT abdomen and pelvis protocol	Dual pancreas protocol
Intravenous contrast material; rate	No	150 mL generic nameIsovue 300; 3 mL/sec	175 mL generic name Isovus 300; 4mL/sec
Oral contrast material	No	No	16 oz. tap water immediately prior to scanning
Phases of imaging	Single (unenhanced)	Single (portal venous phase (60-70 seconds post-contrast))	Triple (unenhanced, arterial phase (20-50 seconds post-contrast), pancreatic phase (40-70 seconds post-contrast))
Section thickness (mm)/ interval (mm)	5 / 5	5 / 5	Arterial phase: 2.5 / 2.5 Unenhanced, pancreatic phase: 5 / 5
Advantages	Obtained rapidly (no wait for IV catheter placement or serum creatinine level)	Can evaluate vessel patency and parenchymal enhancement; Lower radiation dose than dual pancreas protocol	Most sensitive CT protocol for detection of pancreatic adenocarcinoma
Disadvantages	Cannot evaluate parenchymal enhancement (ex. Evaluation of necrosis); cannot evaluate vessel patency	Less sensitive for detection of pancreatic adenocarcinoma as compared to images acquired in the pancreatic phase of enhancement	Higher radiation dose than single phase protocol

hypervascular malignancies (e.g. islet cell tumors and hypervascular metastases such as that from renal cell cancers and melanoma). Pancreatic phase images provide the greatest sensitivity for detection of pancreatic adenocarcinomas, which are hypoenhancing tumors and can sometimes be similar in appearance to the surrounding normal pancreatic parenchyma.

A disadvantage of multiphase protocols is the increase in radiation dose to the patient. Each phase of imaging results in an approximate radiation dose of 10 mSv for the average adult patient. For each abdominal CT scan, the estimated lifetime attributable risk of death from cancer has been reported to be between 0.01% and 0.02%[1] for young adults. Risks are higher in children. Therefore, multiphase imaging of the pancreas should be reserved for the evaluation of suspected pancreatic malignancies.

Basic postprocessing techniques include the creation of multiplanar reformations (MPRs) in the sagittal and/or coronal plane from the acquired axial images. An isotropic data set is required to generate high-quality MPRs. Multidetector CT (MDCT) machines that are capable of acquiring 0.625-mm thin sections (example: 16- and 64-MDCT) can acquire isotropic data sets. If one creates multiplanar reformations from thicker slice sections (e.g. 5 mm) the images are quite blurry.

Maximal intensity projection (MIP) images display a slab of data in a single image and are created by taking the brightest pixel in a given anterior posterior location and displaying these brightest pixels in a single coronal image. MIP technique is frequently used with magnetic resonance cholangiopancreatography (MRCP) where source images are acquired in the axial plane and are then displayed in a single coronal MIP image which displays the entire biliary system.

More advanced postprocessing techniques include the creation of curved multiplanar reformations whereby, most commonly, a single vessel or perhaps the main pancreatic duct is laid out. Such postprocessing techniques are relatively more labor intensive and require an independent 3D workstation at many institutions.

SPECIFIC MDCT APPLICATIONS

The two major MDCT applications in pancreatic imaging are the (1) characterization of pancreatic lesions, and the (2) evaluation of pancreatitis and its complications. MDCT imaging of congenital pancreatic abnormalities will also be discussed.

MDCT Characterization of Pancreatic Lesions

Pancreatic lesions can be characterized as primarily cystic or primarily solid based on CT attenuation values. With picture archiving and communication systems (PACS), a region of interest can be drawn within a given lesion, and the mean attenuation value within the region of interest will be displayed. In general, cystic lesions have attenuation values of 0–10 Hounsfield units (HU) at enhanced CT. Complicated cystic lesions (e.g. containing blood products or proteinaceous material) may measure slighter greater (e.g. 17–18 HU). The attenuation value of a cystic lesion should increase by fewer than 10 HU when postcontrast images are compared to precontrast images. An attenuation increase of 10–20 HU after administration of intravenous contrast material is indeterminate, and an increase in attenuation of 20 HU is evidence of enhancement. Lesions that measure at least 1 cm in size can be reliably characterized as cystic or solid at MDCT while smaller lesions are often too small to characterize given volume averaging with surrounding structures. Differential diagnoses for cystic and solid pancreatic masses are provided in Tables 2 and 3.

Cystic lesions

With increased use of CT imaging, improved MDCT technology, and the resultant higher resolution images, cystic lesions of the pancreas are being identified at MDCT with increasing frequency and often incidentally. Unsuspected pancreatic cysts were identified at 16-MDCT in 2.6% of patients in a recent series.[2]

Table 2

Solitary pancreatic cystic lesion: Differential diagnosis	
Benign	Pseudocyst
	Dilated ductal side branch
	True, epithelial-lined cyst
	Mucinous (macrocystic) adenoma
	Serous (microcystic) adenoma
Malignant	Intraductal papillary mucinous neoplasm
	Mucinous (macrocystic) adenocarcinoma
	Serous (microcystic) adenocarcinoma
	Solid and pseudopapillary epithelial neoplasm

Table 3

Solitary pancreatic solid lesions: Differential diagnosis

Hypoenhancing (relative to normal pancreatic parenchyma)	Primary adenocarcinoma
	Metastatic disease
	Lymphoma
	Ectopic splenic tissue
	Solid and pseudopapillary epithelial neoplasm
	Focal autoimmune pancreatitis
Hyperenhancing (relative to normal pancreatic parenchyma)	Islet cell tumor (example: insulinoma, gastrinoma)
	Hypervascular metastasis (example: renal cell carcinoma, some breast cancers)

The differential diagnosis of a cystic pancreatic lesion is given in Table 2. While some of these cystic lesions have characteristic appearances as will be discussed below, frequently these lesions cannot be distinguished at MDCT and a list of differential possibilities will be provided in the radiology report. Helpful discriminators for each of these lesions will be described below.

Pseudocyst

Pseudocysts are the most frequently encountered cystic lesions of the pancreas. At histology, pseudocysts are well-defined round or oval collections of fluid with a clearly identifiable fibrous capsule but without an epithelial lining. At CT, a diagnosis of pseudocyst can be rendered with confidence if a prior CT study is available which shows acute pancreatitis (e.g. pancreatic enlargement with peripancreatic inflammatory changes), and a follow-up study shows a new, well-defined fluid collection/cystic lesion. Roughly 4–6 weeks is needed for the fibrous capsule to form around the pseudocyst.

At CT, a pseudocyst often appears as a uniform, low-attenuation fluid collection with a thin wall that may enhance after administration of IV contrast material. The appearance of a pseudocyst at imaging varies with the cyst content as hemorrhagic and proteinaceous material can increase the attenuation of fluid at CT.[3] Secondary infection or communication with bowel can result in air within a pseudocyst. Without prior studies for comparison, pseudocysts may be indistinguishable from cystic neoplasms at imaging.[4] At aspiration, the amylase level of pseudocyst fluid is almost always much higher than the fluid in cystic neoplasms.

Serous (microcystic) adenoma

Serous (microcystic) adenomas are benign neoplasms, more common in women in their 7th decade of life, and represent 1–2% of all pancreatic neoplasms.[5–7] These lesions may have a characteristic honeycomb appearance composed of multiple (usually >6), small (usually <2 cm) cysts, often with a central scar which may be calcified. The classic honeycomb appearance with a calcified, central stellate scar can be considered to be diagnostic (Figure 2).[7,8] At CT, microcystic adenomas can be primarily water, soft-tissue, or mixed density, and have a margin ranging from poorly defined to a thin well-defined capsule. At aspiration, microcystic adenomas contain intracellular glycogen but no mucin, a feature central in differentiating this lesion from a mucinous cystic tumor on percutaneous aspiration biopsy.[5]

Mucinous (macrocystic) adenoma

At MDCT, mucinous (macrocystic) adenomas appear as a unilocular or multilocular cystic mass. In contradistinction to serous (microcystic) adenomas, mucinous (macrocystic) adenomas generally are composed of fewer than six cysts, and the cysts may be larger than 2 cm in size. Mucinous (macrocystic) adenomas do not have a central scar, may have peripheral calcifications, and are most commonly located in the body or tail of the pancreas. Mucinous cystadenomas cannot be distinguished from mucinous cystadenocarcinomas at imaging.

Intraductal papillary mucinous neoplasm

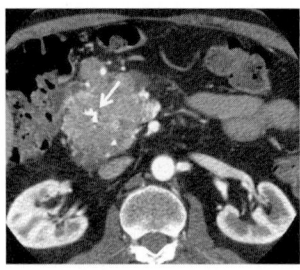
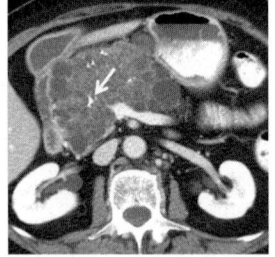
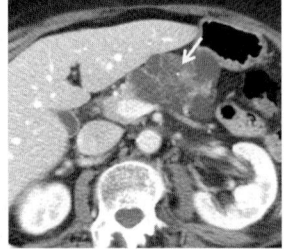

Figure 2. Serous (microcystic) pancreatic adenomas centered in (a) the pancreatic head, (b) neck and (c) body at contrast-enhanced CT. Note the honeycomb appearance with multiple small cysts and a calcified central scar (arrow).

Intraductal papillary mucinous neoplasm (IPMN) can be divided into main duct and branch duct types. IMPNs secrete an excessive volume of mucin into the pancreatic ducts, which produces progressive dilatation of the main pancreatic duct and cystic ectasia of the branch pancreatic ducts. Main duct IPMN presents as diffuse or segmental dilatation of the main pancreatic duct that can be difficult to differentiate from ductal dilatation caused by an obstructing tumor or stricture at CT. On the other hand, a branch duct type IPMN can appear as a multilocular cystic lesion. These tumors all have malignant potential. MRCP may be helpful in demonstrating the communication of a side branch tumor with the main pancreatic duct. ERCP is the definitive diagnostic test, and classic findings include a bulging papilla excreting mucin.

Dilated ductal side branch

A dilated ductal side branch can also appear as a cystic pancreatic lesion at CT and is seen in the setting of a prior episode(s) of pancreatitis. Other findings that favor the diagnosis of a dilated side branch include other findings of chronic pancreatitis such as pancreatic parenchymal calcifications and irregularity of the main pancreatic duct. Pancreatic parenchymal calcifications are more readily detectable at CT rather than MRI. On the other hand, MRI with MRCP is superior to CT for evaluation of irregularities of the pancreatic duct. Establishing that a cystic lesion communicates with the main pancreatic duct favors the diagnosis of a dilated side branch or of a side branch intraductal papillary mucinous neoplasm, which will also communicate with the pancreatic duct. MRI with MRCP can be helpful in determining if a cystic lesion communicates with the pancreatic duct; as such a determination may be below the resolution of CT imaging.

True, epithelial-lined cyst

True, epithelial-lined pancreatic cysts are rare, most often unilocular, and are usually associated with several syndromes. A helpful discriminator is the identification of other syndromic lesions, such as renal cysts in the setting of autosomal dominant polycystic kidney disease, or renal cell carcinomas and hemangioblastomas in the setting of von Hippel Lindau disease. At CT, true cysts appear as well-defined, thin-walled fluid-filled masses of variable sizes.

Cystosis associated with cystic fibrosis

Pancreatic cystosis is a rare manifestation of cystic fibrosis and is thought to be caused by ductal protein precipitation leading to ductal dilatation. Pancreatic cystosis is defined as macrocysts (>1 cm) of varying sizes scattered throughout the pancreas. These cysts can be so numerous and large that most of the pancreas is replaced. A discriminator is marked fatty replacement of the pancreas indicative of cystic fibrosis.

Approach to the cystic pancreatic lesion

Some diagnoses can be rendered with certainty at MDCT (e.g. pancreatic pseudocyst if the lesion is new and prior imaging confirms a prior episode of acute pancreatitis). Some diagnoses can be suggested with a reasonable degree of certainty (e.g. serous (microcystic) adenoma with a classic honeycomb appearance and a calcified central scar). However, for many cystic pancreatic lesions, a differential diagnosis will be given if the lesion is too small to characterize or if it has imaging features that overlap with several entities. If the differential list includes a dilated ductal side branch or IPMN, MRI/MRCP may be helpful to establish whether or not the lesion communicates with the main pancreatic duct. When a diagnosis cannot be made with certainty with CT or MRI, further evaluation with EUS, ERCP or follow-up CT or MRI may be helpful if resection is not planned.

Solid lesions

A lesion can be characterized as solid at CT if it enhances by >20 HU when pre and postcontrast images are compared. In general, if only postcontrast images are available and a pancreatic lesion measures >40 HU at contrast-enhanced CT, it is most likely solid, although hyperdense cysts (hemorrhagic or proteinaceous) can measure up to 60–70 HU. Hyperdense cysts can be distinguished from solid masses by lack of enhancement when pre- and postcontrast images are compared.[9]

Once a pancreatic lesion is determined to be solid, an assessment should be made of whether the lesion is hyperenhancing (enhancing more avidly than normal pancreatic parenchyma) or hypoenhancing (enhancing less avidly than normal pancreatic parenchyma). The differential diagnosis of a solid, hypoenhancing pancreatic mass (e.g. adenocarcinoma, metastatic disease, focal chronic pancreatitis) is quite different from the differential diagnosis of a hyperenhancing solid pancreatic mass (e.g. islet cell tumor and hypervascular metastasis, such as from renal cell carcinoma). The differential diagnosis of a hypo- or hypervascular solid pancreatic lesion is provided in Table 3. Helpful discriminators are described below.

Pancreatic adenocarcinoma

Pancreatic adenocarcinoma is the fourth leading cause of cancer death in the United States and the eighth leading cause of cancer death worldwide.[10] Pancreatic adenocarcinomas appear as hypoenhancing masses at CT, frequently with upstream pancreatic ductal dilatation and pancreatic parenchymal atrophy (Figure 3a). Masses are found in the pancreatic head approximately 60% of the time, in the body 15%, in the tail 5%, and diffusely throughout 20%.[11] For detection of most tumors, MDCT has a sensitivity of 86 to 97%.[12,13] Ductal dilatation with abrupt tapering may be the only finding in some cases of early pancreatic cancer. Small pancreatic tumors can be difficult to identify at CT. In particular, pancreatic head and uncinate process adenocarcinomas can be obscured by streak artifact in patients with biliary stents.

Contrast-enhanced CT can be used to evaluate the patency of adjacent vascular structures and whether or not neighboring structures are involved with tumor. Normally, a fat plane is visible around vessels such as the

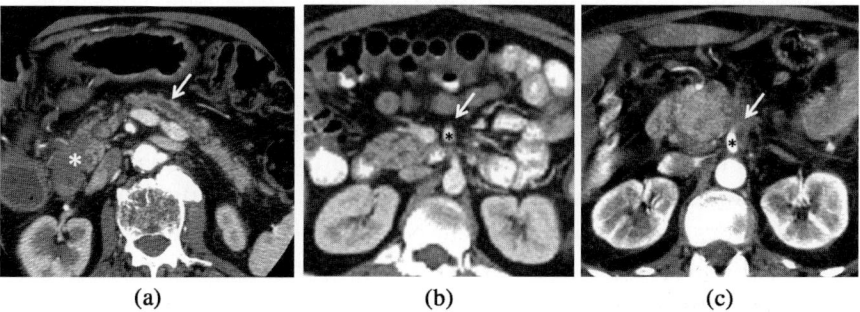

Figure 3. Pancreatic adenocarcinoma, vascular encasement. Intravenous contrast-enhanced CT images. (a) Hypoenhancing pancreatic head mass (*) with upstream pancreatic ductal dilatation (arrow). Mass was found to be a pancreatic adenocarcinoma at surgery. (b) Note clear fat plane (arrow) around the superior mesenteric artery (*) in this normal patient. (c) Loss of fat plane (arrow) around the superior mesenteric artery (*) indicates tumor involvement.

superior mesenteric artery (Figure 3b). Loss of this fat plane is suspicious for tumor involvement (Figure 3c). Tumors with over 180 degrees of vascular involvement are usually deemed unresectable.[14] The involvement of major arteries or occlusion of major veins indicates unresectability. Other indications that the tumor may not be resectable include tissue invasion of adjacent organs, liver metastases, and peritoneal carcinomatosis. CT has a reported accuracy of 77% in determining whether a pancreatic adenocarcinoma is resectable.[15]

Focal chronic pancreatitis

Focal chronic pancreatitis can mimic pancreatic adenocarcinoma at CT as it can appear as a hypoenhancing mass.[16] Establishing distinguishing features for chronic pancreatitis and adenocarcinoma is an area of active radiologic research.

Islet cell tumors

Islet cell or neuroendocrine tumors are hyperenhancing lesions. Unlike pancreatic adenocarcinomas, islet cell tumors are often not associated with upstream pancreatic ductal dilatation or parenchymal atrophy. In addition to an islet cell tumor, the differential diagnosis for a hypervascular pancreatic mass includes hypervascular metastases, such as from renal cell carcinomas, melanoma, thyroid cancer, some breast cancers, and neuroendocrine tumors.

Pancreatic splenosis

Accessory splenic tissue can occur in the pancreas, most frequently the pancreatic tail, on a congenital basis, or due to prior trauma. Pancreatic splenosis will appear as an enhancing round mass with enhancement characteristics similar to the spleen. Nuclear medicine studies (damaged red blood cell study or sulfur colloid liver spleen scan) can be used to confirm the diagnosis of accessory splenic tissue within the pancreas.

Dorsal ventral differential fat deposition

Fat deposition within the dorsal and ventral pancreatic anlages can vary, and sometimes this variable fat deposition can mimic a mass. However, the preservation of the normal architecture of the pancreas is a clue to the diagnosis of differential fat deposition. MRI with in- and out-of-phase imaging can be helpful in differentiating focal pancreatic fat deposition from a true mass.

Pancreatic lymphoma

Lymphoma involves the pancreas most commonly by direct extension from peripancreatic lymphadenopathy. Imaging findings include a focal tumor that is well-circumscribed with homogeneous attenuation that enhances weakly. A bulky, hypoenhancing mass with no or minimal dilatation of the pancreatic duct favors lymphoma over adenocarcinoma. Lymphadenopathy below the level of the renal veins is seen with lymphoma but not with pancreatic adenocarcinoma.

Metastases to the pancreas

Metastases to the pancreas are unusual and are present in only 3–12% of patients with advanced malignancy. The most common tumors are melanoma and carcinomas of the kidney, lung, and breast. Pancreatic metastases are typically round with smooth, discrete margins. They are found with equal frequency in all portions of the pancreas. As described above, metastases from hypervascular primary malignancies (e.g. renal cell carcinoma, thyroid cancer, neuroendocrine tumors, melanoma) appear as hyperenhancing masses at CT. Metastases from hypovascular primary malignancies frequently appear hypovascular at CT.

CT Evaluation of Pancreatitis and its Complications

Though the diagnosis is made clinically, acute pancreatitis can be diagnosed at CT based on the presence of peripancreatic inflammatory changes. Inflammation of the pancreas damages acinar tissue and leads to focal disruption of small ducts, resulting in leakage of pancreatic juices.

Intravenous contrast-enhanced CT is key for evaluation of complications of pancreatitis as pancreatic necrosis is only visible as an area of decreased perfusion of the pancreas at contrast-enhanced CT. Other complications of pancreatitis such as hemorrhage can also be diagnosed at CT (Figure 4a). Blood products appear as high density material at CT. As discussed above, pseudocysts can also be diagnosed at CT. The presence of air within a peripancreatic fluid collection indicates communication

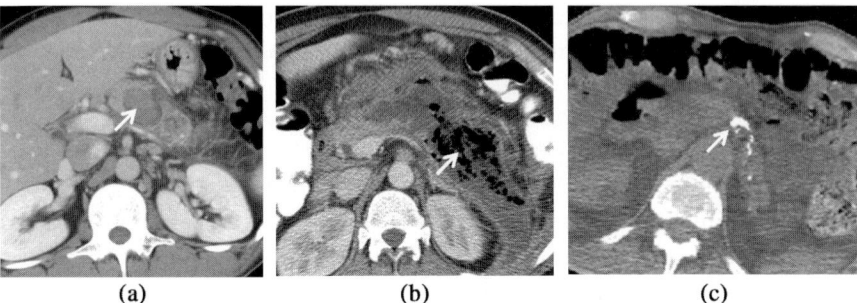

Figure 4. Complications of pancreatitis. (a) Intravenous contrast-enhanced CT image demonstrates high density material (arrow) within a pancreatic fluid collection indicating hemorrhage. (b) Intravenous contrast-enhanced CT image demonstrates peripancreatic inflammatory changes indicating acute pancreatitis as well as extraluminal air in the pancreatic body and tail (arrow) indicating either infection with gas-producing organisms or communication with the GI tract. (c) Noncontrast CT image demonstrating coarse pancreatic parenchymal calcifications (arrow) in a patient with chronic, calcific pancreatitis.

with bowel, sequelae of recent intervention, or perhaps the presence of gas-forming organisms (Figure 4b). Thrombosis of the splenic vein and other peripancreatic vessels can occur as a result of the inflammatory process and can be seen as distended vessels with low-attenuation thrombus which fail to enhance on venous phase scans. Coarse, dystrophic calcifications, often with pancreatic ductal dilatation and parenchymal atrophy, are seen with chronic calcific pancreatitis (Figure 4c).

Oral contrast material can also help in the assessment of complications of pancreatitis. For example, contrast-opacified bowel loops are more readily distinguished from fluid collections than nonopacified bowel loops.

Congenital Abnormalities

Pancreatic divisum is the most common congenital pancreatic ductal variant and occurs in 4–14% of people.[17] Pancreatic divisum anatomy occurs when the dorsal and ventral pancreatic ducts fail to fuse during fetal development. This failure of fusion results in the drainage of the pancreas head via the major papilla by the duct of Wirsung, and drainage of the body and tail by the duct of Santorini via the minor papilla. The anomaly is found with increased frequency in patients with recurrent episodes of pancreatitis. Abnormal pancreatic ductal anatomy is readily visualized with magnetic resonance cholangiopancreatography (MRCP) and endoscopic retrograde cholangiopancreatography (ERCP). If the major papilla is cannulated at ERCP, only the ventral duct will become opacified. MRCP is a non-invasive method which when used to diagnosis pancreatic divisum will show non-communication between the dorsal and ventral ducts.[18] Annular pancreas is a more rare congenital abnormality of the pancreas and occurs in approximately 1 in 20,000 newborns. Annular pancreas can be diagnosed at CT by seeing a ring of pancreatic tissue encircling the entire circumference of the D2 portion of the duodenum. In some cases, the pancreatic duct itself is visible encircling the duodenum.

OTHER IMAGING MODALITIES
MRI

Specific scenarios in which information gained at MRI may be additive to CT include the evaluation of pancreatic ductal anatomy and the determination of whether a cystic pancreatic lesion communicates with the pancreatic duct. Also, subcentimeter low attenuation lesions that are too small to confidently characterize as cystic or solid at CT can sometimes be diagnosed as cystic or solid at MRI. Disadvantages of MRI include greater cost and more limited availability at most institutions. Also, obtaining high quality MRI images is more technologist dependent than obtaining high-quality MDCT images with current scanner technology.

Standard MRI sequences include T1- and T2-weighted images. The signal of the cerebrospinal fluid (CSF) can be used to determine if a sequence is T1- or T2-weighted. If the CSF is "dark" (black), the sequence is T1-weighted. If the CSF is "bright" (white), the sequence is T2-weighted.

Pathology is frequently dark at T1-weighted imaging. However, pathologically bright T1 signal (e.g. T1 bright signal within a focal lesion) can help narrow the differential diagnosis as a relatively limited number of substances such as fat, melanin, protein, gadolinium, and some stages of blood products have intrinsic T1-bright signal. T2-weighted images are helpful for detecting fluid and inflammation, which appear bright at T2-weighted MRI (simple fluid is dark in T1-weighted sequences). Both T1- and T2-weighted sequences can be obtained with and without fat saturation. If the subcutaneous fat appears black, the sequence was obtained with fat saturation/suppression.

Magnetic resonance cholangiopancreatography (MRCP) can be helpful for evaluating pancreatic ductal anatomy. MRCP sequences are acquired as heavily T2-weighted images and are usually displayed as both thin sections and as a slab maximal intensity projection (MIP) image. Please see above for discussion of MIP imaging. Since MRCP images are heavily T2-weighted, all fluid will appear bright including fluid in the pancreatic duct, biliary system and gastrointestinal tract.

No statistically significant difference has been demonstrated between MRI with MRI angiography and CT with CT angiography in the staging of pancreatic adenocarcinoma with vascular invasion.[19] MRCP has been shown to have a sensitivity of 84% and 97% for the detection of pancreatic tumors.[20] MRI with MRCP has been shown to be at least as accurate as ERCP for pancreatic duct morphology.[20]

EUS

Endoscopic ultrasonography (EUS) can be used to characterize lesions of the pancreas and obtain tissue biopsies. This technique provides real-time cross-sectional images of the gastrointestinal wall and adjacent soft tissue structures. It is useful for the detection of pancreatic and periampullary tumors, particularly small lesions (<20mm). Tumors typically appear as an inhomogeneous solid mass with irregular borders and appear hypoechoic to normal pancreatic parenchyma. At ultrasound, simple cysts appear as anechoic (black) structures with increased through transmission (white deep to the lesion).

Endoscopic ultrasound is an important technique in the diagnosis and local tumor staging of pancreatic cancer. It can be helpful for determining tumor size, location, and vascular or lymph node involvement. EUS is more sensitive than CT for detection of tumors smaller than 3cm in diameter, but helical CT is more accurate for T-staging and equivalent for N-staging.[21,22]

Transabdominal Ultrasound

Although the pancreas is usually visible at transabdominal ultrasound, the pancreas is frequently at least partially obscured by bowel gas. Transabdominal sonography is therefore not recommended as a first-line screening test for primary pancreatic pathology.

REFERENCES

1. Brenner DJ, Hall EJ. Computed tomography-an increasing source of radiation exposure. *N Eng J Med* 2007; 357(22):2277–2284.
2. Laffan TA, Horton KM, Klein AP, *et al.* Prevalance of unsuspected pancreatic cysts on MDCT. *Am J Roentgenol* 2008; 191(3):802–807.
3. Thoeni RF, Blankenberb F. Pancreatic imaging. Computed tomography and magnetic resonance imaging. *Radiol Clin North Am* 1993; 31(5):1085–1113.
4. Warshaw AL, Compton CC, Lewandroski K, *et al.* Cystic lesions of the pancreas: new clinical, radiologic, and pathologic observations in 67 patients. *Ann Surg* 1990; 212:432–443.
5. Compton C. Serous cystic tumors of the pancreas. *Semin Diagn Pathol* 2000; 17:43–55.
6. Lundstedt C, Dawiskiba S. Serous and mucinous cystadenomas/cystadenocarcinomas of the pancreas. *Abdom Imaging* 2000; 25:201–206.
7. Procacci C, Graziani R, Bicego E, *et al.* Serous cystadenoma of the pancreas: report of 30 cases with emphasis on imaging findings. *J Comput Assist Tomogr* 1997; 21(3):373–82.
8. Sarr MG, Kendrick ML, Nagorney DM, *et al.* Cystic neoplasms of the pancreas: benign to malignant epithelial neoplasms. *Surg Clin North Am* 2001; 81: 497–509.
9. Suh M, Coakley FV, Qayyum A, *et al.* Distinction of renal call carcinomas from high-attenuation renal cysts at portal venous phase contrast-enhanced CT. *Radiology* 2003; 228(2):330–334.
10. Anderson KE, Mack T, Silverman D. Cancer of the pancreas. In: D. Schottenfield, JF Fraumeni (eds). *Cancer Epidemiology and Prevention*, New York, Oxford University Press, 3rd edition, 2006.
11. Clark JR, JM, Choyke PL, Grant EG, *et al.* Pancreatic Imaging. *Radiol Clin North Am* 1985; 23(3):489–501.
12. Agarwal B, A-HE, Molke KL, *et al.* Endoscopic ultrasound-guided fine needle aspiration and multidetector spiral CT in the diagnosis of pancreatic cancer. *Am J Gastroenterol* 2004; 99:844–850.
13. Fletcher JG, WM, Farrell MA, Fidler JL, *et al.* Pancreatic malignancy: value of arterial, pancreatic, and hepatic phase imaging with multi-detector row CT. *Radiology* 2003; 229:81–90.
14. Lu DS, RH, Krasny RM, *et al.* Local staging of pancreatic cancer: criteria for unresectability of major vessels as revealed by pancreatic-phase, thin-section helical CT. *AJR Am J Roentgenol* 1997; 168(8):1439–1443.

15. Valls C, AE, Sanchez A, Fabregat J, *et al.* Dual-phase helical CT of pancreatic adenocarcinoma: assessment of resectability before surgery. *AJR Am J Roentgenol* 2002; 178(4):821–826.
16. Kim T, MT, Takamura M, Hori M, *et al.* Pancreatic mass due to chronic pancreatitis: correlation of CT and MR imaging features with pathologic findings. *Am J Roentgenol* 2001; 177(2):367–371.
17. Yu J, Turner, MA, Fulcher, AS, *et al.* Congenital anomalies and normal variants of the pancreaticobiliary tract and the pancreas in adults: part 2, Pancreatic duct and pancreas. *Am J Roentgenol* 2006; 187(6):1544–1553.
18. Chalazonitis NA, *et al.* Pancreas divisum: magnetic resonance cholangiopancreatography findings. *Singapore Med J* 2008; 49(11):951–954.
19. Arslan A, BT, Geitung JT. Pancreatic carcinoma: MR, MR angiography and dynamic helical CT in the evaluation of vascular invasion. *Eur J Radiol* 2001; 38(2):151–159.
20. Adamek HE, *et al.* Pancreatic cancer detection with magnetic resonance cholangiopancreatography and endoscopic retrograde cholangiopancreatography: a proscpective controlled study. *Lancet* 2000; 356:190–193.
21. Dewitt J, DB, Chriswell M, McGreevy K, *et al.* Comparison of endoscopic ultrasonography and multidetector computed tomography for detecting and staging pancreatic cancer. *Ann Intern Med* 2004; 141(10):753–763.
22. Volmar KE, VR, Routbort MJ, Creager AJ. Pancreatic and bile duct brushing cytology in 1000 cases: review of findings and comparison of preparation methods. *Cancer* 2006; 108(4):231–238.

ACUTE PANCREATITIS 37

Mayur B. Patel* and Theodore N. Pappas[†]

INTRODUCTION AND HISTORY

"Acute pancreatitis is the most terrible of all the calamities that occur in connection to the abdominal viscera. The suddenness of its onset, the illimitable agony which accompanies it, and the mortality attendant upon it, render it the most formidable of catastrophes".

— B. Moynihan, 1925

This often quoted description of acute pancreatitis is still appropriate in the 21st century. It reflects a morbid, and often mortal condition, described as early as Alexander the Great's death secondary to necrotizing pancreatitis in 323 BC. Clinicopathologic differentiation between pancreatitis and other diseases did not begin until the late 15th century, when postmortem examinations emerged. In 1652, Dutch physician and anatomist Nikolaus Tulp recorded the first portmortem description of necrotizing pancreatitis. The ability of pancreatic secretion to digest proteins, carbohydrates, and fat was elucidated by French physiologist Claude Bernard in 1856. Reginald Huber Fitz, a pathologist at the

---

*Vanderbilt University School of Medicine, Nashville, TN 37212 USA
[†]Duke University School of Medicine, Duke University Medical Center 3479, Durham, NC 27710 USA

Massachusetts General Hospital, published in the 1889 Boston Medical and Surgical Journal, a clinical- and pathology- based classification system for acute pancreatitis, thus allowing clinicians to make an antemortem diagnosis. He held an antisurgical stance and felt fatalities could not be prevented by operative intervention. Pancreatic autodigestion was postulated as the underlying pathophysiological mechanism by Hans Chiari in 1896. Eugene Lindsay Opie proposed the common channel hypothesis in 1901, a theory where ampullary obstruction by gallstones causes bile reflux into the pancreatic duct sparking pancreatic autodigestion.

The treatment for acute pancreatitis has alternated between surgical and conservative management. Successful operative management of necrotizing pancreatitis was reported by Werner Koerte in 1894. Aided by the advancements in anesthesia but impeded by accurate diagnosis, the first quarter of the 20th century was heralded by surgical intervention as the treatment of choice for acute pancreatitis and was advocated by surgical stalwarts such as Arthur W. Mayo Robson, Johann von Mikulicz, and Lord Moynihan, despite mortality rates exceeding 50%. In 1929, Elman at Barnes Hospital in St. Louis, Mo, demonstrated that serum amylase measurements were a reliable and simple diagnostic test for acute pancreatitis. It was found that for acute pancreatitis, mild and conservative treatment was superior to surgical intervention. The middle of the 20th century was dominated by conservative management, though this methodology was also extended to the treatment of severe acute pancreatitis. This nonselective strategy did not significantly improve mortality rates, especially in subset populations of severe acute pancreatitis.

The latter half of the 20th century was marked by a pendulum swing toward surgery, usually initiated within 48 hours of worsening symptomology. More than 75% required re-operation due to postoperative infection and hemorrhage; however, mortality rates were lower, secondary to break-throughs in surgical metabolism and fluid resuscitation. Louis Hollender of Strasburg exemplified Europe's experiences of resection combined with necrosectomies and lavage. Conservative approaches, such as debridement and closed passive drainage with Penrose drains, were practiced in the United States. The 1970s was marked by utilization of sump drainage combined with cholecystectomy, gastrostomy, and feeding jejunostomy. This triple ostomy approach was advocated by a group at Massachusetts General Hospital (MGH), as was reoperation for late sepsis to remove infected necrotic tissues.

As more histological examinations of pancreatic specimens became available, it was clear that a necrotizing process was present in the majority

Table 1. Ranson's criteria.

At admission	During initial 48 hours
Age > 55 years	Hematocrit decrease >10%
White blood cell count > 16,000/μL	Blood urea nitrogen increase >5 mg/dL
Serum glucose > 200 mg/dL	Calcium <8 mg/dL
Serum lactate dehydrogenase > 350 IU/L	PaO_2 <60 mm Hg
Aspartate aminotransferase > 250 IU/L	Base deficit >4 mEq/L
	Fluid sequestration >6 L

Score 0 to 2: 3% mortality & severe pancreatitis unlikely
Score 3 to 4: 16% mortality & severe pancreatitis likely
Score 5 to 6: 40% mortality
Score 7 to 8: 100% mortality

of severe acute pancreatitis cases. The histologic necrosis was found to be patchy and sometimes superficial, and did not correlate with necrosis estimated at the time of surgery, leading to more extensive resections than necessary. This recognition of pathological severity was followed by the development of severity scoring systems, first provided by John Ranson in 1974 (Table 1). He combined a set of clinical and laboratory values that highly correlated with severity of illness and mortality. Diagnostic modalities continued to improve throughout the late 20th century, and it was noted in 1984 by Leena Kivisaari, a Helsinki University Hospital radiology resident, that necrotic pancreas failed to opacify during intravenous contrast-computed tomography (CT). In the 1980s, necrotizing pancreatitis was not extensively resected and was replaced by necrotic debridement and lesser sac lavage, which was advocated by Hans Beger from the University of Ulm, as well as Andrew Warshaw from MGH. Sterile and infected necrosis were dealt with similarly, however still with a significant reoperation rate (20–40%) for infection and/or hemorrhage. To this point in time, none of the reported experiences for sterile pancreatic necrosis directly compare surgery to nonoperative management.

Differentiation of sterile necrosis and its associated systemic inflammatory response from infected necrosis was markedly facilitated in 1987 by SG Gerzof from Brigham Hospital who demonstrated the diagnostic precision and safety of CT-guided fine needle aspiration (FNA) with gram stain and culture. Infected necrosis thus gained its own identity, but mortality rates remained high. Open packing, which is characterized by delayed sequestrectomy, planned re-operation with an accompanying open abdomen, and retroperitoneal lavage, decreased mortality rates consistently to 17% in individual series from University of California in Sacramento and the Mayo Clinic, as well as combined data from world centers, as reported by Bradley.

Today, significant variations in patient presentation, choice of operative technique, and operation on sterile necrosis still occurs, however, regionalization to expert hands has resulted in considerable improvement over previous mortality results. The issue of timing between early (<1week) and delayed procedures (>2weeks) still occurs; however, utilizing the delayed procedure affords an easier debridement, clearer demarcation between necrotic and viable tissues, and a decreased metabolic insult to the patient. The only level I-randomized clinical trial addressing time management of infected pancreatic necrosis was published in 1997 by J Mier, who showed signficantly lower surgical morbidity and mortality rates with delayed debridement procedures.

The late 20th century and early 21st century are marked by a myriad of interventional methods and associated clinical trials for severe acute pancreatitis, involving alternative methods to access the retroperitoneum employing laparoscopy, endoscopic, and/or interventional radiology techniques. Many of these methods are successful, however, they require multiple re-iterations. Medical therapies involving protease inhibitors in attempts to interrupt pancreatic necrosis and autodigestion are seemingly limited by lack of positive data, perhaps due to limited intravenous antiprotease half-life. Accordingly, investigators are amassing an experience with continuous regional arterial infusion of antiproteases in the setting of necrotizing pancreatitis, however this research is limited primarily to Japan. Immune modulation therapies involving tumor necrosis factor(TNF)-α and platelet-activating factor (PAF) receptor antagonism, such as Lexipafant, have not garnered enough data for clinical effectiveness either.

Aside from the clinical challenges of diagnosis and treatment, the terminology in describing acute pancreatitis and its complications has been in relative disarray until the late 20th century. The landmark 1992 Atlanta symposium, consisting of an international group of 40 renowned workers on acute pancreatitis, devised a clinical classification system (Table 2), easing communication and progress in the management of this

Table 2. Atlanta classification.

	Defintion
Acute pancreatitis	An acute inflammatory process of the pancreas with variable involvement of other regional tissues or remote organ systems.
	Associated with raised pancreatic enzyme levels in blood and/or urine.
Severity	
Mild acute pancreatitis	Associated with minimal organ dysfunction and an uneventful recovery; lacks the features of severe acute pancreatitis. Usually normal enhancement of pancreatic parenchyma on contrast-enhanced CT.
Severe acute pancreatitis	Associated with organ failure and/or local complications such as necrosis, abscess, or pseudocyst.
Predicted severity	Ranson score ≥ 3 or APACHE II score ≥ 8.
Organ failure and systemic complications	
Shock	Systolic blood pressure <90 mmHg
Pulmonary insufficiency	$PaO_2 \leq 60$ mmHg
Renal failure	Creatinine $\geq 177\,\mu mol/L$ or $\geq 2\,mg/dL$ after rehydration
Gastrointestinal bleeding	500 mL in 24 h
Disseminated intravascular coagulation	Platelets $\leq 100,000/mm^3$, fibrinogen $<1\,g/dL$ and fibrin-split products $>80\,\mu g/L$
Severe metabolic disturbances	Calcium $\leq 1.87\,mmol/L$ or $\leq 7.5\,mg/dL$
Local complications	
Acute fluid collections	Occur early in the course of acute pancreatitis, are located in or near the pancreas and always lack a granulation of fibrous tissue. In about half of patients, spontaneous regression occurs. In the other half, an acute fluid collection develops into a pancreatic abscess or pseudocyst.
Pancreatic necrosis	Diffuse or focal area (s) of nonviable pancreatic parenchyma, typically associated with peripancreatic fat necrosis; nonenhanced pancreatic parenchyma $>3\,cm$ or involving more than 30% of the area of the pancreas.

(*Continued*)

Table 2. (*Continued*)

	Defintion
Acute pseudocyst	Collection of pancreatic juice enclosed by a wall of fibrous or granulation tissue, which arises as a result of acute pancreatitis, occurring at least 4 weeks after onset of symptoms, is round or ovoid and most often sterile; when pus is present, lesion is termed a "pancreatic abscess".
Pancreatic abscess	Circumscribed, intra-abdominal collection of pus, usually in proximity to the pancreas, containing little or no pancreatic trauma; often 4 weeks or more after onset; pancreatic abscess and infected pancreatic necrosis differ in clinical expression and extent of associated necrosis.

disease. Since the Atlanta symposium, nearly half of the published articles utilize alternative definitions of predicted severity, actual severity, as well as organ failure. Large variations still exist for descriptors and management of local complications.

EPIDEMIOLOGY

Acute pancreatitis is the third most common gastrointestinal disorder requiring hospitalization in the U.S., and affects approximately 233,000 individuals annually, of which 20% have severe acute pancreatitis. The incidence of acute pancreatitis is increasing worldwide, surmised from population-based studies in England, Denmark, Netherlands, Sweden, and the US. This is partially due to the almost routine pancreatic enzyme testing and CT use in emergency room patients presenting with abdominal pain resulting in heightened diagnosis of milder cases. Certainly, the increase in cholelithiasis and obesity plays a major role in this increase in incidence, although obesity does not appear to be a risk factor for necrosis. An intake of more than two drinks per day, irrespective of pancreatitis etiology, may increase the risk for necrosis.

While mild acute pancreatitis has a mortality rate of less than 1%, severe acute pancreatitis is marked by a 10% mortality with sterile necrosis and a 25% mortality with infected necrosis. Although overall mortality rates for severe acute pancreatitis have decreased over the past century, those with advanced age continue to have higher mortality rates. Of those who do die, 65% die within 2 weeks, and 80% die within 4 weeks.

ETIOLOGIES

In the Western world, 85% of pancreatitis has an identifiable cause with gallstone pancreatitis accounting for 38% of acute pancreatitis. Gallstones can be recovered in the stool within a week of onset of illness in up to 90% of patients with gallstone pancreatitis. Patients with biliary colic rarely pass gallstones. Transient ductal obstruction at the ampulla, common bile duct, and/or pancreatic duct promotes pancreatitis by increasing ductal pressure and subsequent unregulated activation of pancreatic autodigestion.

Alcohol abuse is related to 36% of acute pancreatitis cases. The acinar cell is considered the main target of damage by ethanol, as caused by proteinaceous plugging of small pancreatic ductules. But, the correlation between alcohol and pancreatitis also involves a combination of environmental and genetic factors, such as mutation of the cationic trysinogen gene (PRSS1) and serine peptidase inhibitor, Kazal type I (SPINK 1).

Up to 10% of acute pancreatitis cases are idiopathic and remain unknown. Pancreatic divisum has been associated with idiopathic acute pancreatitis and is three to fourfold higher in patients with recurring bouts of acute pancreatitis than in unaffected controls. It is a common congenital anatomical anomaly present in 7% of autopsy series, and results from failure of fusion between the dorsal and ventral ductal systems. Of those with divisum, only 5% have ductal hypertension from inadequate drainage of the independent ductal systems resulting in pancreatitis. Tumors, such as intraductal papillary mucinous neoplasms, whose main tumor mass or associated mucous, may result in another etiology of pancreatic ductal obstruction.

Iatrogenic causes related to medications, and instrumentation of the duct are another set of causes of pancreatitis, although the former is considered a rare event (0.1%). Drugs with strong associations include azathioprine, sulfonamides, valproic acid, estrogens, furosemide, 5-aminosalicylic acid compounds, corticosteroids, and octreotide. The endoscopic retrograde cholangiopancreatography (ERCP) procedure results in up to 70% of patients having asymptomatic hyperamylasemia. Risk factors for post-ERCP pancreatitis include young age, female sex, number of attempts for papillary cannulation, poor emptying after pancreatic duct opacification, and treatment for sphincter of Oddi dysfunction. High risk patients may have decreased rates of post-ERCP pancreatitis with the use of temporary pancreatic ductal stenting. Certainly, shock states in the perioperative period associated with prolonged periods of hypotension can also theoretically result in pancreatitis as a consequence of ischemia-reperfusion injury to the pancreas, but this is rare due to the robust vascular supply of the pancreas.

Penetrating trauma results in more pancreatic injury than blunt trauma. Blunt injury associated with deceleration may cause crush injury to the gland across the spine resulting in pancreatic ductal disruption and its complications, — this is often associated with a delay in diagnosis.

Infections account for less than 1% of acute pancreatitis, and tend to be mild. Various viral infections associated with acute pancreatitis are more common in children. Bacterial causes have been reported but are even more rare than viruses. Worldwide, *Ascaris lumbricoides*, a parasitic roundworm, has been known to cause pancreatitis by migration in and out of the duodenal papilla.

Metabolic derangements, such as hypercalcemia and hypertriglycerdemia are rare. Hypercalcemia also causes <1% of pancreatitis and can be associated with primary hyperparathyroidism, excessive vitamin D, familial hypercalcuric hypercalcemia, and total parenteral nutrition.

Autoimmune pancreatitis is a newly described entity and also extremely rare, but is associated with young patients who have inflammatory bowel disease, primary sclerosing cholangitis, and primary biliary cirrhosis. The specific criteria for diagosis include a focal mass in the pancreatic head by CT, irregular narrowing of the proximal pancreatic duct by ERCP, elevated serum IgG4 levels, and an infiltration of IgG4-containing plasma cells in the pancreas. Uniquely, steroids are the mainstay of therapy.

PATHOPHYSIOLOGY

The pathogenesis of acute pancreatitis is caused by inappropriate conversion of the pancreatic proenzyme trypsinogen to its active form, trypsin. The precise mechanisms responsible for this activation remain unclear, however work in multiple animal models has suggested that stimuli prevent appropriate export of zymogen granules from the acinar cells, leading to fusion with intracellular lysosomes and activation of trypsin by lysosomal enzymes such as cathepsin B. Intracellular conversion of trypsinogen to trypsin initiates a cascade of activation of other zymogens, leading to cellular autodigestion. Once activated, these pancreatic enzymes are responsible for autodigestion of pancreatic and peripancreatic tissues and damage to the microvasculature supplying the gland.

The process of pancreatic necrosis occurs relatively early in the disease process, within the first 24 to 48 hours, and in at least two-thirds of patients, it remains stable throughout the course of the illness. As a result of the acute pancreatic injury, a range of enzymes are released into the bloodstream, including trypsinogen, amylase, lipase, phospholipase A2, trypsinogen-activating peptide, and polymorphonuclear cell elastase. In addition, injury to the pancreatic parenchyma stimulates the production of inflammatory cytokines such as interleukin (IL)-1 and TNF-α. Some of the pancreatic damage may be caused directly by the inflammatory response itself, as TNF-α has been shown to cause acinar cell apoptosis. The release of these cytokines triggers an inflammatory cascade, resulting in the production of additional cytokines including IL-2, IL-6, IL-8, IL-10, bradykinin, and PAF. Humans studies indicate the proinflammatory cytokines seem to be confined to the splanchnic circulation, while anti-inflammatory cytokines are more prevalent systemically.

The end point of this inflammatory cascade is the systemic inflammatory response syndrome (SIRS), characterized by loss of vascular tone and systemic vascular resistance and increased capillary permeability with third-spacing of plasma volume, all leading to hypotension and hyperdynamic cardiovascular response. If unchecked, SIRS may produce acute respiratory distress syndrome (ARDS) or multiorgan dysfunction syndrome (MODS), both with significantly high mortality.

This profound inflammatory response marks the early (<2 weeks) phase of severe pancreatitis, usually necrotizing. It is the body's own inflammatory reaction to the initial injury that produces most of the early morbidity and mortality, and is sometimes marked by organ failure. Up to 50% of those with severe acute pancreatitis develop organ failure within 72 hours and 20% present with MODS at hospital admission. Most who develop organ failure are suffering from necrotizing pancreatitis. There is a strong correlation between clinical severity and extent of pancreatic necrosis, especially those with >50% necrosis by contrast-enhanced CT. Furthermore, those who worsen clinically are likely suffering from infected pancreatic necrosis. The second, late-phase (>2 weeks) can be marked by infectious complications of gland necrosis and the sequelae of organ failure.

DIAGNOSIS

Pancreatitis is marked by severe, steady upper abdominal pain, with fairly sudden onsent without a prodrome, radiating to the lower thoracic region, and is often associated with nausea and vomitting. Tenderness, guarding, and a diffuse peritonitis picture can be present in severe cases, but usually without the board-like quality of a perforated viscus. Initial history should query for history of alcohol use, recent biliary instrumentation or procedures, and a detailed list of medications. Physical signs such as Cullen's sign (periumbilical ecchymosis) and Grey–Turner's sign (flank ecchymosis) occur in less than 3% of patients are associated with a greater than 30% mortality. Differential diagnosis includes acute cholecystitis, perforated peptic ulcer, mesenteric ischemia, and bowel obstruction or perforation.

Elevations of serum amylase and lipase (>3 times normal) support the diagnosis of pancreatitis; however, modest elevations of pancreatic enzymes may be observed in other intra-abdominal emergencies. The elevations and normalization of enzymes do not correlate with severity, but, in general, tend to peak early and decline over 3–4 days. Hyperamylasemia tends to peak occur earlier, while lipase remains elevated longer in the initial course of illness. The half-life of amylase is shorter than the half-life of lipase, and, lipase has a slightly greater sensitivity and specificity and greater overall accuracy than amylase. Other tests such as urinary trypsinogen activation peptide, serum and urinary trypsinogen, C-reactive protein and procalcitonin have diagnostic and prognostic potential but are less widely available and not recommended. Increased levels of serum alanine aminotransferase (ALT) up to three times its normal value is indicative of gallstone pancreatitis, and a meta-analysis has shown ALT >150 IU/L has a senstivity of 96% for gallstone pancreatitis, as opposed to other etiologies. However, a biliary etiology should not be excluded when liver function tests are normal since 15–20% of patients with biliary pancreatitis can have normal lab work due to microlithiasis being more prevalent in this condition. If hypertriglyceridemia or hypercalcemia is suspected, the testing must occur early in the clinical presentation, as their levels decline during the hospitalization, which commonly includes fasting and intravenous fluid resuscitation. A history of triglyceride levels >1000 mg/dL (11.3 mmol/L) is suggestive of an etiology.

Plain films are neither sensitive or specific, although suggestive findings such as a localized ileus of the small bowel, a "sentinel loop", may be visible. Ultrasonography can be used to detect gallstones and also to image an edematous, swollen gland, but this is limited by patient factors related to obesity and local bowel gas patterns. Notably, ultrasound has a false negative rate of 1.5%, which is important to keep in mind when considering a diagnosis of "idiopathic" pancreatitis. Contrast-enhanced CT is useful for differentiating pancreatitis from other intra-abdominal conditions, and can delineate local complications, as well as necrosis. Infection may manifest as gas bubbles within necrotic tissue on CT (Figure 1). An admission CT may also serve as a baseline for future comparison, but if possible, delaying the CT for 72 hours may allow evolving necrosis to be imaged.

Initially, concerns existed that iodinated contrast administration could worsen pancreatic necrosis however, this has not been borne out in animal models or in clinical studies. The pancreas enhances maximally with intravenous contrast to 120 Hounsfield units (HU) from its baseline

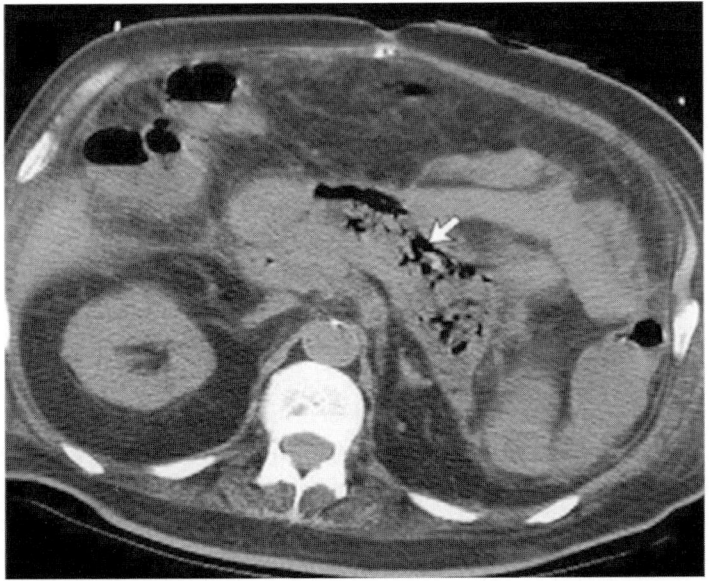

Figure 1. Necrotizing pancreatitis. The white arrowhead demonstrates a necrotizing infection of the midbody and tail of the pancreas and accompanying gas bubbles, suggestive of infection.

attenuation of 40 HU. In mild acute pancreatitis, in which the parenchymal capillary network remains intact, there remains good uniform enhancement. With severe or necrotizing pancreatitis, areas of pancreas can demonstrate decreased or no enhancement. Improvements in contrast bolus technique and imaging acquisition have revealed subtle, previously unapparent findings, related to edema and ischemia. Newer CT techniques under research include dynamic perfusion multidetector CT, in which pancreatic perfusion color maps and blood volume can be calculated.

The current clinical definition of pancreatitis requires two of the three following features: (1) abdominal pain suggestive of pancreatic origin, (2) level of serum amylase or lipase greater than or equal to three times normal, and (3) characteristic findings on contrast-enhanced CT. Furthermore, the Acute Pancreatitis Classification Working Group met to revise definitions set forth in the Atlanta Symposium in May 2007 (Table 3).

Up to 57% of patients with acute pancreatitis will have a fluid collection on CT, with 39% having two collections, and 33% with three or more collections. Fluid collections are ill-defined initially, and managed

Table 3. Two classification schemes, 1992 versus 2007.

Atlanta Symposium (1992)	Acute Pancreatitis Working Group (2007)
< 4 Weeks After Onset of Pancreatitis	
Acute fluid collection (AFC)	Acute peripancreatic fluid collection (APFC)
	Sterile
	Infected
	Post-necrotic pancreatic/peripancreatic fluid collection (PNPFC)
Pancreatic necrosis (sterile)	Sterile
Infected pancreatic necrosis	Infected
> 4 Weeks After Onset of Pancreatitis	
	Pancreatic pseudocyst
Pancreatic pseudocyst	Sterile
Pancreatic abscess	Infected
	Walled-off pancreatic necrosis (WOPN) (is a mature PNPFC with defined wall)
	Sterile
	Infected

conservatively. They evolve over time and may enlarge, cause pain, become infected, and/or compress adjacent organs requiring intervention. Fluid collections with high levels of pancreatic enzymes are usually associated with pancreatic duct disruptions and may eventually form pseudocysts, ascites, or pleural effusions.

FNA under CT guidance with analysis by gram stain coupled with bacterial and fungal culture can assist with determining infected necrosis. Bacteriological analysis usually reveals gram-negative microbes deriving from intestinal translocation, such as Escherischia coli (40%), Enterococcus (18%), and Klebsiella (18%), and is monomicrobial 75% of the time. Although in recent years, increased incidence of gram-positive organisms are being isolated. Infected pancreatic necrosis necessitates surgical debridement, while sterile necrosis is managed best nonoperatively. This dichotomy of treatment strategies based on the presence of infection has led to the widespread advocacy for early FNA of the necrotic pancreas.

Although early necrosectomy was historically advocated, as previously mentioned, delayed surgical intervention (>2 weeks) is associated with reduced mortality and morbidity and is the current standard of care, even in the setting of infected necrosis.

An argument against routine FNA is that during the 2-week delay, most patients who have sterile necrosis will improve clinically, while those who have infected necrosis will not. Examination of the data from two studies advocating FNA shows that the mean time from presentation to surgery in patients who had positive aspirates was 3–4 weeks, while the mean total length of hospital stay in those patients with negative aspirates, or sterile necrosis, was no different. In these studies, patients undergoing FNA were treated only with prophlyactic antibiotics for several weeks regardless of their aspiration data. Surgical debridement was performed for those with positive FNAs or those without clinical improvement and signs of ongoing sepsis. Few surgeons would withhold surgical intervention based on a negative FNA in the face of clinical deterioration. Unless the results of the FNA push the clinician to intervene earlier or withhold antibiotics pending the result, it remains unneccessary. There is no evidence that use of FNA reduces mortality, and it has been the authors' practice to avoid aspiration and rely exclusively on clinical evaluation to guide surgical intervention with good results.

Magnetic resonance cholangiopancreatography (MRCP), ERCP, and endoscopic ultrasound can help detect small bile stones as a cause of pancreatitis. MRI is difficult to perform in the acute setting related to patient instability, agitation, and renal function depression. MRCP has been shown to have greater than 90% sensitivity and specificity for choledochlithiasis and can delinate other etiologies of biliary obstruction. ERCP may help define ductal anatomy to guide further intervention and provide early ductal clearance of stones.

SEVERITY PREDICTION AND OUTCOME

Given no single biomarker can predict the course of pancreatitis, a number of physiologic scoring systems have been developed, including Ranson's criteria (Table 1). This system was developed in 1974, and still remains a commonly employed severity scoring system to predict outcome on admission and at 48 hours. The Acute Physiology and Chronic Health Evaluation II (APACHE II) measures 12 distinct variables designed to predict mortality on admission, which generally is performed on a retrospective analysis or using an online calculator, given its relative complexity. Other less often used physiologic scoring systems exist, such as the Glasgow (Imrie), as do organ dysfunction scoring systems, such as Multiple Organ Dysfunction Score and the Sequential Organ Failure Assessment.

Infected necrosis and fungal superinfection are two of the most striking independent predictors of outcome, along with early multiorgan dysfunction syndrome involving at least two organs. Age >70 and obesity (body mass index >30 kg/cm^2) are also significant risk factors for morbidity.

Given the diagnostic dependency on imaging, CT findings have been linked to mortality and complications. The Balthazar CT severity index is the most commonly known radiologic scoring system (Table 4, 5). Points

Table 4. Balthazar CT severity index.

CT grade	Descriptor	Points	Necrosis	Extra points
A	Normal pancreas	0	0	0
B	Pancreatic enlargement	1	0	0
C	Pancreatic/peripancreatic fat inflammation	2	<30%	2
D	Single peripancreatic fluid collection	2	30–50%	4
E	Two or more fluid collections/ retroperitoneal air	4	>50%	6

Table 5. Relationship between severity scores and outcomes.

Index	Score			
Ranson's Score	0–2	3–4	5–6	7–8
% Survival and intensive care > 7 d	1	24	53	—
% Death	3	16	40	100
% Death or intensive care > 7 d	4	40	93	100
CT Severity Index	0–3	4–6	7–10	
% Complications	8	35	92	
% Death	3	6	17	

are given for grades of inflammation A through E, and for percentage of gland necrosis. For example, a severity score of 7–10 yields a 17% mortality rate and 92% complication rate.

EARLY MANAGEMENT

Maintenance of adequte intravascular volume and end-organ perfusion is the key to managing pancreatitis. This initial resuscitation period usually stratifies those with mild acute pancreatitis from severe acute pancreatitis requiring advanced hemodynamic monitoring and resuscitation according to the Surviving Sepsis Campaign guidelines. Unless active hemorrhage is present, deep venous thrombosis prophylaxis with heparin or lovenox should be provided. Gastric ileus or severe perigastric inflammation may require nasogastric tube decompression, but this should not preclude enteral nutrition. Most treatment guidelines advocate early enteral feeding in patients with pancreatitis, regardless of severity, based on at least six randomized trials showing decreased infectious rates, reduced hospital stay, and lowered need for surgical intervention, compared to total parenteral nutrition (TPN). Post-ampullary feeding does not stimulate pancreatic exocrine function, and maintains the normal enteric barrier to gram-negative flora. TPN should be reserved for intolerance of distal enteral feeding after a 7-day trial, at the risk for central venous catheter infections, particularly fungal.

Empiric antibiotic use remains unquestioned in severe necrotizing pancreatitis with systemic manifestations of organ failure. Typically, carbapenems and quinolones have been the most studied. However, two large placebo controlled double-blind trials in 2004 by Isenmann[5] (n = 76) and in 2007 by Dellinger[3] (n = 100) have failed to show a benefit to prophlyaxis with regard to infection or mortality rates in cases of severe pancreatitis. Both studies have been criticized for being underpowered due to discordance between a 40% expected infection rate against actual infection rates (17%, 12%). Furthermore, each study had a significant crossover of placebo patients receiving intravenous antibiotics of some kind (46%, 54%). Late fungal infection has been correlated with antibiotic prophylaxis and may increase mortality fourfold, independent of APACHE II severity.

Mild biliary acute pancreatitis is dealt with biliary ductal clearance and cholecystectomy, usually during the index admission, to avoid a recurrence of increased severity. In the setting of persistent biliary obstruction and acute pancreatitis due to suspected or confirmed gallstones, urgent ERCP should be performed within 72 hours of onset of symptoms. If ERCP is unavailable or not technically feasible, other biliary clearance/drainage procedures may be required. Laparoscopic to open cholecystectomy conversion rates up to 15% are expected, and up to 44% of those managed nonoperatively can expect to have recurrent pancreatitis within 6 months that is more severe and with higher morbidity and mortality than the index episode.

Based on a few randomized controlled clinical studies, a small subset of patients with severe acute pancreatitis related to biliary etiologies may have decreased mortality associated with early ductal clearance, if they fail to improve within 24 hours of admission, and have demonstrable ductal obstruction, which is cleared by ERCP within 48 hours. Cholecystectomy is still preferably performed in the same hospital admission, but sometimes requires outpatient delay for severe retroperitoneal inflammation and patient recovery.

Surgical intervention for severe necrotizing pancreatitis should be delayed if physiologically possible for >2 weeks and is indicated for the following groups:

- Unrelenting clinical deterioration despite maxmial intensive care,
- Infected necrosis,
- Sterile necrosis without clinical improvement.

Mier[6] performed the first randomized clinical trial comparing early pancreatic resection and debridement within 72 hours versus delayed surgery at 11 days and demonstrated a decreased mortality rate between groups (56% versus 27%). In fact, this trial was terminated because of the high mortality rate for the patients undergoing early surgery. Other indications, such as hemorrhagic pancreatitis, ischemia or perforation of the small or large bowel, and/or abdominal compartment syndrome can occur at any time and may necessitate emergency operation.

Three generic approaches to open surgical debridement of infected pancreatic necrosis exist with numerous minor technical modifications reported in the literature. Evidenced-based comparison between them are not possible given the variability intrinsic to the disease process and institutional technical experience. All of the procedures revolve around debridement and necrosectomy are coupled with the following:

- Closed suction drainage and primary abdominal closure.
- Immediate continuous lesser sac lavage and primary abdominal closure.
- Packing with planned re-exploration, lavage, and secondary abdominal closure.

Pancreatic debridement and necrosectomy is generally performed with blunt finger dissection, stopping once bleeding tissue is encountered in an effort to spare the viable remainder of the gland and to avoid catastrophic hemorrhage. Formal pancreatic resection is associated with higher morbidity than organ-sparing debridement. Extension of the necrosis into the retroperitoneal pericolic gutters or mesentery is common, and this should be explored gingerly with blunt dissection. Involvement of the large bowel, particularly the transverse mesocolon, has been shown to be a particularly morbid complication. If feasible, cholecystectomy should be performed, irrespective of etiology. Some authors have advocated the placement of a feeding jejunostomy tube. Given the high incidence of postoperative enterocutaneous fistula, however, it has been the authors' practice to avoid even intentional enterotomies. Following debridement of the necrotic tissue, the cavity should be drained with several large-bore closed-suction drains, such as silastic (Davol) drains, which can be used for postoperative irrigation and drainage. Even if all necrotic material is not completely removed, the abdomen may be closed. Continuous closed lavage may be performed postoperatively and consists of local irrigation of saline until effluent is clear of necrotic debris. Open abdomen management, with or without marsupialization, timed with return trips to the operating room for dressing changes, has fallen out of favor, likely because the delay in surgical intervention has promoted organization of the necrotic tissue to facilitate complete debridement at the time of initial laparotomy. Recurrent collections may be drained percutaneously after the manual operative removal of the necrotic parenchyma. Clinical sepsis does not subside in the first postoperative day, but usually in the first postoperative week.

Minimally invasive methods utilize alternative approaches and instrumentation of the retroperitoneum and include video-assisted retroperitoneal debridement (VARD), laparoscopic transperitoneal necrosectomy, and endoscopic drainage. These procedures aim at infection control, rather than complete necrotic tissue removal, and may blunt the physiologic response of an intervention, but often patients manifest persistent sepsis and require 3–4 procedures. The VARD approach avoids peritoneal contamination, but is limited in detecting colonic ischemia or dealing with the biliary system. In addition, the retrieval channel is limited in its ability to extract debris and may require multiple additional procedures. Laparoscopic transperitoneal necrosectomy has the advantage of assessing the peritoneal cavity with the simultaneous drawback of transperitoneal contamination. Subsequent laparoscopic procedures are rarely possible due to intra-abdominal adhesions and inflammation. Endoscopic drainage involves a transenteric drainage route usually coupled with internal stenting to maintain patency. This method avoids an external pancreatic fistula, however intraperitoneal procedures cannot be performed. The necrosis must be walled off and endoscopically accessible. Other difficulties of minimally invasive methodology are associated with necrosis behind the pancreatic head, which involves risks of massive bleeding if the portal vein is damaged during debridement. Hospital mortality remains around 15–20%, irrespective of open or minimally invasive methods.

Percutaneous drainage of infected pancreatic necrosis may decrease clinical toxicity and postpone surgical drainage until at least the third week of illness. Using large-bore drainage catheters, atypical for most interventionalists and interventional procedures, is required to effectively allow removal of necrotic, inspissated debris. Periodic upsizing and adjunctive interventional or surgical therapies are often required. Certainly, there are patients who may have been cured by this methodology alone, however, literature is sparse regarding percutaneous drainage for infected necrosis, and the appropriate patient population has yet to be defined.

Complications such as intestinal fistulazation and hemorrhage along the drain tract are possible, but certainly the associated mortality rate of percutaneous drainage is low.

A randomized multicenter trial called Minimally Invasive Step Up Approach versus Maximal Necrosectomy in Patients with Acute Necrotising Pancreatiting (PANTER) was recently published in April 2010. Eighty-eight patients recruited from 2005 to 2008 over 19 Dutch hospitals were randomly assigned to undergo primary surgical necrosectomy with postoperative closed lavage or a step-up approach to treatment. The step-up approach initially involved percutaneous drainage, and if this failed twice, it was followed by VARD with postprocedural lavage. Sixty-nine percent of the open necrosectomy group sustained major complications (multiple organ failure, perforation, fistula, bleeding or death), against 40% in the step-up approach group. Mortality was similar between groups (19 vs. 16%), but multiple organ failure occurred less often in the step-up approach (12% vs. 40%). Notably, 35% of the step-up approach only required percutaneous drainage as a mono-intervention. These patients also had a lower incisional hernia rate (7% vs. 24%), new-onset diabetes (16% vs. 38%), and hospital costs (by 12%).

Pancreatic abscess, an ill-defined entity recently reclassified, is an indication for surgical intevention; however, it can be managed by percutaneous methods alone, if the drain is of sufficient caliber and clinical status improves. Pancreatic abscess generally develops > 4 weeks following onset of pancreatitis, and involves a more polymicrobial infection. Without clinical improvement, or association with any significant necrotic pancreatic burden, open surgical drainage is preferred. Overall, the mortality and hospital course is less acute than that of infected pancreatic necrosis.

Pancreatic pseudocysts also usually require 4 weeks to form and are typically free of solid debris. They form due to pancreatic ductal disruption, either from acute or chronic pancreatitis. They can cause local symptoms of pain, gastric ileus, or gastric outlet obstruction may require percutaneous, endoscopic, transpapillary, or surgical drainage depending on ductal integrity and imaging. The results of endoscopic and surgical drainage are the best and are currently comparable. Superinfection or bleeding usually forces a decision to intervene. In the past, the criteria of pseudocyst persistence for 6 weeks and/or 6-cm diameter necessitated intervention. This is not necessarily required, and continued observation is safe with little risk of infection, bleeding, malignancy, or rupture.

Complications following debridement of necrotizing pancreatitis remain common and include pancreatic or enterocutaneous fistula, wound infection, and wound dehiscence and hernia. Operative approaches to these complications can easily result in failure caused by ongoing inflammation in the retroperitoneum impacting the dissection, and by decreased integrity of tissues resulting in their failure to hold sutures. Fistulae occur in up to 30% of patients undergoing laparotomy, and initially they should be managed conservatively, with surgical repair deferred until such time as the pancreatitis has resolved completely. Bleeding is a rare complication but associated with mortality rates in excess of 50%. Most high volume centers initially manage bleeding complications angiographically. Angiography is 96% sensitive in identifying the source of hemorrhage, and embolization is feasible and successfully controls hemorrhage in approximately 60% of patients. Surgical exploration for management of hemorrhage is reserved for angiographic failure. Wound infection and dehiscence must be treated more aggressively, although resultant hernias are dealt with months after the acute illness. Endocrine and exocrine insufficiencies of the pancreas are also relatively common. Despite the high incidence of morbidity, the long-term quality of life for patients requiring debridement approaches that of patients who have chronic pancreatitis.

Another complication worth mentioning is ductal necrosis, particularly related to midgland pancreatic necrosis. This entity is sometimes referred to as disconnection of the main pancreatic duct. This problem is difficult to diagnose by CT or MRCP and requires ERCP to demonstrate contrast extravasation during pancreatography. The disconnected duct and associated pancreatic fluid collections, pseudocysts, or necrosis are unlikely to resolve with conservative drainage methods. Usually this requires surgery in the form of distal pancreatectomy or median segment pancreaticojejunostomy if the distal gland is thought to have significant pancreatic function.

REFERENCES

1. Bollen TL, van Santvoort HC, Besselink MG, et al. Dutch Acute Pancreatitis Study Group. The Atlanta Classification of acute pancreatitis revisited. *Br J Surg* 2008; 95(1):6–21.
2. Bradley EL 3rd, Dexter ND. Management of severe acute pancreatitis: a surgical odyssey. *Ann Surg* 2010; 251(1):6–17.

3. Dellinger EP, Tellado JM, Soto NE, et al. Early antibiotic treatment for severe acute necrotizing pancreatitis: a randomized, double-blind, placebo-controlled study. *Ann Surg* 2007; 245(5):674–683.
4. Haney JC, Pappas TN. Necrotizing pancreatitis: diagnosis and management. *Surg Clin North Am* 2007; 87(6):1431–1446, ix.
5. Isenmann R, Rünzi M, Kron M, et al. German Antibiotics in Severe Acute Pancreatitis Study Group. Prophylactic antibiotic treatment in patients with predicted severe acute pancreatitis: a placebo-controlled, double-blind trial. *Gastroenterology* 2004; 126(4):997–1004.
6. Mier J, León EL, Castillo A, et al. Early versus late necrosectomy in severe necrotizing pancreatitis. *Am J Surg*. 1997; 173(2):71–75.
7. Nathens AB, Curtis JR, Beale RJ, et al. Management of the critically ill patient with severe acute pancreatitis. *Crit Care Med.* 2004; 32(12):2524–2536.
8. Navaneethan U, Vege SS, Chari ST, Minimally invasive techniques in pancreatic necrosis. *Pancreas* 2009; 38(8):867–875.
9. Sandrasegaran K, Tann M, Jennings SG, Disconnection of the pancreatic duct: an important but overlooked complication of severe acute pancreatitis. *Radiographics* 2007; 27(5):1389–1400.
10. van Santvoort HC, Besselink MG, Bakker OJ, et al. Dutch Pancreatitis Study Group. A step-up approach or open necrosectomy for necrotizing pancreatitis. *N Engl J Med* 2010; 22;362(16):1491–1502.
11. Whitcomb DC. Clinical practice. Acute pancreatitis. *N Engl J Med* 2006; 18; 354(20):2142–2150.

CHRONIC PANCREATITIS 38

Jack Haney* and
Eugene P. Ceppa[†]

INTRODUCTION

Chronic pancreatitis is a condition of irreversible and progressive injury to the pancreas ultimately resulting in diminished exocrine and endocrine function. Clinically, it is characterized by the hallmarks of epigastric pain, malabsorption and diabetes. The incidence of chronic pancreatitis varies, from 10–15 cases/100,000 in western countries to 114–200/100,000 in India. Etiologic factors for the development of chronic pancreatitis vary, but in industrialized nations 70–80% of cases are caused by chronic alcohol consumption, usually after 6–12 years of heavy intake. Other etiologies include chronic pancreatic duct obstruction from gallstones, strictures or anatomic abnormalities including pancreatic divisum. Other causes include hypertryglyceridemia, hypercalcemia, so-called tropical pancreatitis, and autoimmune pancreatitis.[1–5]

PATHOPHYSIOLOGY

Morphologically, chronic pancreatitis is characterized by gland fibrosis, acinar and islet cell destruction and atrophy, and distorted or obstructed ducts. Calcification of the gland and the formation of stones within the

---

*Duke University School of Medicine, Durham, NC 27710 USA
[†]Indiana University School of Medicine, Indianapolis, Indiana, USA

ducts are also characteristic. Current understanding of the pathophysiology rests on a model of progressive injury to pancreatic parenchyma from recurrent escalating episodes of pancreatic necroinflammation.[2] Acute inflammatory attacks are associated with progressive destruction, eventually resulting in irreversible changes including acinar atrophy and gland fibrosis. Pancreatic stellate cells — morphologically similar to hepatic stellate cells, the principle effectors of hepatic fibrosis and cirrhosis — appear to play a critical role in stimulating the synthesis of extracellular matrix proteins and initiating gland fibrosis.[3] These stellate cells may be stimulated directly by chronic ethanol exposure and are activated by inflammatory cytokines during episodes of necroinflammation.

As the leading cause, much of the research in the pathophysiology has focused on the detrimental effects of alcohol. Although not completely understood (Figure 1), acinar cell physiology is altered by chronic exposure of alcohol: destabilization of acinar cytoplasmic granules, premature release of granule contents (trypsinogen, lipase, and amylase), and an increase in degranulated acinar cells from digestive enzyme secretion. All

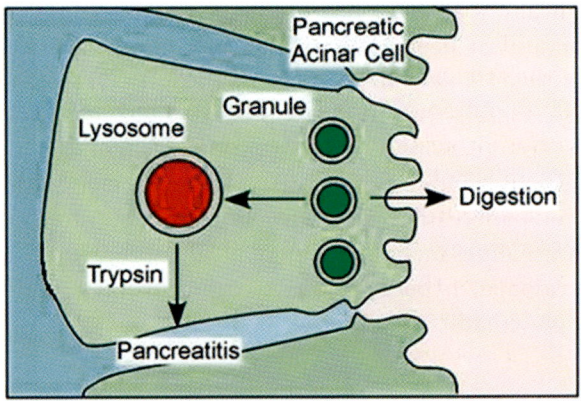

Figure 1. Representation of a pancreatic acinar cell which in physiologic settings releases zymogens stored in granules into pancreatic ducts to undergo activation within the lumen of the duodenum via enterokinase. It is believed that in a pathophysiologic setting, acinar cell granules become destabilized, granule contents are released prematurely and activated by the presence of lysosomal peptidases (cathepsin B). Consequently, activation of various isoforms of trypsins within the pancreatic acinar cell and parenchyma in general is thought to lead to autodigestion.

of these findings are suggestive of autodigestion leading to irreversible pancreatic parenchymal injury.

Furthermore, metabolism of alcohol by acinar cells results in toxic metabolites that produce oxidative stress and cell damage.[2] Alcohol metabolites such as cholesteryl esters and fatty acid ethyl esters increase the fragility of the containing organelles. Alcohol also reduces glycoprotein GP2 content within the zymogen granule membranes, further destabilizing them. This increased fragility of the containing structures significantly increases the likelihood of premature intracellular activation and autodigestive injury. Alcohol intake has been shown to increase acinar mRNA expression for the production of trypsinogen, chymotrypsinogen, lipase and lysosomal cathepsin B. In order to protect against autodigestion, pancreatic enzymes are produced by acinar cells in the form of zymogens or inactive precursor enzymes. They are secreted in membrane-bound organelles and activated after secretion by the cleavage of the serine protease trypsinogen to active trypsin, by lysosomal cathepsin B or by the duodenal enzyme enteropeptidase. Once activated, trypsin activates additional proteolytic enzymes. Trypsin also possesses autocatalytic activity, so cleavage of only a small amount of trypsinogen will stimulate an accelerating catalytic activation of enzymes. Acinar cell granules also possess intracellular serine–protease inhibitor to counterbalance intragranular trypsin activity to protect against acinar cell autodigestion. Various trypsin isoforms exist by way of slight genetic alterations or splice variants which confers an endogenous resistance to serine protease inhibitors; these isoforms are thought to be upregulated in settings of pancreatitis and may be the principal culprits in the parenchymal autodigestion associated with pancreatitis in both an acute and chronic setting. Acinar cells metabolize alcohol by oxidative and non-oxidative pathways. However, primary acinar cell metabolism of alcohol occurs as a result of increased intracellular oxidant stress. Alcohol oxidation increases generation of reactive oxygen species and decreases antioxidant defenses, raising the level of oxidant stress within the cell. 4-Hydroxynonenol (aldehydes) and palmitoleic acid (fatty acid ethyl esters) are examples of generated reactive metabolites that directly cause acinar cell injury, possibly by increasing levels of the transcription factor NF-κB, leading to increased inflammatory cytokine expression.[4]

The cumulative result of chronic alcohol exposure is an increase in proteolytic enzyme production in the setting of a weakened containment structure, significantly tipping the balance towards the risk of autoactivation and autodigestive damage.

A second mechanism inducing the changes of chronic pancreatitis is that of pancreatic duct obstruction. Obstruction of the pancreatic outflow results in duct hypertension and ultimately autoactivation of digestive enzymes at the acinar level and is the mechanism for gallstone pancreatitis. Repeated or chronic duct obstruction ultimately leads to escalating episodes of necroinflammation and chronic pancreatitis. This may be a result of repeated transient obstruction from biliary stones, or from chronic scarring and stricture formation as a result of repeated duct trauma and inflammation. It may also result from chronic obstruction secondary to an obstructing pancreatic or duodenal mass. Congenital outflow obstruction, notably from pancreatic divisum, also leads to risk of chronic pancreatitis. In pancreatic divisum, the dorsal and ventral pancreatic ducts fail to fuse properly, resulting in 70% of pancreatic parenchyma draining through the dorsal duct and minor papilla. While this congenital abnormality has been found in up to 7% of patients in autopsy studies, the majority of patients will remain asymptomatic. A minority will suffer from repeated attacks of pancreatitis, putting them at risk for developing chronic pancreatitis.

Tropical pancreatitis refers to an observed subtype described within India, sub-Saharan Africa and the Caribbean, predominantly affecting patients under the age of 25 and characterized radiographically by abundant ductal calcifications and clinically by a very high incidence of endocrine and exocrine insufficiency. Suggested etiologic factors include malnutrition, dietary intake of cyanogenic glycosides, viral or parasitic infections, or increased oxidative stress burden secondary to low intake of antioxidants.[4] A definitive mechanism has yet to be determined.

Autoimmune pancreatitis is a rare condition characterized pathologically by lymphocytic infiltrates and pancreatic fibrosis in the absence of gland calcifications, elevated IgG4 and the presence of autoantibodies including anti-carbonic anhydrase, anti-lactoferrin, antinuclear antibodies, and rheumatoid factor.[4] The condition is rare and the IgG4 antibodies may be responsible for other sclerosing manifestations within the retroperitoneum, biliary tree or kidneys. As with most autoimmune disorders, autoimmune pancreatitis does appear to respond to steroid therapy.

GENETICS

A minority of chronic alcohol consumers develop chronic pancreatitis, leading researchers to investigate other environmental or genetic susceptibility triggers. Tobacco use has been identified as a major risk factor, reducing trypsin inhibitory capacity and enhancing autoactivation. Research into the genetic mechanisms underlying susceptibility to chronic pancreatitis has identified several predisposing risk factors. Loss-of-function mutations within the serine–protease inhibitor, kazal type I (SPINK1) — a pancreatic trypsin inhibitor which protects against intrapancreatic activation — have been linked to increased sensitivity, identified in 5.8% of alcoholic patients with chronic pancreatitis, compared to 0.8% in alcoholics without chronic pancreatitis and 1% of controls.[3] Mutations in cationic trypsinogen, referred to as serine–protease 1 (PRSS1) have been shown to convey gain-of-function increases in proteolytic activity and linked with increased risk of chronic pancreatitis. Conversely, protective mutations within anionic trypsinogen PRSS2 have been found less commonly in patients with alcoholic pancreatitis (0.8% vs. 3.4%).

CLINICAL MANIFESTATIONS

Clinically, chronic pancreatitis is characterized by abdominal pain and heralded by exocrine and endocrine insufficiency ("pancreatic burnout"). The pain in chronic pancreatitis is classically epigastric, radiating to the back. It may be episodic (type A) or continuous (type B). Abdominal pain may be confounded by recurrent attacks of acute pancreatitis, pancreatic pseudocysts, portal or splenic vein thrombosis, biliary obstruction, or gastric or duodenal ulceration. While the precise mechanisms mediating the chronic pain are unknown, several mechanisms have been explored. Chronic pancreatitis appears to be associated with the concept of nociception. Pancreatic sensory neurons perceive a pain-inducing stimulus which is relayed centrally to the dorsal root ganglia (DRG) and this is defined as nociception; the DRG sends signals further centrally but a reflex arc exists, stimulating various neurons at the level of the viscera and this is defined as pain. In the setting of chronic pancreatitis, there is an increased number and size of intrapancreatic sensory nerves.[6] Duct obstruction and hypertension appears to play a role. Transient receptor potential (TRP) channels are calcium ion channels located on the proximal sensory neurons that when activated by certain stimuli, propagate an action potential towards the DRG. An entire family of TRP channels exists with similar cellular structure and intracellular pathways, yet distinct agonists; these TRP channels within the pancreas have been shown to respond to changes in high temperatures, low pH, capsaicin (V1) (Figure 2), osmotic pressure (V4), and cold temperatures and reactive oxygen species like hydroxynonenal (A1).

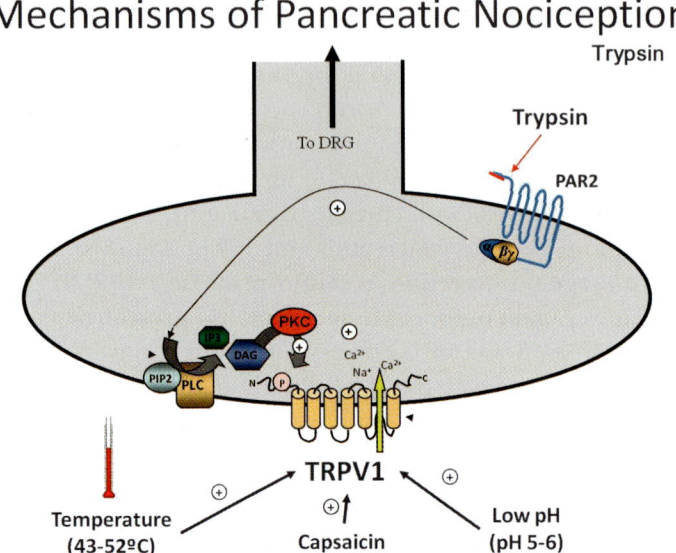

Figure 2. This schematic serves as an example of the role of TRP channels on sensory neurons. In this case, the relationship of TRPV1 and PAR2 on the pancreatic sensory neuron is depicted. When noxious stimuli such as high temperatures, capsaicin, and low pHs are present, TRPV1 allows entry of extracellular calcium to induce an action potential towards the dorsal root ganglion in the central nervous system (CNS). Nociception occurs when "pain" sensory neurons are activated sending a signal to the CNS, while pain sensation is the reciprocating signal back towards the viscera. Trypsin cleaves the extracellular domain of PAR2 which is present on sensory neurons initiating an intracellular cascade that ultimately sensitizes TRPV1 to lower its threshold for activation. Thus, in the setting of pancreatitis with an abundance of trypsin within the pancreatic parenchyma, the noxious stimuli in order to stimulate TRPV1 on nociceptive neurons are lowered leading to more sensation of pain.

Experimental evidence has shown reproduction of pain with injections to increase duct pressures by greater than 25 mm H_2O. Conversely, dropping duct pressures by at least 10 mm H_2O improves clinical pain, resulting in enthusiasm for surgical drainage procedures, especially in the setting of a dilated and obviously obstructed duct. Futhermore, trypsins and other proinflammatory mediators[7] appear to sensitize TRP channels in lowering the threshold required to activate these channels. Autoactivation of pancreatic exocrine enzymes also appears to mediate pain, as trypsin has been shown to cause pain by activating protease-activated receptor 2 (PAR 2) in various animal models including rats and mice. Ultimately, the pain of chronic pancreatitis often dissipates coincident with pancreatic burnout and the onset of exocrine and endocrine insufficiency, again supporting a role for exocrine secretions mediating the symptoms.

Endocrine and exocrine insufficiency generally occurs with the loss of 90% of responsible pancreatic tissue. Lipase secretion decreases more rapidly than protease or amylase secretion, resulting in the onset of steatorrhea and fat malabsorption. Fat malabsorption also results in deficiencies in the fat-soluble vitamins A, D, E, and K. Diabetes, classified as Type IIIc, is characterized by the destruction of both insulin- and glucagon-producing islet cells, resulting in a fragile diabetic state where the loss of glucagon aggravates hypoglycemic episodes. Ultimately the combination of fat malabsorption and diabetes results in the malnutrition and weight loss that characterize the disease. Duct obstruction and inflammation may result in leaks and pseudocyst formation in as many as 25% of patients. These pseudocysts are associated with pain as they expand and in 5–10% of cases can cause duodenal or biliary obstruction by mass effect, necessitating surgical or endoscopic drainage.

DIAGNOSIS

The diagnosis of chronic pancreatitis rests primarily on the presence of the classic clinical symptoms in the setting of an appropriate history of recurrent acute pancreatitis in patients of any age group. Rarely will patients present without a history of prior acute attacks, in which case a history of appropriate risk factors should be elucidated. Patients with chronic pancreatitis may have slightly elevated or normal serum levels of amylase and lipase, reflecting the chronicity of the condition and pancreatic parenchymal burnout. Confounding and reversible sources of epigastric pain should be ruled out, including acute pancreatitis, gastric or duodenal ulceration, and biliary colic or cholecystitis.

Although rarely performed by clinicians, qualitative and quantitative serologic tests exist to measure pancreatic exocrine function. The "gold standard" secretin-stimulation test is rarely performed as it requires invasive measurement of stimulated pancreatic secretions from the duodenum.[1] Alternative metrics include measuring fecal elastase or serum trypsinogen, with deficiencies of each indicative of exocrine insufficiency.

Steatorrhea, may be documented by either elevated acid steatocrit on a random stool sample or defined by >6g of fecal fat excretion per day repeated over a 3-day test.

Diagnostic imaging of the pancreas is the primary method of confirming clinical suspicion of chronic pancreatitis. Review of cross sectional imaging focuses not only to confirm the diagnosis by identifying calcifications, parenchymal fibrosis and ductal strictures, but also findings that would alter operative planning by evaluating associated sequelae such as pseudocysts or atrophy and arterial anatomy to define extent of disease. Both computed tomography (CT) (Figures 3a, 3b) and magnetic resonance imaging (MRI) yield high-quality images of pancreatic parenchyma. MRI with additional MRCP images (Figure 4) provides pancreatic duct assessment without the risk of stimulating acute pancreatitis.[1] Alternatively, both endoscopic ultrasound (EUS) and endoscopic retrograde cholangiopancreatography (ERCP) are valuable especially in cases of diagnostic uncertainty providing an opportunity for tissue diagnosis and therapeutic intervention. EUS provides excellent resolution of both parenchymal changes and ductal anatomy with low risk of complications, and established EUS criteria for the diagnosis are well-published.[9] ERCP provides the highest-quality evaluation of pancreatic ductal anatomy and offers the

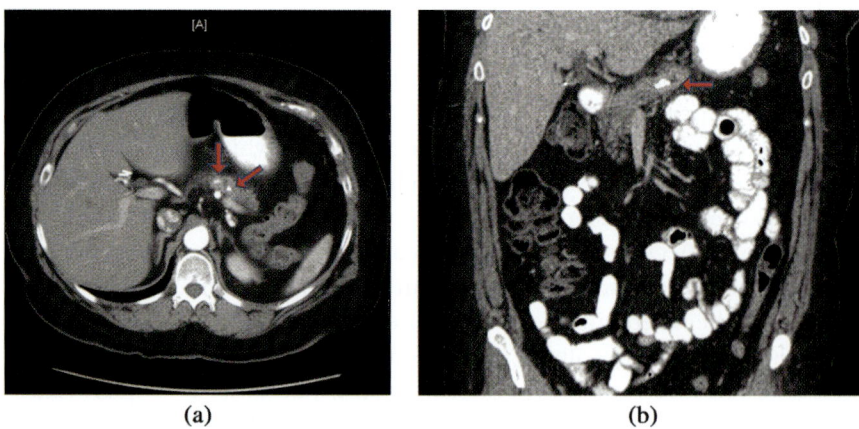

Figure 3. (a) CT axial image representative of chronic pancreatitis with two distal pancreatic duct stones (red arrows) and slightly dilated pancreatic duct in between. (b) CT coronal reconstruction image representative of chronic pancreatitis with a large pancreatic duct stone (red arrow).

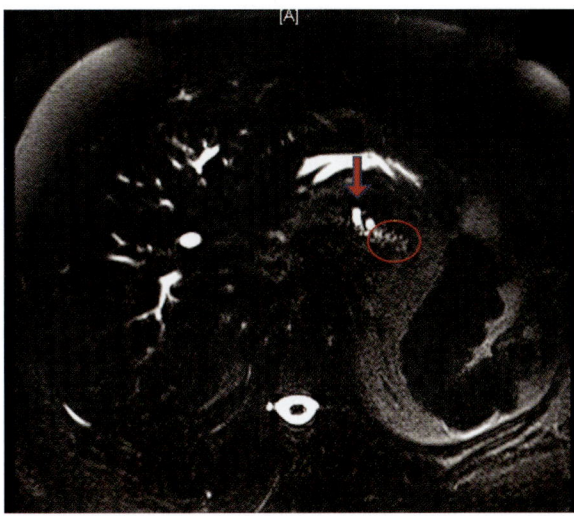

Figure 4. MRCP axial image representative of chronic pancreatitis with pancreatic duct stones (red arrow) and pancreatic parenchymal calcifications (red oval).

opportunity for intervention, but does carry a 10% risk of postprocedural pancreatitis. Ultimately, the diagnosis is usually made by the combination of appropriate clinical symptoms, history, and radiographic confirmation of pancreatic damage.

MANAGEMENT

Management principles for chronic pancreatitis center on pain control, avoidance of further pancreatic damage, replacement of pancreatic function, and nutritional support. Once the diagnosis is made, reversible triggers need to be ruled out. Pain control frequently requires significant narcotic analgesia, but importantly includes abstinence from alcohol and tobacco. Avoidance of alcohol has been clearly shown to improve pain control.[1-3] Tobacco smoking has been shown to have an additive effect to alcohol, not only in increasing the risk of developing chronic pancreatitis, but also in developing associated pancreatic neoplasia. Tobacco is also independently associated with much of the increased mortality of this group, thus its cessation should likewise be emphasized. Reducing pancreatic exocrine stimulation with exogenous enzymes has also been shown to improve pain control.[5] Exocrine secretion is stimulated by cholecystokinin

(CCK)-releasing peptide in the duodenum, which is itself degraded by pancreatic serine proteases. In the absence of sufficient protease activity, increased CCK stimulation worsens pain. Replacement of protease activity via exogenous enzymes has been shown to improve pain symptoms. Non-enteric–coated enzymes are more effective at reducing pain but are susceptible to gastric acid, thus require additional treatment with acid suppression therapy. Acid suppression also raises duodenal pH and lessens stimulation for exocrine secretion. Pain control may also improve with surgical management including resection of the chronically inflamed parenchyma or decompression of an obstructed pancreatic duct. Chapter 50 discusses the role of surgery in the management of chronic pancreatitis.

In addition to pain control, management of chronic pancreatitis includes the treatment of pancreatic insufficiency. Management of exocrine dysfunction includes both the adoption of a low-fat diet and the replacement of exocrine enzymes, typically 25,000–50,000 units of lipase per meal, but frequently titrated higher for effect. Patients specifically require education about the maintenance of a truly low-fat intake as the sources of hidden fats in our heavily processed diets are ubiquitous. Dietary modifications include the supplementation of fat-soluble enzymes A, D, E, and K. Patients with chronic pancreatitis frequently present with significant weight loss from a combination of pain-induced food fear and malabsorption. This often requires aggressive nutritional supplementation, potentially from postpancreatic feeds if pancreatic stimulation still produces significant pain. Patients who experience endocrine insufficiency require insulin supplementation for their diabetes. The goal of management should not be for strict and narrow blood glucose control, as the insufficiency induces a brittle state in which glucagon insufficiency confers an acute clinical risk of hypoglycemia.

OUTCOMES

While the course of chronic pancreatitis is unpredictable, the natural history is nevertheless of lessening or resolving pain over a period of years. At 10 years following the onset of symptoms, approximately half of the patients will still have some episodes of pain, while at 15 years one-quarter still have pain, and 75% of these patients experience less than one episode per year.[10] By 20 years, nearly all patients have had resolution of their pain which highlights the evolution of the disease process by coinciding with pancreatic burnoutheralding the onset of more advanced medical problems.

The 10 year mortality rate for patients with chronic pancreatitis is 30%, and at 20-years the mortality rate is 55%. Based on the average age of onset, this represents a three-to fourfold increase in mortality and implies a 10–20-year loss of life expectancy.[10] Prognostic factors include age at diagnosis, tobacco smoking, continued use of alcohol and the presence of concomitant liver cirrhosis. Population studies have found that nearly one-quarter of patients with chronic pancreatitis will develop a neoplasm at 20 years following diagnosis, but only 4% of these will be of pancreatic origin, again confirming the independent risks of the associated activities, in particular chronic alcohol and tobacco consumption. The risk of developing pancreatic cancer is in general 2% per decade.

CONCLUSION

In summary, chronic pancreatitis is the consequence of repeated, escalating episodes of pancreatic inflammation, characterized by the scarring and fibrosis of the pancreatic parenchyma. This produces a clinical syndrome of recurrent epigastric pain and may progress to malabsorption and weight loss as a consequence of pancreatic exocrine insufficiency and manifestations of poor blood glucose control from endocrine insufficiency. In the western world, the leading cause is chronic alcohol consumption, but additional etiologies include those resulting in chronic obstruction of the pancreatic duct. The hallmarks of management are behavioral and diet modification, particularly the abstinence from alcohol or tobacco and low fat diets, in addition to pain control, exocrine and endocrine replacement, and nutritional support. The natural history is one of gradually improving pain, but the condition conveys a significant increase in long-term morbidity and mortality.

REFERENCES

1. Braganza JM, Lee SH, McCloy RF, et al. Chronic pancreatitis. *Lancet* 2011; 377(9772):1184–1197.
2. Witt H, Apte MV, Keim V, et al. Chronic pancreatitis: challenges and advances in pathogenesis, genetics, diagnosis, and therapy. *Gastroenterology* 2007; 132(4):1557–1573.

3. Tattersall SJ, Apte MV, Wilson JS. A fire inside: current concepts in chronic pancreatitis. *Intern Med J* 2008; 38(7):592–598.
4. Vonlaufen A, Wilson JS, Apte MV. Molecular mechanisms of pancreatitits: current opinion. *J Gastroenterol Hepatol* 2008; 23(9):1339–1348.
5. Gupta V, Toskes PP. Diagnosis and management of chronic pancreatitis. *Postgrad Med J* 2005; 81:491–497.
6. Demir IE, Tieftrunk E, Maak M, *et al.* Pain mechanisms in chronic pancreatitis: of a master and his fire. *Langenbecks Arch Surg* 2011; 396(2):151–160.
7. Ceppa E, Cattaruzza F, Lyo V, *et al.* Transient receptor potential ion channels V4 and A1 contribute to pancreatitis pain in mice. *Am J Physiol Gastrointest Liver Physiol* 2010; 299(3):G556–571.
8. Ceppa EP, Lyo V, Grady EF, *et al.* Serine proteases mediate inflammatory pain in acute pancreatitis. *Am J Physiol Gastrointest Liver Physiol* 2011; 300(6):G1033–1042.
9. Gourgiotis S, Germanos S, Ridolfini MP. Surgical management of chronic pancreatitis. *Hepatobiliary Pancreat Dis Int* 2007; 6(2):121–133.
10. Talamini G, Bassi C, Butturini G, *et al.* Outcome and quality of life in chronic pancreatitis. *JOP* 2001; 2(4):117–123.

CYSTIC NEOPLASMS OF THE PANCREAS   39

Eugene P. Ceppa* and
Douglas S. Tyler†

INTRODUCTION

Management of primary cystic neoplasms of the pancreas remains controversial. This underscores the heterogeneity of pancreatic cystic lesions and the diversity of opinions of experienced surgeons. In 1978, Compagno and Oertel made the first distinction between serous and mucinous cystic neoplasms of the pancreas.[1,2] Since that time, a great interest in further classifying these cystic lesions both histologically and clinically has ensued. Cystic lesions of the pancreas can be categorized as benign, inflammatory, or malignant. The various forms of primary cystic neoplasms are distinct by way of presentation, appearance on diagnostic imaging, histology, and overall prognosis. The importance of further investigation of cystic lesions of the pancreas has increased over time as these lesions are recognized more frequently in symptomatic and asymptomatic patients due to the increased use of cross-sectional imaging. This chapter will review in detail primary cystic neoplasms of the pancreas, the suggested management, and the most current debates ongoing in the literature.

---

*Indiana University School of Medicine, Indiana polis, Indiana, USA
†Duke University Medical Center, Durham, NC 27710 USA

Epidemiology

Pancreatic cysts comprise 15% of all pancreatic tumors. These cysts are predominantly pseudocysts (60%) as well as simple cysts, primary cystic neoplasms and solid tumors with cystic degeneration (Table 1). Ten to twenty percent of cysts are primary cystic neoplasms of the pancreas; adenocarcinoma is eventually diagnosed in 1–5% of all cysts. Pancreatic cancer is the fourth leading cause of death from cancer in both sexes combined. Although the ratio of mortality to incidence in pancreatic adenocarcinoma

Table 1. Pancreatic cystic lesions.

Histologic appearance	Pancreatic cyst type
1. No epithelial lining	Pancreatic pseudocyst
2. Epithelial lining	Serous cystadenoma
	Intraductal papillary mucinous neoplasm
	Mucinous cystic neoplasm
	Mucocele
	Von Hippel Lindau pancreatic cysts
3. Degenerative changes	Solid pseudopapillary neoplasm
	Cystic ductal adenocarcinoma
	Cystic neuroendocrine tumors (islet cell)
	Cystic mesenchymal neoplasm
	Metastases
4. Squamous lining	Lymphoepithelial cysts
	Epidermoid cysts
	Dermoid cysts
	Squamoid cysts of pancreatic duct
5. Acinar cell lining	Acinar cell adenoma
	Acinar cell adenocarcinoma
6. Endothelial lining	Lymphangioma
7. Rare cyst forms	Cystic hamartoma
	Duplication cyst
	Endometriotic cyst
	Congenital cysts
	(Cystic fibrosis, polycystic kidney disease)

is 98%, cystic neoplasms have a much better prognosis highlighting the importance of distinguishing cystic lesions from solid lesions.

There is no formal classification of cystic lesions of the pancreas. Cystic lesions have been categorized in the past based on gross histologic appearance as unilocular, multilocular (microcystic vs. macrocystic), and cystic with solid component. Unilocular cysts consist of primarily pseudocysts and simple cysts. Multilocular microcystic lesions consist of only serous cystadenoma; meanwhile multilocular macrocystic lesions include intraductal papillary mucinous neoplasm, mucinous cystic neoplasm, and acinar cell cystadenonoma. Cystic lesions with solid components can include macrocystic neoplasms as well as solid pseudopapillary neoplasm, pancreatic neuroendocrine tumors, ductal pancreatic adenocarcinoma, cystic teratoma, and metastases. However, this method is inconsistent in that neoplasms can fall into more than one category. More simply, pancreatic cysts can be differentiated pathologically into pseudocysts, primary cystic neoplasms, and retention cysts. The focus of this chapter will be on pancreatic pseudocysts and the most common primary cystic neoplasms of the pancreas.

Pancreatic pseudocysts develop as a result of pancreatic inflammation and necrosis. Pseudocysts are found within or outside of the pancreas and lack an epithelial lining which distinguishes them from primary cystic neoplasms. The behavior of the distinct forms of primary cystic neoplasms ranges widely, thus each has several distinguishing features. The primary cystic neoplasms include serous cystadenoma (SCA), mucinous cystic neoplasms (MCNs) and intraductal papillary mucinous neoplasms (IPMNs). The distinction of SCA — which have extremely low malignant potential — from MCN or IPMN — which have a definite malignant potential — is paramount.

DIAGNOSTIC EVALUATION

Clinical Presentation

Cystic lesions of the pancreas are typically asymptomatic frequently identified by cross-sectional imaging for other reasons. However, some patients become symptomatic when the mass effect of the neoplasm applies pressure to adjacent organs. The most common presenting symptoms include vague abdominal pain associated with early satiety. Pancreatitis (pancreatic duct obstruction) is commonly seen as well. Additionally, symptoms consistent with biliary duct obstruction (jaundice) and other symptoms such as back pain, weight loss, anorexia, and steatorrhea are less frequent. These more rare symptoms are more suggestive of a pancreatic cyst adenocarcinoma.

Diagnostic Imaging

Currently, radiographic imaging is a critical component of diagnosis of cystic lesions of the pancreas; in certain cases, they possess characteristic features sufficient to classify them as pancreatic pseudocyst, SCA, or mucinous neoplasm. However, adjuncts to cross-sectional imaging, such as endoscopic retrograde cholangiopancreatography (ERCP), endoscopic ultrasound (EUS) with cyst fluid analysis by way of fine needle aspiration (FNA) and, more recently, positron emission tomography (PET), are frequently employed to more accurately characterize these lesions with respect to subtype and risk of malignancy. The study of choice is a contrast-enhanced triphasic multidetector computed tomography (CT), while EUS serves as the primary adjunct for further cyst classification.

Computed Tomography

The primary aims of contrast-enhanced dynamic thin-section CT are to diagnose and/or stage pancreatic cystic lesions. Abdominal CT is frequently indicated in the workup of patients with abdominal pain, nausea, vomiting, or weight loss. Patients with obstructive jaundice, as suggested by history, laboratory evaluation, or biliary ductal dilatation, may also be initially evaluated with ERCP. However, in patients in whom malignancy is suspected, cross-sectional imaging should ideally precede biliary stenting, as this may obscure subtle findings. If any imaging study suggests a pancreatic lesion (cyst or mass), dynamic, thin-section, contrast-enhanced CT is indicated to detect hepatic or peritoneal metastases and to define the extent of the lesion with respect to the celiac axis, superior mesenteric artery, and superior mesenteric vein/portal vein confluence. Contraindications include allergy to iodinated intravenous contrast and renal insufficiency are relative contraindications to CT, because contrast enhancement is needed to distinguish the pancreatic mass from the adjacent normal parenchyma. Dynamic gadolinium-enhanced magnetic resonance imaging is a good alternative study in patients with this allergy.

The technique consists of intravenous contrast-enhanced dynamic CT with 3-mm sections done in two phases: pancreatic and portal venous. Pancreatic images are acquired about 40 seconds after injection of contrast (at 5 mL/s), and portal venous phase images of the liver are acquired about 60 seconds after intravenous contrast is given. Axial images of cystic lesions found within the pancreas are examined for size and density and are described by location, unilocular versus multilocular, and the presence of septations.

Computed tomography is the preferred and primary method of diagnosis of cystic lesions of the pancreas. However, the estimated accuracy of CT for the diagnosis of malignant transformation of cystic lesions is quite poor. Findings of malignancy include the presence of a solid mass, diffuse involvement of the gland, and dilatation of the main pancreatic duct more than 10 mm. If malignancy is suspected, an assessment is made regarding involvement of the celiac axis, superior mesenteric artery, superior mesenteric vein/portal vein confluence, regional lymph nodes, and extrapancreatic spread of disease. Assessment of vascular involvement includes the presence or absence of normal pancreas or a fat plane between the tumor and major regional vessels, the extent and convexity of the interface between the tumor to the superior mesenteric/portal venous (SMV/PV) confluence, and thrombosis or occlusion of adjacent vessels.

Endoscopic Retrograde Cholangiopancreatography

Endoscopic retrograde cholangiopancreatography (ERCP) is used to image the biliary and pancreatic ductal system. In patients with biliary or pancreatic ductal abnormalities on either ultrasound or cross-sectional imaging, ERCP can be used to define the anatomy of the problem and to obtain ductal brushings, biopsy samples, or fluid aspirates for diagnosis. ERCP is unnecessary, however, in all patients who have a diagnosis of a pancreatic cystic lesion. In patients with recurrent pancreatitis, mucinous features and a dilated pancreatic duct by CT, ERCP can be both diagnostic and therapeutic for IPMNs. Contraindications previously included patients with altered anatomy due to previous foregut surgery that limited access to the duodenum, although more recently, spiral enteroscopy has now made these patients candidates for ERCP.

A side-viewing endoscope is advanced to the second portion of the duodenum leading to cannulation of the papilla of Vater. Contrast is administered, and fluoroscopic images are obtained to define the biliary and pancreatic ductal anatomy. Ductal brushings, bile, and pancreatic juice may be obtained for cytologic analysis to optimize the yield of malignant cells. Transampullary retrograde pancreatic duct stenting is generally performed endoscopically using temporary plastic stents to diminish the associated risk of postprocedural pancreatitis.

Factors that are predictive of a malignant process include stricture location in the head or neck, jaundice, and patient age, while factors that predict a nonmalignant process include history of pancreatitis, presence of multiple strictures, pancreatic duct stones, pseudocyst, pancreatic divisum, irregular side branches, and irregular pancreatic duct morphology. In patients with malignant biliary or pancreatic ductal strictures, the yield of endoscopic brushings has been estimated to be as high as 70%. For diagnostic imaging, magnetic resonance cholangiopancreatography (MRCP) may represent a non-invasive alternative to ERCP. Therapeutic ERCP decompresses the malignant obstruction in more than 95% of cases. However, complications can occur in up to 15% of patients following ERCP including pancreatitis (5%), cholangitis (4%), cardiopulmonary complications (2%), hemorrhage (1%), and perforation (1%).

Endoscopic Ultrasonography

Computed tompography and EUS have become useful complementary techniques in the diagnosis of pancreatic cystic lesions. CT and MRI are limited in detection of pancreatic lesions smaller than 2 cm, but EUS is more reliable capable of detecting lesions as small as 5 mm and provides an opportunity for FNA and cyst fluid analysis. EUS is less reliable in the detection of regional lymph node metastasis and vascular involvement. Potential complications of EUS include viscous perforation, bleeding, and, rarely, acute pancreatitis.

A high-frequency ultrasound probe is introduced through a side-viewing endoscope that is advanced into the duodenum. Pancreatic cystic lesions collectively possess a heterogeneous group of findings by EUS. Some lesions may be simple unilocular cysts and others complex multilocular cysts. The sensitivity of EUS for the detection of pancreatic cystic neoplasms exceeds 90%. Yet, distinguishing benign from malignant cysts is poor by imaging features only. Also, it is unreliable for assessment of liver, peritoneal or transverse mesocolon involvement. The addition of FNA biopsy to EUS has substantially improved the poor specificity. The addition of FNA adds a 3% risk of pancreatitis to the procedure. EUS with FNA biopsy is a safe and accurate method of tissue diagnosis.

F-18 Fluorodeoxyglucose Whole Body Positron Emission Tomography

F-18 fluorodeoxyglucose positron emission tomography (PET) is performed to identify both the primary lesion and potential metastatic deposits through the detection of sites of increased glucose uptake. The role of PET in the management of pancreatic cystic lesions is undetermined. False-positive results may occur in the setting of pancreatitis, and PET scanning does not provide accurate information on the relationship of the lesion to the adjacent vascular structures. Therefore, the information provided by PET in addition to CT rarely changes the clinical management of patients with suspected or recently diagnosed pancreatic cystic lesions. For patients who have undergone resection of pancreatic neoplasms, PET may be useful for detecting local, regional and extra-abdominal recurrence, where CT findings are often nonspecific. Contraindications include hyperglycemia and active inflammatory processes which may contribute to false-negative and false-positive results, respectively, on PET.

PATHOLOGY

A true cyst defined by a cavity lined by a layer of epithelium in this case includes the multilocular cysts as well as simple unilocular cysts. Pseudocysts have no true epithelial lining and consequently compose the majority of the grossly unilocular cysts. The various forms of cystic neoplasms of the pancreas have features in terms of presentation, diagnostic imaging, and cyst fluid analysis that distinguish one from another.

Pancreatic Pseudocysts

Pancreatic pseudocysts account for approximately 60% of all pancreatic cystic lesions. Pseudocysts are fluid-filled cavities with no epithelial lining that typically develops following a bout of pancreatitis (secondary to alcohol or gallstones). The pathogenesis of pseudocyst formation is the inflammation and necrosis of pancreatitis leading to disruption of the pancreatic duct and parencyhma. This results in pancreatic enzymes leaking outside of the gland and solubilizing peripancreatic fat. The space where this acute pancreatic fluid collection forms is commonly in the lesser sac. The walls of pseudocysts consist of surrounding organs (greater omentum, pancreas, stomach and transverse mesocolon). In addition, the wall contains fibrous and granulation tissue. The fluid collection consists of necrotic cells, hemolyzed blood, pancreatic enzymes, and neutrophils that over time produce granulation tissue resulting in the development of a fibrotic pseudocapsule.

There are numerous reports of primary cystic neoplasms being confused for pancreatic pseudocysts. This highlights the importance of history as well diagnostic imaging in the diagnosis of cystic lesions of the pancreas. Although pseudocysts can take on many forms and be associated with any part of the pancreas, pseudocysts are typically identified by CT alone (Figure 1). In cases in which diagnostic imaging is not able to distinguish between cystic neoplasms and pseudocysts, cyst fluid analysis by way of EUS with FNA is thought to be the best option (Table 2). EUS shows a cyst with a thick wall and intra-cystic floating debris. A pseudocyst is suspected in patients with a cyst that contains enzyme-rich fluid or demonstrates continuity with the pancreatic duct by ERCP in the setting of recent pancreatitis and an elevated amylase concentration (Figure 2). Malignant degeneration

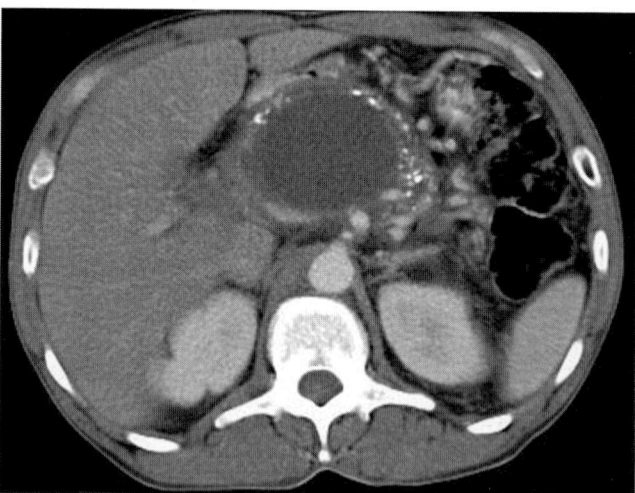

Figure 1. Computed tomography of pancreatic pseudocyst. Characteristic extra-pancreatic extension of pseudocyst is seen on the cyst lesion.

Table 2. Cyst fluid analysis of pancreatic cystic lesions.

Cyst type	Cytology	Viscosity	Cyst fluid CEA (ng/ml)	Cyst fluid amylase
Pseudocyst	Histiocytes	Low	<200	High
Serous	Glycogen	Low	<0.5	Low
Mucinous	Mucinous	High	>200	Low
IPMN	Mucinous	High	>200	High

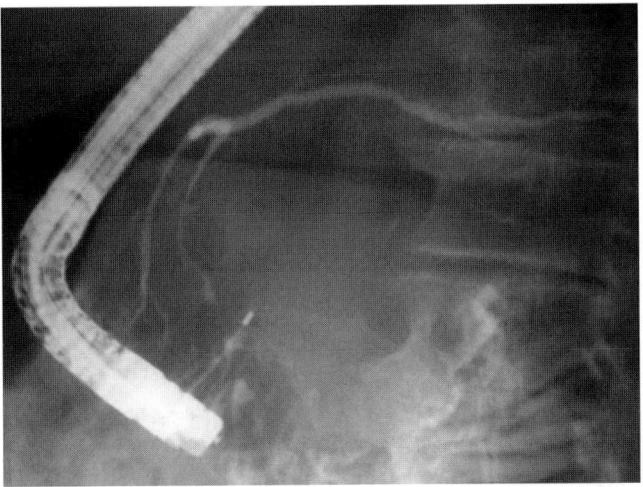

Figure 2. Pancreatogram in the setting of pancreatic pseudocyst. The image demonstrates a space occupying lesion that alters the orientation of the pancreatic duct.

of pancreatic pseudocysts has not been reported in the literature. Nevertheless, biopsy of the pseudocyst wall is important to confirm the diagnosis and prevent mistaking a pseudocyst for a MCN.

The treatment of pseudocysts is predicated on the presence of symptoms and size. Asymptomatic lesions are more common and are observed since most acute pseudocysts will resolve spontaneously. Pseudocysts that are less than 4 cm or located within the pancreatic parencyhma are more likely to resolve without intervention. To guide management of asymptomatic pseudocysts larger than 4 cm, many surgeons follow the patient expectantly for 6 weeks following diagnosis before considering intervention for pseudocysts. Chronic pseudocysts larger than 4 cm persisting for longer than 6 weeks rarely resolve thus necessitating an intervention. Furthermore, the treatment of chronic pseudocysts greater than 4 cm has been found to decrease long-term complications such as biliary obstruction, hemorrhage, infection, or rupture as a result of untreated lesions. Thus, pseudocysts that are symptomatic or increasing in size or persistently greater than 4 cm are treated primarily with drainage (endoscopic vs. external vs. internal), although resection via distal pancreatectomy for distal lesions is an alternative. Internal drainage procedures are favored over external drainage due to a high rate of persistent pancreaticocutaneous fistulas with external drainage. Internal drainage procedures include cystduodenostomy, cystgastrostomy, or cystjejunostomy; choosing among the different procedures relies on cyst location and surgeon preference. The outcomes for open internal drainage procedures includes a reported mortality less than 3%, morbidity of 25%, and up to 90% have resolution of their pseudocyst without recurrence. Reports of laparoscopic drainage procedures cite similar outcomes except for a lower rate of morbidity. Open drainage and laparoscopic drainage have shown a higher primary success rate (81%, 88%) as compared to endoscopic drainage (51%).[3] However, endoscopic drainage has been shown to have a lower complication rate (16%) and comparable overall success rate by accounting for re-intervention (85%).

Serous Cystadenoma

Serous cystadenomas (SCA), also known as serous cystic neoplasms, microcystic cystadenomas, and glycogen-rich cystadenomas, is generally a benign cystic tumor with only eight reported cases of malignancy (serous cystadenocarcinomas) in the literature.[4] These tumors have a predilection for women (F:M = 2:1) and commonly found in patients with a mean age of 60 (Table 3). Some complain of vague symptoms of abdominal pain and nausea. Symptomatic cysts are commonly larger than 6 cm in size and can be larger than 20 cm in some instances at the time of diagnosis. Yet, many patients have no symptoms and are incidentally found on cross-sectional imaging studies for other indications.

Diagnosis is primarily made by CT which reveals a low-density mass with multiple small cysts divided by septae; a central stellate calcification in a sunburst pattern is identified in 30% of cases (Figure 3). They are found predominantly in the head or body of the pancreas and are typically not involved with the pancreatic duct. MRI shows similar features as CT but

Table 3.

Cyst type	Cyst location	Age (decade)	Gender (M:F)	Pancreatic duct communication	Distinctive feature
Pseudocyst	Body/Tail	3rd–4th	3:1	Yes	Recent pancreatitis
Serous	Head/Body	6th	1:2	No	Central stellate calcification (CT)
Mucinous	Body/Tail	4th–5th	1:8	No	Ovarian stroma (Pathology)
IPMN	Head	6th–7th	1-1.5:1	Yes	Mucin in ampulla (ERCP)

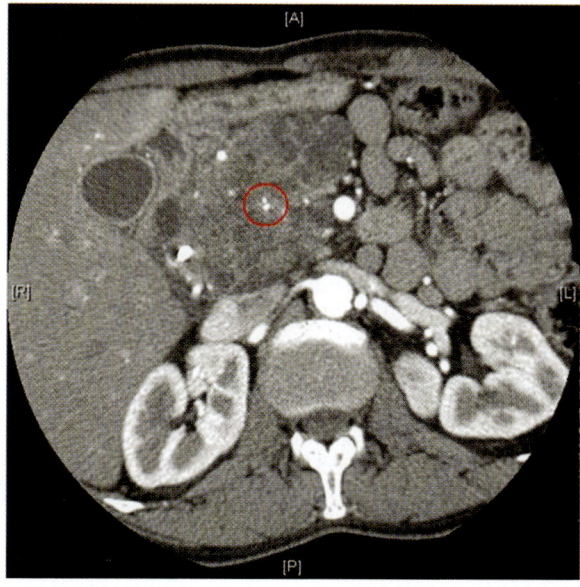

Figure 3. Computed tomography of a serous cystadenoma. A large microcystic lesion is seen with multiple septae and a central calcification, all of which are characteristic findings of a SCA.

with less definition; T2-weighted signals show hyperintense fluid filled cysts and septae. The most characteristic finding by EUS is the presence of vascular proliferation within and surrounding the cysts. Although uncommon, cyst fluid analysis by way of EUS with FNA reveals no evidence of mucin, and cytology with glycogen-rich cells, low viscosity, low CEA, and low amylase. This constellation of cyst fluid analysis is an alternative method to distinguish SCA from mucinous lesions.

The cell of origin is thought to be the pancreatic centroacinar cell. SCA possess numerous glycogen-rich cuboidal or flat epithelial-lined cysts some with fibrous septae dividing the locules. The locules range in size from 1 mm to 2 cm. The morphology of the cyst ranges from 70% polycystic, 20% honeycomb and less than 10% macrocystic features. These cysts typically do not require resection. However, cysts that are symptomatic or are increasing in size over time are then considered for surgery either via a cyst enucleation or formal pancreatic resection. After resection, these cysts do not recur.

Mucinous Cystic Neoplasm

Mucinous cystic neoplasms (MCNs) are considered pre-malignant lesions. They do carry a predilection for occurring in perimenopausal females (F:M = 8:1) and being located in the distal pancreas. Fifty percent of patients are asymptomatic thus are incidentally discovered. Those with symptoms present with nonspecific complaints of abdominal pain or pancreatitis.

On cross-sectional imaging, they can appear like a pseudocyst. CT scan provides anatomical detail and spatial resolution of the mucinous lesions as well as evaluating for distant disease (Figure 4). However, to distinguish between types of mucinous lesions, typically EUS is necessary providing detail regarding the relationship of the duct to the cyst. MCNs have no gross connection to the pancreatic duct which is one distinguishing feature. EUS also provides access for FNA of cyst fluid allowing for chemical analysis and cytology.

MCNs on gross appearance are multilocular cysts with varying sizes. The cyst wall is thick and fibrotic possessing a papillary, trebeculated pattern. Cyst contents predominantly contain mucin, but blood, purulence and water have been found as well. Histologically, MCNs have three distinct layers: (1) the innermost layer consists of tall, mucin-producing columnar epithelial cells with possible hyperplasia, dysplasia, carcinoma *in situ*, or invasive adenocarcinoma; (2) the middle layer possesses dense mesenchymal ovarian-like stroma; (3) the outermost layer is hyalinized connective

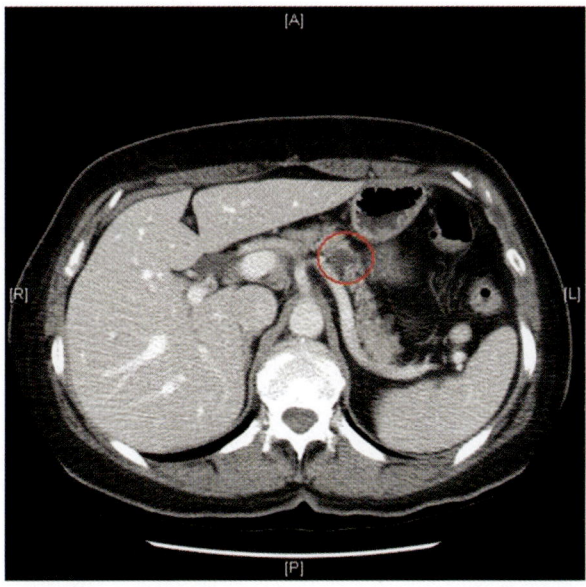

Figure 4. Computed tomography of a mucinous cystic neoplasm. A cyst is found in the body of the pancreatic parenchyma.

tissue. The ovarian-like stroma is virtually pathognomonic for this entity.[5] The growth of these cysts may be influenced by hormones as luteal-type cells are found in the stroma which expresses progesterone receptors.

Surgery is recommended on the basis that these cystic lesions can progress into an adenocarcinoma which carries a poorer prognosis. Most MCNs are distal lesions thus requiring a distal pancreatectomy. One-quarter of these patients will have malignant cells on the final surgical pathology. Five-year survival is approximately 70% overall, but the majority of the long-term survivors had no malignant elements on the surgical pathology. Mucinous cystadenocarcinoma represents mucinous neoplasms that have progressed to adenocarcinoma and tend to be bulky lesions with irregular borders. They are less invasive as pancreatic ductal adenocarcinoma and have a reported 5-year survival as high as 63%.

Intraductal Papillary Mucinous Neoplasm

Once intraductal papillary mucinous neoplasms (IPMN) were first classified and distinguished from MCNs in 2000, they were considered rare

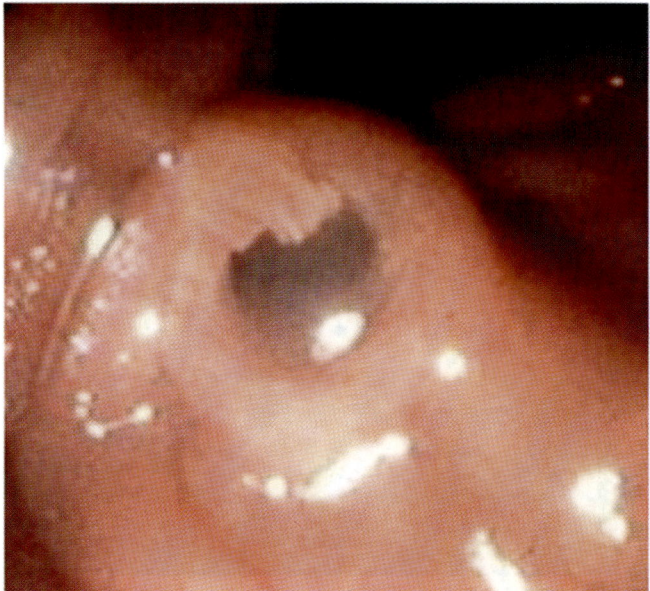

Figure 5. Endoscopic photograph of the ampulla of Vater. This image is characteristic for IPMN in that mucin is seen extruding from the ampulla.

lesions. However, since then, the recognition of IPMNs has increased over the last decade. IPMNs like MCNs are considered premalignant lesions based upon clear examples of malignant transformation of these lesions. IPMNs are defined as cystic dilatation of the pancreatic duct with papillary projections of mucin-secreting ductal epithelium. The mucin can be copious causing ductal obstruction and cystic dilation of the pancreas resulting in the development of pancreatitis. Furthermore, mucin production can be so exaggerated that it protrudes through the ampulla of Vater, seen at the time of ERCP, which is pathognomonic for IPMNs (Figure 5).

IPMNs have a slight predominance in males and are more frequently seen in older patients. Symptomatic patients can present with pancreatitis primarily from pancreatic duct obstruction with mucin. Other symptoms include abdominal pain, diabetes, jaundice, and weight loss. IPMNs can be found throughout the pancreas with multicentric disease, yet they are primarily found in the head of the pancreas. Thirty percent of patients with IPMNs have a metachronous or synchronous malignancy outside of the pancreas.

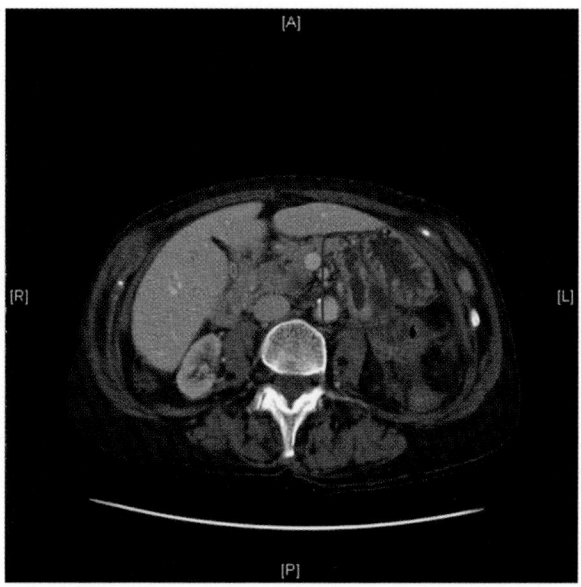

Figure 6. Computed tomography of an intraductal pancreatic mucinous neoplasm. A cystic dilatation of the pancreatic duct is suggestive of IPMN.

Cross-sectional imaging may reveal evidence of a cystic mass, pancreatic duct dilatation, or pancreatitis (Figure 6). Typically, these lesions are greater than 1 cm in size and are a visible mass by CT. ERCP is particularly helpful in diagnosing IPMNs in that the presence of extrusion of mucus from the ampulla or pancreatic duct, dilated pancreatic duct, and pancreatic duct filling defect are virtually diagnostic. The pancreatic ducts are commonly seen as dilated and tortuous with multiple papillary excrescences (Figure 7). Histologically, three distinct patterns are seen in the mucin-producing epithelium of the dilated, cystic pancreatic duct: intestinal (like a villous adenoma), pancreatic (papillae lined with cuboidal cells), or gastric-type epithelium.

IPMNs have macroscopic variation between main-duct or branch-duct types. Specifically, main-duct refers to cystic dilatation of the main pancreatic duct, while branch-duct most commonly refers to the uncinate branch of the pancreatic duct. This distinction has been made because many believe that there exists a biologic difference associated with disparate long-term prognosis. Macroscopically, main-duct type are distributed in

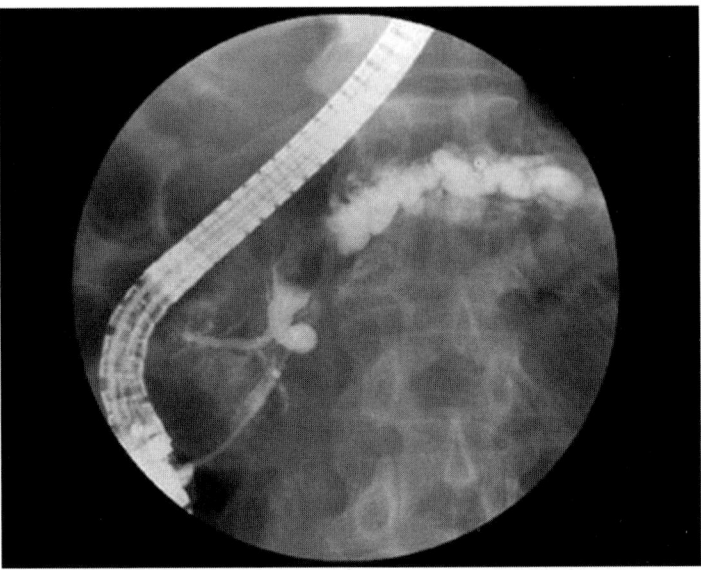

Figure 7. Pancreatogram of an IPMN. The elongated cystic dilatation of the pancreatic duct is characteristic of IPMN.

segmental or diffuse patterns, meanwhile branch-duct type are found in the head and uncinate process as a localized mass.

Resection is frequently the recommendation for IPMN. Thirty percent of all IPMNs harbor an adenocarcinoma. Adenocarcinoma found in the setting of IPMNs has a much more favorable prognosis when compared to typical pancreatic ductal adenocarcinoma. Most studies report a 5-year survival of 60–70% following resection. The prevalence of malignancy in main-duct IPMNs is 70%, while branch-duct IPMNs is 25%. In general, simple forms of main-duct (small, cystic, lacking nodularity) and branch-duct type typically are benign and carry a better prognosis.[5] A subgroup of branch-duct IPMNs that were asymptomatic, size <3 cm, no mural nodules (by EUS), and failed to grow in size over interval cross-sectional imaging had an exceedingly low rate of malignancy; this may be the only subgroup of IPMNs that may not require resection.

The presence of IPMN at surgical margins is not uncommon especially due to the presence of multifocal disease. Options include further resection until the pancreatic margin is free of IPMN; some authors have proposed creation of a pancreaticogastrostomy in the setting of pancreaticoduodenectomy to allow for endoscopic surveillance. Total pancreatectomy has been suggested as an option for treatment of IPMNs due to its multifocal nature, yet caution should be used when considering the significant morbidity of a total pancreatectomy.

Solid Pseudopapillary Neoplasm

Solid pseudopapillary neoplasms (SPN) are a cystic lesion of the pancreas occurring in young females which is completely unique to the pancreas. These lesions present with abdominal symptoms when large; on cross-sectional imaging, SPN can be confused with pseudocysts because of a mix of solid and cystic components. The cysts present are consistent with cystic degeneration and necrosis; the cavity contains blood, macrophages, and necrotic tissue. The cyst wall takes on a pseudopapillary pattern that gives it its moniker. The cell type of origin is not clearly defined to any native cell type that is found in the pancreas. Furthermore, the cells commonly express both progesterone and estrogen receptors highlighting the female predilection. A very small percentage of these patients can present with metastasis following anatomical resection, thus all of these lesions undergo pancreatectomy. Eighty percent of patients with SPN are cured with resection.

CONTROVERSIES IN MANAGEMENT

The evaluation and management of pancreatic cystic lesions continues to evolve. High quality cross-sectional imaging allows us to differentiate primary cystic neoplasms from pseudocysts, retention cysts or solid tumors with cystic degeneration. Most surgeons agree with how a pancreatic cystic lesion should be treated (Table 4), but the principal question is when a primary cystic lesion of the pancreas should be treated? The focus of surgeons and gastroenterologists has been on distinguishing primary cystic neoplasms with malignant potential (MCNs and IPMNs) from cystic neoplasms with no or very low malignant potential (SCA).[4] For healthy patients with a long life expectancy, the diagnosis of a mucinous neoplasm is considered an indication for resection. However, for many of our patients — particularly elderly patients with incidentally identified cystic lesions — the risks of resection may exceed the risks of malignancy. Therefore, there has been increasing focus on distinguishing mucinous neoplasms with a high

Table 4. Traditional treatment of cystic lesions of the pancreas.

Location	Pseudocyst	SCA*	MCN	IPMN	Malignancy
Head	Drainage	Observe	Rare	Resection (PD)	Resection (PD)
Body	Drainage	Observe	Resection (DP)	Resection (DP)	Resection (DP)
Tail	Resection	Observe	Resection (DP)	Resection (DP)	Resection (DP)

*Symptomatic — enucleation vs. resection (PD or DP).
Abbreviations:
PD — Pancreaticoduodenectomy.
DP — Distal Pancreatectomy.

risk of being malignant (or becoming malignant in the future) from those with a low risk of malignancy.

The debate surrounding size criteria as an indication for resection is of particular interest. Pancreatic cyst size has generally been considered to be one of the most important risk factors, with very low rates of malignancy associated with tumors less than 3 cm.[6] A recent review of patients undergoing serial cross-sectional imaging and subsequent resection failed to show a significant relationship between cyst size and malignancy,[7] but several studies focusing only on patients who underwent resection ultimately concluded that size matters in decision making. For example, SCA ≥ 4 cm were recommended to be removed based solely on these particular lesions having an accelerated rate of growth but not due to symptoms or malignancy.[8] SCA are typically removed only if symptomatic considering less than 10 reported cases of serous cystadenocarcinoma.[4] In fact, SCA can grow to become quite large (greater than 20 cm) with no increased risk of malignancy.

MCNs have also been discussed with size criteria recommendations. One series reported a 17.5% malignancy rate in resected MCNs and found a correlation that 92% of malignant tumors were greater than 6 cm in size; the remaining malignant lesions that were less than 6 cm all had solid components on imaging. The recommendation was that any tumor greater than 4 cm or had solid components required resection. Other series have reported the presence of malignant MCNs in tumors less than 4 cm without solid components.[9] One important consideration for the treatment of MCNs is that the majority of these lesions reside in the body/tail of the pancreas, thus many are candidates for laparoscopic distal pancreatectomy which possesses a lower associated morbidity and mortality compared to open distal pancreatectomy as well as pancreaticoduodenectomy.[10]

IPMNs have also been shown that preoperative cyst size is as a significant predictor for malignancy.[8] Yet, other studies have found that 70% of malignant IPMNs were less than 3 cm in size.[9] The primary issue is that size is one component in making a decision for resection. The recommendation should be tailored towards the primary cystic lesion risk of developing malignancy, the presence of symptoms as a result of the lesion, and the feasibility of the patient tolerating a resection. Age as a risk factor has been supported by some,[7] but not by others.[9] Symptoms have also not been consistently associated with malignancy, yet patients suffering from symptoms related to the cystic neoplasm warrant resection regardless of the cyst type.

Due to these considerations, the management of cystic lesions of the pancreas remains controversial. Although many authors previously proposed that almost all cystic lesions should be resected, most recent studies have supported a more selective approach to resection.[7,9] Proposed selection criteria for resection have included age, symptoms, cyst size, cyst growth, suspicious features on imaging (e.g. solid components, septations, pancreatic ductal dilatation, biliary ductal dilatation), cyst fluid analyses (e.g. presence of mucin, high viscosity, elevated carcinoembryonic antigen (CEA) levels, and presence of K-*ras* mutations), and serum tumor markers (CEA, CA 19-9). Elevated CEA or CA 19-9 is suggestive of malignancy in the presence of a known pancreatic cyst and would lead surgeons to favor resection over observation.

Endoscopic diagnostic modalities are useful adjuncts to cross-sectional imaging. ERCP has a significant albeit limited role; it's primarily role is as a diagnostic modality reserved for patients who present with biliary duct or pancreatic duct dilatation without an associated lesion on cross-sectional imaging. It also serves a therapeutic role for biliary decompression in jaundiced patients. However, it is the most sensitive diagnostic modality to identify a direct communication between the pancreatic duct and a cyst.[6] IPMN has certain findings exclusive to ERCP that are considered pathognomonic. Mucus protruding through either the papilla or pancreatic duct correlates highly with the diagnosis of IPMNs. MRCP may be superior to ERCP in identifying IPMNs by improved visualization of the extent of ductal involvement and internal architecture.

EUS appears to be the most valuable endoscopic modality by allowing for high-resolution imaging of the pancreas and acquisition of tissue and fluid by FNA. Controversy exists regarding the ability of EUS to distinguish benign from malignant lesions based on cyst morphology alone. IPMNs are readily detectable by EUS with a high sensitivity, but EUS alone fails in distinguishing benign and malignant lesions. The presence of mucin or mucinous cells by FNA, however, is highly specific for mucinous neoplasms. Furthermore, the degree of cytologic atypia seen by FNA in IPMN has been shown to be predictive of malignancy. The combination of EUS and FNA is the most promising in predicting lesions requiring resection with reported sensitivities and specificity of 97% and 100% respectively. However, this ability of cytology to predict malignancy and guide resection has been brought into questions by similar studies with less convincing results, and overall its role still remains unclear. Aspirated cyst fluid analysis has been reported to improve diagnostic accuracy by measurement of tumor markers (CA15-3, CA19-9, CA72-4, CA-125, CEA); CEA — with a cutoff of 192 ng/ml — had the highest sensitivity (73%) and specificity (84%) in differentiating mucinous versus non-mucinous cysts. More recently, molecular studies of cyst fluid have shown that K-ras mutations, a common tumor suppressor gene mutation, are more prevalent in malignant lesions.

CONCLUSION

The debate regarding appropriate evaluation and management of primary cystic neoplasms of the pancreas continues among surgeons. The landscape continues to change as cross sectional imaging, endoscopic techniques, and surgical outcomes continue to improve. We support a selective operative management of pancreatic cysts lesions based on symptoms, cyst features, and operative risk to the patient.

REFERENCES

1. Compagno J, Oertel JE. Mucinous cystic neoplasms of the pancreas with overt and latent malignancy (cystadenocarcinoma and cystadenoma). A clinicopathologic study of 41 cases. *Am J Clin Pathol* 1978; 69(6):573–580.
2. Compagno J, Oertel JE. Microcystic adenomas of the pancreas (glycogen-rich cystadenomas): a clinicopathologic study of 34 cases. *Am J Clin Pathol* 1978; 69(3):289–298.
3. Melman L, Azar R, Beddow K, *et al.* Primary and overall success rates for clinical outcomes after laparoscopic, endoscopic, and open pancreatic cystgastrostomy for pancreatic pseudocysts. *Surg Endosc* 2009; 23(2):267–271.
4. King JC, Ng TT, White SC, *et al.* Pancreatic Serous Cystadenocarcinoma: a case report and review of the literature. *J Gastrointest Surg* 2009; 13(10):1864–1868.

5. Tanaka M, Chari S, Adsay V, *et al.* International consensus guidelines for management of intraductal papillary mucinous neoplasms and mucinous cystic neoplasms of the pancreas. *Pancreatology* 2006; 6(1–2):17–32.
6. Sahani DV, Saokar A, Hahn PF, *et al.* Pancreatic cysts 3 cm or smaller: How aggressive should treatment be? *Radiology* 2006; 238(3):912–919.
7. Spinelli KS, Fromwiller TE, Daniel RA, *et al.* Cystic pancreatic neoplasms: observe or operate. *Ann Surg* 2004; 239(5):651–657; Discussion 657–659.
8. Tseng JF, Warshaw AL, Sahani DV, *et al.* Serous cystadenoma of the pancreas: tumor growth rates and recommendations for treatment. *Ann Surg* 2005; 242(3):413–419; Discussion 419–421.
9. Ceppa EP, De la Fuente SG, Reddy SK, *et al.* Defining criteria for selective operative management of pancreatic cystic lesions: does size really matter? *J Gastrointest Surg* 2010; 14(2):236–244.
10. Kooby DA, Hawkins WG, Schmidt CM, *et al.* A multicenter analysis of distal pancreatectomy for adenocarcinoma: Is laparoscopic resection appropriate? *J Am Coll Surg* 2010; 210(5):779–785.

PERIAMPULLARY CANCER 40

Diana L. Diesen*
and Theodore N. Pappas[†]

INTRODUCTION

Periampullary carcinoma refers to cancer arising from the pancreas, ampulla of Vater, bile duct, or duodenum. The most common type of this tumor includes pancreatic adenocarcinoma while others include ampullary adenocarcinoma, cholangiocarcinoma, and duodenal adenocarcinoma. Depending on the location, these masses may be asymptomatic or may present with jaundice and/or duodenal obstructive symptoms. The evaluation of these patients includes a detailed history and physical, laboratory data, radiological evaluation, and endoscopy with biopsy. Treatment, depending on clinical staging, often includes a combination of chemotherapy and surgical intervention. In this chapter, we will break down periampullary carcinoma into pancreatic adenocarcinoma, ampullary adenocarcinoma, cholangiocarcinoma, and duodenal adenocarcinoma.

TYPES OF PERIAMPULLARY CARCINOMAS

Pancreatic Adenocarcinoma

Pancreatic cancer is the fourth leading cause of cancer death in the US with 31,800 deaths in 2005. The incidence of pancreatic cancer rose in the early

---

*UT Southwestern Medical Center, Dallas TX 75235, USA
[†]Duke University Medical Center, Durham, NC 27710 USA

part of the 20th century but has been relatively stable since 1970 with a slight increase in the past 10 years (8 cases per 100,000 people). This incidence is similar to that seen in Europe. There is a lower incidence of pancreatic cancer in India and the Middle East. Unfortunately, pancreatic cancer is particularly fatal with a yearly mortality approaching the yearly incidence.

The cause of pancreatic cancer is unknown. Demographic factors that have been associated with the condition include age >60, male gender (relative risk 1.35), and African-American races (30–40% higher). Mean age at time of diagnosis is 60–65 years. Other risk factors include Ashkenazi Jewish heritage, cigarette smoking, diabetes mellitus, chronic pancreatitis, obesity, sedentary lifestyle, and exposure to carcinogens. There are genetic conditions that also have increased risk of pancreatic cancer including hereditary pancreatitis, hereditary nonpolyposis colorectal cancer (HNPCC), hereditary breast and ovarian cancer, familial atypical multiple mole melanoma syndrome, Peutz–Jeghers syndrome (PJS), and ataxia-telengiectasia.

Ampullary Adenocarcinoma

Ampullary carcinoma is a rare tumor noted in 6 per one million people per year. It is more common (200- to 300-fold more) in patient with familial polyposis syndromes such as familial adenomatous polyposis (FAP), PJS, or hereditary nonpolyposis colorectal cancer (HNPCC). Upper GI adenomas will be found in up to 90% of FAP patients. Due to the incidence of ampullary lesions in these patients, routine surveillance is recommended. Lesions may be detected during surveillance before symptoms present and ideally before adenomas develop malignant transformation. Inherited polyposis ampullary lesions are usually diagnosed in patients greater than 40 years of age though sporadic lesions are more common in patients greater than 60 years of age. Patients with symptoms may present with abdominal pain, jaundice (50–70%), pancreatitis, nausea, vomiting, weight loss and less commonly purities, cholangitis, and/or sepsis. Ampullary adenocarcinoma tends to present earlier than other cancers due to location. These lesions tend to be less aggressive and since they present earlier, they are more amenable to surgical resection with a resection rate up to 80%. Factors affecting poor prognosis include presence of lymph node metastasis, perineural invasion, and poor tumor differentiation.

Benign lesions may be locally excised either endoscopically or with local ampullectomy. If these lesions are malignant per biopsy endoscopically or during ampullectomy, patient should receive a pancreaticoduodenectomy. Survival for ampullary carcinoma is the highest of all of the periampullary cancers with a 30–70% 5-year survival for ampullary cancer depending on the series.

Cholangiocarcinoma

Cholangiocarcinoma originate from the epithelial cells in the bile duct and may be intrahepatic, perihilar, or extrahepatic in location. Cholangiocarcinoma is rare in the United States but more common in Asian countries. It is associated with a variety of chronic inflammatory conditions of the bile duct including sclerosing cholangitis, parasitic infestation, fibropolycystic liver disease, cholelithiasis, hepatolithiasis, toxic exposure (Thorotrast), Lynch syndrome, biliary papillomatosis, chronic liver disease, diabetes, obesity, and HIV infection. Distal bile duct cancer accounts of 25% of cholangiocarcinomas and present clinically similarly to pancreatic cancer. Classification of cholangiocarcinomas is described by the Bismuth–Corlette classification or the TNM staging classification (Table 5). The diagnosis of cholangiocarcinoma is more likely with a preoperative workup demonstrating an isolated bile duct stricture with normal pancreatic duct.

Duodenal Adenocarcinoma

Duodenal adenocarcinoma is a rare condition thought to be from malignant transformation of a duodenal polyp. Duodenal carcinoma represent < 0.5% of all gastrointestinal tract cancers but does account for 45% of all small bowel cancers. Duodenal carcinomas may occur throughout the duodenum. Because it is so rare, little is known about risk factors, tumor staging, prognostic value of nodal status, or degree of differentiation. Duodenal adenocarcinoma is more common in patients with FAP, HNPCC, and PJS to the point where surveillance endoscopy is recommended for these patients. In patients with FAP, duodenal cancer is the second most common cancer next to colon cancer in this population. Other suggested risk factors for duodenal adenocarcinoma include chronic inflammatory states, alcohol, refined sugar, red meat, salt-cured, smoked foods, and possibly tobacco. Surgical resection is the only potential curative treatment. Benign tumors of the duodenum may be treated with duodenectomy. Malignant lesions of the duodenum should be treated with pancreaticodudodenectomy.

DIAGNOSTIC EVALUATION

History and Physical

Patients with tumors of the periampullary region are more likely than other pancreatic cancer patients to present with symptoms. (Table 1) The typical presentation would be painless jaundice from obstruction of the ampulla or bile duct. Patients may also complain of intermittent epigastric pain, dark urine, light stools, and/or pruritis. Up to 25% also have common bile duct stone due to stasis. These pancreatic lesions may eventually cause compression of the celiac plexus causing abdominal and/or back pain.

In 20% of patients with pancreatic cancer, new-onset diabetes mellitus is observed; thus, a new onset of DM in an elderly patient may prompt further evaluation of the pancreas. Also a new diagnosis of pancreatitis in

Table 1. Presenting symptoms.

Asymptomatic	Pruritis
	Dyspepsia
Jaundice	Nausea
Gastric outlet obstruction	Vomiting
Pain (epigastric, abdominal, back)	Anorexia
Malabsorption	Fatigue
Steatorrhea	Duodenal obstruction
Diarrhea	Anemia
Weight loss	Failure to thrive
General malaise	Supraclavicular adenopathy (Virchow's nodes)
New-onset diabetes	Ascites
Dark urine	Palpable hepatic metastases periumbilical lymphadenopathy (sister Mary Joseph's nodules)
Light stools	Drop metastases surrounding the perirectal region (Blumer's shelf)

an elderly patient should also prompt evaluation of the pancreas as this may be a sign of ductal obstruction from mass compression especially if the patient does not have a history of gallstones, ethanol use, or elevated triglycerides.

If the lesion is large enough, the patient may present with gastric outlet obstruction manifested by nausea, vomiting, dyspepsia, and/or epigastric pain. If on the other hand, the pancreatic duct is obstructed, the patient may present with exocrine insufficiency leading to malabsorption, steatorrhea, diarrhea, weight loss, and general malaise. Thirty percent of patients present with anemia, heme-positive stools, or upper GI bleed. If the disease is more advanced, patients may present with fatigue, weight loss, anorexia, anemia, purities, and failure to thrive. Patient's with metastatic disease may also have enlarged left supraclavicular adenopathy (Virchow's nodes), ascites, palpable hepatic metastases periumbilical lymphadenopathy (Sister Mary Joseph's nodules), or drop metastases surrounding the perirectal region (Blumer's shelf).

Laboratory Evaluation

Laboratory values to obtain when concerned about periampullary carcinoma include complete blood count, basic chemistry, liver function panel, amylase, lipase, albumin, and serum carbohydrate antigen 19–9 (CA 19–9). The elevation in liver function is dependent on the degree of obstruction of the common bile duct. Hyperglycemia may be seen. Anemia is common. Malnutrition may be noted either due to malabsorption or tumor burden. Vitamin deficiency especially fat-soluble vitamins may be noted along with elongation of prothrombin time. Elevating in CA19–9 may be seen particularly in patients with pancreatic adenocarcinoma but this is neither a sensitive the or specific marker. Approximately 15% of patients do not secrete CA 19–9 and it may not elevate in the early stages of the disease.

Radiology

Ultrasound (US)

Right upper quadrant US often the initial study ordered for patients presenting with jaundice and/or abdominal pain. While US is most sensitive for evaluating gallbladder pathology, other more ominous signs of advanced periampullary adenocarcinoma may be seen such as hepatic metastases, peripancreatic and hilar lymphadenopathy, and ascites. It is not useful in evaluating the periampullary region specifically.

Computed tomography (CT)

Multidetector spiral CT is the most useful diagnostic tool to diagnose and stage patients with peripancreatic carcinoma. CT is able to give details about mass characteristics, proximity to adjacent structures, presence of tissue planes between structures, possible invasion of adjacent structure, lymphadenopathy, hepatic metastases, peritoneal dissemination, pulmonary involvement, and/or ascites. Figure 1 demonstrates the moderate intrahepatic and advanced common bile duct dilatation down to the ampulla, consistent with the history of an ampullary carcinoma. Pancreatic ductal dilation is also present.

Magnetic resonance imaging (MRI)

MRI like CT is able to provide tumor characteristics, proximity to adjacent structures, vascular, hepatic, or pulmonary involvement. MRI is particularly helpful when delineating hepatic structures. MRCP may also be performed at the same time which may be used to image the biliary tree and pancreatic duct. It has the advantage of being non-invasive but does not have any therapeutic options. If a distal bile duct obstruction is suspected but no mass is seen on CT scan, cholangiography may be helpful. Figure 2 demonstrates an MRI showing an obstructing mass in the region the duodenum/ampulla of Vater with associated marked dilation of the biliary and pancreatic ducts. This patient also had mass in the anterior left hepatic lobe and inferior right hepatic lobe which have an appearance most suggestive of hemangiomas.

Endoscopic retrograde cholangiopancreatography (ERCP)

ERCP provides both diagnostic and therapeutic options. ERCP images may confirm the diagnosis of a pancreatic or periampullary mass. During the procedure, brushings or biopsy of the mass may be obtained as well as decompression of the biliary tree. The decision of stent placement depends on the likelihood of surgical resection. The classic finding of a long irregular stricture in the pancreatic duct with distal dilation or a

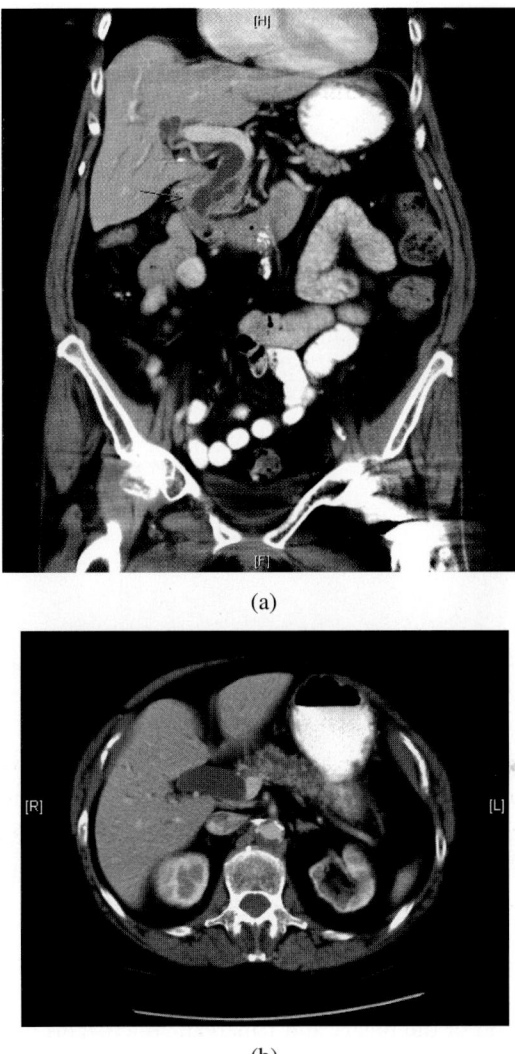

Figure 1. CT images of a patient with ampullary adenocarcinoma. These images demonstrate moderate intrahepatic and advanced common bile duct dilatation down to the ampulla, consistent with the history of an ampullary carcinoma. The pancreatic duct is also dilated.

cutoff of both the pancreatic duct and distal bile duct are pathognomonic of pancreas cancer. The observation of an irregular structure of the bile

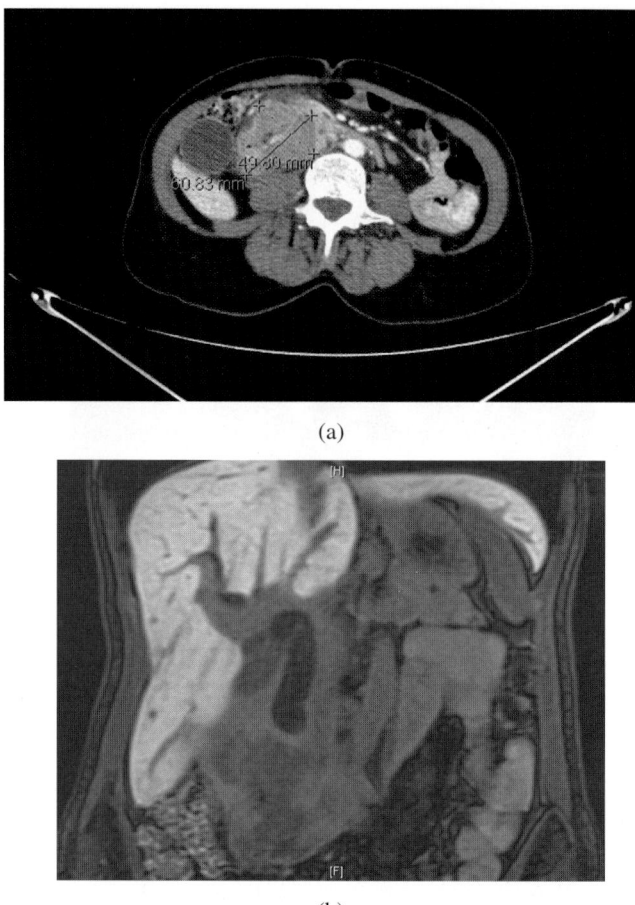

Figure 2. MRI and CT scans of duodenal adenocarcinoma. This MRI demonstrates the obstructing mass in the duodenum/ampulla of Vater region with associated marked dilation of the biliary and pancreatic ducts. This patient also had an anterior left hepatic lobe and inferior right hepatic lobe masses with an appearance most suggestive of hemangiomas.

duct with normal pancreatic duct is pathognomonic for cholangiocarcinoma. With the advancement of CT and MRI, ERCP is rarely needed to diagnosis a periampullary mass. It does allow for biopsy and stent placement if needed.

Percutaneous transhepatic cholangiography (PTC)

Percutaneous transhepatic cholangiography provides excellent definition of the biliary anatomy. Visualization of the pancreatic duct and the most distal portion of the extrahepatic bile duct is not optimal. If the patient has biliary obstruction and drainage is necessary, a percutaneous biliary drain may be inserted after the cholangiogram allowing the drainage of the proximal biliary tree. PTC is not routinely performed because it is invasive and may result in complications including bleeding.

Positron emission tomography (PET)

The role of PET in periampullary carcinoma is not clear. Some studies suggest it is useful in assessing for metastatic disease but its prognostic value is undetermined.

Endoscopy and Endoscopic Ultrasound (EUS)

After CT scan for initial diagnosis, most ampullary and duodenal mass are examined with endoscopy. Endoscopy allows visualization of the mass as well as biopsy of the lesion. During endoscopy, EUS is performed to properly assess for lymphadenopathy and local invasion. EUS may assess the duodenum, ampulla, head of the pancreas, and uncinate process of the pancreas. The EUS probe placed in the stomach allows visualization of the pancreatic body and tail. EUS may also be used to assess for vascular involvement. With EUS, fine needle biopsy may also be performed.

Pathology

Due to the variety of lesions that present in the periampullary region, tissue diagnosis is critical for determining management decisions, and assessing prognosis. Usually biopsy may be performed with minimal risk of complication via endoscopy or ERCP. Some centers advocate neoadjuvant chemoradiation for pancreatic adenocarcinoma which requires a tissue diagnosis. This is not the approach taken by all centers. Others advocate that a patient with a resectable mass by preoperative imaging may be taken directly to resection. Biopsy is also necessary in patients that are unresectable for appropriate diagnosis before palliative chemoradiation may be performed.

DIFFERENTIAL DIAGNOSIS

The differential diagnosis of a periampullary mass includes both benign and malignant lesions (Table 2).

MANAGEMENT OPTIONS

In order to assess for resectability, staging is necessary. For each of the tumors included (pancreatic adenocarcinoma, ampullary, cholangiocarcinoma, duodenal carcinoma), there is a TNM definition and staging from the American Joint Committee on Cancer (AJCC) (Tables 3–6). Based on staging, patients are divided into operative and nonoperative candidates. Stage four patients of all groups are considered unresectable and should be referred for operative or nonoperative palliation.

Resectable

Surgical resection remains the only potentially curative therapy for the treatment of periampullary lesions. Unfortunately, few patients are resectable at the time of diagnosis. Curative resection is based on the extent of disease. The standard treatment is usually pancreaticoduodenectomy.

Table 2. Differential diagnosis to periampullary carcinoma.

Benign	Malignant
Adenoma	Carcinoid
Lipoma	Sarcoma
Leiomyomas	Lymphoma
Fibroma	Melanoma
Hemangiomas	Metastatic disease
Leiomyofibromas	Renal cell
Lymphangiomas	Melanoma
Neurogenic tumors	

Table 3. TNM staging system for exocrine and endocrine tumors of the pancreas.

Primary tumor (T)	
TX	Primary tumor cannot be assessed
T0	No evidence of primary tumor
Tis	Carcinoma *in situ*
T1	Tumor limited to the pancreas, 2 cm or less in greatest dimension
T2	Tumor limited to the pancreas, more than 2 cm in greatest dimension
T3	Tumor extends beyond the pancreas but without involvement of the celiac axis or the superior mesenteric artery
T4	Tumor involves the celiac axis or the superior mesenteric artery (unresectable primary tumor)
Regional lymph nodes (N)	
NX	Regional lymph nodes cannot be assessed
N0	No regional lymph node metastasis
N1	Regional lymph node metastasis
Distant metastasis (M)	
M0	No distant metastasis
M1	Distant metastasis

Anatomic stage/prognostic groups

Stage 0	Tis	N0	M0
Stage IA	T1	N0	M0
Stage IB	T2	N0	M0
Stage IIA	T3	N0	M0
Stage IIB	T1	N1	M0
	T2	N1	M0
	T3	N1	M0
Stage III	T4	Any N	M0
Stage IV	Any T	Any N	M1

AJCC Cancer Staging Manual, Seventh Edition (2010) published by Springer New York, Inc.

Table 4. TNM staging for ampullary carcinoma.

Primary tumor (T)	
TX	Primary tumor cannot be assessed
T0	No evidence of primary tumor
Tis	Carcinoma *in situ*
T1	Tumor limited to the ampulla of Vater or sphincter of Oddi
T2	Tumor invades duodenal wall
T3	Tumor invades pancreas
T4	Tumor invades peripancreatic soft tissues or other adjacent organs or structures other than pancreas
Regional lymph nodes (N)	
NX	Regional lymph nodes cannot be assessed
N0	No regional lymph node metastasis
N1	Regional lymph node metastasis
Distant metastasis (M)	
M0	No distant metastasis
M1	Distant metastasis

Anatomic stage/prognostic groups			
Stage 0	Tis	N0	M0
Stage IA	T1	N0	M0
Stage IB	T2	N0	M0
Stage IIA	T3	N0	M0
Stage IIB	T1	N1	M0
	T2	N1	M0
	T3	N1	M0
Stage III	T4	Any N	M0
Stage IV	Any T	Any N	M1

AJCC Cancer Staging Manual, Seventh Edition (2010) published by Springer New York, Inc.

In most cases, preoperative biliary decompression is unnecessary and results in increased postoperative complications. Patients with biliary sepsis or significant time delay before surgery (perhaps due to malnutrition) may benefit from endoscopic biliary decompression with a plastic stent. If

Table 5. TNM staging system for distal cholangiocarcinoma.

Primary tumor (T)

TX	Primary tumor cannot be assessed
T0	No evidence of primary tumor
Tis	Carcinoma *in situ*
T1	Tumor confined to the bile duct histologically
T2	Tumor invades beyond the wall of the bile duct
T3	Tumor invades the gallbladder, pancreas, duodenum, or other adjacent organs without involvement of the celiac axis, or the superior mesenteric artery
T4	Tumor involves the celiac axis, or the superior mesenteric artery

Regional lymph nodes (N)

NX	Regional lymph nodes cannot be assessed
N0	No regional lymph node metastasis
N1	Regional lymph node metastasis

Distant metastasis (M)

M0	No distant metastasis
M1	Distant metastasis

Anatomic stage/prognostic groups

Stage 0	Tis	N0	M0
Stage IA	T1	N0	M0
Stage 0IB	T2	N0	M0
Stage IIA	T3	N0	M0
Stage IIB	T1	N1	M0
	T2	N1	M0
	T3	N1	M0
Stage III	T4	Any N	M0
Stage IV	Any T	Any N	M1

AJCC Cancer Staging Manual, Seventh Edition (2010) published by Springer New York, Inc.

Table 6. TNM staging system for small bowel cancer.

Primary tumor (T)	
TX	Primary tumor cannot be assessed
T0	No evidence of primary tumor
Tis	Carcinoma *in situ*
T1a	Tumor invades lamina propria
T1b	Tumor invades submucosa
T2	Tumor invades muscularis propria
T3	Tumor invades through the muscularis propria into the subserosa or into the nonperitonealized perimuscular tissue (mesentery or retroperitoneum) with extension 2 cm or less*
T4	Tumor perforates the visceral peritoneum or directly invades other organs or structures (includes other loops of small intestine, mesentery, or retroperitoneum more than 2 cm, and abdominal wall by way of serosa; for the duodenum only, invasion of pancreas or bile duct)
Regional lymph nodes (N)	
NX	Regional lymph nodes cannot be assessed
N0	No regional lymph node metastasis
N1	Metastasis in 1–3 regional lymph nodes
N2	Metastasis in >4 regional lymph nodes
Distant metastasis (M)	
M0	No distant metastasis
M1	Distant metastasis

Anatomic stage/prognostic groups			
Stage 0	Tis	N0	M0
Stage I	T1	N0	M0
	T2	N0	M0
Stage IIA	T3	N0	M0
Stage IIB	T4	N0	M0
Stage IIIA	Any T	N1	M0
Stage IIIB	Any T	N2	M0
Stage IV	Any T	Any N	M1

Note: cTNM is the clinical classification, pTNM is the pathologic classification.
* The nonperitonealized perimuscular tissue is, for jejunum and ileum, part of the mesentery and, for duodenum in areas where serosa is lacking, part of the interface with the pancreas.
AJCC Cancer Staging Manual, Seventh Edition (2010) published by Springer New York, Inc.

endoscopic decompression is not possible, percutaneous transhepatic biliary drainage is performed.

Pancreaticoduodenectomy is the treatment of choice for pancreatic adenocarcinoma. Patients with local ampullary masses may be treated with ampullectomy but if adenocarinoma is found on pathology, a pancreaticoduodenectomy is recommend. Duodenal carcinoma may be treated with a resection of the duodenum and part of the pancreatic head with the creation of pancreticoduodenostomy with anastomosis of the pancreatic head (including the CBD and pancreatic duct) to either the distal duodenum or jejunum.

If pancreaticoduodenectomy is the operation of choice, the procedure may be partial vs. total pancreatectomy, classic vs. pylorus preserving, and standard vs. extended pancreaticoduodenectomy. We tend to favor a laparoscopic exploration followed by a pylorus preserving partial pancreatectomy with standard lymph node dissection due to decreased complications. A laparoscopic exploration allows for identification of potential metastatic disease to the peritoneum or the liver prior to laparotomy. Laparoscopy is positive in up to 20% of patients with periampullary cancer. For further dissection of pancreaticoduodenectomy, please refer to Chapter 46.

Pancreaticoduodenectomy is associated with a mortality rate of 2–4% and a complication rate of 31–50%. The most common complications include: delayed gastric emptying 14%, wound infection 7%, pancreatic fistula 5%, reoperation 3%, bile leak 2%, cholangitis 3%, wound infection 7%, intra-abdominal abscess 3%, pneumonia 1%, and pancreatitis 1%. These numbers vary based on type of operation performed and patient's preoperative functional status.

Adjuvant/neoadjuvant chemoradiation

After surgical resection, patients should receive chemoradiation. The 5-year survival for all patients with pancreatic cancer is only 3% and with surgical resection is only 10–20%. The first randomized controlled trial examining the role of adjuvant therapy for pancreatic cancer was reported by the Gastrointestinal Tumor Study Group (GITSG) by Kalser & Ellenbery in 1985. Chemotherapy with 5-FU was found to increase survival from 11 months with surgery alone to 20 months with surgery and chemotherapy. The European Study Group for Pancreatic Cancer (ESPAC-1) found that adjuvant chemotherapy had a survival benefit while chemoradiation had a deleterious effect of survival. Many clinical trials are underway exploring the benefits of various chemotherapy regimens (5-FU, gemcitabine, leucovorin, cisplatin, and interferon alfa) and well as radiation.

While neoadjuvant chemoradiation is not the gold standard, it has become increasingly more common. The advantage to neoadjuvant chemoradiation includes assessment of the biology of the tumor (aggressiveness overtime) as well as possible shrinkage of the tumor to allow for more effective resection. Those patients with more aggressive tumor biology that manifests metastatic disease after chemotherapy would thus avoid an operation that would likely be of little benefit. Preoperative chemotherapy would eliminate the risk of delayed or incomplete treatment. Also since radiation efficacy is dependent on oxygenation, it is thought that radiation may be more effective when given before the tissue is disrupted by surgery. While studies have not found a survival benefit of neoadjuvant chemoradiation, the debate is ongoing.

Unresectable:

Operative palliation

Many patients with periampullary lesions will be found to have unresectable disease at the time of diagnosis. For these patients, palliation of obstructive jaundice, gastric outlet obstruction, and pain are the goals of treatment.

Obstructive jaundice may be palliated in one of three ways including: endoscopically during ERCP, percutaneously via PBD, or surgically with biliary bypass. Endoscopic placement of stents is tolerated well with minimal discomfort to the patient and avoids the complications inherent in percutaneous drainage or surgical bypass including hemobilia, bile leakage, or wound infection. Endoscopic stents are available in both metal and plastic. Plastic stents tend to be smaller and may require periodic changing. Self-expanding metallic stents may be larger but may eventually fail due to tumor in growth. When examining this population comparing stent vs. operative bypass, the patients with endoscopic stent placement have fewer complications and hospitalizations.

Gastric outlet obstruction is also a complication in these patients resulting in significant discomfort due to chronic nausea and vomiting.

The interventions available for this complication include percutaneous endoscopic gastrostomy tube for drainage, duodenal stent, and/or gastrojejunostomy. Initial reports are that gastroduodenal stents are initially successful in 80–90% of patients with gastric outlet obstruction but that gastrojejunostomy provides a more durable relief of obstructive symptoms.

Fifty to ninety percent of patients with unresectable pancreatic cancer experience severe pain. Pain management initially starts with systemic narcotics and neuroleptics. Pain service consultations are often helpful. In some patients, percutaneous or endoscopic celiac plexus block improves pain control.

Chemoradiation

The GITSG defined a 5-FU–based chemoradiation regime as the most conventional option for treatment of locally advanced pancreatic cancer. 5-FU–based chemoradiation produces a twofold increase in median survival (42 weeks vs. 22 weeks) compared to radiation alone. Gemcitabine is the standard chemotherapy for locally advanced and metastatic adenocarcinoma of the pancreas showing some decreased time to progression and improved survival compared to 5-FU. GITSG also found that patients with unresectable pancreatic cancer benefited from 5-FU and radiation over radiation therapy alone. Studies examining various chemotherapy regimens (5-FU, gemcitabine, leucovorin, cisplatin, and interferon $-\alpha$) as well as radiation are ongoing.

OUTCOMES

The general survival for patient with periampullary carcinoma depends on location, stage, and other patient characteristics (Table 7). For pancreatic cancer, overall survival is $\sim 25\%$ at 1- year and 6% at 5-year survival with a median survival of 4–24 months depending on stage. Factors that portend a favorable prognosis include patients who have undergone resection with tumors $<3\,cm$, negative lymph nodes, blood loss $<750\,mL$, well or moderately differentiated tumor, or postoperative chemoradiation. When assessing resectable periampullary cancer as a group, the survival was 15% for pancreas, 39% for ampullary, 27% for distal bile duct, and 59% for duodenal adenocarcinoma. Survival was improved for well-differentiated tumors,

Table 7. Outcomes.

Type	Stage/Category	5-yr survival
Pancreatic adenocarcinoma	I	13%/11%
	II	6%/5%
	III	2.7%
	IV	1
Ampullary adenocarcinoma	I	84%
	II	70%
	III	27
	IV	0
Distal bile duct cholangiocarcinoma	Total	18
	Resectable	32
	Nonresectable	0
Duodenal adenocarcinoma	I	85
	II	52
	III	20
	IV	5

negative margins, and negative lymph nodes. Some studies suggest patients with node-positive cancer may have better outcomes after extended lymphadenectomy with 1- and 5-year survival being 78% and 25% for stand resection vs. 76% and 31% for extended lymphadenectomy.

REFERENCES

1. *AJCC Cancer Staging Manual.* 7th edition. Springer New York, NY. 2010.
2. Beger HG, Treitschke F, Gansuage F, Harada N, Hiki N, Mattfeldt T. Tumor of the ampulla of Vater: experience with local or radial resection in 171 consecutively treated patients. *Arch Surg* 1999; 134(5):526–532.
3. Haller DG. New perspectives in the management of pancreas cancer. *Semin Oncol* 2003; 4(Suppl 11):3–10.
4. Hines, Heber. Periampullary cancer. In: Am Cameron, JL Cameron (eds). *Cameron: Current Surgical Therapy.* 9th edition, Mosby. 2008.
5. Jang J, Kim S, Park D, *et al.* Actual long-term outcome of extrahepatic bile duct cancer after surgical resection. *Ann Surg* 2005; 241(1):77–84.

6. Kalser MH, Ellenberg SS. Pancreatic cancer. Adjuvant combined radiation and chemotherapy following curative resection. *Arch Surg* 1985; 120(8):899–903.
7. Nakakura Y. Periampullary and pancreatic tumors. In: W Jargin (ed). *Blumgart: Surgery of the Liver, Biliary Tract and Pancreas*, 4th edition, Saunders. 2006.
8. Neoptolemos JP, Stocken DD, Friess H, Bassi C, Dunn JA, Hickey H, Beger H, Fernandez-Cruz L, Dervenis C, Lacaine F, Falconi M, Pederzoli P, Pap A, Spooner D, Kerr DJ, Büchler MW. (2004) European Study Group for Pancreatic Cancer. A randomized trial of chemoradiotherapy and chemotherapy after resection of pancreatic cancer. *N Engl J Med* 350(12):1200–10.
9. Schulick, Cameron. Pancreatic and periampullary carcinoma. In: CJ Yeo (ed). *Yeo: Shackelford's Surgery of the Alimentary Tract*, 6th edition, Saunders. 2007.
10. Tempero M, Arnoletti JP, Ben-Josef E, Bhargava P, Casper ES, Kim P, Malafa MP, Nakakura EK, Shibata S, Talamonti M, Wang H, Willett C. (2007) Pancreatic adenocarcinoma. Clinical Practice Guidelines in Oncology. *J Natl Compr Canc Netw* 5(10):998–1033.
11. Sohn TA, Yeo CJ, Cameron JL, Koniaris L, Kaushal S, Abrams RA, Sauter PK, Coleman J, Hruban RH, Lillemoe KD. (2000) Resected adenocarcinoma of the pancreas-616 patients: results, outcomes, and prognostic indicators. *J Gastrointest Surg* 4(6):567–79.

PANCREATIC NEUROENDOCRINE TUMORS   41

Tamarah Westmoreland* and John Olson

INTRODUCTION

Pancreatic neuroendocrine tumors (PNETs) encompass a group of rare tumors that have their origin in embryonic endodermal cells that give rise to islet cells of Langerhans.[1] The overall incidence of pancreatic neuroendocrine tumors is 1 per 100,000 and represents 1–2% of all pancreatic tumors.[2] The peak age at diagnose is between 30 and 60 with a male predominance.[3] PNETs increasingly are being diagnosed do to widespread use of abdominal imaging including CT and MRI. Asymptomatic PNETs have been identified in autopsy series in up to 10% of patients, suggesting there may be a reservoir of silent PNETs that are not diagnosed.[4] Malignancy can be difficult to initially determine, but a mitotic count >20/10 high power fields or a Ki-67 proliferation index of >20% is accepted as an aggressive malignancy.[5] The majority of PNETs are sporadic, but they may also be associated with certain genetic syndromes, such as MEN-1, von Hippel-Lindau disease, neurofibromatosis 1, and tuberous sclerosis.[5]

In MEN-1, PNETs normally comprise multiple pancreatic microadenomas and represent approximately 10% of PNETs.[5] Only a minority of

---

*University of Mississipi Medical Center, Jackson MS 39216 USA

these tumors are functional. When there is a suspicion for MEN-1 based on family history, age of patient, and organ involvement, tests for hyperprolactemia and primary hyperparathyroidism should be performed. Screening for PNETs in the setting of MEN-1 includes assessing for biochemical markers and imaging studies, such as endoscopic ultrasound.

Von Hippel–Lindau (VHL) syndrome is an autosomal dominant inherited syndrome that results in hemangioblastomas of the brain, spinal cord, and eye, renal cell carcinoma, pheochromocytoma, and pancreatic lesions. The majority of the pancreatic lesions in these patients represent simple cysts while only 11% of these patients truly have PNETs.[3]

Neuroendocrine tumors are characterized by their ability to produce the specific neuroendocrine markers chromogranin, synaptophysin, or neuron-specific enolase.[2] These tumors can be divided into functional or nonfunctional tumors depending on whether they produce an active peptide that results in a clinical syndrome. The incidence of functional neuroendocrine tumors is 2% of all gastrointestinal tract tumors.[6] Nonfunctional tumors have been reported to represent 30–40% of all neuroendocrine tumors; however, their true incidence is difficult to determine because they are not associated with a clinical syndrome.[3] Furthermore, the majority of the nonfunctional PNETs are discovered incidentally on imaging for other reasons.

Classification of PNETs can be challenging because of the number of originating sites. The WHO has adopted the following three categories as classification for PNETs:

1. Well-differentiated endocrine tumor: (i) benign and (ii) uncertain malignant potential.
2. Well-differentiated endocrine carcinoma: low-grade malignant.
3. Poorly differentiated endocrine carcinoma: high-grade malignant.[7]

A benign tumor is defined as ≤2 cm, mitotic count <2 per 10 HPF, and proliferation index <2%.[3] The staging system was developed by the American Joint Committee on Cancer and the International Union Against Cancer.[8] The following details the current staging system:

TNM staging for PNETs

T — primary tumor (for any T, add (m) for multiple tumors)
    TX Primary tumor cannot be assessed
    T0 No evidence of primary tumor
    T1 Tumor limited to the pancreas and size ≤ 2 cm

T2 Tumor limited to the pancreas and size >2 cm
T3 Tumor extends beyond the pancreas, but without involvement of the celiac axis or the superior mesenteric artery
T4 Tumor involves the celiac axis or the superior mesenteric artery (unresectable)
N — regional lymph nodes
NX Regional lymph node cannot be assessed
N0 No regional lymph node metastasis
N1 Regional lymph node metastasis
M — distant metastases
MX Distant metastasis cannot be assessed
M0 No distant metastases
M1 Distant metastasis (indicates the presence of any single or multiple metastases at any distant anatomical site including non-regional nodes)

Stage Ia	Stage Ib	Stage IIa	Stage IIb	Stage III	Stage IV
T1, N0	T2, N0	T3, N0	T1–3, N1	T4, any N, M0	Any T, N, M1[3]

Diagnosis of PNETs is frequently delayed due to their nonspecific clinical syndromes. As a result, more than 75% of the patients present with metastatic disease to the liver or less frequently the bone.[9] Preoperative imaging with CT of the abdomen and pelvis and MRI of the liver and pancreas are very helpful in identifying the primary tumor as well as any metastatic disease.[6] Figure 1 is a CT image demonstrating a pancreatic

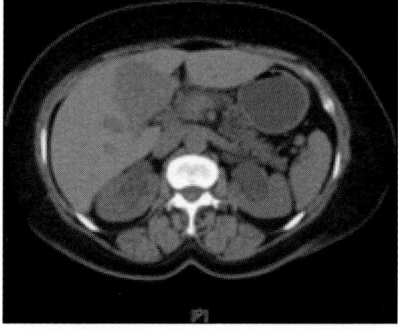

Figure 1. CT image of a pancreatic neuroendocrine tumor in the head of the pancreas with disease in the liver.

neuroendocrine tumor with disease in the liver. The most sensitive imaging study to localize most pancreatic neuroendocrine tumors is the indium-111 somatostatin receptor scintigraphy because of the high expression of the somatostatin subtypes.[6] PET scanning utilizing 5-hydroxytryptophan labeled with ^{11}C has identified greater than 95% of PNETs.[9]

There are multiple different subtypes of pancreatic neuroendocrine tumors. Each of these will be discussed separately. Below is a table that summarizes the PNET characteristics.

Tumor	Secreted hormone	Presentation	Malignancy
Insulinoma	Insulin	Hypoglycemia, reversible symptoms with glucose administration	<10%
Gastrinoma	Gastrin	Diarrhea, hypergastrinemia, gastric acid hypersecretion, peptic ulcer disease	60%
Glucagonoma	Glucagon	Necrolytic migrating erythematous dermatitis, diabetes, DVT, depression	80%
VIPoma	VIP	Watery diarrhea, hypokalemia, achlorhydria	65%
Ppoma	PP	Mass effect	>50%
Somatostatinoma	Somatostatin	Flushing, diarrhea, cardiac valvular disease, bronchospasms	>50%
ACTHoma	ACTH	Cushing Syndrome	>95%
Carcinoid	Serotonin (5-HIAA)	Flushing, diarrhea, cardiac valvular diseases, bronchospasms	60–80%

INSULINOMA

Insulinoma is the most common type of sporadic functional islet cell tumor. Patients with insulinoma normally present in the 5th and 6th decade of life with a female preponderance (3:2).[9] Patients with familial syndromes involving insulinoma (e.g. MEN-1, VHL) present earlier, usually in the 3rd decade of life.[9] Most patients are symptomatic due to hyperinsulinism and hypoglycemia. These symptoms include hunger, fatigue, and weakness which are worsened with a 72-hour fast. Most insulinomas (90%) are benign and management centers on proper diagnosis, preoperative localization, and surgical resection of the offending tumor should be sought.[9]

Diagnosis of insulinoma revolves around a hyperinsulinemic (insulin >5 pU/ml) and hypoglycemic (glucose <50 mg/dL) syndrome. Patients can develop symptoms of Whipple's Triad, which includes symptoms of hypoglycemia (hunger, sweating, tachycardia), blood glucose levels less than 50 mg/dl, and relief of symptoms with glucose administration.[10] Furthermore, signs of neuroglycopenia (anxiety, tremor, confusion, and obtundation) are present. A supervised 72-hour fast which involves observing a patient for hypoglycemia while obtaining serum samples of glucose, insulin, proinsulin, and C-peptide.[1] This supervised fast will also identify those patients with factitious hypoglycemia and postprandial reactive hypoglycemia. As part of the evaluation, patients should be screened for manifestations for MEN-1, including primary hyperparathyroidism and prolactinoma, foregut carcinoid, and VHL.

Preoperative localization of insulinomas can be quite difficult. Ultrasound, CT, and MRI have been utilized but have a low sensitivity ranging from 7% to 46%.[9] Endoscopic ultrasound has recently been found to be more helpful in identifying intrapancreatic tumors with a sensitivity of 75–86%.[9] Moreover, there has been a small amount of evidence that portal venous sampling of insulin as well as arterial sampling of insulin after stimulation with calcium gluconate is beneficial.[9] Insulinomas do not significantly express somatostatin receptors; therefore, somatostatin receptor scintingraphy is not helpful in localizing these tumors. Even with all these measures, there are 20–60 % of insulinomas that are not identified preoperatively.[9] Intraoperative ultrasound in addition to surgical exploration by an experienced pancreas surgeon is likely the most effective manner in localizing the insulinoma.[9]

Treatment of localized insulinoma is surgical resection. Preoperatively, hypoglycemia is initially managed medically or with diet. Patients are instructed to eat frequent small meals, and may require intravenous dextrose administration to maintain normoglycemia. Pharmacologic approaches to reduce insulin secretion include verapamil and diazoxide.[11] For surgical resection, the entire pancreas should be mobilized with a wide kocherization and separation of the transverse mesocolon from the inferior border of the pancreas. The entire pancreas then should be examined visually and with bimanual palpation. These tumors are normally solitary small encapsulated reddish brown masses that can be located throughout the pancreas.[9] Intraoperative ultrasound can be beneficial in localization as well as resection. These tumors are usually amenable to enucleation; however, resection may be required as in the case of MEN-1. If there are multiple tumors throughout the gland, careful resection with preservation of as much pancreas as possible is warranted. Complete pancreatectomy is never indicated for insulinomas. Malignancy is determined at the time of surgery by the presence of involved lymph nodes or liver metastases. If a malignant insulinoma is present, debulking can help palliate the symptoms of hypoglycemia.[12] Greater than 95% of patients are cured with surgical resection. Liver resection in conjunction with pancreas resection has been shown to offer an improved survival.[12]

GASTRINOMA

Gastrinomas represent the second most common overall functional islet cell tumor and the most common function pancreatic tumor in MEN-1.[9] They are a rare cause of peptic ulcer diasease representing only 0.1%.[9] However, in patients with recurrent peptic ulcer disease, gastrinoma can represent up to 2%.[9] The male to female ratio is 2:1, and the age at diagnosis is approximately 50 years.[9] This tumor presents with uncontrollable peptic ulcer disease, which is known as Zollinger–Ellison (ZE) syndrome. In ZE syndrome, the gastrin hormone is secreted in excessive amounts, which then stimulates gastric acid secretion resulting in peptic ulcer disease. The majority of these patients present with duodenal ulceration at the time of diagnosis.[9] The diagnosis of ZE syndrome is confirmed by measuring a fasting gastrin hormone greater than 100 pg/ml with a basal gastric acid output (BAO) of 15 meq/h or greater than 5 meq/h in patients with previous ulcer surgery.[9] Patients should not be using any antisecretory medications approximately 1 week before the test to prevent false-positive gastrin values. Fasting hypergastrinemia without elevated BAO can be seen in atrophic gastritis, renal failure, and patients taking H_2-receptor antagonists or proton pump inhibitors.[1] Furthermore, fasting hypergastrinemia with elevated BAO can be seen in retained gastric antrum syndrome, gastric outlet obstruction, and in antral G-cell hyperplasia. If the diagnosis remains uncertain, a secretin stimulation test can be performed. In this test, the diagnosis of ZE syndrome is confirmed with an increase in the serum gastrin level greater than 200 pg/ml after secretin administration.[13] Patients with other conditions do not have the gastrin elevation.

The majority of gastrinomas are slow growing tumors; however, 60% of these tumors may be malignant.[9] Two–thirds of the tumors are sporadic, with the remainder representing the familial form of the disease, specifically MEN-1 syndrome.[1] In this syndrome, gastrinomas can be multifocal with 50% of patients presenting with metastases to the lymph nodes, liver, or distant organs.[9] Hyperparathyroidism is the most common problem in this group of patients. When these patients have both hyperparathyroidism and ZE syndrome, it has been shown that resection of the parathyroid hyperplasia may reduce the hypergastinemia end organ effects.[2,9] As a result, when there is any question of MEN-1 syndrome, the patients should first be examined for hyperparathyroidism. Some of the gastrinoma tumors in patients with MEN-1 syndrome are not functional which can lead to a low cure rate. However, the 10-year survival rate is 90–100%.[9] Patients with MEN-1 syndrome have been shown to have a better 20-year survival compared to those patients with sporadic gastrinomas.[9]

Localization of the gastrinoma tumor can be very challenging. CT scan can be helpful but has difficulty in visualizing any tumors smaller than 1 cm.[9] The best imaging test is the somatostatin receptor scintigraphy which has a specificity of 80–95%.[6] Moreover, MRI, intraoperative and endoscopic ultrasound are also beneficial.

Though there are multiple choices in medical therapy for peptic ulcer disease, the treatment of gastrinoma remains surgical, offering potential cure. These patients should be treated with H_2-receptor antagonists or proton pump inhibitors preoperatively. The entire pancreas should be visualized to allow for bimanual palpation and intraoperative ultrasound. If there is difficulty in preoperative localization, one should examine the gastrinoma triangle, which consists of a line joining the cystic and common bile duct, the junction of the second and third portion of the duodenum, and the junction of the neck and body of the pancreas.[9] Approximately 80% of gastrinomas are located within this triangle. Moreover, a duodenotomy should be performed to better visualize and palpate the duodenum. Encapsulated tumors can be resected with enucleation; however, larger tumors may require a segmental resection such as a distal pancreactectomy or Whipple operation. If the gastrinoma is not located, which can occur in

5–8% of patients, a highly selective vagotomy should be performed.[9] Distant metastases are a large determinant of the 5-year survival, which approaches 40%.[9] These patients may also benefit from debulking large tumors; furthermore, resection of hepatic metastases may offer a survival advantage.

VASOACTIVE INTESTINAL PEPTIDE TUMOR

Vasoactive intestinal peptide tumor (VIPoma) normally presents with voluminous watery diarrhea (>1 L/ day), hypokalemia, and achlorohydria or hypochlorhydria with a slight female preponderance.[9] Fasting VIP levels greater than 200 pg/ml confirms the diagnosis of VIPoma.[1] Duodenal VIPomas have been reported; however, approximately 90% of these tumors arise in the tail of the pancreas.[9] These tumors are normally solitary and have an average size of 3 cm.[9] They can be localized with CT scan, and early metastases are common.

Preoperatively, these patients require fluid resuscitation to correct their electrolyte disorder. Treatment with octreotide can dramatically reduce the volume of diarrhea and serum VIP levels.[1] Intraoperative ultrasound is beneficial in locating these tumors as is bimanual pancreatic palpation.[9] A distal pancreatectomy is normally sufficient as the majority of these tumors are located in the tail of the pancreas. If the tumor is not located, examination of the retroperitoneum, adrenals, and autonomic chain is needed. Surgical debulking of unresectable disease assists in alleviating symptoms.[1]

GLUCAGONOMA

Glucagonoma tumors are quite rare representing only 0.2 cases per million per year.[9] Because of the excessive glucagon, the patients present with the "4D" syndrome: diabetes mellitus, deep vein thrombosis, depression, and dermatitis.[1] The dermatitis, a characteristic pruitic rash named necrolytic migratory erythema, results from an amino acid deficiency, zinc deficiency, or increased glucagon.[1] It is normally located in the pretibial, perioral, and intertriginous areas. Patients also report anemia, weight loss, painful glossitis, and pulmonary emboli.[9]

Diagnosis of glucagonoma is confirmed with an elevated serum glucagon level greater than 500 pg/ml.[1] Octreotide has been shown to be beneficial in reducing glucagon levels and improving malnutrition and rash.[9] The majority of these tumors present late and are, therefore, large and easily seen on CT scan. Furthermore, metastasis to the liver at presentation is common. Glucagonomas are almost always found within the tail of the pancreas.[9] As a result, a distal pancreatectomy with liver resection of metastases is normally the operative choice with only 30% of cases having a complete resection.[1]

SOMATOSTATINOMA

Somatostatinomas are rare tumors that can present with the even rarer somatostatinoma syndrome which consists of steatorrhea, cholelithiasis, diabetes mellitus, and achlorhydria.[1] Located in the head of the pancreas and duodenum, greater than 75% of these tumors present with early metastases.[9] Duodenal somatostatinomas are frequently seen in von Recklinghausen syndrome or VHL.[1] A pancreaticoduodenectomy is normally required for these tumors with no metastases. With a complete resection, the 5-year survival rate is 100%.[9] However, even with metastatic disease, the 5-year survival rate approaches 60%.[9]

NONFUNCTIONAL PNETs

The majority of PNETs are nonfunctional tumors.[1] These tumors do not produce hormones clinically, but they can release peptides, such as chromogranin A, pancreatic polypeptide, pancreastatin, and human chorionic gonadotropin.[1] Symptoms are normally a result of local invasion. Treatment is similar to the functional PNETs consisting of surgical resection and/or chemotherapy.[1]

ADVANCES IN TREATMENT OF PANCREATIC NEUROENDOCRINE TUMORS

The outcome of patients with malignant pancreatic neuroendocrine tumors who have failed current treatment has been dismal. In 2011, two teams of researchers have provided hope for this group of patients. One group of researchers studied the tyrosine kinase inhibitor, sunitinib. With a daily dose of 37.5 mg, the progression-free survival was 11.4 months as compared to 5.5 months in the placebo group.[14] This study was terminated early because of the increase in deaths and adverse events in the placebo group. A second group of researchers investigated the mTOR inhibitor, everolimus. The progression-free survival was 11 months in the treatment arm and 4.6 months in the placebo arm using a daily dose of 10 mg. Furthermore, at 18 months 34% of patients receiving everolimus had progression-free survival as compared to 9% in placebo.[15] Though these studies may lead to many questions, they offer optimism to patients with this difficult to treat disease.

REFERENCES

1. Batcher E, Gianoukakis A. Pancreatic neuroendocrine tumors. *Endocrine Research* 2011; 36(1):35–43.
2. Metz DC. Gastrointestinal neuroendocrine tumors: pancreatic endocrine tumors. *Gastroenterology* 2008; 135:1469–1492.
3. Asa SL. Pancreatic endocrine tumors. *Modern Pathology* 2011; 24:66–77.
4. Kimura W, Morioka Y. Clinical pathology of endocrine tumors of the pancreas. Analysis of autopsy cases. *Dig Dis Sci* 1991; 36:933–942.
5. Kulke MH, Picus J, Pommier R, et al. Evolving diagnostic and treatment strategies for pancreatic neuroendocrine tumors. *J Hematol Oncol* 2011; 4(29).
6. Tkacz, DHJN, et al. Gastroenteropancreatic neuroendocrine tumors: multimodality imaging features with pathological correlation. *Jpn J Radiol* 2011; 29:85–91.
7. Kloppel G, PA, Heitz PU. The gastroenteropancreatic neuroendocrine cell system and its tumors: the WHO classification. *Ann NY Acad Sci* 2004. 1014:13–27.
8. Edge SB, Carducci MA, et al. AJCC Cancer Staging Manual, 7th edition, New York, Springer. 2009.
9. Abood GJ, Malhotra D, Shoup M. The Surgical and Systemic Management of Neuroendocrine Tumors of the Pancreas. *Surg Clin N Am* 2009; 89:249–266.
10. Whipple AO, FV. Adenoma of islet cells with hyperinsulinism: a review. *Ann Surg* 1935; 101:1299–1335.
11. Goode PN, FJ, Anderson J, Johnston ID, et al. Diazoxide in the management of patients with insulinoma. *World J Surg* 1986; 10:586–592.
12. Sarmiento JM, HG, Rubin J, Ilstrup DM, et al. Surgical treatment of neuroendocrine metastases to the liver: a plea for resection to increase survival. *J Am Coll Surg* 2003; 197(1):29–37.
13. Berna MJ, HK, Serrano J, Gibril F, et al. Serum gastrin in Zollinger-Ellison syndrome: I. Prospective study of fasting serum gastrin in 309 patients from the

National Institutes of Health and comparison with 2229 cases from the literature. *Medicine,* 2006; 85:295–330.
14. Raymond E, Dahan L, Raoul J, *et al.* Sunitinib Malate for the Treatment of Pancreatic Neuroendocrine Tumors. *N Eng J Med,* 2011; 364(6):501–513.
15. Yao JC, Shah MH, Ito T, *et al.* Everolimus for Advanced Pancreatic Neuroendocrine Tumors. *N Eng J Med,* 2011; 364(6):514–523.

UNUSUAL PANCREATIC NEOPLASMS   42

James Padussis* and Douglas S. Tyler[†]

INTRODUCTION

Pancreatic ductal adenocarcinoma (PDA) accounts for the vast majority of all pancreatic neoplasms. Other frequently seen and well-described pancreatic neoplasms include pancreatic neuroendocrine tumors (PET) and cystic neoplasms of the pancreas. There are other distinctive neoplasms of the pancreas, however, which display a wide range of symptoms, biological behaviors, and outcomes. These include solid pseudopapillary tumors, acinar cell carcinoma, squamous cell carcinoma, pancreatic lymphoma, and metastatic lesions of the pancreas. These tumors are becoming more frequently documented in the literature and recognized more often, and at earlier stages, due to the increased sensitivity and utilization of diagnostic imaging. Therefore, the correct identification and treatment of these less common neoplasms of the pancreas is becoming increasingly important.

SOLID PSEUDOPAPILLARY TUMORS OF THE PANCREAS

Initially reported by Franz in 1959, solid pseudopapillary tumor (SPT) has historically been described by multiple names, most of which have been

---

*Duke Weight Loss Surgery Center, Durham, NC 27704 USA
[†]Duke University Medical Center 3118, Durham, NC 27710 USA

descriptive of the cystic and papillary nature of these tumors. In 1996, the World Health Organization classified these tumors as SPT and further defined malignant SPT as tumors with angioinvasion, perineural invasion, or deep invasion of the surrounding pancreatic parenchyma. The number of patients diagnosed with SPTs of the pancreas has increased over the last decade, which may be related to the improved characterization of the clinicopathologic features of these tumors.

SPTs account for 0.13–2.7% of pancreatic tumors and 5.54–12% of pancreatic cystic neoplasms. They typically occur in young women. In a review of 718 patients described in the literature over a 70-year period, more than 90% of affected patients were female, with a mean age at presentation of 22 years. Additionally, only 6% of patients were greater than age 50 and a disproportionate amount involved African–American and Asian women.

SPTs are generally of low malignant potential, and in the review by Papavramidis they found a 2- and 5-year survival rate of 97% and 95%, respectively. Metastases (5% to the liver) or local invasion into the duodenum, portal vein, or spleen were seen in 19.5%, whereas recurrent disease occurred in 6.6%. Despite metastases or locally advanced disease, patients may still experience long-term survival.

Patients with SPTs present with common but nonspecific abdominal complaints including discomfort, nausea, or an increase in abdominal girth. Tumors may also be discovered as a palpable mass on routine physical examination in the asymptomatic patient or incidentally on imaging studies performed for other indications. There have been rare reports of pancreatitis, bile duct obstruction, and tumor rupture with hemoperitoneum. Laboratory studies are often not helpful in diagnosis as it is uncommon for patients to have elevations in pancreatic or hepatic enzymes and tumor-specific serum markers have not been identified. Normal serum levels of alpha protein (AFP), carcinoembryonic antigen (CEA), carbohydrate antigen 19-9 (CA19-9), and cancer antigen 125 (CA-125) have been found in small series of patients.

SPTs may be found throughout the pancreas but are slightly more predominant in the pancreatic tail. They are usually larger than 6 cm at the time of diagnosis and may be as large as 30 cm. Findings on standard imaging studies are often characteristic of these tumors. Abdominal ultrasound shows a heterogeneous, encapsulated mass with solid echogenic and cystic hypoechoic components as well as peripheral calcifications, posterior enhancement, and displacement of surrounding structures. Computed tomography (CT) imaging shows a well-defined, low-attenuation mass with peripheral enhancement and complex cystic components with areas of necrosis and internal hemorrhage. Magnetic resonance imaging (MRI) shows variable signal intensity on T1-weighted images and high signal intensity on T2-weighted images.

Fine-needle aspiration cytology may be useful when routine imaging is inconclusive and diagnostic uncertainty exists. One circumstance in which this is especially important is when the differential diagnosis includes both SPTs and PETs and the tumor is large and bulky requiring a technically difficult or extended resection. In contrast to SPTs, preoperative tumor reduction may occur in PETs as the response rate to combination chemotherapy (5-flourouracil, doxorubicin, and streptozocin) is up to 39%. Characteristic cytologic features of SPTs include branching papillary fronds composed of fibrovascular stalks covered by cuboidal or cylindrical cells, high cellularity, uniform cellular appearance, intracytoplasmic inclusions, and nuclear folds. The immunohistochemical (IHC) staining pattern of these tumors is unlike that of any other pancreatic tumor. The majority of SPTs show staining for vimentin, neuron-specific enolase, CD10, CD56, and alpha-1 antitrypsin. Keratins, chromogranin, synaptophysin, endocrine, and pancreatic enzymes are generally not expressed or are found only focally allowing for differentiation from epithelial, neuroendocrine, and acinar cell tumors.

SPTs exhibit a genetic profile distinct from that of PDA. They do not contain mutations in *k-ras*, do not harbor genetic abnormalities in *DPC4*, and few have *p53* mutations. Moreover, unlike PDA, abnormalities of the adenomatous polyposis coli *(APC)*/β-catenin pathway have been shown in the majority of SPTs. Nuclear accumulation of β-catenin has been found in 95% to 100% of SPTs, with the majority having activating mutations in exon 3. Furthermore, cyclin D, a downstream effector of β-catenin, was over-expressed in over 50% of specimens analyzed, suggesting that aberrant cell cycle signaling through the APC/β-catenin pathway may be responsible for tumorigenesis in SPTs. Similar findings have also implicated this pathway in other tumor types including colorectal and gastric cancer.

Surgical resection is the mainstay of therapy, including the resection of adjacent organs or metastatic disease when possible. Pancreaticoduodenectomy or distal pancreatectomy is performed most commonly, although in Japan up to 35% of SPTs originating in the pancreatic head have been treated with enucleation. A minority of tumors present with lymph node metastases, and, therefore, complete lymphadenectomy may not be essential. More than 95% of patients with SPTs are cured with complete surgical resection, and the rate of recurrence is low. Metastatic disease may occur in up to 10–20% of patients. When present, metastases are most often identified in the liver, mesentery, and peritoneum. Limited data would suggest that metastasectomy can result in a favorable outcome, with some patients surviving greater than 5 years.

Because these tumors are so rare and surgical resection is generally successful, standard systemic treatment regimens have not been established. There are anecdotal case reports describing success with cisplatin, 5-fluorouracil, and gemcitabine whereas others have found no response to multiple agents. It has also been suggested that these tumors are radiosensitive, and there is one report of a patient with an unresectable tumor treated with 40 Gy over 6 weeks whose tumor responded; the patient remained asymptomatic at the 3-year follow-up. Although the majority of these tumors are considered to be of low malignant potential, a recent report of two cases of aggressive SPTs noted death of the patients at 6 and 16 months after diagnosis. In these cases, a high mitotic index and extensive tumor necrosis was noted. These findings might help distinguish a more virulent form of SPT and lead to a more aggressive postoperative treatment course.

ACINAR CELL CARCINOMA

Acinar cells make up the majority of the pancreas, yet acinar cell carcinoma (ACC) accounts for only 1–2% of all pancreatic tumors. ACC is characterized by the systemic release of pancreatic enzymes including trypsin, chymotrypsin, amylase, and lipase, although the serum levels are not always elevated. ACC is twice as common in men than women, and the disease usually occurs in the 5th to 7th decade of life, although there have been several case reports of ACC in children. Tumors tend to be uni-focal, slightly more predominant in the head of the pancreas and are often large at diagnosis, ranging from 10 to 15 cm in diameter. ACCs have an aggressive biological behavior with overall survival only slightly better than PDA. Metastatic disease is seen in up to 50% of patients at presentation, most commonly in the liver and lymph nodes.

Patients with ACC may be asymptomatic or may present with non-specific symptoms such as abdominal pain, bloating, postprandial vomiting, or a change in bowel habits. Presenting signs may include a palpable abdominal mass, elevated liver enzymes, and jaundice. The lipase hypersecretion syndrome is found in approximately 15% of patients and is a paraneoplastic syndrome characterized by subcutaneous nodules, eosinophilia, and arthralgias secondary to the hypersecretion of lipase. The subcutaneous nodules associated with this syndrome tend to be widely distributed, erythematous, and painful and may be misinterpreted as erythema nodosum or metastases. Often, the peripheral joints are involved secondary to periarticular fat necrosis.

There are no specific laboratory studies that are of high sensitivity for the diagnosis of ACC. Serum lipase levels are elevated in less than 25% of patients, and levels do not appear to correlate with extent of disease or prognosis. Serum tumor markers such as CA 19-9, AFP, and CEA are variably expressed. Serum AFP, when elevated, does not predict the development of liver metastases but is useful for diagnosis and as a marker for evaluating recurrent disease and response to treatment.

Although imaging studies are not diagnostic of ACC, these tumors are often exophytic, hypovascular, and well marginated on CT scan and MRI. Chiou *et al.* evaluated the clinical and radiologic manifestations of 10 patients with ACC and found a well-defined capsule in 6, internal foci of calcifications in 5, and a central hypodense area in 8. PDA rarely have calcifications (2%) and do not commonly have a central hypodensity; therefore, a diagnosis of ACC should be considered in patients with these radiographic findings. Other pancreatic tumors with a central hypodense area on imaging include neuroendocrine tumors, which are usually hypervascular, or SPTs, which tend to be more heterogeneous and complex. Intratumoral hemorrhage makes the diagnosis of ACC less likely.

Cytologically, ACC consists of highly cellular, loosely cohesive clusters of cells, usually with the characteristic acinar formation. The tumor cells have abundant granular cytoplasm with prominent nucleoli. Although FNA biopsy can usually differentiate PDA from ACC, in small studies it has been difficult to separate ACCs from PETs based on cytology alone. However, if there is adequate tissue, IHC studies can assist in the differentiation of ACC from other pancreatic tumors. These tumors show a unique IHC staining pattern for products of exocrine pancreatic secretion including trypsin, lipase, amylase, phospholipase, and chymotrypsin. Furthermore, most tumors stain diffusely for AAT and do not stain for CEA and mucicarmine, which distinguishes them from PDA. Unlike typical pancreatic adenocarcinoma, the genetic mutations in K-*ras*, *p*53, and S*mad* are uncommonly found but there seem to be alterations in the adenomatous polyposis coli-*b*-catenin pathway, similar to colorectal cancer.

Surgery is the treatment of choice for ACC if the tumor is localized and resectable. In the most comprehensive series to date reported by Holen *et al.*, 39 patients treated for ACC had a median survival of 19 months. There is clearly a stage-specific survival with more advanced disease associated with a worse prognosis. In the same series, the 16 patients with localized resectable disease had a median survival of 38 months, whereas the 19 patients with metastatic disease survived only 14 months. Unfortunately, those who underwent surgical resection had a high rate of recurrence; of 18 patients who underwent surgery with curative intent, 13 (72%) recurred, including 5 (56%) of 9 after an R0 resection and 3 (75%) of 4 after an R1 resection. Most recurrences occurred at distant sites, suggesting that local control can be achieved, but hematogenous metastases drive the poor prognosis.

The aggressive natural history of ACC and the frequent finding of distant metastases suggest that systemic therapy is a logical treatment approach. There are case reports of mixed success with various chemotherapeutic agents, the most commonly used being 5-flourouracil, streptozocin, cisplatin, and doxorubicin. However, no single regimen has proved most successful.

PRIMARY LYMPHOMA OF THE PANCREAS

Primary pancreatic lymphoma (PPL) is exceedingly rare, comprising less than 0.5% of pancreatic tumors. The majority of PPLs are diffuse large-cell lymphomas of intermediate to high grade. The disease occurs more often in men than women and usually presents in the 5th to 6th decade of life. PPL should be differentiated from secondary involvement of the pancreas by lymphoma, which may occur in up to one-third of patients with non-Hodgkin's lymphoma.

Unfortunately, the clinical presentation will usually not accurately distinguish those patients with PPL from other types of pancreatic masses because B-type symptoms such as fever and night sweats are uncommon. Patients may present with nonspecific complaints of abdominal pain, weight loss, nausea, and vomiting. Jaundice, pancreatitis, diarrhea, gastric outlet obstruction, and small bowel obstruction have also been reported. Laboratory studies are often nondiagnostic. Both pancreatic enzymes and markers of hepatic function may be abnormal. Serum levels of lactate dehydrogenase (LDH) may be elevated in up to 50% of cases, and increases in CA 19-9 may also occasionally be associated with PPL.

CT imaging often reveals a large, homogenous pancreatic head mass with or without associated lymphadenopathy. Extrapancreatic extension is common, and the tumors may encroach on the mesenteric vessels. Less commonly, there may be a mass in the body or tail of the pancreas, and, rarely, there is diffuse involvement of the entire pancreas. Although difficult to differentiate from PDA, lymphoma should be suspected in the presence of a large bulky tumor with rapid growth and/or the presence of multifocal regional adenopathy.

FNA biopsy can be performed under EUS guidance; however, an expert cytopathologist will be needed to secure a diagnosis of PPL. Biopsies show hypercellular specimens with discohesive cells with round nuclei, prominent nucleoli, mitoses, karyorrhexis, and a monoclonal pattern of immunoglobulin light-chain expression by flow cytometry. Immunophenotyping with a panel of IHC antibodies including CD 20 also help with diagnosis.

In patients with a pancreatic mass, the diagnosis of PPL is crucial because chemotherapy, not surgery, is the cornerstone of treatment. The most common chemotherapeutic regimen includes cyclophosphamide, doxorubicin, vincristine, and prednisone. Complete remission can be expected with multidrug chemotherapy in 63–77% of patients with diffuse large B-cell lymphoma. More recently, rituximab (a monoclonal antibody directed against the CD 20 antigen) has been combined with cyclophosphamide, doxorubicin, vincristine, and prednisone resulting in improved response rates of up to 85% and long-term survival for patients with diffuse large B-cell lymphomas. Furthermore, radiolabeled antibodies (90 Y-Ibritumomab and 131 I-tositumomab) are now in clinical trials and may contribute to better outcomes.

Surgery may be indicated when a preoperative diagnosis cannot be made or if treatment with chemotherapy/chemo-radiation therapy is not successful. Some authors have argued that pancreatectomy in conjunction with adjuvant chemotherapy and radiation therapy may improve survival in patients with resectable PPL as the morbidity of pancreatectomy continues to decrease. However, with newer systemic agents, the potential benefits of surgery are likely to be quite modest.

METASTATIC LESIONS OF THE PANCREAS

Although uncommon, the pancreas may serve as a site for distant metastases and when these metastases present as an isolated pancreatic mass, questions regarding diagnosis and treatment may arise. Almost any tumor type may metastasize to the pancreas, but in an analysis in an autopsy database, the majority of tumors found were lymphomas, and carcinomas of the stomach, kidney, and lung. A review of resection for metastases to the pancreas found renal cell carcinoma to be the most frequent primary histopathology (62%), followed by non-small cell lung cancer, melanoma, and sarcoma. In this series, postoperative morbidity was 25%, mortality was 6%. The median survival of patients with resected pancreatic metastases from solid tumor sites other than renal cell carcinoma (RCC) is approximately 2 years, whereas those with resected RCC have a 5-year survival of 68% to 75%.

The prolonged disease free interval between the initial cancer and pancreatic recurrence can be quite prolonged (median 2.6–7.5 years). Hiotis *et al.* found that approximately one-third of the metastatic tumors evaluated were clinically suspected to be primary pancreatic neoplasms. The clinical presentation is similar to other pancreatic tumor types with potential for pain, jaundice, nausea/vomiting, weight loss, and gastrointestinal hemorrhage. These findings demonstrate the difficulty in diagnosing pancreatic metastases and emphasize the need to consider metastatic disease to the pancreas in the workup of any pancreatic tumor and particularly in patients with a history of prior malignancy.

Metastatic RCC appears on CT scans as a large hypervascular spherical mass with well-defined margins and a central area of low attenuation, which can be confused with other hypervascular lesions of the pancreas such as PET but is easily differentiated from the hypodense PDA. A tissue biopsy is helpful if the diagnosis is uncertain, the patient has a history of non-RCC malignancy, or a nonoperative approach is planned. In the majority of patients with a history of RCC, the CT findings are so characteristic that a biopsy is often unnecessary.

Most patients with pancreatic metastases likely possess additional sites of disease even if not apparent on physical examination. Therefore, a thorough staging evaluation should be performed in all patients with suspected or biopsy-proven metastatic disease to the pancreas. Patients with isolated RCC metastases may experience a prolonged disease-free course after pancreatectomy. Retrospective reviews suggest that resection of RCC metastatic to the pancreas can greatly benefit a carefully selected group of patients, and 5-year survivals of up to 75% have been shown even in the presence of synchronous metastatic disease in other sites. The goal of therapy should be complete tumor resection with negative margins and preservation of pancreatic parenchyma when possible to prevent insulin dependence.

In conclusion, the most common neoplasm affecting the pancreas is ductal adenocarcinoma but there are a host of less common pancreatic neoplasms with distinct clinical and biological behaviors. Although relatively rare, more of these lesions will be seen as diagnostic imaging continues to become more frequent and sensitive. Accurate and timely identification of a pancreatic neoplasm coupled with a knowledge of its biological behavior and therapy will be essential in order to offer patients the optimal therapy.

PANCREAS AND ISLET CELL TRANSPLANTATION 43

Keri E. Lunsford* and
Bradley H. Collins*

CLINICAL PROBLEM OF DIABETES MELLITUS

Diabetes mellitus poses an increasing public health threat worldwide. In 2007, the Center for Disease Control and Prevention listed diabetes as the third leading cause of disease and the seventh leading cause of death in the United States. The American Diabetes Association estimates that almost 26 million people have some form of diabetes in the United States, accounting for more than $116 billion in healthcare service costs annually [National Diabetes Fact Sheet, 2011]. The majority of these costs result from inpatient care of diabetic patients who account for more that 4 million hospital visits and 25 million days of hospital stay each year. Specifically, Type I diabetes mellitus, due to irreversible autoimmune destruction of pancreatic β cells, accounts for 5–10% or all cases of diabetes. Normal control of glucose homeostasis is, thus, replaced by daily monitoring of blood glucose and exogenous administration of insulin.

Despite insulin therapy for diabetic patients, persistent metabolic derangements, particularly persistent hyperglycemia, result in serious long-term complications. These complications are responsible for the high rate of morbidity and mortality and increasing costs of medical treatment of diabetic patients. Persistent hyperglycemia results in microangiopathy due

---

*Duke University Medical Center, Department of Surgery, Durham, NC 27710 USA

to glycosylation of nucleic acids, lipids, and collagen in blood vessel walls. Eventually, microangiopathy causes end-organ damage, including cardiovascular disease, cerebral vascular disease, nephropathy, retinopathy, and peripheral vascular disease.

In 1993, the Diabetes Control and Complications Trial (DCCT) Research Group reported that tight control of blood glucose through multiple daily injections of insulin decreases and delays long-term complications in Type I Diabetes by 35–70%.[1] Thus, in current treatment protocols for Type I diabetes mellitus, a major objective is stringent glycemic control. Despite the significant decrease in long-term complications of diabetes offered by tight glucose regulation, increased control of blood glucose is associated with a greater than threefold increased risk of hypoglycemic episodes, including both seizures and coma. This risk is compounded by the absence of autonomic symptoms associated with falling blood glucose or "hypoglycemic unawareness". Hypoglycemic unawareness occurs because the physiologic changes associated with diabetes lower the threshold for autonomic symptoms in response to hypoglycemia. Thus, despite the beneficial effects of intensive insulin therapy, hypoglycemic unawareness remains one of the most frightening and immediately life-threatening complications of diabetes. Exogenous insulin therapy remains the major therapeutic option for the treatment of diabetes, but it does not completely substitute for the glycemic control afforded by native pancreatic islets.

CLINICAL TRANSPLANTATION FOR THE TREATMENT OF TYPE 1 DIABETES MELLITUS

Currently, pancreatic β cell replacement therapy offers the only definitive cure for Type I diabetes. This can be accomplished either through transplantation of the whole pancreas or through transplantation of isolated pancreatic islet cells. Since the first vascularized whole pancreas transplant in December of 1966 by Drs. Richard Lillehei and William Kelly at the University of Minnesota, pancreas transplantation has evolved from a highly experimental procedure with a high rate of failure to a commonly performed procedure with excellent long-term outcomes. From 2000 to 2005, vascularized whole pancreas transplants had 1- and 5-year graft survivals of 80.1% and 50.6% when transplanted alone and 86.2% and 72.5% when performed in combination with kidney transplanta. Despite the relatively high success rate of pancreas transplantation, this major surgical procedure is performed in a physiologically compromised patient population and is associated with significant morbidity and mortality. Combined kidney and pancreas transplantation (or pancreas transplant alone) in Type I diabetic patients significantly decreases the risk of diabetic nephropathy in renal allografts or native kidneys and increases the general health of recipients by preventing and even reversing progression of diabetic sequellae. Thus, the risks of the major surgical procedure combined with the relative shortage of acceptable donor pancreata provide the major barriers for pancreas transplantation as a widespread cure for Type I diabetes mellitus.

Since the mid-1960s and the first report of pancreatic islet isolation and transplantation in rats, the transplantation of isolated pancreatic islets of Langerhans has been considered a potential therapeutic modality and cure for Type I diabetes mellitus. Similar to vascularized pancreas transplantation, pancreatic islet transplantation replaces the patient's physiologic glucose control and insulin production that is lost due to the pathology of Type I diabetes. In addition, islet cell transplantation is relatively non-invasive as it is performed by either percutaneous or open portal venous injection with subsequent islet engraftment in the liver. Under current protocols, the procedure is usually performed multiple times in order to achieve the optimal mass of islets required for successful reversal of diabetes.

Clinical studies have shown a slow reversal of long-term diabetic sequellae following whole organ pancreas transplantation. However, long-term sequellae of IDDM are often extensive by the time the risks of surgical intervention are justified. Theoretically, this reversal of long-term diabetic sequellae also applies to transplantation of isolated pancreatic islet cells. Animal models demonstrate that islet transplantation prevents and in some cases even reverses long-term complications of IDDM, such as diabetic retinopathy, nephropathy, and neuropathy. Clinical trails have also shown a decrease in diabetic vasculopathy resulting from successful islet transplantation. As pancreatic islet cell transplantation is much less invasive than whole pancreas transplantation, earlier intervention could theoretically be justified, thus preventing long-term complications of diabetes.

CLINICAL PANCREAS TRANSPLANTATION

Indications for Transplantation

Transplantation of vascularized pancreas allografts is currently the treatment of choice for endocrine cell replacement therapy and offers the

Table 1. Reason for pancreatic transplantation.[a]

Reason for transplantation	% of pancreas transplants
Type I diabetes mellitus	83.0%
Type II Diabetes mellitus	4.7%
Retransplant/allograft failure	4.0%
Pancreatectomy prior to pancreas transplant	0.1%
Diabetes secondary to chronic pancreatitis without	< 0.1%
Diabetes secondary to cystic fibrosis without pancreatectomy	< 0.1%
Pancreatic cancer	< 0.1%
Bile duct cancer	< 0.1%
Other cancers	< 0.1%
Other/Not reported	5.6%

[a] Data according to the Organ Procurement and Transplantation Database for all pancreas transplants occurring between January 1, 1988 and October 31, 2009.

only current definitively curative option for patients with Type I diabetes mellitus. Unlike transplantation of the liver, heart, or lungs, pancreas transplantation is not a life-saving procedure. It can, however, significantly improve the quality of life of diabetic patients. In addition, patients with extremely brittle diabetes benefit as life-threatening hypoglycemic unawareness is no longer factor.

The most frequent indication for pancreas transplantation is Type 1 diabetes. Of the 23,055 pancreas transplants performed between 1988 and 2009, 83% of patients had Type 1 diabetes mellitus. Currently, however, eight indications are recognized for pancreas transplant (Table 1). Among these, the most second common reason for pancreas transplant is Type 2 diabetes mellitus. Studies evaluating efficacy of pancreas transplantation for Type 2 diabetics suggest achievement of long-term normoglycemia in these patients.[2] This has led advocates to promote pancreas transplantation for Type 2 diabetics; however, studies are largely retrospective and underpowered. Further evaluation is necessary before Type 2 diabetes is accepted as an absolute indication for pancreas transplantation.

Due to operative morbidity and risks of immunosuppression, the vast majority of pancreas transplants are performed in combination with kidney allografts. Pancreas transplantation benefits uremic type I diabetic patients with secondary sequellae of diabetes mellitus (retinopathy, vasculopathy, and neuropathy) or patients with hypoglycemic unawareness. Specifically, diabetic patients with a glomulorular filtration rate (GFR) less then 20 mL/min/1.73 m^2 are generally candidates for kidney–pancreas transplantation. In most cases, a single decreased donor serves as the source for both the kidney and pancreas allograft (CPK: combined pancreas-kidney). In cases where a living donor is available, a kidney from a living donor may be transplanted either simultaneously with a deceased donor pancreas, or more commonly, pancreas transplantation occurs after kidney transplantation (PAK: pancreas-after-kidney). Living donor partial pancreas transplant techniques have also been described, but due to donor operative morbidity, the practice is not common.

For nonuremic diabetic patients with severe hypoglycemic unawareness but minimal proteinurea and stable renal function, pancreas transplantation alone (PTA) is an option. The need for future renal transplantation is unlikely in patients with glomulorular filtration rates (GFR) of 80–100 mL/min/1.73 m^2; however, the cumulative effects of immunosuppression with calcineurin inhibitors is an independent risk factor for deterioration of renal function posttransplant. Thirty percent of PTA recipients require a future renal transplant given approximately 10 years of exposure to immunosuppressants. In addition, cumulative allograft and patient survival for PTA is inferior to that observed for CPK. Thus, PTA is generally reserved for select candidates.

Donor Considerations

Deceased donors

Because pancreas transplantation is not a life-saving operation, surgeons exhibit considerable caution when evaluating deceased donors. Fairly young donors are preferred (<50 years of age) because pancreatic fibrosis can occur with aging. Trauma victims with evidence of upper abdominal injury, such as a retroperitoneal hematoma, usually are not considered because possible pancreatic parenchymal or duodenal injury that could result in fatal recipient complications. Prolonged donor hypotension and use of high doses of vasopressors are relative contraindications due to possibility of postoperative pancreatitis. Massive donor resuscitation can result in pancreatic edema, the identification of which during organ recovery usually leads to turning down of the pancreas for whole organ transplantation; however, these organs may be used for islet cell harvest. Abnormalities found during organ recovery such as induration or glandular calcifications are also relative contraindications. Absolute contraindications to pancreas recovery include donor sepsis, an active malignancy (except controlled, non-melanoma skin cancers), and HIV.

Living donor

Although not common, partial pancreata may be obtained from living donors. Donors who are less then 50 years old, with high β cell reserve, and low body-mass index (BMI <27 kg/m^2) may be considered as appropriate donors. Adequate β cell reserve of the donor should be assessed by demonstrating a greater than threefold increase in serum insulin concentrations with arginine and glucose stimulation tests.

Pre-Operative Recipient Evaluation

Candidates for pancreas transplantation undergo rigorous preoperative evaluation and cardiac risk stratification. The patient's age, BMI, past medical history, past surgical history, and social history should be evaluated. Evaluation of past medical history should include determination of coronary artery disease as well as of long-term sequellae of diabetes. History of malignancy in the past 5 years or of substance abuse within <6 months are absolute contraindications. Ideal candidates have a BMI less than 30 kg/m^2. Patients of any age may be eligible, providing their comorbidities are not contraindicative. In general, allograft rejection rates are lower in older than younger recipients; however, postoperative complications increase in patients over 50 years.

The most common causes for postoperative morbidity following pancreas transplantation are cardiac complications and postoperative infection. At a minimum, recipients without history of cardiac disease should undergo a routine ECG and echocardiogram or exercise-stress testing. However, asymptomatic diabetic patients with end-stage renal disease (ESRD) have a 40% prevalence of coronary artery disease (CAD), and the 2-year cardiac and all-cause mortality of diabetic patients with CAD is worse than in their nondiabetic counterparts.[3] Risk of asymptomatic CAD is greatest in diabetic, Caucasian patients with ESRD who have a smoking history, who are older than 47 years old, and with a BMI >25.[4]

Transplant candidates with these risk factors may best be served by undergoing pre-emptive preoperative cardiac catheterization with possible intervention.

Operative Techniques

A variety of surgical techniques for vascularized whole pancreas transplantation exist, and the technical aspects of the procedure are covered in detail in Chapter 51. Donor pancreata are recovered as part of the multivisceral organ harvest from a deceased donor. Following the exposure of the infrarenal and suprahepatic aorta, the superior mesenteric artery (SMA) is exposed and encircled with heavy umbilical tape. The lesser sac is entered and the pancreas is inspected. The donor pancreas should ideally be free of fatty infiltration, hematoma, calcifications, or excessive edema. The duodenum is flushed with antibiotic-iodine–containing solution. Aortic and portal cannulation (via the inferior mesenteric vein, IMV) is performed, and the vascular system is rapidly flushed with cold perfusate. After approximately 1L of cold perfusate has been flushed through the aorta, the ligatures on the SMA are tightened to avoid excessive distention of the pancreas. The duodenum is stapled proximally just below the pylorus and distally below the pancreatic head. As perfusion is completed and the portal vein is transected, the pancreas is sharply divided from its retroperitoneal attachments, using the spleen as a handle to avoid manipulation of the pancreas. The IMV is ligated near the inferior border of the pancreas, and the SMA is divided near its origin at the aorta. The organ is then packed for transport on ice in cold perfusion solution along with the harvested donor's iliac artery and vein, which are used in back-table donor organ preparation.

Prior to transplantation, meticulous back-table preparation of the donor pancreas is required. The spleen is removed, and the pancreas is divested of excess fat. The pancreas vasculature is reconstructed with a Y-graft of the donor internal iliac artery anastomosed to the SMA and donor external iliac artery anastomosed to the splenic artery in order to create a single arterial inflow tract to the pancreas. The duodenal staple lines are oversewn for additional reinforcement against leakage.

Many variations for pancreas implantation exist; however, these all seek to address the vascular inflow and outflow and the exocrine drainage of the pancreas. The pancreas may be placed intraperitoneally or extraperitoneally in the iliac fossa. Vascular inflow and outflow is established with the systemic circulation (generally via the right iliac artery and vein) or via the portal circulation (generally via a tributary of the portal vein). Theoretically, drainage via the systemic circulation circumvents the first-pass metabolism of insulin by the liver, resulting in systemic hyperinsulinemia. This may result in accelerated atherosclerosis by increasing systemic LDL and VLDL levels; however, the effect has not been proven. Portal venous drainage of the pancreas results in more physiologic insulin levels. Exocrine pancreatic drainage is established either by enteric or bladder anastomosis. Bladder drainage is established via duodenocystostomy and has the benefits of allowing for early detection of graft rejection through monitoring of urinary amylase. In addition, the pancreas may be placed totally extraperitoneal; however, recipients are prone to excessive loss of bicarbonate and must be carefully monitored for dehydration. Patients are also prone to cystitis and urethritis due to the irritating effects of pancreatic secretions. Alternatively, the pancreas may be drained enterically, via a duodenojejunostomy, duodenoiliestomy, or Roux-en-Y duodenojejunostomy. This allows for enteric reabsorption of pancreatic secretions; however, detection of allograft malfunction may be delayed.

Immunosuppressive Therapies

Transplantation of the pancreas requires implantation of the C loop of the duodenum to facilitate the management of exocrine secretions. The intestine is generally considered more immunogenic than other solid organs due to its lymphocyte burden, so the trend has been to utilize fairly rigorous recipient immune suppression. Patients are generally induced with anti-CD25 monoclonal antibody (e.g. daclizumab, basiliximab). Polyclonal preparations such as rabbit anti-thymocyte globulin are also utilized. Recipients receive bolus corticosteroids prior to surgery. Triple maintenance immunosuppression is standard and includes a calcineurin inhibitor (tacrolimus or cyclosporine), an antimetabolite (mycophenolate), and low-dose prednisone. Some centers employ steroid-sparing protocols to limit effects of chronic corticosteroids.

Adequate immune system suppression is more art than science, and clinicians seek to achieve a balance that prevents rejection, but does not induce significant infectious complications. Serum levels of calcinuerin inhibitors are useful in dosing; while, antimetabolites are often dosed by side effects.

Post-Operative Monitoring of Allograft Function

Following transplantation, pancreas transplant recipients are monitored closely in an ICU or step-down unit. Pancreas allograft function may be assessed by serial blood glucose measurements. After discontinuation of insulin infusion and establishment of euglycemia post-transplant, any elevated blood glucose level results in investigation for causes of allograft dysfunction, including graft thrombosis, anastomotic leak, or acute rejection. Imaging studies are urgently performed to evaluate for surgical complications. Ultrasound evaluation of the transplanted organ can provide rapid insight into the vascular flow of the organ and must be considered at onset of any postoperative derangement. If the patient is a CPK recipient, creatinine elevation may provide insight into early rejection. This may be monitored by percutaneous renal biopsy. If PTA or PAK was performed, percutaneous pancreas biopsy may be required. Unfortunately, early rejection events are usually asymptomatic and go undetected until they proceed to overt hyperglycemia and immunologic islet destruction. Bladder drainage does allow for earlier detection of allograft rejection through monitoring of urinary amylase levels; however, the procedure has fallen out of favor due to associated complications.

The ability to monitor the immune status of a patient following the transplantation of any solid organ continues to be a problem in the clinical setting. Allograft acceptance or rejection is generally monitored by assessment of the functional status of the graft. These measurements are often not very sensitive to ongoing immunologic damage to the allograft. A significant amount of immune damage may occur before clinically detectable functional deterioration is evident. Investigations of peripheral immune monitoring for solid organ allografts has yielded some promising results for the forewarning of acute rejection responses. These include monitoring of cytokine production by peripheral blood leukocytes, monitoring of alloantibody production, and measurements of cellular immune activation. Early detection of immunologic graft loss requires additional study in order to minimize graft damage through the early treatment of asymptomatic rejection.

Table 2. Major procedure-related complications following pancreas transplant.

Complication following pancreas transplantation
Anastomotic leak
Arterial or venous thrombosis
Bleeding
Allograft pancreatitis
Infection
Malignancy
Acute rejection
Chronic rejection
Drug toxicity

Clinical Complications

Although the overall morbidity of pancreas transplantation has declined with improved immunosuppressive and antibiotic therapy, pancreas transplantation is prone to technical complications and failure. In fact, the rate of technical complications is generally felt to be higher with pancreas transplantation than with most other vascularized solid organ allografts. Complications for pancreas transplantation include thrombosis, pancreatitis, anastomotic leak, rejection, infection, and bleeding (Table 2).

Graft thrombosis

Graft thrombosis is one of the most devastating events that can occur following pancreas transplantation. Donor factors, such as prolonged cold ischemia time, old age, and death due to cerebrovascular accident, as well as recipient factor, such as pancreatitis, rejection, hypotension, and ischemia-reperfusion injury, can contribute to the genesis of allograft thrombosis. Thrombosis may occur in either the arterial or the venous system. Arterial thrombosis of the SMA is heralded by painless rising serum glucose combined with falling serum amylase. This generally results in nonviability of the duodenal segment. Graft removal is often required following SMA thrombosis, even if the splenic artery remains patent. Venous thrombosis results in pancreatic swelling and symptomatic abdominal pain. Biochemical derangements include elevation in both serum glucose and amylase. Ultrasound evaluation of the transplanted pancreas is useful for the detection of both arterial and venous thrombosis. In the case of arterial thrombosis, arterial flow is not detectable. Venous thrombosis is suggested by high pancreatic arterial resistive indices in the absence of detectable venous flow. The incidence of pancreatic thrombosis may be decreased by routine perioperative anticoagulation; however, this results in an increased risk of postoperative bleeding complications.

Allograft pancreatitis

Allograft pancreatitis is generally a mild and self-limited complication resulting from ischemia-reperfusion injury or pancreatic handling. However, similar to pancreatitis in the naïve pancreas, the sequellae may be severe. It presents as peripancreatic pain and transient serum amylase elevation. Treatment is generally supportive; however, peripancreatic fluid collections, necrosis, superinfections, or fistulas may develop in severe pancreatitis. Drainage or debridement may become necessary should these complications develop. In bladder-drained recipients, post-transplant pancreatitis may also be caused by urinary reflux into the pancreatic duct. Cases not responsive to supportive therapy with self-catheterization and alpha-adrenergic therapy may require enteric conversion.

Anastomotic leak

Anastomotic leakage is a potentially life-threatening complication. The leakage of enterically drained pancreata has the potential for intraperitoneal spillage of enteric contents, and typically presents and fever, leukocytosis, and abdominal pain without alterations in glucose homeostasis. Peripancreatic abscesses or pancreaticocutaneous fistulae may result. Early leakage after transplant is typically a result of technical complications or duodenal segment ischemia; whereas, late leaks result from rejection, infection, or ischemia. Early treatment with broad-spectrum antibiotics, including fungal coverage, is critical, and surgical exploration should be performed. Intraoperative management may include combination of wide drainage, primary repair, and Roux diversion or transplant pancreatectomy. In the case of bladder drainage, leaks will typically present in the first 3 months's following transplant, and two-thirds will respond to prolonged bladder drainage with a foley catheter. Resistant cases require anastomotic revision or enteric conversion.

Bleeding

Gastrointestinal bleeding following pancreas transplant typically results from duodenal mucosa reperfusion injury or from a bleeding vessel at the staple line. Perioperative anticoagulation may exacerbate bleeding; however, discontinuation of the anticoagulant is often effective. Patients with enteric drainage present with melanotic stools, and patients with bladder drainage demonstrate hematuria.

Clinical Outcomes

The survival advantage afforded by pancreatic transplantation has been the subject of considerable recent debate. The most recent data from the U.S. Organ Procurement and Transplantation Network and the Scientific Registry of Transplant Recipients reports 10 year unadjusted patient survival as 70.1% for CPK, 65.4% for PAK, and 73.3% for PTA and 10 year unadjusted pancreatic allograft survival as 52.9% for CPK, 34.6% for PAK and 26.3% for PTA (Figure 1). The most common cause of allograft loss after 10 years was the death of the recipient (53%) followed by chronic allograft rejection (33%).[5] CPK transplantation appears to afford a 60% survival advantage to Type I diabetic patients when compared to diabetic recipients of kidney transplant alone.[6] Furthermore, CPK transplant recipients are estimated to have a lifetime gain of 15 years over Type I diabetic patients on the waiting list for a transplant.[7]

It is unclear, however, whether patient survival is improved by CPK over living donor kidney transplant alone. Recipients of living donor kidney transplants have similar patient and superior kidney allograft survival rates compared to CPK recipients; however, both patient and graft survival are worse for recipients of deceased donor kidney transplants compared to CPK transplantation.[8] Thus, it may be preferable to perform living-related kidney transplantation should a suitable donor be available to avoid the morbidity and mortality associated with the wait for a CPK.

In comparison to CPK transplant, PTA into nonuremic diabetic recipients results in significant risks of morbidity and mortality to the recipient without clear-cut to long-term survival advantages. Several studies have evaluated the effect of PTA on long-term patient survival. A study by

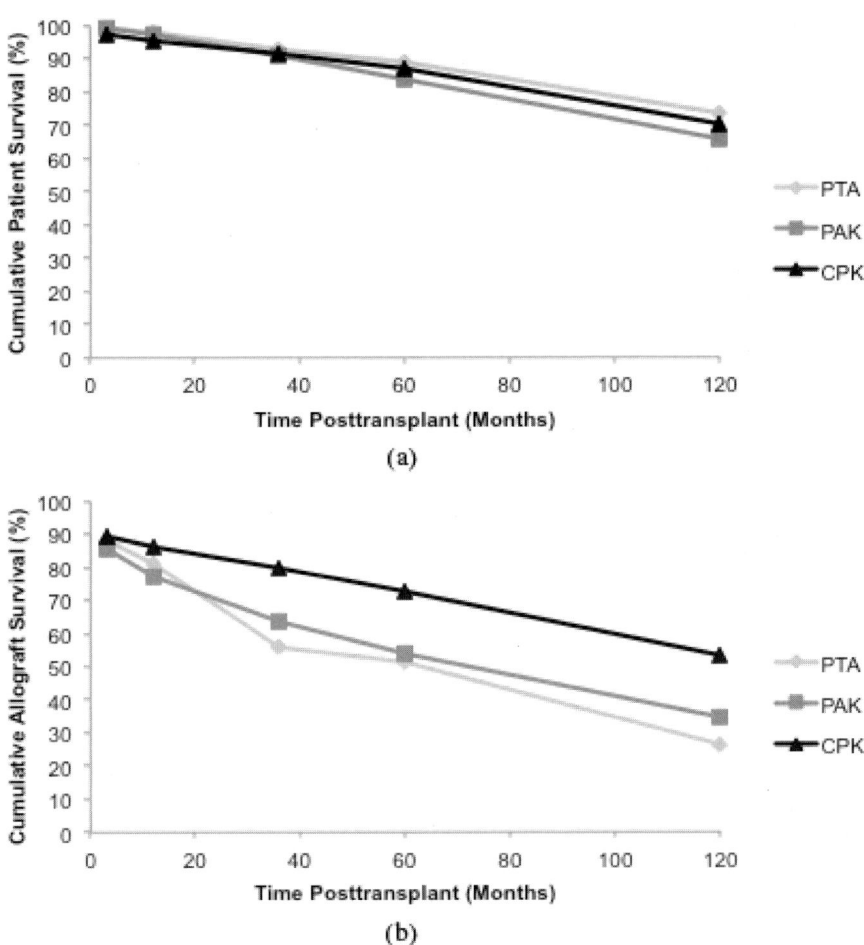

Figure 1. Patient and pancreatic allograft survival following pancreatic transplantation. (a) Patient survival and (b) pancreas allograft survival from decreased donors. Primary pancreas transplants from deceased donors during Jan 1, 1997, to Dec 31, 2006. PAK, pancreas after kidney transplantation; PTA, pancreas transplantation alone; CPK, combine pancreas and kidney transplantation. Data as reported by the U.S. Organ Procurement and Transplantation Network and the Scientific Registry of Transplant Recipients.

Venstrom *et al.* found that pancreas transplant alone increased mortality in comparison to diabetic patients awaiting transplantation receiving conventional insulin therapy.[9] However, significant bias may have resulted from patients who were listings at several transplant centers. A second study by Gruessner *et al.* accounted for the problem of multiple listings in the data by counting these patients only once. Through analysis of the 4-year survival data, they found that mortality was not increased by PTA, PAK, or CPK in comparison to nonuremic diabetic patients. Only survival of patients receiving CPK, however, was improved.[10] Thus, although there is no definitive advantage over conventional insulin therapy for pancreas transplant in nonuremic diabetic patients, the treatment remains the primary therapy available to achieve durable insulin independence in this patient population. Patients with extremely brittle diabetes should be considered for the procedure.

CLINICAL ISLET TRANSPLANTATION

Unlike vascularized pancreas transplantation, pancreatic islet transplantation is a minimally invasive alternative that can theoretically replace the patient's physiologic glucose homeostasis mechanisms. Despite the initial advent of experimental islet transplant techniques in the 1960s and the first successful human islet transplant in 1974 at the University of Minnesota, initial clinical results with islet transplantation were dismal. Between 1990 and 1999, 1-year pancreatic islet cell allograft survival was limited to 8%. The failure of clinical islet transplantation was attributed to (1) the use of diabetogenic agents such as glucocorticoids for immunosuppression, (2) primary early loss of transplanted islet mass, (3) high metabolic demands on transplanted islets, and (4) recurrence of autoimmunity.

More recent advances in islet isolation and purification have increased the number, purity, and viability of islets available for transplantation. In 1999, the Edmonton trial utilized high-dose, corticosteroid-free immunosuppression in combination with the infusion of multiple doses of islets heterotopically engrafted to the liver. This resulted in a majority of patients remaining insulin independent at one year post-transplant.[11] One of the major barriers to short-term islet allograft survival prior to this study was the diabetogenic effect of immunosuppressive therapies. The steroid-free immunosuppressive therapy with tacrolimus and sirolimus used in the Edmonton trial demonstrated substantially less toxicity to transplanted islets and, therefore, minimized the incidence of early islet allograft failure.

The advent of this protocol and the promising short-term clinical outcomes stimulated resurgence in interest in clinical pancreatic islet

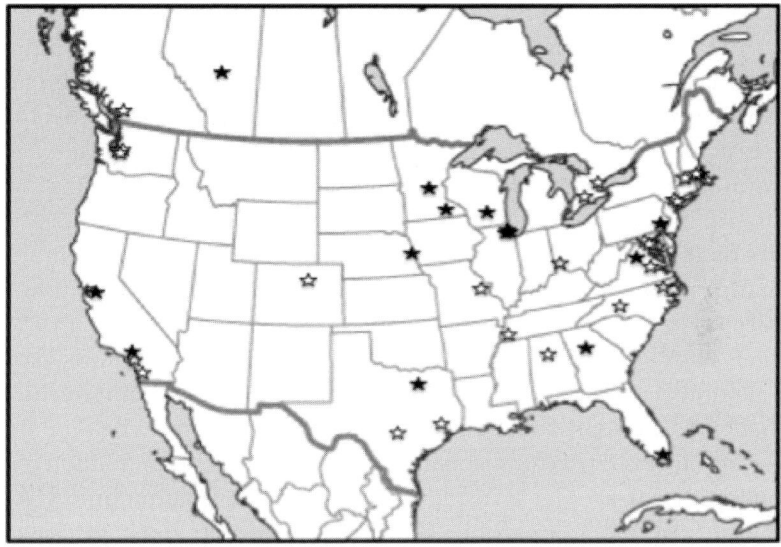

Figure 2. North American Islet Transplant Centers. Registered islet transplant centers according to the Collaborative Islet Transplant Registry Database as of 2010 (http://citregistry.org/). Centers with active protocols are indicated by ★, and centers with inactive protocols are indicated by ☆.

transplantation over the past decade. Between 1999 and 2009, a total of 32 medical centers in North America performed at least one clinical islet transplant (Figure 2). However, enthusiasm for islet transplantation has waned somewhat since the initial reported success of the Edmonton group given progressive loss of insulin independence among a number of recipients. As of 2010, only 16 centers reported active islet transplant protocols (Figure 2).

Indications for Transplantation

The majority of clinical islet transplants are currently performed as part of experimental clinical trials. Patient qualification criteria for these trials include: age between 18 and 65 years, confirmed Type I diabetes mellitus for more than 5 years, and very poor glycemic control. Poor glycemic control is generally defined as frequent episodes of hypoglycemic unawareness requiring medical intervention, wide variations in blood glucose despite intensive insulin regimen, or consistent elevation of HgA_{1C} levels >8. In some cases, progression of secondary complications of diabetes despite intensive insulin therapy is considered an inclusion factor.

Given the experimental nature of the procedures, most protocols have very strict exclusion criteria. Most commonly, these include severe cardiovascular disease, active substance abuse within 6 months, major psychiatric illness, active infection (including hepatitis B, hepatitis C, HIV, or tuberculosis), obesity (BMI >28), untreated proliferative retinopathy, pregnancy, intent of future pregnancy or fatherhood, failure to demonstrate effective contraceptive method, very high insulin requirements (>0.7 IU/kg/day), HgA_{1C} >12, and untreated hyperlipidemia. In addition, patients must demonstrate medical compliance and an understanding of the risks and benefits of the procedure.

Several forms of islet transplantation are available to patients. The first option is for *de novo* islet transplantation (islet transplant alone, ITA) for which the risks of undergoing immunosuppression must be balanced against the benefits of potential insulin independence. A second option is available to recipients of previous solid organ transplants with stable renal function. This requires reinduction immunosuppressive therapy; however, patients are already stabilized on chronic immunosuppression. This most commonly occurs following prior renal transplant (islet-after-kidney, IAK). Next, patients may undergo a simultaneous islet-kidney transplant (SIK) during which the renal transplant is performed followed by transplantation of islets from the same donor on postoperative day 1. Finally, patients requiring partial or total pancreatectomy for non-oncologic reasons (e.g. chronic pancreatitis, insulinoma, or trauma) may undergo islet autotransplantation. This results in up to a 55% rate of complete insulin independence at 1 year immunosuppression is unnecessary since islets are autologous.

Donor Considerations

In general, criteria for donors selected for islet transplantation are the same as those for other organs donated during multivisceral recovery, and the surgical technique is the same as that described for pancreas transplant. Specifically, islet donors must be nondiabetic and have normal sodium levels. In general, pancreata are offered for pancreas transplantation prior to being offered for islet donation. Ideal donors are less than 50 years of age;

however, older age and obesity are not absolute contraindications to islet donation. In fact, the yield of islets is greater from obese and older donors, given increased ease of separating islets from acinar tissue. At the present time, islets are transplanted from deceased human donors primarily; however, isolation of islets from non–heart-beating donors and living donors has been utilized successfully and may further expand the donor pool.

Islet Isolation and Transplantation

Following recovery of donor organs, the pancreas is sent to an approved islet isolation facility for further processing and islet isolation prior to transplantation (Figure 2). The pancreas is perfused and transported on ice in cold preservation solution. On arrival at the isolation facility, the harvested pancreas is divested of excess adipose tissue, the spleen, and the duodenum. The main pancreatic duct is cannulated, and Liberase®, a highly purified combination of collagenase and thermolysin, is infused into the pancreatic duct until the pancreas is completely distended. The pancreas is then cut into multiple pieces, which are transferred to the Ricordi chamber for further mechanical and chemical digestion. The temperature of the chamber is slowly increased to 37°C while the digesting pancreas is gently agitated. Once 50% of islets have been released from the surrounding acinar tissue, islets are washed clean of the enzymatic solution and purified from the digested acinar tissue by COBE centrifugation. Islet-containing layers are then stained with dithizone, collected together, washed, counted, and resuspended for transplantation or culture (Figure 3). Islets may be cultured prior to transplantation, shipped to another facility for transplant, or directly implanted into the recipient. Islets constitute approximately 1.3% of the total volume of the pancreas, about 50% of which is recovered during purification. This translates into approximately 300,000–600,000 islet equivalents (IEQ) from each pancreas after purification.

The islet transplantation procedure occurs most commonly in interventional radiology; however, a laparoscopic or open approach may also be utilized. Induction immunosuppressive therapies are initiated. Under ultrasound or fluoroscopic guidance, a 4-French catheter is inserted into the portal vein. Portal pressures are monitored initially and throughout the procedure to ensure portal vein patency. Highly concentrated islets resuspended in approximately 150 ml of heparin-containing solution are

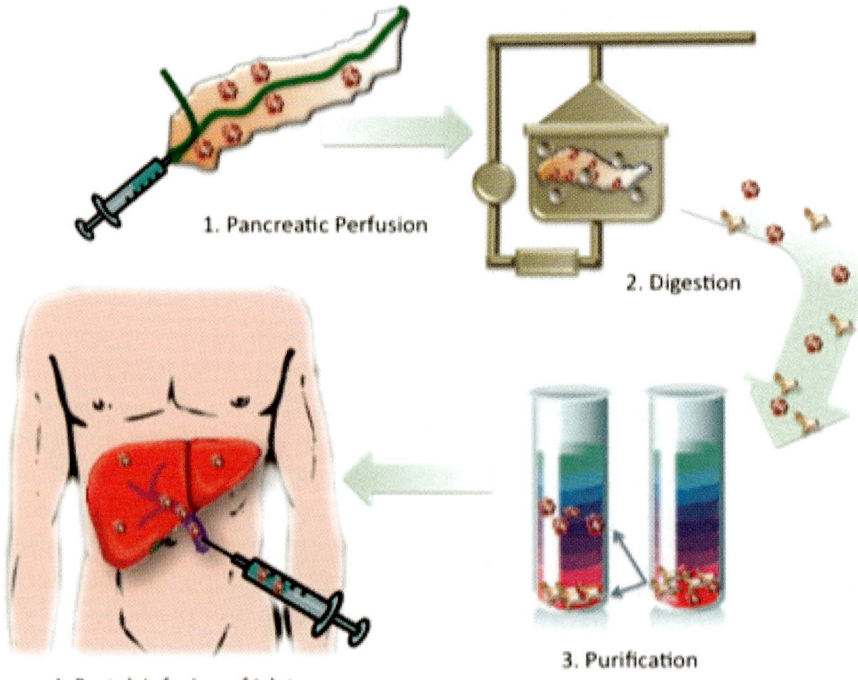

Figure 3. Human islet isolation and transplantation technique. Following harvest of the donor pancreas, the organ is transported to an approved islet isolation facility in cold preservation solution. There, (1) the pancreatic duct is infused with collagenase solution, after which (2) it is further mechanically and chemically digested in the Ricordi chamber. Digested pancreas is collected from the Ricordi chamber, washed, and (3) purified on a continuous gradient via COBE centrifugation. Purified islets are quantitated and (4) infused for engraftment in the liver by portal venous injection.

then slowly infused into the portal vein to engraft islets into the liver. On average, 427,000 IEQs (6000–7000 IEQs/kg) are infused during each procedure. According to the guidelines setup by the Edmonton trial, infusions of less than 5,000 IEQs/kg are not acceptable for transplant, and a minimum total islet volume of 10,000 IEQs/kg is necessary to achieve insulin independence.

Following percutaneous infusion, the catheter is withdrawn and the venotomy is closed with sealant. Patients are observed in the hospital for 1–2 days following islet infusion during which time they are transitioned to maintenance immunosuppression. Blood glucose is monitored to evaluate for efficacy of transplantation; however, optimal islet allograft function is often delayed. In many cases, multiple infusions of islets are necessary for patients to achieve durable insulin independence: 75% of patients transplanted receive a second islet infusion, and 25% of patients transplanted require a third infusion. On average, approximately 28 weeks elapse between first and second islet infusions.

Clinical Complications

Although islet transplantation is a minimally invasive procedure, it does carry an intrinsic risk for both procedure-related and immunosuppressive-related complications. The incidence of serious clinical complications related either to islet infusion or to immunosuppression is reported to be 66%. Of these, 27% are related to the islet allograft infusion. The most common complication seen following islet allograft infusion is post-infusion elevation of liver enzymes. Intra-abdominal or hepatic hemorrhage and portal vein thrombosis are the most serious complications reported and are the second and third most commonly reported events, respectively (Table 3).

Post-Operative Monitoring of Islet Allograft Survival

At present, the primary method of monitoring islet allograft survival following transplantation is the serial evaluation of patient's fasting blood glucose. Complete insulin independence is the measurement of successful

Table 3. Major procedure-related complications during the first year following islet transplantation.[16]

Complication following islet transplantation	% Total
Elevated Liver Function Tests	41.2%
Hemorrhage	20%
Portal vein thrombosis	7.4%
Abdominal pain	2.9%
Hypoglycemia	1.5%
Anemia	0.7%

engraftment; however, partial success may result in a decrease in the patients overall insulin requirements. Following transplantation, patients are also monitored for C-peptide, HgA_{1C}, and autoantibodies. In addition, patients may receive glucose tolerance testing. Complete loss of graft function is indicated by absence of detectable C-peptide following transplantation.

Clinical Outcomes

Historically, the progressive loss of metabolic function has been the major drawback for islet transplantation, with many patients maintaining islet allograft function for only a short time after transplant.[12,13] Despite advances in immunosuppressive therapy and isolation technique resulting in improved short-term islet engraftment, subsequent follow-up to the initial Edmonton trial suggested islet allografts remain vulnerable to loss late following transplantation. Tracking of long-term patient outcomes from this initial series demonstrated that 6 of 15 patients with graft survival greater than 1 year subsequently developed partial graft failure as demonstrated by the need for exogenous insulin. Three patients subsequently developed complete loss of islet allograft function as demonstrated by the absence of detectable C-peptide secretion. Furthermore, using the stringent criteria of the American Diabetes Association, 11 of 17 patients have developed overt diabetes.[14]

The CITR has recently reported long-term follow-up data for 412 islet allograft recipients who were transplanted between 1999 and 2008.[15] Three hundred and forty-seven patients received islet transplant that did not have a previous renal transplant (84%, ITA), and 65 patients received islet transplant following a previous renal transplant (16%, IAK). The rate of insulin independence following a single initial infusion of islets was about 11–15% with an additional 8–12% of patients retaining detectable C-peptide levels without reinfusion. The majority of patients (74%) receive at least two infusions of islets. Despite multiple infusions, however, only 70% of patients ever achieve insulin independence. The rate of insulin independence was not durable. Of patients who achieved insulin independence, 70% of ITA and 62% of IAK recipients remain insulin independent at 1 year following transplant. This falls to 42% of ITA and 24% of IAK recipients attaining insulin independence at 3 years post-transplant. Overall, this translates to a percentage of insulin independence in all ITA recipients of 55% at 6 month, 47% at 1 year, 27% at 3 years, and

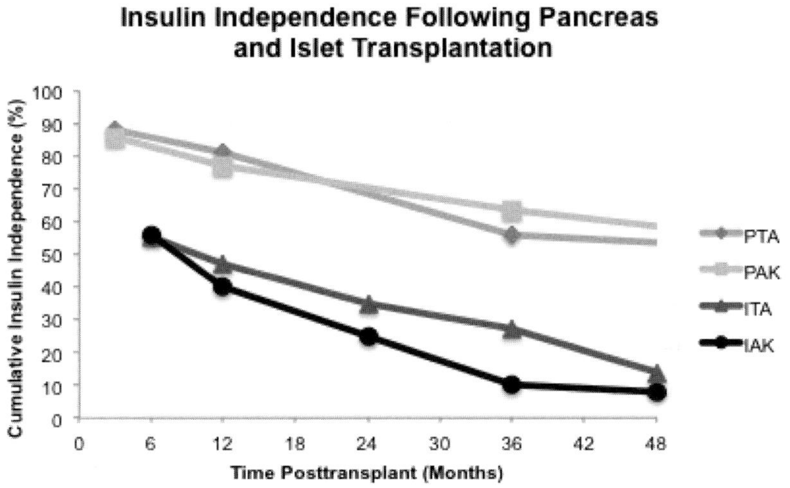

Insulin Independence Following Pancreas and Islet Transplantation

Figure 4. Insulin independence following pancreas or islet transplantation.

16% at 4 years following last islet infusion (Figure 4). Furthermore, 42% of ITA patients have no detectable C-peptide at 4 years following transplantation. For IAK recipients, overall rates of insulin independence are 56% at 6 months, 40% at 1 year, 10% at 3 years, and 8% at 4 years following last islet infusion (Figure 4). Despite significantly worse results for islet transplantation in comparison to pancreas transplantation (Figure 4), these results represent a significant improvement over the 8% rate of insulin independence at 1 year for islet transplant between 1990 and 1999.

Graft survival of vascularized pancreas transplant alone (PTA) or pancreas after kidney (PAK) transplant in comparison to insulin independence following islet transplant alone (ITA) or islet after kidney (IAK) transplant. In the case of pancreas transplant, graft survival is defined as insulin independence. Data as reported by the U.S. Organ Procurement and Transplantation Network and the Scientific Registry of Transplant Recipients and the Collaborative Islet Transplant Registry (CITR).

FUTURE CONSIDERATIONS FOR PANCREAS AND ISLET CELL TRANSPLANTATION

Currently, demand for donor organs far outweighs the supply; thus, patients risk decline of their initial health status due to microvascular effects of diabetes while awaiting solid organ or cellular transplantation. Clearly, the donor organ shortage will need to be addressed if transplantation is to become a viable alternative on a much larger scale. Transplantation of porcine islets may prove to be one source of additional donor tissue. At present, investigations are underway to genetically engineer pig tissues so that they are not recognized as xenogenic by human hosts; as the immune response to xenogenic tissues is much more difficult to suppress than that to allogeneic tissues. In addition, stem cell therapy may offer a source by which patient's own tissues may be genetically engineered into new islets or into cells with beta cell function. Finally, improved glycemic control for diabetics may not even involve transplantation. Improved technologies may allow for development of implantable insulin pumps with all the function of native pancreatic islets.

REFERENCES

1. The effect of intensive treatment of diabetes on the development and progression of long-term complications in insulin-dependent diabetes mellitus. The Diabetes Control and Complications Trial Research Group. *N Engl J Med* 1993; 329(14):977–986.
2. Nath DS, Gruessner AC, Kandaswamy R, *et al.* Outcomes of pancreas transplants for patients with type 2 diabetes mellitus. *Clin Transplant* 2005; 19(6):792–797.
3. Herzog CA, Ma JZ, Collins AJ. Long-term survival of renal transplant recipients in the United States after acute myocardial infarction. *Am J Kidney Dis* 2000; 36(1):145–152.
4. Ramanathan V, Goral S, Tanriover B, *et al.* Screening asymptomatic diabetic patients for coronary artery disease prior to renal transplantation. *Transplantation* 2005; 79(10):1453–1458.
5. Gruessner AC, Sutherland DE. Pancreas transplant outcomes for United States (US) and non-US cases as reported to the United Network for Organ Sharing (UNOS) and the International Pancreas Transplant Registry (IPTR) as of June 2004. *Clin Transplant* 2005; 19(4):433–455.
6. Tyden G, Bolinder J, Solders G, *et al.* Improved survival in patients with insulin-dependent diabetes mellitus and end-stage diabetic nephropathy 10 years after combined pancreas and kidney transplantation. *Transplantation* 1999; 67(5):645–648.

7. Ojo AO, Meier-Kriesche HU, Hanson JA, et al. The impact of simultaneous pancreas-kidney transplantation on long-term patient survival. *Transplantation* 2001; 71(1):82–90.
8. Young BY, Gill J, Huang E, et al. Living donor kidney versus simultaneous pancreas-kidney transplant in type I diabetics: an analysis of the OPTN/UNOS database. *Clin J Am Soc Nephrol* 2009; 4(4):845–852.
9. Venstrom JM, McBride MA, Rother KI, et al. Survival after pancreas transplantation in patients with diabetes and preserved kidney function. *JAMA* 2003; 290(21): 2817–2823.
10. Gruessner RW, Sutherland DE, Gruessner AC. Mortality assessment for pancreas transplants. *Am J Transplant* 2004; 4(12):2018–2026.
11. Shapiro AM, Lakey JR, Ryan EA, et al. Islet transplantation in seven patients withtype 1 diabetes mellitus usisng a glucocorticoid-free immunosuppressive regimen. *N Engl J Med* 2000; 343(4):230–238.
12. Oberholzer J, Triponez F, Mage R, et al. Human islet transplantation: lessons learned from 13 autologous and 13 allogeneic transplantations. *Transplantation* 2000; 69:1115–1123.
13. Roep BO, Stobbe I, Duinkerken G, et al. Auto and alloimmune reactivity to human islet allografts transplanted into Type I diabetic patients. *Diabetes* 1999; 48:484–490.
14. Ryan EA, Lakey JR, Paty BW, et al. Successful islet transplantation: continued insulin reserve provides long-term glycemic control. *Diabetes* 2002; 51(7):2148–2157.
15. Center CC. (Collaborative Islet Transplant Registry. Sixth Annual Report. Rockville, MD: The EMMES Corporation; 2009.

INTERVENTIONAL TECHNIQUES

44

Stephen Philcox* and Paul Jowell[†]

INTRODUCTION

Endoscopic modalities such as endoscopic retrograde cholangiopancreatography (ERCP) and endoscopic ultrasound (EUS) and radiologically guided percutaneous procedures are commonly utilized in the treatment of symptoms and complications of acute and chronic pancreatitis and are often helpful in the management of pancreatic cystic lesions and cancer. The advantages of utilizing these techniques is that they are generally associated with lower mortality and morbidity compared to surgery and either patients may be managed on an outpatient basis or the treatment results in shortened inpatient stays.

PANCREATITIS

Acute Pancreatitis

Acute pancreatitis is an acute inflammatory process of the pancreas with variable involvement of other regional tissues or remote organ systems.

---

*John Hunter Hospital, New Lambton Heights NSW, Australia
[†]Division of Gastroenterology, Duke University Medical Center, Durham, NC 27710 USA

Table 1. Causes of pancreatitis.

Gallstones*
Alcohol
Autoimmune disorders
Cancer, including occult malignancies and premalignant conditions such as intraductal papillary mucinous neoplasm (IPMN)*
Chronic pancreatitis*
Drugs
Hereditary
Metabolic abnormalities (hypertriglyceridemia, hypercalcemia)
Sphincter of Oddi dysfunction (SOD)*
Structural or congenital abnormalities (e.g. pancreas divisum)*
Trauma*

The entries with an asterisk are amenable to endoscopic therapy and will be discussed below.

The underlying process is generally reversible and the gland returns to normal once the injury resolves although this may not occur in severe pancreatitis with necrosis or acute recurrent pancreatitis. Chronic alcohol use or gallstones are responsible for 75–80% of cases of acute pancreatitis in Western countries. Alternative causes are shown in Table 1.

Supportive therapy in a medical intensive care or step-down unit is generally all that is required in mild-moderate acute pancreatitis regardless of etiology with a focus on identifying and managing precipitating causes, aggressive intravenous fluid resuscitation, avoidance of oral intake and analgesia. With increasing severity as determined by set clinical scoring systems such as APACHE II or Ranson's criteria, or a stable or rising hematocrit despite adequate fluid resuscitation, assessment for pancreatic necrosis and CBD stone retention should be undertaken, antibiotic therapy may need to be implemented and early jejunal enteral feeding commenced.

Gallstone Pancreatitis

Evidence of biliary obstruction or signs of cholangitis are well-accepted indications for urgent ERCP, although the benefit of performing ERCP and sphincterotomy (ES) simply in the setting of acute gallstone pancreatitis remains controversial with some trials showing no morbidity or mortality benefit where others have. One possible explanation for the differences in study results may relate to patient selection. In contrast, early ERCP with ES in patients with predicted severe acute pancreatitis secondary to gallstones compared with predicted mild pancreatitis has been shown to provide a significant reduction in complication rates with no mortality benefit.

Is it gallstone pancreatitis?

A history of biliary colic and imaging studies such as ultrasound or magnetic resonance cholangiopancreatography (MRCP) demonstrating the presence of gallstones, common bile duct (CBD) stones or CBD dilatation is strongly suggestive of gallstone pancreatitis. Any liver function test or pancreatic enzyme rise in the first 24–48 hours has a positive predictive value of 31% for retained CBD stones and 21% PPV for complications. This represents a four- and three-fold increase in risk, respectively compared to those patients without this rise. Furthermore, an ALT greater than or equal to 150 U/L predicts a 95% probability of gallstone pancreatitis and a bilirubin greater than 1.5 mg/dL (25 μmol/L) on day 2 of admission has also been associated with an increased likelihood of retained CBD stones.

In summary, ERCP and ES should be performed in patients with predicted severe acute pancreatitis secondary to gallstones. Patients with obstructive jaundice or cholangitis should have ERCP and ES independent of the presence of acute pancreatitis. Cholecystectomy is recommended prior to discharge, although in those patients who have undergone ERCP and ES and are elderly or sick, this decision may be deferred.

Microlithiasis ("Biliary sludge")

In those patients who experience acute recurrent pancreatitis, microlithiasis and sludge may account for up to two-thirds of cases. Episodes of recurrent acute pancreatitis are as high as 61% in conservatively treated patients and cholecystectomy reduces pancreatitis rates towards the levels seen in the general population. ERCP and ES is as effective, but they do not eliminate the risk of cholecystitis or cholangitis. Therefore, ERCP and ES should be recommended for patients who are high-risk surgical candidates or refuse cholecystectomy. ERCP and ES is often required in patients with evidence of retained CBD stones following cholecystectomy.

Congenital abnormalities of biliary and pancreatic anatomy

Pancreas divisum is the most common congenital variant of pancreatic duct anatomy and occurs in 5–10% of the general population. Pancreatitis is thought to be due at least in part to relative outflow obstruction at the site of the minor papilla; however, a recent article by Garg *et al.* reported an increased incidence of SPINK1 and CFTR gene polymorphisms in patients with idiopathic pancreatitis and pancreas divisum, offering an additional or alternative potential mechanism. Several studies have shown long-term benefit with endoscopic stenting of the dorsal pancreatic duct and minor papilla sphincterotomy. A recent systematic review comparing endoscopic and surgical therapy of pancreas divisum showed no difference with either modality with an overall response rate of 69% and 74%, respectively. The weight of evidence suggests that patients with an acute recurrent pancreatitis presentation respond more favorably than those with chronic pain or pain without evidence of acute or chronic pancreatitis with symptom relief achieved in 80%, <70% and <55% respectively.

A less common congenital anomaly that may predispose to acute pancreatitis is the Todani Type III choledochal cyst or choledochocele. Anomalous pancreaticobiliary drainage is felt predispose to acute pancreatitis that can also respond to sphincterotomy.

Duodenal duplication cysts or diverticulae rarely are implicated in recurrent pancreatitis and may be managed with a needle-knife endoscopically.

Cystic neoplasm

Cystic tumors may present with acute recurrent pancreatitis and abdominal pain. Pancreatitis is most often caused by ductal obstruction with mucin or mass effect, papillary projections from the pancreatic duct wall or secondary ductal strictures. Stent placement at ERCP may assist in bypassing the obstruction but is not usually helpful if the obstruction is caused by mucin as this tends to block the stent. More detailed discussion concerning the malignant potential of cystic lesions is provided in a later section.

Sphincter of Oddi dysfunction (biliary and/or pancreatic)

Sphincter of Oddi dysfunction (SOD) refers to an abnormality in sphincter contractility resulting in intermittent biliary and/or pancreatic duct

Table 2. Comparison of the Milwaukee and Rome III SOD classification systems.

Sphincter dysfunction type	Milwaukee classification	Rome III revision
All require typical biliary-pancreatic pain to be present		
Type I	1. Bil, ALP, ALT/AST ≥1.5–2 × ULN or amylase/lipase ≥1.5–2 × ULN 2. CBD ≥12 mm or PD ≥6 mm in head/5 mm in body 3. Prolonged biliary drainage ≥45 min or pancreatic drainage >9 min	1. Biochemistry >2 × ULN on 2 or more occasions or amylase/lipase ≥1.5–2 × ULN 2. CBD >8 mm on ultrasound PD ≥6 mm in head/5 mm in body
Type II	Positive findings for 1 or 2 of type I	Positive findings for 1 or 2 of type I
Type III	No abnormalities other than typical pain	No abnormalities other than typical pain

Note: SOD, sphincter of Oddi; Bil, total bilirubin; ALT, alanine transferase; AST, aspartate transferase; ULN, upper limit of normal; CBD, common bile duct; PD, pancreatic duct.

obstruction. This diagnosis should be considered when no other cause of acute recurrent pancreatitis has been identified, particularly in a patient with prior cholecystectomy; it may account for as many as one-third of these patients.

The majority of patients with type I SOD by either classification schemes probably have papillary stenosis and experience either complete or partial resolution of symptoms after either biliary ES in the case of biliary SOD, or dual ES in the case of pancreatic SOD. Manometry ideally should be performed in those patients type II SOD in order to identify patients with a resting basal pressure >40 mmHg (~ 60%) who are most likely to benefit from ES. Type III patients are the least likely group to benefit from ES (~ 10%) and all efforts should be made to avoid performing invasive procedures in these patients. Non-invasive tests such as a CCK-HIDA scan or secretin-MRI may be of benefit in helping to exclude the diagnosis and suggest the presence of a functional bowel disorder such as irritable bowel syndrome or functional dyspepsia.

The incidence of post-manometry pancreatitis has been reported to be 17% compared with 5% for ERCP without manometry, with recent studies suggesting the increased rate is probably not due to manometry itself, but more likely relates to the high risk patient group undergoing this procedure. These patients are typically young females with normal liver function tests and pancreatic duct anatomy and no bile duct stones demonstrated on imaging or cholangiogram. To help reduce the risk, the recommendation from the NIH Statement that these patients are best managed in a high-volume center with extensive experience in performing manometry and ERCP.

Chronic Pancreatitis

Chronic pancreatitis is a syndrome involving progressive inflammatory changes in the pancreas that result in permanent structural damage, which leads to impairment of exocrine and endocrine function. Abdominal pain is a dominant symptom in pancreatitis, and may be persistent or intermittent, is often postprandial and may be associated with nausea and vomiting. The diagnosis may be confirmed by non-invasive imaging studies including CT and MRI/MRCP; however, EUS is the most accurate investigation and can provide information on severity.

While alcohol is the most common cause of chronic pancreatitis in developed countries, obstruction is also implicated. Causes of obstruction include (post-traumatic) ductal strictures, stones, pseudocysts, mechanical or structural changes in the pancreatic sphincter, and periampullary tumors. Obstruction of the main pancreatic duct is felt to either primarily cause pain or predispose to attacks of acute pancreatitis superimposed on chronic pancreatitis. Relief of outflow obstruction is the goal of interventional techniques and may apply to both the pancreatic duct and the bile duct.

Pancreatic duct strictures

Strictures are thought to result from inflammation or fibrosis around the main pancreatic duct. Significant reductions in pain scores following pancreatic duct stenting have been reported although response rates have varied from 46% to 94%. One long-term multicenter study showed surgery was eventually required in 24% of patients despite an initial response to stenting in 84% and there was no associated improvement in pancreatic function. Stent patency and post-treatment duct diameter do not seem to be associated with clinical response rates.

There are complications associated with stenting the pancreatic duct including pain, pancreatitis, infection, stent migration or occlusion, duodenal erosions, stone formation, ductal perforation, post-sphincterotomy bleeding (if performed) and stent-induced ductal damage. These latter concerns may be unfounded as the changes appear to improve over time and are of unproven clinical significance, particularly in patients with advanced chronic pancreatitis; however, pending definitive studies, stent-induced strictures should still be considered a potential problem.

Pancreatic duct stones

Pancreatic duct stones are generally difficult to remove, as they may be large, are hard and spiculated, may be multiple and are often associated with strictures. Usually some form of lithotripsy is required prior to attempting endoscopic removal and the most effective appears to be extracorporeal shock-wave lithotripsy (ESWL), although mechanical and electrohydraulic lithotripsy are also used. This has the effect of fragmenting or pulverizing stones and reducing stone burden. Stones that do not respond as well to endoscopic therapy are those located diffusely throughout the duct or predominantly in the tail, those impacted behind tight strictures or in the prepapillary region, or stones associated with complex parenchymal disease. Endoscopic therapy is varied but includes pancreatic sphincterotomy, dilatation of pancreatic duct strictures, balloon and basket stone extraction, and pancreatic duct stenting.

Biliary obstruction

Recurrent inflammation can lead to fibrosis around the bile duct and subsequent stricture formation or the presence of a chronic pseudocyst may cause extrinsic compression of the duct. In similar fashion, an acute pseudocyst may compress the duct, or alternatively, edema secondary to acute pancreatic inflammation can also sometimes cause duct compression. Duct obstruction can lead to abnormal liver function tests, frank jaundice or even cholangitis.

Very tight strictures may require balloon or catheter dilatation of the duct to facilitate access to the biliary tree. As these are usually fibrotic strictures, this alone is usually insufficient to maintain duct patency and a plastic stent is generally placed to relieve the obstruction. The ERCP is then repeated every 3 months for at least 12 months, often placing additional stents during each procedure in an effort to dilate the duct back to a normal diameter. Recent series have described success with the use of covered metal stents in benign disease as the covering deters tissue ingrowth into the stent and subsequently permits its removal. These may be left in for much longer with the benefit of exposing the patient to fewer procedures; however, further studies are required to fully assess this indication. Despite these options, biliary bypass surgery is still sometimes required.

Celiac plexus blockade

The management of pain in patients with pancreatic cancer and chronic pancreatitis is challenging. Medical approaches utilize medications including acetaminophen, tramadol and opiates in addition to pancreatic enzyme supplementation, antioxidants and octreotide with varying efficacy achieved. Endoscopic stenting of strictures and stone removal have also shown some benefit as has extracorporeal shock-wave lithotripsy (ESWL) of intraductal stones and surgery for selected patients. As the celiac plexus mediates pain signals from the pancreas, it has also been targeted with both neurolysis (using alcohol for patients with cancer) and neural blockade (steroid agent) in an effort to reduce oral analgesia requirements. Each of these techniques includes the concurrent injection of a local anesthetic, usually bupivicaine. Approaches to the celiac plexus include percutaneous, surgical and endosonographic guidance and although there have been no comparative studies, the results of a variety of studies would suggest there are no significant differences in efficacy between each technique.

One recent meta-analysis of EUS-guided management for pain secondary to pancreatic cancer demonstrated a good or excellent response rate in patients with 85% of patients who underwent bilateral injection and 46% with a unilateral injection. Relief of pain lasts up to 3 months following the procedure. Pain secondary to chronic pancreatitis was relieved in 60% of patients. Complications are rare with the most commonly reported complication being diarrhea.

PANCREATIC CYSTS

Pseudocysts are the most common cystic lesion in the pancreas accounting for 90% of all cysts and should be suspected in patients with a history of pancreatitis, a lack of septae, loculations, solid components or cyst wall calcifications on cross-sectional imaging, absence of PD communication at MRCP or ERCP and a high amylase level on FNA (see below).

The most common cystic lesions after pseudocysts include mucinous cystadenoma and cystadenocarcinoma (MCN), mucinous duct ectasia or intraductal papillary mucinous neoplasm (IPMN), serous cystadenoma (SCN), papillary cystic neoplasm, congenital or simple cysts, cystic adenocarcinoma and cystic islet cell tumors.

MCN is the most frequent cystic tumor accounting for around 50% of the non-pseudocyst lesions and are most commonly found in women in their mid-50s with two-thirds of lesions located in the body and tail. SCN may be diagnosed on morphological characteristics alone with an accuracy of 92–96%. Characteristic features include the presence of microcystic compartments (<3 mm), central fibrosis or calcification, and a highly vascular stroma.

Mucin-producing tumors have high malignant potential (with larger size being more concerning) and should generally be considered for surgical management. Efforts to distinguish this type of tumor from other benign tumors have been generally unsatisfactory; imaging studies including CT, MRI or EUS can suggest the diagnosis as can the analysis of cyst fluid usually obtained by EUS-guided FNA. Cytology has the highest specificity, followed by elevated CEA levels particularly in combination with low amylase levels; however, sensitivity is poor resulting in a low negative predictive value.

Pseudocysts

Pancreatic pseudocysts (PPs) are fluid collections arising in or adjacent to the pancreas enclosed by a fibrous capsule and lack a true epithelial lining. The fluid in a PP arises from a disruption to the pancreatic duct or side branches and the cause of injury is inflammatory, most commonly secondary to acute or chronic pancreatitis, trauma (including post-surgical), and ductal obstruction due to stricture or stone. PPs are found in 10–30% of patients with chronic pancreatitis, the majority (~70%) of which are associated with alcohol abuse. In contrast, PPs complicate only 5–15% of patients with acute pancreatitis.

It is estimated that 30–60% of acute PPs may resolve spontaneously within 4–6 weeks, although resolution rates appear to be lower in patients with chronic PPs, multiple cysts, larger cysts (>5 cm) or cysts that increase in size on follow-up examination, pseudocyst location in the tail of the pancreas, thicker pseudocyst wall, lack of communication with the pancreatic duct, an associated proximal stricture of the pancreatic duct, biliary or postoperative etiology of pancreatitis, extent of necrosis greater than 25–30%, and extra-pancreatic development in patients with chronic alcoholic pancreatitis.

There are a variety of potential complications associated with PPs. Pain is the most commonly reported symptom, and acute complications include bleeding (usually from splenic artery pseudoaneurysm), infection, and rupture. Chronic complications encompass gastric outlet obstruction, biliary obstruction and thrombosis of the splenic or portal veins with development of gastric varices. Management of pancreatic necrosis will be discussed separately (see below).

Drainage

Indications

The two main indications for intervention are the presence of symptoms such as pain, fever and jaundice or the presence of complications (infection, bleeding, gastric outlet or biliary obstruction) and should only be considered after 4–6 weeks to permit the cyst an opportunity to resolve spontaneously and to allow maturation of the pseudocyst wall, thereby minimizing the risk of perforation and peritonitis.

Pre-procedural planning

Pre-procedural planning can assist in reducing the risks associated with the procedure:

(1) Exclude alternative diagnoses with a good history, physical and appropriate cross-sectional imaging. EUS can also assist in this regard.
(2) Thorough review of cross-sectional imaging and/or EUS images to determine:
- Does the PP communicate with the main pancreatic duct?
- Does the cyst contain solid debris?

- Is the cyst wall accessible from the stomach or proximal duodenum?
- Is the cyst wall less than 10 mm in thickness?
- Is there evidence of portal hypertension and/or varices?

(3) Assess for appropriateness of moderate sedation and consider general anesthesia
(4) Check and correct any coagulopathy

Techniques

Prophylactic antibiotics are indicated regardless of approach.

Percutaneous drainage

This is achieved by percutaneous placement of a pigtail catheter into the pseudocyst under CT or US guidance with subsequent connection to an external collecting system. The catheter is then removed once output is minimal, which usually takes 2–3 months. This modality appears to be most useful in patients with normal ductal anatomy and least helpful in patients with duct disruption, strictures or chronic pancreatitis. Relapse rates range from 20% to 1%. The most common complications are pain and infection, which can occur in a third of patients, with persistent fistula, bleeding, superficial skin infections and drain occlusion also problematic. This approach is probably best reserved for collections not adjacent to the gastric or duodenal wall, those that do not communicate with the pancreatic duct or as an adjunct for patients who have failed endoscopic or surgical treatment.

Transpapillary drainage

Placing a stent (usually 5- or 7-Fr) or nasopancreatic catheter across the pancreatic duct with or without pancreatic sphincterotomy is recommended when the fluid collection communicates with the main pancreatic duct. The proximal end of the stent may be placed within the PP or can be used to bridge a main duct disruption. The stent can also bypass obstructive processes such as strictures or stones that contribute to cyst recurrence — these may be treated more definitively subsequent to stent removal. Cysts over 6 cm are less likely to respond to this treatment and the stent may cause ductal scarring. Stents may be replaced every 4–6 weeks with resolution observed at a median 10 weeks in one study.

Transmural drainage

Access into the PP is obtained either via puncturing the duodenal or stomach wall. This may be achieved using a duodenoscope or a therapeutic linear EUS scope. There are clear theoretical advantages to direct visualization with EUS including assessing the contents of the cyst, selection of site of entry into the cyst, identification and avoidance of varices or pseudoaneurysms and the opportunity to obtain a prepuncture fluid sample in cases where the diagnosis is uncertain. If EUS is unavailable, a bulge seen endoscopically reflecting extrinsic compression is helpful to localize the cyst, or fluoroscopic techniques such as needle indentation of a communicating cyst once contrast has been injected via the pancreatic duct may be used.

In our institution, cyst puncture is predominantly achieved under EUS guidance. We use a 19G Cook EUS-FNA needle using the Seldinger technique via a Pentax linear array EUS scope. We initially confirm intracystic localization with aspiration of cyst contents and advance a 0.035" guidewire into the cyst. The position of the wire is then confirmed by observing it coiling within the cyst under EUS/fluoroscopic imaging.

Once wire position is satisfactory, the needle is then removed and an 8–10 mm through-the-scope (TTS) balloon dilator is passed along the wire and used to dilate the tract. Occasionally, this is initially unsuccessful and a cautery needle-knife may be required to open the fistula tract sufficiently to permit entry of the balloon; this step has been associated with an increased risk of bleeding. Once dilation has been achieved, a second wire is then passed into the cyst using the inner catheter of the Cook Fusion stent deployment system. The presence of two wires permits deployment of multiple stents whilst maintaining continuous access to the cyst; however, the disadvantage is that all but the final stent need to be a maximum of 7Fr in diameter; we usually insert three 3–4 cm 7-Fr double-pigtail stents. Alternatively, one or more 10-Fr stents may be deployed by sequentially regaining access to the pseudocyst or using a double channel fistulotome. If infection is present, further dilatation of the tract is performed and a nasocystic drain placed alongside the stents to permit continuous lavage until the infection has resolved.

Repeat cross-sectional imaging is obtained 4 weeks following the procedure to assess for resolution of the pseudocyst. Stents are then removed within two weeks of cyst resolution which is seen in up to 92% of pseudocysts associated with chronic pancreatitis and 74% of those associated with acute pancreatitis.

Complications

Bacterial colonization is to be anticipated and infection is the most common complication of endoscopic PP drainage. Other complications include serious bleeding that may be secondary to tract dilatation, blood vessel perforation or trauma to pseudoaneurysms, stent migration, pancreatitis and perforation. The morbidity rates are 12–20%; however, the mortality of endoscopic therapy is very low (<0.5%).

Comparison of endoscopic and laparoscopic approaches

Superior rates of resolution of pseudocysts have been demonstrated with the laparoscopic approach compared with endoscopic, which may be secondary to the larger stoma created at surgery. In addition, the recurrence rates of 14% in those treated endoscopically over a mean follow-up period of 24 months are significantly higher than the 2.5% achieved laparoscopically. Conflicting morbidity data has been reported, so at this stage it is unclear which is the safer procedure; mortality rates appear to be comparable. These approaches are likely to be complementary depending upon local expertise, with the laparoscopic approach perhaps more suitable for large pseudocysts or those situated beyond the reach of the endoscopic approach.

Pancreatic Necrosis Debridement

Several clinical scoring systems have been validated in acute pancreatitis, with the most commonly used APACHE II score ≥ 8 correlating with severe pancreatitis. Necrosis as identified on contrast-enhanced CT (CECT) has been shown to correlate with the severity of acute pancreatitis with a mortality rate as high as 23% and a complication rate up to 92% in patients with necrosis of greater than 30% of the pancreas.

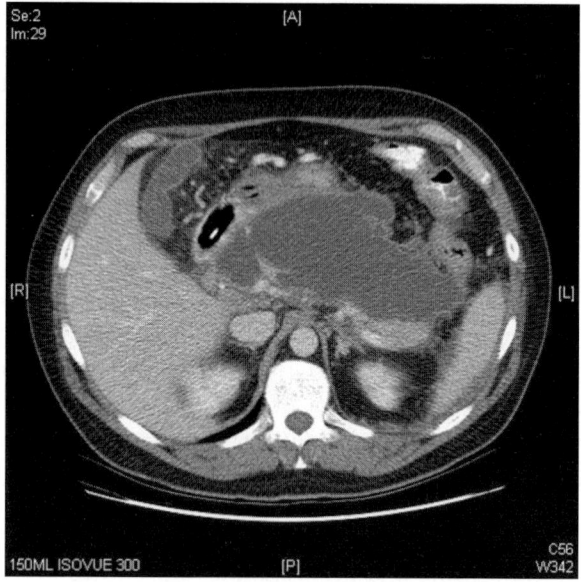

Figure 1. Organized necrosis.

Surgical and minimally invasive necrosectomy

Open surgical management of pancreatic necrosis is associated with high morbidity (13–53%) and mortality (6–25%), particularly if attempted early. Retroperitoneal necrosectomy, often using a nephroscope via a percutaneously created tract in patients with infected necrosis, is also associated with a high mortality rate of 16%, need for multiple procedures and a 13% conversion rate to open operation. There are limited published data on laparoscopic necrosectomy, which appears to require fewer attempts but still is associated with a mortality rate of 7% and an 11% conversion to open operation.

Endoscopic necrosectomy

Endoscopic necrosectomy has gained momentum during the past decade after the initial report published by Baron *et al*. Over time, the original technique has evolved into direct endoscopic-guided mechanical debridement in addition to endoscopic lavage and nasobiliary irrigation. The tract

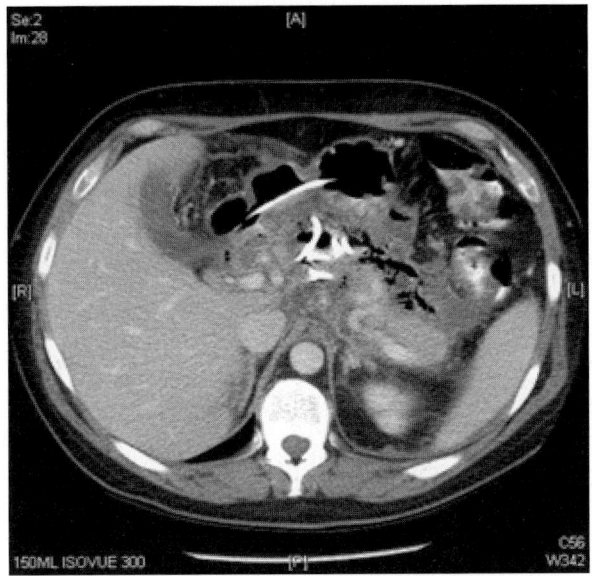

Figure 2. Stents within the necrosis.

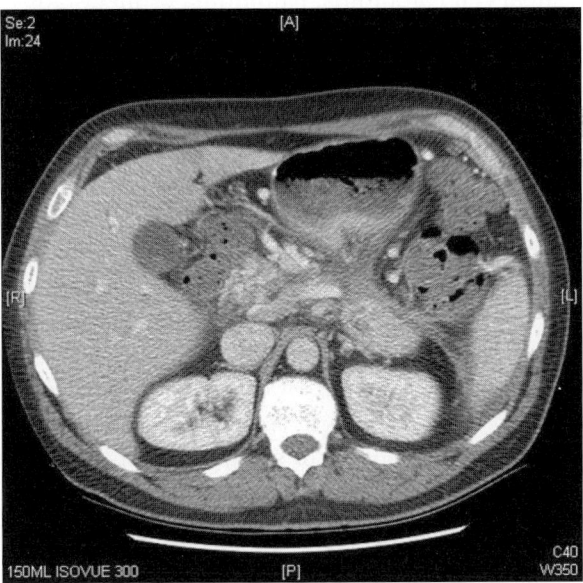

Figure 3. Resolution of necrosis.

is sequentially dilated to 15–20 mm, usually over a number of sessions, with placement of pigtail stents and a nasocystic drain with irrigation should infection be felt to be present. When the tract has been sufficiently dilated, a therapeutic gastroscope is advanced into the cyst and the necrotic tissue is treated with both targeted lavage via a spray catheter or similar, and with mechanical debridement using a variety of accessories such as Roth net basket, Dormia basket, snares and rat-tooth forceps. This procedure needs to be repeated until healthy non-necrotic tissue is encountered which takes 2–10 sessions.

Success rates of 80–93% with a complication rate of 5–7% are being achieved in experienced tertiary referral centers, with low associated mortality rates of around 5%. A close interdisciplinary relationship involving interventional endoscopists, surgeons and interventional radiologists is crucial to managing this subset of ill patients.

SOLID PANCREATIC LESIONS

Solid lesions identified on imaging most commonly represent adenocarcinoma; however, other neoplasms should be considered such neuroendocrine tumors, small cell carcinoma, lymphoma or metastatic deposits from other primary tumors such as renal cell, colon or breast cancer. Occasionally, benign conditions may also have this appearance with the most common being focal pancreatitis or autoimmune pancreatitis.

Fine Needle Aspiration Biopsy

A tissue diagnosis is helpful in guiding treatment options. EUS-FNA is the preferred technique for obtaining tissue with sensitivity up to 90% and specificity of 99%. Percutaneous CT or US-guided techniques are a reasonable alternative; however, the advantages of EUS-FNA are that it may be used for smaller lesions, there is a lower risk of needle tract seeding and peritoneal carcinomatosis, and it appears to be more cost-effective. In addition, EUS-FNA permits the option of sampling lymph nodes, the left lobe of the liver and ascites during a single procedure.

It is generally accepted FNA should be obtained in patients who are poor surgical candidates and in those who are not resectable in order to make a tissue diagnosis to help guide treatment. What is less clear is the benefit of FNA in those who are good surgical candidates and appear to have resectable disease. A recent literature review by Hartwig *et al.* recommended proceeding primarily with surgical resection followed by adjuvant chemotherapy without obtaining preoperative FNA due to concerns regarding the relatively high false negative rate at EUS-FNA of 10–15%. This approach leads to a 5–30% 5-year survival rate depending upon stage.

The low resectability rate found after staging laparoscopy of 15–20%, the poor long-term outcomes following pancreaticoduodenectomy and the small subset of patients found to have benign disease at laparotomy has led to the assessment of the benefit of neoadjuvant chemoradiotherapy, which can help in selecting patients who are likely to progress before surgery is performed. This approach requires pretreatment EUS-FNA for tissue diagnosis. Recent studies have demonstrated a 25–35% reduction in the EUS-FNA false-negative rate by repeating the FNA, leading to a false negative rate approaching 5–10%.

Similar resectability and survival have been demonstrated and studies are ongoing that will hopefully settle the debate regarding these different management approaches.

Biliary Obstruction

Obstructive jaundice or cholangitis is a common initial presentation in patients with a solid pancreatic lesion and is the result of obstruction usually via extrinsic compression of the bile duct or direct infiltration of tumor into the bile duct as it passes through the head of the pancreas. Occasionally, porta hepatis lymphadenopathy may also obstruct the proximal bile duct via extrinsic compression. ERCP is the mainstay procedure in this situation. These tumors often cause very tight biliary strictures, which may necessitate balloon dilatation of the duct to facilitate access to the biliary tree. If a tissue diagnosis has not been made prior to the procedure, a brush is usually then passed into the duct to obtain cells for cytological analysis. Balloon dilatation is often employed in an attempt to disrupt the lining of the bile duct, which increases the yield of brushing. Finally, a stent is then placed into the bile duct in order to relieve the obstruction. A plastic stent is usually placed if the tumor is felt to be potentially resectable or if the patient is unlikely to survive longer than 3 months. Metal stents are placed in patients with unresectable tumors who are likely to survive more than 3 months as these stents have a low migration rate and can remain patent for up to 12 months. These stents may be bare metal (usually Nitinol) or include a covering of a thin flexible membrane that may be partial or full. The uncovered stent is preferable in patients who still have a gallbladder in order to reduce the risk of obstructing the cystic duct with the subsequent potential risk of cholecystitis, or those with hilar strictures so as to permit maximum bile drainage, whereas a covered stent should be used in all other patients with obstruction below the hilum, to reduce the rate of tissue ingrowth into the stent, thereby prolonging the life of the stent.

Occasionally, biliary access cannot be obtained at ERCP and the percutaneous route may be employed under radiological guidance. Despite comparable success rates, however, complications of pain, loss of access, infections and patient preference have led to seeking alternative methods of gaining access. Recent work has demonstrated efficacy with rendezvous procedures utilizing both EUS and ERCP to access the biliary tree; this is achieved by accessing the biliary tree with an EUS-guided FNA needle either from the stomach or first part of the duodenum, and utilizing this access to pass a wire into the bile duct. Once this has been achieved, the echoendoscope can be exchanged for a duodenoscope, which can then load the wire in a retrograde fashion via a catheter and the ERCP can proceed as normal. Despite these options, biliary bypass surgery is still sometimes required.

Should access to the papilla be compromised due to duodenal obstruction secondary to tumor infiltration in patients who are not surgical candidates or decline surgery, alternative access to the biliary tract should be obtained first, as indicated in the previous paragraph (most commonly via the percutaneous route), followed by the endoscopic placement of an enteral stent to effectively bypass the obstruction. Obtaining internal biliary drainage initially avoids the potential complication of obstructing the major papilla by the enteral stent, which would necessitate external drainage with a percutaneous catheter and collection bag.

SUMMARY

Interventional techniques, particularly endoscopic, are increasingly being utilized in the management of pancreatic pathology due to the ease of access, equivalent or superior success rates compared with other techniques, and relatively low complication rates.

REFERENCES

Adler DG, Lichtenstein D, Baron TH, *et al.* The role of endoscopy in patients with chronic pancreatitis. *Gastrointest Endosc* 2006; 63:933–937.

Baillie J. Endoscopic therapy in acute recurrent pancreatitis. *World J Gastroenterol* 2008; 14:1034–1037.

Baron TH, Harewood GC, Morgan DE, *et al.* Outcome differences after endoscopic drainage of pancreatic necrosis, acute pancreatic pseudocysts, and chronic pancreatic pseudocysts. *Gastrointest Endosc* 2002; 56:7–17.

Cohen ME, Slezak L, Wells CK, *et al.* Prediction of bile duct stones and complications in gallstone pancreatitis using early laboratory trends. *Am J Gastroenterol* 2001; 96:3305–3311.

Hartwig W, Schneider L, Diener MK, *et al.* Preoperative tissue diagnosis for tumours of the pancreas. *Br J Surg* 2009; 96:5–20.

Isayama H, Nakai Y, Togawa O, *et al.* Covered metallic stents in the management of malignant and benign pancreatobiliary strictures. *J Hepatobiliary Pancreat Surg* 2009; 16:624–627.

Jacobson BC, Baron TH, Adler DG, *et al.* ASGE guideline: The role of endoscopy in the diagnosis and the management of cystic lesions and inflammatory fluid collections of the pancreas. *Gastrointest Endosc* 2005; 61:363–370.

Liao Z, Gao R, Wang W, *et al.* A systematic review on endoscopic detection rate, endotherapy, and surgery for pancreas divisum. *Endoscopy* 2009; 41:439–444.

Melman L, Azar R, Beddow K, *et al.* Primary and overall success rates for clinical outcomes after laparoscopic, endoscopic, and open pancreatic cystgastrostomy for pancreatic pseudocysts. *Surg Endosc* 2009; 23:267–271.

Puli SR, Reddy JB, Bechtold ML, *et al.* EUS-guided celiac plexus neurolysis for pain due to chronic pancreatitis or pancreatic cancer pain: a meta-analysis and systematic review. *Dig Dis Sci* 2009; 54:2330–2337.

Talreja JP, Kahaleh M. Endotherapy for pancreatic necrosis and abscess: endoscopic drainage and necrosectomy. *J Hepatobiliary Pancreat Surg* 2009; 16:605–612.

van Santvoort HC, Besselink MG, de Vries AC, *et al.* Early endoscopic retrograde cholangiopancreatography in predicted severe acute biliary pancreatitis: a prospective multicenter study. *Ann Surg* 2009; 250:68–75.

SURGICAL TECHNIQUES: WHIPPLE   45

Rebekah R. White* and Eugene P. Ceppa[†]

INTRODUCTION

The most common indication for pancreaticoduodenectomy is pancreatic ductal adenocarcinoma. However, other periampullary cancers (ampullary adenocarcinoma, cholangiocarcinoma, and duodenal adenocarcinoma), pancreatic tumors (cystic neoplasms and neuroendocrine tumors), and sequelae from chronic pancreatitis are also potential indications for pancreaticoduodenectomy (PD). The morbidity and mortality associated with this procedure are paramount in the discussion with patients requiring PD, since even high-volume centers report morbidity as high as 50% and mortality up to 5%. In addition to the surgeon, other medical specialists (including gastroenterologists, radiologists, and pathologists) and the medical facility itself (including nurses and ancillary services) all play a role in achieving the best possible outcomes.

DIAGNOSTIC EVALUATION

Preoperative imaging is critical for PD, and both radiologic and invasive imaging studies provide details that assist surgeons in preoperative

---

*Duke University Medical Center, Department of Surgery, Durham, NC 27710 USA
[†]Indiana University School of Medicine, Department of Surgery, Indianapolis, Indiana USA

planning. Transabdominal ultrasonography, computed tomography (CT), endoscopic retrograde cholangiopancreatography (ERCP), angiography, endoscopic ultrasound (EUS), magnetic resonance imaging (MRI), positron emission tomography (PET), and laparoscopy all have potential roles in the diagnosis and staging of pancreatic and periampullary neoplasms. The vast majority of patients undergoing PD are for suspected malignant disease, and imaging is used to evaluate for local tumor extension and distant metastasis to determine if the patient has resectable disease. At the time of presentation, malignant disease will actually be resectable in less than one-quarter of patients. Therefore, the first goal of management is to identify those patients who have localized disease and are potential candidates for resection. Cross-sectional imaging, usually CT or MRI, may demonstrate distant metastatic disease to the liver, peritoneum, or — less often — lungs. Cross-sectional imaging may also demonstrate clear evidence of local vascular involvement that precludes resection, such as thrombosis of the portal vein/superior mesenteric vein (PV/SMV) confluence or involvement of the celiac axis or superior mesenteric artery (SMA). Whether disease that involves the PV/SMV confluence without thrombosis should be resected used to be controversial, but vein resection with reconstruction is now performed at most high-volume centers for patients in whom an R0 (margin negative) resection cannot otherwise be achieved.

For patients with unresectable disease, histologic diagnosis can usually be achieved by either percutaneous image-guided or EUS-guided needle biopsy, and these patients are managed nonoperatively with chemotherapy and/or radiation therapy. The role of surgery in the palliation of patients with unresectable periampullary cancer has decreased with improvements in endoscopic stenting (see Chapter 46). For patients with potentially resectable disease, preoperative histologic diagnosis is necessary only for patients being considered for neoadjuvant (preoperative) therapy. Otherwise, preoperative diagnosis may be useful for counseling patients but is not essential if surgery is planned, as a negative biopsy does not reliably exclude cancer. Similarly, when preoperative imaging studies reveal a mass consistent with a pancreatic cancer, intraoperative biopsy is not generally warranted.

SURGERY

Staging laparoscopy is recommended for patients who do not require open surgical palliation in order to rule out occult metastatic disease prior to laparotomy for resection. Although modern dynamic contrast-enhanced CT is highly accurate for predicting local resectability, it remains limited in its ability to detect small (<1 cm) deposits of metastatic disease. With the combination of high quality cross-sectional imaging and staging laparoscopy, open abdominal exploration now has a limited role in the assessment of resectability, and nontherapeutic laparotomy should be an uncommon occurrence. In patients with potentially resectable disease, the goal of treatment is complete resection of all gross disease with negative microscopic margins. The most common surgical procedure performed for pancreatic and peri-pancreatic neoplasms is the standard (modified Whipple) pancreaticoduodenectomy. This procedure is discussed in detail, as are important modifications to this procedure, including the pylorus-preserving pancreaticoduodenectomy, extended (or regional) pancreatectomy, and vascular resection.

Staging Laparoscopy

Despite the technological advances of multiphase computed tomography and dynamic magnetic resonance imaging, these techniques do not detect small (<1 cm) superficial peritoneal and hepatic metastases from pancreatic adenocarcinoma. Laparoscopy spares up to 20% of patients with pancreatic carcinoma unnecessary laparotomy because it accurately identifies low-volume metastases that preclude resection.

Indications

Laparoscopy is indicated prior to laparotomy for attempted resection in patients with radiographic evidence of resectable disease. Laparoscopy may also be indicated to exclude distant metastatic disease in patients with radiographically localized disease being considered for neoadjuvant therapy or palliative chemoradiation.

Contraindications

Patients with previous abdominal surgery who have extensive adhesions that preclude safe laparoscopic access to the peritoneal cavity are not candidates for laparoscopic staging. Patients with obvious signs of unresectable disease on staging dynamic computed tomography do not need to undergo laparoscopy in the absence of symptoms that can be palliated laparoscopically (e.g., biliary or gastric bypass). Patients with symptoms that will require open surgical palliation — due to surgeon preference or patient factors — regardless of metastatic disease also do not need to undergo laparoscopy.

Technique

Staging laparoscopy is conducted under general anesthesia. Laparoscopic exploration is conducted to identify signs of unresectable disease. Hepatic, peritoneal, and organ surfaces are inspected for signs of metastases, and biopsy samples are obtained accordingly. The region of the ligament of Treitz is examined to evaluate the presence of extrapancreatic extension of tumor with involvement of the mesocolon. Some surgeons routinely examine the lesser sac for evidence of regional metastases. With extended laparoscopy, the foramen of Winslow is examined for enlarged portal lymph nodes, and biopsy samples are obtained if indicated. Laparoscopic ultrasonography has been described in combination with extended laparoscopy as a way to evaluate for regional lymph node involvement and local vascular invasion.

Interpretation

Signs of unresectable disease include distant spread to the liver, bowel serosa, or peritoneum, encasement of the portal or superior mesenteric vein or artery, invasion of the celiac axis or the hepatic artery, mesocolon involvement, and gross celiac or portal nodal metastases. Encroachment without encasement of the portal or superior mesenteric vein is not considered a contraindication to resection. Patients lacking these aforementioned signs can proceed to laparotomy.

Efficacy

The yield of laparoscopy depends on the quality of the preoperative imaging as well as the patient population and is higher in patients with locally advanced tumors and tumors of the body or tail. The combination of multiphase, thin-section dynamic computed tomography and laparoscopy should result in a less than 10% rate of unresectable disease at laparotomy, which is much better than the 30–50% rate historically associated with exploration for pancreatic cancer.

Complications

Staging laparoscopy may be associated with complications of pneumoperitoneum, hernia, and iatrogenic injury of abdominal structures.

Pancreaticoduodenectomy

Goals

Resection is the only potentially curative treatment option for localized periampullary cancer. The goal of pancreaticoduodenectomy is complete resection of the malignant lesion in an effort to prolong patient survival if not cure the disease.

Indications

Pancreaticoduodenectomy for pancreatic adenocarcinoma is indicated in patients in whom complete resection can be attained. The timing of surgery should be considered carefully if the patient's overall medical health or nutritional status is poor, coagulation is impaired, or biliary sepsis is present.

Contraindications

Pancreaticoduodenectomy is contraindicated in patients with distant metastasis and in patients with locally advanced disease such as arterial (celiac, hepatic, or superior mesenteric artery) involvement or major venous (superior mesenteric or portal vain) occlusion. Because cancers involving the superior mesenteric–portal venous confluence may be resected completely with vascular repair or reconstruction, contiguity to major veins or partial encirclement without complete encasement is not an absolute contraindication to resection. Most surgeons regard gross regional lymph node disease as a marker for systemic disease and do not proceed with resection when it is encountered. Microscopic regional lymph node metastasis may be considered a relative contraindication to resection, and the extent to which normal-appearing regional lymph nodes should be evaluated prior to resection may depend on patient factors such as age and comorbid conditions.

Technique

Pancreatic surgeons at the M.D. Anderson Cancer Center have divided pancreaticoduodenectomy into six well-defined surgical steps: (1) mobilization of the right colon, entrance into the omental bursa, and exposure of the third and fourth portions of the duodenum and superior

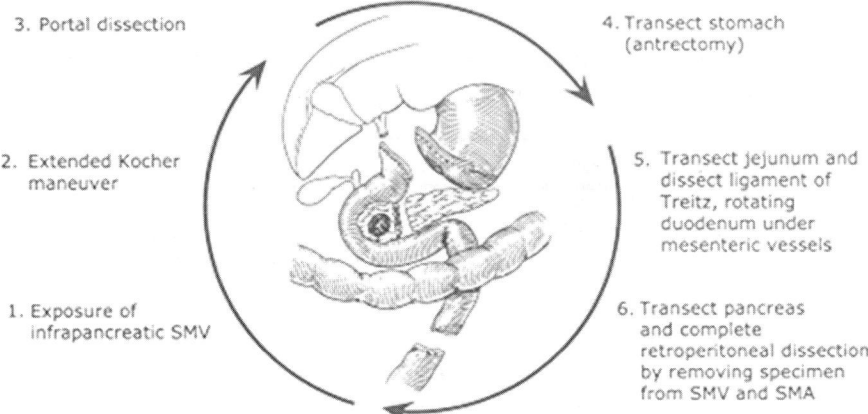

Figure 1. Steps of the pancreaticoduodenectomy. (1) SMV exposure. (2) Kocher maneuver. (3) Hepatoduodenal dissection. (4) Antrectomy. (5) Ligament of Trietz dissection. (6) Pancreatic neck transection. Figure is a reprint from Tyler, D.S. and D.B. Evans. (1994) Reoperative pancreaticoduodenectomy. *Ann Surg* 219(2): 211–221. Permission was granted from Annals of Surgery *via* J.B. Lippincott Company.

mesenteric vein; (2) extensive mobilization of the duodenum (Kocher maneuver); (3) dissection of the porta hepatis; (4) transection of the stomach; (5) transection of the proximal jejunum and division of its mesentery; and (6) transection of the pancreas and retroperitoneal dissection to remove the tumor-bearing specimen from the superior mesenteric artery (Figure 1).[1] These are all necessary components of the extirpative portion of the procedure. If resectability is in question, the area of concern is often addressed first, so that the remaining steps can be avoided in the patient discovered to have locally advanced disease.

Resection

Pancreaticoduodenectomy begins with assessment of resectability. If no distant metastases or gross regional lymph-node metastases are present and the base of the transverse mesocolon lacks evidence of direct tumor extension, the hepatic flexure and right colon are mobilized, exposing the third and fourth portion of the duodenum and superior mesenteric vein. An extended Kocher maneuver is performed to allow complete palpation of the duodenum and head of pancreas and identification of the left renal vein.

The gastrocolic omentum is divided, and the lesser sac is entered. Division of the middle colic vein is performed routinely by some surgeons to help expose the superior mesenteric vein. Gentle dissection is performed immediately anterior to the superior mesenteric vein at the inferior margin of the pancreatic neck to determine whether the tumor involves the confluence of the superior mesenteric and portal veins. Any resistance in developing this plane of dissection should halt further mobilization of the pancreatic neck inferiorly, because injuries to the retropancreatic portal vein can be very difficult to control.

Dissection of the porta hepatis in the hepatoduodenal ligament is begun. The gallbladder is dissected free of the liver. The common hepatic duct is divided just superior to the cystic duct. The common bile duct is mobilized inferiorly and the common hepatic artery is retracted medially, exposing the anterior surface of the portal vein. The gastroduodenal artery is divided, and the plane between the anterior surface of the portal vein and pancreatic neck is developed further. During the portal dissection, the surgeon should consider the possibility of an accessory or replaced right or common hepatic artery and limit unintentional injury or ligation of the aberrant vessel.

If the patient is undergoing standard pancreaticoduodenectomy, an antrectomy is performed along with a segmental omentectomy. A pylorus-preserving Whipple procedure resects the duodenum 2 cm distal to the pylorus (see "PPPD"). The jejunum just beyond the ligament of Treitz is divided, along with its supporting mesentery. The mobilized jejunum and fourth portion of the duodenum are delivered beneath the superior mesenteric vessels to the patient's right side. The pancreatic neck is divided over the portal vein. The pancreatic head and uncinate process are dissected off of the superior mesenteric and portal veins; these vessels are then retracted medially to expose the superior mesenteric artery, from which the pancreatic attachments are separated. If limited lateral venous involvement is identified, it can be managed with either tangential or segmental resection of the portal vein and/or superior mesenteric vein (see "Extended Resection").

Reconstruction

To complete the reconstruction, three anastomoses must be made: pancreaticojejunostomy or pancreaticogastrostomy, choledochojejunostomy, and gastrojejunostomy. The order in which these are performed is a matter of surgeon preference. The jejunum is typically delivered through the transverse mesocolon, and the pancreas is mobilized off of the splenic vein. A two-layer pancreaticojejunal anastomosis is made end-to-end or end-to-side with fine interrupted absorbable monofilament suture, approximating pancreatic duct-to-jejunal mucosa. An end-to-side choledochojejunostomy is performed in one layer by using continuous or interrupted absorbable monofilament suture. In standard pancreaticoduodenectomy, the stomach is anastomosed to a loop, or roux limb, of jejunum brought anterior to the transverse colon. The gastrojejunal anastomosis is accomplished in an end-to-side manner. The jejunum should lie in a roughly transverse manner along the greater curvature of the stomach once the anastomosis is complete.

Due to the risk of pancreatic leak, the placement of intraperitoneal drains at the time of resection has been considered routine practice. However, a prospective randomized trial compared no intraperitoneal drain placement with placement of a standard closed suction drain at the choledochojejunal and pancreaticojejunal anastomosis after pancreatic resection.[2] No significant difference was observed between groups in overall morbidity or mortality; however, patients who received a drain were more likely to develop intra-abdominal fluid collection, fistula, and abscess. Thus, the conclusion of this trial was that routine drainage did not benefit and may harm patients undergoing pancreatic resection. The placement of a feeding jejunostomy tube is an option for enteral access for nutrition in case of postoperative complications. This also is dependent on surgeon preference and carries a unique set of risks.

Efficacy

Although resection has long been considered the only potentially curative treatment option for pancreatic cancer, only one trial has actually compared resection to nonsurgical therapy in a randomized fashion. A small Japanese trial compared radical resection (20 patients) to chemoradiation (22 patients) in patients with resectable pancreatic cancer and demonstrated significantly better one-year (62% vs. 32%, $p<0.03$) and mean survival (greater than 17 vs. 11 months, $p = 0.04$ in the resection group).[3]

These results are comparable to those of several, larger non-randomized studies. In one of the largest published series, over 600 patients from Johns Hopkins Hospital, 1- and 5-year survival rates after potentially curative pancreaticoduodenectomy were 64% and 17%, respectively; median survival was 17 months. Important prognostic factors after potentially curative resection include lymph node status, tumor size, tumor grade, and resection margin status and long.

Complications

The main complications of pancreaticoduodenectomy are abdominal wound infection (10%), delayed gastric emptying (20–40%), pancreatic fistula (10–20%), and intra-abdominal abscess (10–15%). Tertiary referral centers report overall morbidity rates of 40–50%. Five to ten percent of patients require reoperation in the immediate postoperative period because of bleeding, abscess, or dehiscence. Over the last decade, there has been increasing recognition of the relationship between outcomes and pancreaticoduodenectomy volume, particularly hospital volume. Operative mortality rates associated with pancreaticoduodenectomy at high-volume institutions rarely exceed 5%.

In particular, surgeons have sought ways to reduce the likelihood of pancreatic leak, since this complication causes considerable morbidity and mortality. Several retrospective or nonrandomized trials have suggested that pancreaticogastrostomy may be associated with lower rates of leak and morbidity than pancreaticojejunostomy. However, these results have not been substantiated in randomized trials.

Although numerous approaches to the pancreatic anastomosis have been described, few have been studied in randomized trials. A prospective randomized trial at a single institution comparing invagination ("dunking"), end-to-end with duct-to-mucosa, end-to-side pancreaticojejunostomy after classic pancreaticoduodenectomy for resectable periampullary cancer found a lower rate of pancreatic fistula, morbidity and mortality in the duct-to-mucosa group.[4] However, more recently, another prospective randomized, dual-institution trial found that the invagination has a significantly lower rate of pancreatic fistula, morbidity and mortality.[5] The most important variable after a multivariable analysis was the presence of a "soft" gland. Pancreatic duct occlusion rather than anastomosis does not appear to reduce postoperative leaks or complications and may increase the long-term risk of diabetes.

Octreotide inhibits pancreatic exocrine secretions and, in a series of trials that included a range of procedures for both benign and malignant diseases, was shown to decrease pancreatic leak rate and overall morbidity. Subsequent trials including only patients undergoing pancreaticoduodenectomy failed to support a benefit for the routine use of prophylactic octreotide, although its selective use in patients with high-risk glands — soft consistency and/or small ducts — may be justified.[6]

Pylorus-Preserving Pancreaticoduodenectomy

Indications

Surgeons who favor pylorus-preserving pancreaticoduodenectomy (PPPD) cite a decreased incidence of long-term complications, such as nutritional deficiency, marginal ulceration, post-gastrectomy dumping, bile reflux gastritis, and abnormal gastric acid secretion. It is controversial whether these benefits to long-term digestive function may be associated with increased short-term complications. However, PPPD is considered an acceptable alternative to standard PD, particularly for patients with a long life expectancy.

Contraindications

Tumor involvement of the pylorus or first portion of the duodenum is a contraindication to pylorus-preserving pancreaticoduodenectomy. Patients with evidence of tumor encroachment on the first portion of the duodenum or pylorus should undergo the standard Whipple procedure. If there is evidence of ischemia of the retained duodenal cuff, a pylorus-preserving pancreaticoduodenectomy should not be attempted.

Technique

Pylorus preservation involves proximal division of the gastrointestinal tract to preserve the antrum and pylorus. The duodenum is divided 2–3 cm distal to the pylorus. Careful preservation of the blood flow to the proximal duodenum and vagal innervation to the antrum and pylorus must be achieved.

Efficacy

Nonrandomized studies have suggested that PPPD is associated with long-term benefits such as better weight gain, decreased incidence of postgastrectomy syndromes, and improved pancreatic endocrine and exocrine function. Prospective randomized data indicate that standard PD and PPPD are similar in terms of perioperative morbidity, mortality, quality of life, and oncologic outcome.[7,8] Therefore, whether long-term digestive function is better after PPPD remains unproven, but PPPD appears to be a safe and oncologic-equivalent alternative to standard PD for appropriate patients.

Complications

Although one randomized trial demonstrated a significantly higher incidence of delayed gastric emptying after PPPD,[7] the other actually demonstrated a slightly but not significantly higher incidence after standard PD.[8] Those who support standard pancreaticoduodenectomy also point out the theoretically increased incidence of duodenojejunal anastomotic ulceration, although the incidence of this complication seems to be quite low with the routine use of pharmacologic acid suppression.

Extended (Regional) Pancreaticoduodenectomy and Vascular Resection

Indications

Surgeons have proposed wide *en bloc* resection of peripancreatic soft tissue, including that overlying the medial aspect of the right kidney and inferior vena cava, along with nodal stations along the common hepatic artery, superior mesenteric artery, and superior and inferior borders of the body of the pancreas. The rationale for this approach is based on the high incidence of retroperitoneal soft tissue invasion and metastases to these regional nodes. Although vascular resection is not routinely a part of extended pancreaticoduodenectomy, resection of the portal vein (PV) or superior mesenteric vein (SMV) is indicated when necessary to achieve an R0 (margin negative) resection.

Contraindications

Similar to standard pancreaticoduodenectomy, extended pancreaticoduodenectomy is contraindicated in the setting of distant metastatic or locally advanced disease with arterial encasement or major venous occlusion.

Technique

Extended pancreaticoduodenectomy requires an extended Kocher maneuver to the left side of the aorta. The line of pancreatic resection is extended to the left of the superior mesenteric artery and superior mesenteric vein to better visualize these vessels as well as the celiac axis. The peripancreatic soft tissue, including that overlying the medial right kidney and inferior vena cava, is aggressively resected, and the aorta, hepatic, proximal splenic and superior mesenteric arteries and the inferior vena cava are skeletonized for resection of these nodal basins.

Vascular resection consists of either tangential or segmental venous resection as part of the specimen. Division of the splenic vein is one alternative that allows for better visualization of the PV-SMV confluence for difficult lesions as well as simplifying vascular control of the PV confluence. Proximal and distal control of the involved segment is obtained and the resection ensues. Reconstruction of the resected vein specimen depends on size of vein removed; options include primary repair, vein patch, or interposition graft from a saphenous, internal jugular or common femoral vein graft. In patients with preoperative imaging that demonstrates evidence of vein involvement, prepping the vein harvest site at the outset of the procedure allows for convenient harvesting later during the procedure.

Efficacy

Nonrandomized studies from Japan suggested improved survival in patients who underwent more extensive lymphadenectomy. However, Western randomized controlled trials have been unable to demonstrate a survival benefit for extended lymphadenectomy.[9,10]

An Italian multicenter trial compared standard (40 patients) with extended (41 patients) lymphadenectomy plus pancreaticoduodenectomy for pancreatic head adenocarcinoma.[10] Extended resection did not appear to improve the rate of negative microscopic resection margins.

A more recent single-center trial conducted at the Mayo Clinic compared standard (40 patients) to extended (39 patients) lymphadenectomy for pancreatic head adenocarcinoma.[9] Operative time was longer and blood transfusion more likely in the extended lymphadenectomy, but perioperative morbidity and mortality were not significantly different. All previous studies were underpowered to detect a survival difference between groups, particularly since the only patients who theoretically should benefit from extended lymphadenectomy are those who have retroperitoneal nodal metastases not included within a standard lymphadenectomy, who have a complete (R0) resection, and who do not have occult distant metastases. It has been estimated that fewer than 1% of patients meet these criteria, and a definitive study would require a prohibitively large number of patients.

Numerous studies have studied the role of vascular resection, specifically focusing on either portal or superior mesenteric vein resection. Most of these studies reveal that morbidity, mortality, and median survival are not significantly affected by vascular resection. Most have described the use of venous grafts for reconstruction, yet some have published on the successful use of prosthetic graft in this setting. The data for arterial resection and reconstruction has not been as favorable, and thus arterial resection is not performed with nearly as much frequency as venous resection at most high-volume centers. There is a paucity of data and lack of consensus regarding the use of either anticoagulation (heparin, low molecular weight heparin, Coumadin) or anti-platelet therapy (aspirin, Plavix) in the postoperative period for the preservation of PV patency.

SUMMARY

Pancreaticoduodenectomy is a technically challenging operation. However, very acceptable morbidity and mortality rates have been achieved at high volume centers. Preoperative planning including review of comorbid conditions and diagnostic imaging studies is imperative for best results following PD. The technical, intraoperative steps of the procedure are reproducible by experienced surgeons. The most critical and challenging component may be the postoperative management of patients requiring PD. A strong medical system with resources and capable surgeons, intensivists, radiologists, gastroenterologists, and pathologists all contribute to the continued improved outcomes of patients undergoing PD.

REFERENCES

1. Tyler DS, Evans DB. Reoperative pancreaticoduodenectomy. *Ann Surg* 1994; 219(2):211–221.
2. Conlon KC, Labow D, Leung D, *et al.* Prospective randomized clinical trial of the value of intraperitoneal drainage after pancreatic resection. *Ann Surg* 2001; 234(4):487–493; Discussion 493–494.
3. Imamura M, Doi R, Imaizumi T, *et al.* A randomized multicenter trial comparing resection and radiochemotherapy for resectable locally invasive pancreatic cancer. *Surgery* 2004; 136(5):1003–1011.
4. Chou FF, Sheen-Chen SM, Chen YS, *et al.* Postoperative morbidity and mortality of pancreaticoduodenectomy for periampullary cancer. *Eur J Surg* 1996; 162(6):477–481.
5. Berger AC, Howard TJ, Kennedy EP, *et al.* Does type of pancreaticojejunostomy after pancreaticoduodenectomy decrease rate of pancreatic fistula? A randomized, prospective, dual-institution trial. *J Am Coll Surg* 2009; 208(5):738–747; Discussion 747–749.
6. Li-Ling J, and Irving M. Somatostatin and octreotide in the prevention of postoperative pancreatic complications and the treatment of enterocutaneous pancreatic fistulas: a systematic review of randomized controlled trials. *Br J Surg* 2001; 88:190–199.
7. Lin PW, Shan YS, Lin YJ, *et al.* Pancreaticoduodenectomy for pancreatic head cancer: PPPD versus Whipple procedure. *Hepatogastroenterology* 2005; 52(65):1601–1614.
8. Seiler CA, Wagner M, Sadowski C, *et al.* Randomized prospective trial of pyloruspreserving vs. Classic duodenopancreatectomy (Whipple procedure): initial clinical results. *J Gastrointest Surg* 2000; 4(5):443–452.
9. Farnell MB, Pearson RK, Sarr MG, *et al.* A prospective randomized trial comparing standard pancreatoduodenectomy with pancreatoduodenectomy with extended lymphadenectomy in resectable pancreatic head adenocarcinoma. *Surgery* 2005; 138(4):618–628; Discussion 628–630.
10. Pedrazzoli S, Dicarlo V, Dionigi R, *et al.* Standard versus extended lymphadenectomy associated with pancreatoduodenectomy in the surgical treatment of adenocarcinoma of the head of the pancreas: a multicenter, prospective, randomized study. Lymphadenectomy Study Group. *Ann Surg* 1998; 228(4):508–517.

SURGICAL TECHNIQUES: PALLIATIVE SURGERY 46

Jeffrey Nienaber*
and Theodore N. Pappas*

INTRODUCTION

With the majority of pancreatic cancers presenting with either metastatic or unresectable disease, the surgeon should be knowledgeable of the various modalities and techniques of palliative therapy and their respective indications. As most pancreatic tumors develop in the head, palliation is most commonly needed for obstruction of either the biliary or gastrointestinal tract. Pain control is the next most common indication for intervention, often in combination with other palliative procedures. The decision to intervene and the timing and mode of palliation depend on many factors, particularly the patient's level of disease, anticipated survival and comorbid conditions. With advancements in endoluminal and percutaneous interventions as well as chemoradiation therapy, many situations that could previously only be managed operatively are now preferentially managed nonoperatively.

In this chapter, palliative management will be presented from the perspective of the surgeon faced with the decision of how best to palliate the patient's symptoms in the setting of unresectable disease. Sometimes this decision can be made preoperatively. Often, however, some degree of operative exploration is required to determine resectability and decisions must be made intraoperatively. In either case, it is important to know the

---

*Duke University Medical Center, Department of Surgery, Durham, NC 27710 USA

anatomy of the tumor including its location within the pancreas, the tumor size and the direction and degree of growth into surrounding structures.

More importantly, one must know prior to any surgical exploration if the patient is in need of palliation regardless of whether resection is possible or not; i.e. does the patient have biliary or gastrointestinal obstruction or pain referable to the tumor. A plan for how to deal with possible intraoperative findings should be in place prior to surgery in order to properly counsel the patient, request preoperative interventions, avoid poor intraoperative decisions and limit the need for reintervention postoperatively. Biliary obstruction is typically evident clinically by the presence of jaundice or generalized pruritis. Laboratory studies will show hyperbilirubinemia with elevated alkaline phosphatase and imaging studies, most commonly CT or ultrasound, will show dilation of the intra and extrahepatic biliary tree (Figures 1a, 1b). Gastrointestinal or, more specifically, gastric outlet obstruction (GOO, Figures 2a, 2b), typically presents with vomiting and dehydration though nausea, fullness, anorexia and weight loss can be early symptoms as well. Pain referable to the tumor is often a constant dull pain in the epigastric area or in the mid to upper back. Thus, the typical preoperative workup of a history and physical, laboratory studies including liver function tests and an abdominal CT will provide sufficient assessment of the need for palliative therapy. If suspicion for gastric outlet obstruction exists, additional studies including a gastric emptying study and a trial of prokinetic agents may be necessary to evaluate for gastroparesis as not all patients with nausea and vomiting in the setting of a pancreatic head mass have true GOO.

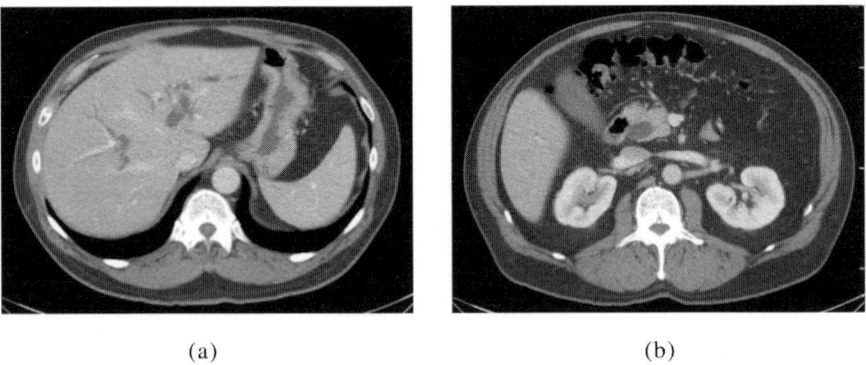

(a)   (b)

Figure 1. (a) Intrahepatic and (b) extrahepatic biliary ductal dilation.

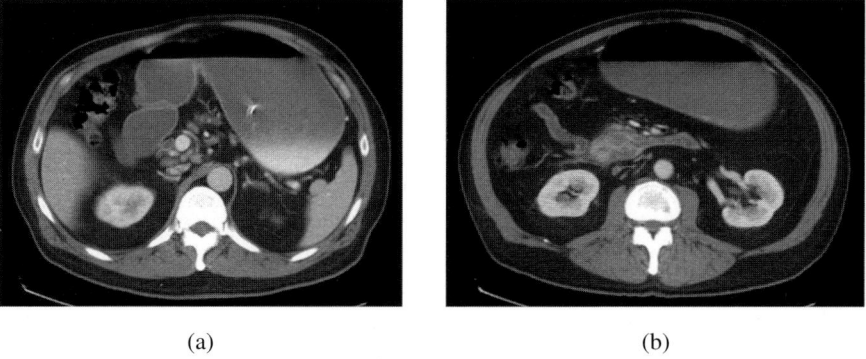

(a) (b)

Figure 2. Gastric outlet obstruction: (a) stomach and proximal duodenum dilated secondary to (b) obstructing pancreatic head mass. (b) Note the decompressed 4th portion of the duodenum.

Three common scenarios leading to palliative therapy for pancreatic head cancer are:

Scenario #1 — Occult metastatic disease identified on exploratory laparoscopy.

Scenario #2 — Open exploration and mobilization performed in preparation for possible pancreaticoduodenectomy only to find the disease to be unresectable.

Scenario #3 — Unresectable or metastatic disease based on preoperative imaging with clinical biliary and/or gastric outlet obstruction.

SCENARIO #1: OCCULT METASTATIC DISEASE IDENTIFIED ON EXPLORATORY LAPAROSCOPY

Many surgeons routinely perform exploratory laparoscopy prior to proceeding with pancreaticoduodenectomy as approximately 20% of patients will have visible metastatic disease, which would contraindicate pancreaticoduodenectomy. With respect to palliation, the question then becomes whether any further surgical intervention should be performed at that time. A study by Espat et al.[1] showed that only 3% of patients deemed unresectable by exploratory laparoscopy required surgical palliation in the future. Furthermore, the general principle in this scenario is to use the least invasive means of palliation available as the anticipated survival for these patients is typically in the order of months. Nonoperative measures such as biliary and duodenal stenting are viewed with increasing favor in this setting. In those instances where surgical palliation is necessary at the time of exploratory laparoscopy, laparoscopic techniques are preferred and will be discussed in this scenario.

There is a fairly strong consensus that if the patient has a patent biliary stent in place upon identifying metastatic disease on laparoscopy, surgical biliary bypass is not recommended. Likewise, if the patient does not have a stent in place and no evidence of biliary obstruction, no biliary intervention is recommended. Rather, the patient should be monitored for the development of biliary obstruction and stenting attempted at that time. Smith et al.[2] have shown that patients can be palliated with biliary stents with less morbidity and procedure-related mortality than surgical bypass, albeit with greater likelihood for re-intervention (of note, teflon stents were used in this trial, published in 1994, rather than metal). Another, subsequent randomized trial[3] showed that metal stents have longer patency rates than plastic stents. Due to lower costs, plastic stents are typically recommended for palliation of patients with estimated survival less than 6 months (e.g. those with liver metastases). Self-expanding metal stents remain the gold standard for the rest and covered or chemotherapeutic-eluting stents show promise for extending patency rates in the future. With such advancements in biliary stenting, the odds of needing to perform a biliary bypass in Scenario #1 or at any point thereafter are very low. Accordingly, open and laparoscopic biliary bypass techniques will be discussed in Scenarios #2 & 3 respectively.

While the incidence of biliary obstruction due to a pancreatic head mass is fairly high (approximately 70%) and expertise in biliary stenting is increasingly widespread, the incidence of gastric outlet obstruction is relatively low (approximately 20%) and expertise in duodenal stenting is more limited. If the patient in Scenario #1 is not exhibiting GOO clinically, no further intervention at this time is indicated. If they are symptomatic, however, palliation is clearly indicated though the mode remains a topic of debate. As with biliary obstruction, nonoperative intervention is associated with less morbidity, though with greater likelihood for reintervention. No large randomized studies comparing duodenal stenting and gastrojejunostomy have been published to date. Small randomized studies and a systematic review[4] have concluded that stenting is associated with earlier oral intake but shorter long-term patency compared with gastrojejunostomy (Figure 3). Thus, the literature suggests that stenting is better for patients

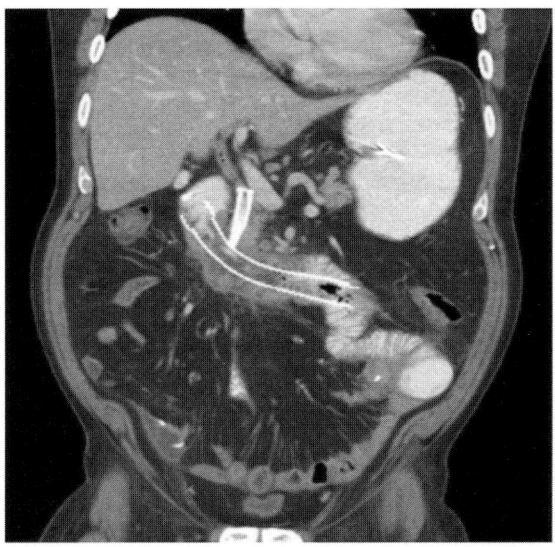

Figure 3. Palliative gastrojejunostomy was performed on this patient following occlusion of a duodenal stent (contrast in the small intestine on this reformatted coronal CT scan is secondary to a patent gastrojejunostomy). A biliary stent is also in place.

with very limited (up to a couple of months) prognosis. At this time, however, unlike with biliary stenting, the patency rates have not been shown to be long enough to justify duodenal stenting rather than gastrojejunostomy at the time of laparoscopic exploration prior to possible pancreaticoduodenectomy. This may certainly change over the next several years as endoluminal therapies continue to evolve.

If the patient has GOO in this scenario, our practice is to perform a gastrojejunostomy during the same procedure. This is preferably performed laparoscopically. Though no large randomized studies have been published, retrospective and small randomized studies such as that by Navarra et al.[5] have shown that laparoscopic gastrojejunostomy has faster time to solid food intake and overall less morbidity compared to open. Our method utilizes a Hassan port at the umbilicus plus three other ports: a 12-mm port below the right costal margin to accommodate a stapler and 5-mm ports below the 12-mm port and in the left upper quadrant at the mid-clavicular line. The greater omentum and transverse colon are retracted cephalad and the ligament of Treitz is identified. A defect is created in the transverse mesocolon near the ligament of Treitz to the left of the middle colic artery and the posteroinferior face of the stomach is pulled through this window. It is important to confirm that the area is prepyloric and, ideally, in the most dependent portion of the stomach. A loop of jejunum 15 cm distal to the ligament of Treitz is identified and approximated to the stomach using stay sutures. The anastomosis is created with a 60 × 3.5 mm GIA stapler after making a gastrotomy and jejunotomy with either electrocautery or a harmonic scalpel. The common enterotomy is closed with another fire of a 3.5-mm stapler. The mesenteric defect is closed with multiple interrupted absorbable sutures connecting the stomach to the transverse mesocolon.

Consideration should be given for concomitant placement of a feeding jejunostomy tube downstream of the anastomosis, which can also be placed laparoscopically. Enteral nutrition is clearly superior to parenteral nutrition and delayed gastric emptying is not an uncommon (up to 20% of cases) complication of gastrojejunostomy limiting progression of oral nutrition. However, while often performed for the purpose of ensuring early enteral nutrition, major complications related to a feeding jejunostomy tube occur in approximately 2% of cases. These include pneumatosis intestinalis, volvulus, bowel obstruction, enterocutaneous fistula and abdominal wall, subcutaneous or intra-abdominal infection. An alternative, which has not been studied in the palliative gastrojejunostomy literature, is a temporary nasojejunal tube. In a study by Abu-Hilal et al.[6] primarily including pancreaticoduodenectomy patients, nasojejunal tubes were associated with fewer postoperative complications compared with feeding jejunostomy tubes. Our practice is to place feeding jejunostomy tubes selectively and we typically do not place feeding jejunostomy tubes in this scenario.

If the surgeon is not skilled in performing a laparoscopic gastrojejunostomy, open gastrojejunostomy is indicated. The anastomosis is essentially the same as for a laparoscopic gastrojejunostomy except that the procedure is performed through an upper midline laparotomy. Alternatives to open gastrojejunostomy, depending on the surgeon's skill set, include combined gastrostomy and jejunostomy tube placement, either laparoscopic or open, or attempted placement of a gastrojejunal tube, typically by gastroenterology or interventional radiology. Again, if the patient is felt to be healthy enough for pancreaticoduodenectomy, gastrojejunostomy is typically the preferred surgical procedure as this is intuitively associated with better quality of life as the patient has fewer dietary limitations and is not necessarily dependent on tubes for nutrition and gastric decompression.

Debate is ongoing regarding optimal anatomy of the gastrojejunostomy. One issue is whether the anastomosis should be in the ante- or retrocolic location. Our preference is for a retrocolic anastomosis to better allow gravity to aid in emptying the stomach. Strong data to back this are lacking, however, though the group at Johns Hopkins cites a slightly decreased incidence of delayed gastric emptying with a retrocolic anastomosis.[7] Another issue is whether to use a roux limb or a loop and this will be discussed under Scenario #2 with biliary bypass options.

Finally, for those that perform open exploration rather than laparoscopic and occult metastatic disease or other indicators of unresectability are identified prior to mobilization, there is no consensus for whether the patient should undergo any further surgery. If the patient has no biliary obstruction or a patent biliary stent and no clinical GOO, many would advocate closing up without any further intervention. Others would favor a prophylactic double bypass (biliary and gastrointestinal), arguing that the much of the morbidity of a double bypass has already been incurred by the laparotomy alone. Finally, others go on a case-by-case basis where one or the other or both bypasses are done selectively if, for example, the patient is fairly robust with a longer than average anticipated survival and tumor anatomy that would place them at higher risk for obstruction in the near future. Again, it is typically preferred to exhaust all reasonable nonoperative options in the setting of biliary obstruction. Data for the prophylactic gastrojejunal bypass point of view will be discussed in Scenario #2.

SCENARIO #2: OPEN EXPLORATION AND MOBILIZATION PERFORMED IN PREPARATION FOR POSSIBLE PANCREATICODUODENECTOMY ONLY TO FIND THE DISEASE TO BE UNRESECTABLE

In this scenario, the patient has already had a laparotomy and some degree of mobilization in preparation for possible pancreaticoduodenectomy, only to find the disease to be unresectable. Again, while some would advocate closing up in the absence of clinical biliary or gastric outlet obstruction, we feel that in most cases, much of the morbidity of either a pancreaticoduodenectomy or a double bypass has already been inflicted. Thus, our practice is typically to perform a double bypass (gastric and biliary) regardless of the patient's symptoms. Lillemoe *et al.*[7] have shown, in a randomized trial of 87 patients, that prophylactic retrocolic gastrojejunostomy reduced the incidence of late GOO. All patients had disease that was found to be unresectable upon exploration, many of whom had metastatic disease (the group's preference was to perform open rather than laparoscopic exploration). Most of these patients were felt to have or be at risk for GOO based on preoperative workup and intraoperative findings, and underwent gastrojejunostomy without inclusion in the trial. The remaining patients who were not felt to be at risk for GOO were randomized to either undergo gastrojejunostomy or not. Between 80% and 90% also underwent concomitant hepaticojejunostomy and/or chemical splanchnicectomy. The authors found that 19% of the patients who did not undergo prophylactic gastrojejunostomy eventually required intervention for GOO, primarily via gastrojejunostomy (one patient underwent duodenal stenting). There were no differences in morbidity, mortality, long-term survival or hospital length of stay, though the procedure took 45 minutes longer with a gastrojejunostomy. A subsequent, multicenter randomized trial in the Netherlands[8] showed similar results. Thus, one argument for performing a prophylactic gastrojejunostomy is that it can be done with equivalent outcomes in this scenario and eliminates the need for reoperation later on when the patient may be in a more morbid state.

Opponents of the prophylactic gastrojejunostomy counter that the incidence of GOO is not as high as that reported in the aforementioned studies and that it can be difficult to distinguish clinically from gastroparesis. Others point out that these studies were performed a decade ago and that duodenal stent capabilities have improved in the interim. Indeed, while most would not advocate for a prophylactic duodenal stent, many would consider it the first line of palliative treatment. Finally, many would argue for preventive gastrojejunostomy only in select patients, though the clinical grounds for this decision are more difficult to define (e.g. what constitutes "impending GOO" based on tumor anatomy, how can survival be accurately predicted).

Oftentimes, the question is simplified based on the amount of mobilization that needs to be done before someone is declared unresectable. If, for example, the common bile duct and stomach are divided only to find that the tumor cannot be separated from the portal vein (even with possible reconstruction), the decision to do a double bypass is fairly simple. Furthermore, there is nonrandomized data to suggest that an R1 (microscopic margin-positive) pancreaticoduodenectomy is associated with improved survival relative to palliative double bypass in high-volume centers.[9] There is currently no consensus on this approach, however, and this study lacks quality of life data to compare the relative palliative value of the two approaches. One must consider that pancreatic cancer is primarily a surgical disease at the present time, and that more aggressive surgical approaches with a realistic intent to cure are typically justified.

Our preference for a standard double bypass is to perform a retrocolic Roux-en-y choledochojejunostomy with retrocolic gastrojejunostomy (Figure 4). This is typically performed through an upper midline laparotomy, though a bilateral subcostal approach is also acceptable. A cholecystectomy is performed. If the common bile duct has already been transected, any stents are removed and the defunctionalized stump is oversewn with polyglyconate suture. The anastomosis is then performed in an end-to-side manner. If the common bile duct is intact, it is preferable to leave it intact and perform a side-to-side anastomosis, again after removing any stents.

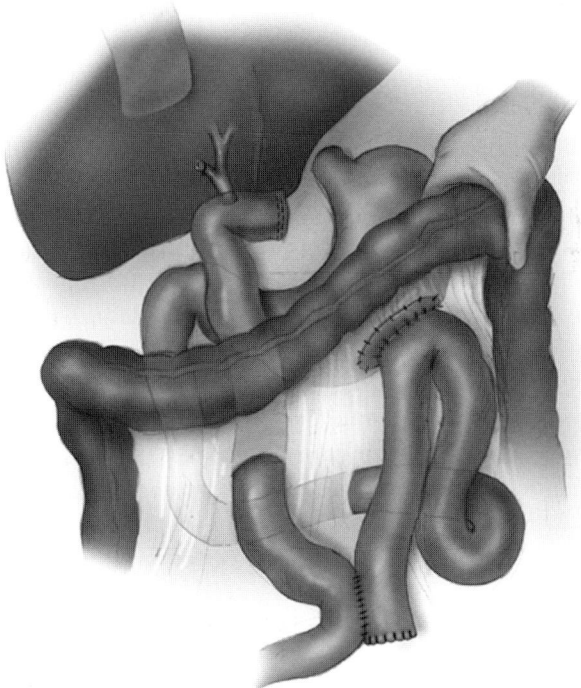

Figure 4. Retrocolic Roux-en-y choledochojejunostomy (right of middle colic artery) and gastrojejunostomy (left of middle colic artery).

To create the Roux limb, the jejunum is transected 30 cm distal to the ligament of Treitz using a GIA stapler. A window is created in the transverse mesocolon to the right of the middle colic artery and the proximal Roux limb is brought through this into the right upper quadrant. The mesentery must be adequately mobilized to avoid tension without compromising the blood flow to the tip of the roux limb. After creating a jejunotomy a few centimeters from the staple line, an end (common bile duct) to side (jejunum), or side-to-side choledochojejunostomy is then performed. The anastomosis is performed using interrupted 3-0 polyglyconate sutures in a "spokes on a wheel" fashion with the knots on the posterior sutures tied inside the lumen and the remaining knots outside. Care is taken to ensure that biliary ductal mucosa is in contact with jejunal mucosa. Interrupted absorbable sutures are then used to close the mesenteric defect by approximating the mesocolon to the jejunum.

The gastrojejunostomy is then performed to the left of the middle colic artery as described in Scenario #1, approximately 15 cm from the ligament of Treitz. Finally, the jejunojejunostomy is performed approximately 50 cm from the end of the choledochojejunal anastomosis in a side-to-side, functional end-to-side manner. This is done by creating a jejunotomy in the Roux limb as well as the distal gastrojejunal limb and connecting the lumens on the antimesenteric border with a 60-mm GIA stapler. The common enterotomy is likewise closed with a GIA or TA stapler. Again, consideration should be given for placing a feeding jejunostomy tube as discussed above. We do not routinely place a feeding tube in this scenario either. A drain is typically placed near the choledochojejunostomy and removed if the output is nonbilious once the patient is tolerating a diet or tube feeding.

There are several alternatives to a Roux-en-y choledochojejunostomy. One would be a loop choledochojejunostomy where the jejunum is left in continuity and is brought through the transverse mesocolon downstream of the gastrojejunal anastomosis and the anastomosis is performed as with a Roux limb. A side-to-side jejunojejunostomy is performed to limit biliary reflux into the stomach. While this saves operating time, a loop is associated with more tension and a higher rate of cholangitis compared to a Roux. A choledochoduodenostomy is another alternative if the anatomy will allow for a side-to-side anastomosis of the common bile duct to the first part of the duodenum. A choledochoduodenostomy is generally avoided if there is concern for impending duodenal obstruction from the tumor, which limits its application in the setting of pancreatic head lesions.

A cholecystojejunostomy, either open or laparoscopic, provides more variable palliation of biliary obstruction than other means. Utilization of this approach requires careful patient selection to achieve acceptable outcomes. Prior cholecystectomy, tumors <1 cm from the hepatocystic junction and hilar obstruction are contraindications to cholecystojejunostomy. Furthermore, the patency of the cystic duct must be confirmed prior to proceeding with the bypass. The laparoscopic procedure can be combined with a laparoscopic gastrojejunostomy and will be discussed in Scenario #3 below. The open approach has largely fallen out of favor and is rarely indicated.

Two other infrequently indicated options for biliary bypass are hepaticojejunostomy and segment III bypass. Hepaticojejunostomy is indicated if there is compromise of the common bile duct or portions of the common hepatic duct either from tumor, lymphadenopathy or fibrosis (infection, radiation therapy). Here, the origin of the common hepatic duct is anastomosed to either a Roux limb or a loop of jejunum similar to a choledochojejunostomy. Segment III or right sectorial duct bypass is indicated when there is compromise of the hepatic duct confluence or the left hepatic duct. Most commonly this is used for Klatskin tumors and indications for the procedure with unresectable pancreatic head lesions are fortunately rare as the procedure carries a higher biliary leak rate compared with aforementioned options. The dilated segment III duct is identified just left of the falciform ligament running along with the segmental portal vein branch within the hepatic parenchyma. The duct is incised over a 1-cm length and anastomosed to a Roux limb or loop similar to a choledochojejunostomy.

SCENARIO #3: UNRESECTABLE OR METASTATIC DISEASE BASED ON PREOPERATIVE IMAGING WITH CLINICAL BILIARY AND/OR GASTRIC OUTLET OBSTRUCTION

In this setting, the patient is clearly not a candidate for resection based on preoperative imaging or comorbidities. Again, endoscopic or percutaneous biliary stenting is the first line of treatment for biliary obstruction. In this scenario, duodenal stenting is often the preferred initial treatment for gastric outlet obstruction. Surgical therapy is considered once patients have failed nonoperative palliative interventions as discussed above, though one must consider whether the patient has an extremely limited life expectancy (e.g. weeks) or comorbidities that would prohibit general anesthesia. In such cases, percutaneous biliary drainage for biliary obstruction or percutaneous gastrojejunostomy tube placement for decompression and feeding may be in order.

The advantage in this scenario relative to Scenarios 1 and 2 is that the surgeon can plan for the most minimally invasive surgical means of palliation prior to going to the operating room. While surgical options can include a laparoscopic or open bypass (either biliary, gastrointestinal or both), the laparoscopic approach is typically preferred, though strong data indicating superiority to open techniques are lacking. Laparoscopic approaches require careful patient selection in this population, specifically with regards to the biliary anatomy as in Scenario #2. If the patient only has gastric outlet obstruction, laparoscopic gastrojejunostomy is preferred, as opposed to laparoscopic double bypass; this technique was discussed in Scenario #1. For patients with isolated biliary obstruction that have failed nonsurgical palliation, laparoscopic biliary bypass is preferred, as opposed to laparoscopic double bypass. If open palliation is required, again our practice is typically to do a double bypass.

For patients deemed appropriate palliative surgery candidates, our preferred technique for laparoscopic biliary bypass utilizes an antecolic loop cholecystojejunostomy with possible concomitant gastrojejunostomy if deemed appropriate.[10] Port placement for cholecystojejunostomy is the same as described in Scenario #1 for laparoscopic gastrojejunostomy. The first step is to confirm patency of the cystic duct with a cholangiogram via the gallbladder. Relative contraindications to proceeding with cholecystojejunostomy are cholangitis, cholelithiasis and tumor involvement of the hepatic duct/cystic duct confluence or hilum. Significant stenosis or near obliteration of the cystic duct is an absolute contraindication. If the cystic duct is patent, a loop of jejunum 30–40 cm distal to the ligament of Trietz is identified and approximated to the gallbladder in an antecolic manner. If a concomitant gastrojejunostomy is to be performed, this loop is used for the gastrojejunostomy and the biliary anastomosis is performed at least 10 cm downstream of the gastrojejunal anastomosis to prevent biliary reflux. Either anastomosis can be done first in this case. A 3-O nylon suture on a Keith needle is brought through the right upper quadrant abdominal wall, brought through the gallbladder and antimesenteric surface of the jejunum sequentially and used for manipulation and stabilization. A jejunotomy and cholecystotomy are made next to each other using electrocautery and a 30-mm by 3.5-mm load GIA stapler is used to create the anastomosis. The common enterotomy can be closed with either another 30-mm GIA stapler or a handsewn closure. The nylon suture is removed and a blake drain is left in place near the anastomosis. The drain is removed if the output is nonbilious once the patient is tolerating a diet.

PALLIATION OF PAIN

Pain alone is an uncommon indication for surgical palliation. Most chronic pain secondary to unresectable pancreatic malignancies can be managed with either nonsteroidal or narcotic pain medication including scheduled long-acting narcotics. From a general surgical standpoint, interventions aimed at alleviating pain are typically done in combination with other palliative procedures, though other interventions can be performed in isolation in the appropriate clinical setting. The primary means of palliation of pain is via splanchnicectomy. This can be done via a laparotomy (chemical splanchnicectomy), thoracoscopically (division of splanchnic nerves) or percutaneously (celiac plexus block, chemical splanchnicectomy).

The celiac plexus is the largest sympathetic plexus. It is located at approximately the level of L1 on both anterolateral surfaces of the aorta less than 1 cm caudal to the celiac axis. It is composed of a dense network of interconnected presynaptic sympathetic nerve fibers derived from the greater, lesser and least splanchnic nerves as well as parasympathetic fibers from the vagus nerve. The peripancreatic afferent sympathetic fibers transmit pain sensation through this plexus. A percutaneous approach either by an anesthesiologist or an interventional radiologist is typically the preferred initial approach for those failing medical management who are not in need of a laparotomy for other reasons. A solution of 50–100% alcohol is injected near the celiac axis using either bony landmarks (e.g. L1 spinous process) or, preferably, CT or ultrasound guidance to identify the origin of the celiac axis more precisely, which makes the treatment more effective. The alcohol solution destroys the nerve fibers and thus alleviates the pain. Pain relief is typically in the order of several months, which, for many patients, is until their natural death. Bulky retroperitoneal lymphadenopathy is a relative contraindication. Complications most commonly can include transient hypotension and diarrhea with more uncommon complications including paraplegia and paresthesias, gastroparesis, chylothorax, pneumothorax, aortic pseudoaneurysm, retroperitoneal hemorrhage and retroperitoneal fibrosis.

While a laparotomy solely for pain relief is almost never indicated, chemical splanchnicectomy is commonly performed along with other open palliative procedures (e.g. biliary and/or gastrointestinal bypass) in some centers. The most definitive study was a prospective randomized trial by Lillemoe et al.,[11] where patients undergoing laparotomy for unresectable pancreatic cancer received an intraoperative injection of either 50% alcohol or saline (control) in the celiac ganglia. The authors found that experimental patients who did not have significant preoperative pain, had either no subsequent pain or a delay in the onset of pain relative to controls. Furthermore, those that did have pain preoperatively experienced significant relief relative to controls. Surprisingly, those in the experimental group who had significant preoperative pain also had significantly improved survival relative to controls with significant preoperative pain. There were no significant postoperative complications related to the treatment. Relief of pain typically lasted 3–4 months. The treatment itself is fairly simple and consists of injection of 50% alcohol on each side of the aorta at the level of the celiac axis using a 20- or 22-guage spinal needle. The celiac axis can be exposed through a window in the gastrohepatic ligament if necessary.

Thoracoscopic splanchnicectomy has also been proposed as a minimally invasive surgical alternative to abdominal approaches, which is particularly attractive in patients who have failed or are not candidates for percutaneous celiac plexus blockade and have no other indications for laparotomy. The greater and lesser splanchnic nerves are divided via a 3-port thoracoscopic technique either unilaterally or bilaterally.[12] Hospital stays are typically 3 days and approximately 84% of patients will have complete pain relief in their remaining lifespan, which is typically no more than several months. Postoperative complications include pleural effusion, intercostal pain, pneumothorax and recurrent abdominal pain.

REFERENCES

1. Espat NJ, *et al.* Patients with laparoscopically staged unresectable pancreatic adenocarcinoma do not require subsequent surgical biliary or gastric bypass. *J Am Coll Surg* 1999; 188:649–657.
2. Smith AC, *et al.* Randomized trial of endoscopic stenting versus surgical bypass in malignant low bile duct obstruction. *Lancet* 1994; 344:1655–1660.

3. Kaassis M, et al. Plastic or metal stents for malignant stricture of the common bile duct? Results of a randomized prospective study. *Gastrointestinal Endoscopy* 2003; 57:178–182.
4. Jeurnink SM, et al. Stent versus gastrojejunostomy for the palliation of gastric outlet obstruction: a systematic review. *BMC Gastroenterology* 2007; 7:18.
5. Navarra G, et al. Palliative antecolic isoperistaltic gastrojejunostomy: a randomized controlled trial comparing open and laparoscopic approaches. *Surg Endosc* 2006; 20:1831–1834.
6. Abu-Hilal M, et al. A comparative analysis of safety and efficacy of different methods of tube placement for enteral feeding following major pancreatic resection. A non-randomized study. *J Pancreas* 2010; 11:8–13.
7. Lillemoe KD, et al. Is prophylactic gastrojejunostomy indicated for unresectable periampullary cancer? A prospective randomized trial. *Ann Surg* 1999; 230:322–330.
8. Van Heek NT, et al. The need for a prophylactic gastrojejunostomy for unresectable periampullary cancer: a prospective randomized multicenter trial with special focus on assessment of quality of life. *Ann Surg* 2003; 238:894–905.
9. Lavu H, et al. Margin positive pancreaticoduodenectomy is superior to palliative bypass in locally advanced pancreatic ductal adenocarcinoma. *J Gastrointest Surg* 2009; 13:1937–1947.
10. Chekan EG, et al. Laparoscopic biliary and enteric bypass. *Semin Surg Oncol* 1999; 16:313–320.
11. Lillemoe KD, et al. Chemical splanchnicectomy in patients with unresectable pancreatic cancer. A prospective randomized trial. *Ann Surg* 1993; 217:447–457.
12. Saenz A, et al. Thoracoscopic splanchnicectomy for pain control in patients with unresectable carcinoma of the pancreas. *Surg Endosc* 2000; 14:717–720.

SURGICAL TECHNIQUES: DISTAL PANCREATECTOMY 47

Jin S. Yoo and Aurora D. Pryor

INTRODUCTION AND OVERVIEW

This chapter will address the preoperative evaluation and the surgical technique of distal pancreatectomy with and without splenic preservation of pancreatic lesions involving the body and tail of the pancreas. Both open and laparoscopic techniques will be described. There are multiple studies that have shown that laparoscopic distal pancreatectomy can be done safely from a patient safety standpoint as well as clinical outcome (Table 1). It is unsurprising that the laparoscopic approach is supplanting the open approach as the initial approach of choice as the benefits of the minimally invasive approach are realized, such as better visualization of the anatomy during the dissection, less postoperative pain, and earlier return to work/activity.

INDICATIONS/CONTRAINDICATIONS

Pancreatic lesions that are located in the body and tail of the pancreas can be treated with a distal pancreatectomy. This includes benign and malignant pancreatic tumors as well as pseudocysts and even chronic pancreatitis with predominant calcified disease in the body/tail of the pancreas. Small (<2 cm), benign tumors can also be treated with a central pancreatic resection or enucleation, but these two procedures are less commonly

Table 1. Results of laparoscopic distal pancreatectomy (studies with patient sample size more than 10 patients only).

Author	N	Median OR time (min)	Median LOS (days)	Conversion (%)	Peri-op mortality (%)	Overall peri-op morbidity (%)	Leak/ fistula (%)
Patterson et al.[1]	13	264 (96–336)	6 (1–26)	15	0	38	23
Park[2]	25	144 (108–420)*	4.4 (2–8)*	8	0	17	4
Farbe[3]	13	280 (180–480)*	5–22	15	0	30	7
Fernandez-Cruz[4]	19	NR	5.7	0	0	NR	15
Mabrut[5]	96	200 (65–400)	7 (3–67)	15	0	42	16
D'Angelica[6]	17	196 (128–235)	5.5 (4–18)	11	0	26	20
DUKE experience	12	221 (135–358)*	4 (2–7)*	16	0	NR	50

*Average value.
NR not reported.

performed. The most common indication (>70%) for laparoscopic distal pancreatectomy is for benign tumors, more specifically cystadenomas and localized neuroendocrine neoplasms like insulinomas. In general, pancreatic malignancy is a contraindication to laparoscopic resection. However, there are data to support that laparoscopic resection of malignant pancreatic lesions can be safely performed without compromising oncologic principles and more importantly, the overall prognosis.[5–8]

SPLENIC PRESERVATION

There are three general approaches to performing a distal pancreatectomy: (1) distal pancreatectomy with *en bloc* splenectomy, (2) distal pancreatectomy with splenic preservation by preserving the splenic vessels, and (3) distal pancreatectomy with splenic preservation by transecting the splenic vessels proximal to the pathology at the line of gland division and then again at the splenic hilum (and leaving the spleen to survive off collateral blood supplies). The rationale for splenic preservation is to preserve the immune function against encapsulated microorganisms (i.e. Hemophilus, Neisseria, and Streptococcus). Those who do not routinely preserve the spleen during distal pancreatectomy argue that even though some studies show that splenic preservation is associated with decreased peri-operative morbidity,[9] especially infectious complications, there are also studies which have found no difference.[9–14] Splenic preservation with the spleen living off its collateral blood supply (i.e. short gastric arteries and the small vessels in the splenocolic ligaments) allows maintenance of the spleen and thus its function while minimizing the complexity added by attempting to preserve the splenic vessels.[15] This approach is easier and takes less operative time than trying to preserve the splenic artery and vein because it avoids the tedious dissection required to gently separate the pancreas off the vessels and ligate all the small branches during the dissection.[16] However, this approach is associated with a higher risk of splenic infarct when compared to preserving the splenic artery and vein. Fortunately, most of these infarcts are asymptomatic and they will resolve over time based on the trauma literature involving splenic artery embolization.[15,17–18] In several of these series, although infarcts occurred after splenic artery embolization for splenic injury, they were multiple, small, peripherally located infarcts which resolved with time.[17] Furthermore, spleens have regenerative potential demonstrated from the pediatric literature following partial splenectomy.[19]

We recommend splenic preservation with splenic vessel division whenever technically possible to decrease the morbidity of the procedure. If the tumor or pancreatic pseudocyst is closely adherent to the spleen, splenic salvage may not be possible for oncologic and technical reasons, respectively. Portal hypertension is another relative contraindication for splenic vessel preservation due to higher risk of major hemorrhage. The technique of splenic preservation detailed here allows for a short operative time with minimal perioperative mortality and blood loss.[16,20]

LAPAROSCOPIC DISTAL PANCREATECTOMY

Patient Positoning and Preparation

After induction of adequate anesthesia and endotracheal intubation, a foley catheter is placed and the patient is positioned in a supine to right semilateral decubitus position. Supine position is recommended for lesions close to the head of the pancreas and the semilateral decubitus position is

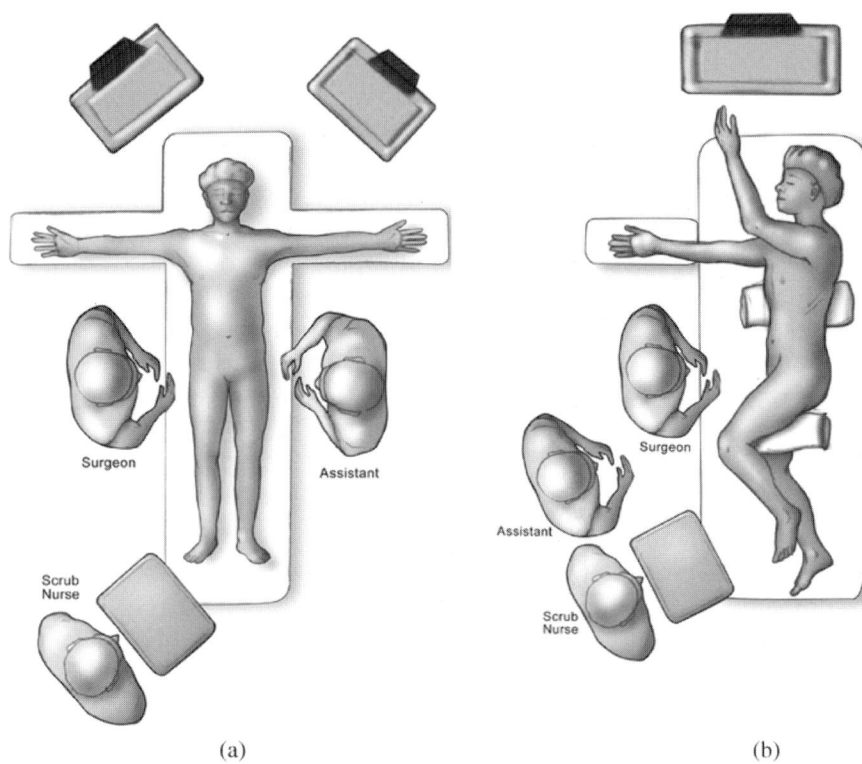

Figure 1. Patient positioning and set-up.

advantageous for lesions away from the head (Figure 1a). Sequential compression devices are placed on each leg for DVT prophylaxis. The abdomen is then prepped and draped in sterile fashion. The surgeon stands on the patient's right side and the assistant stands on the patient's left side. If the patient is positioned in a semilateral decubitus position (Figure 1b), both the surgeon and the assistant stands on the same side.

Positioning of the Laparoscopic Ports (Figure 2)

A 12–15 mm Hasson port is placed at or above the umbilicus and carbon dioxide pneumoperitoneum is created to a pressure of 15 mmHg. A video scope is placed and the abdomen is explored for unsuspecting pathology. The scope may be 30-, or 45-degrees depending on the

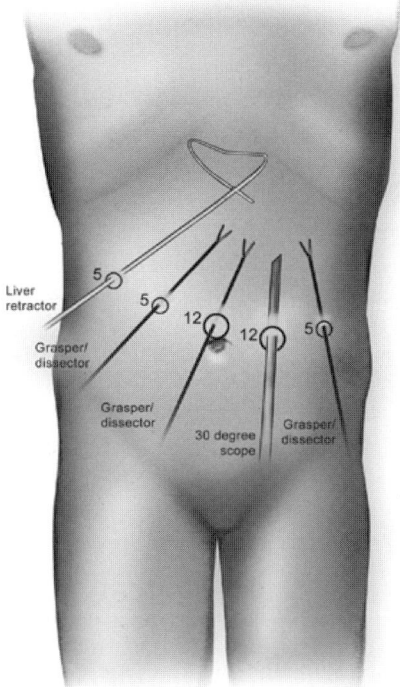

Figure 2. Port positions and the instruments used in those particular ports.

surgeon's preference. We generally choose a 5-mm 45-degree scope to facilitate exposure behind the pancreas and near the splenic hilum. Four 5-mm ports are placed under direct visual guidance. The semicircular port location facilitates interchangeability of instruments and camera. For large tumors (>7 cm), a hand-assisted technique may be employed which requires a 6–7 cm vertical midline incision in-between the xiphoid and the umbilicus to serve as a hand-port site.[6,21] This technique is most appropriate for surgeons learning advanced laparoscopic techniques.

Surgical Technique

The pancreas can be accessed by dissecting through the lesser curvature or through the greater curvature with mobilization of the splenic flexure of the colon in order to enter the lesser sac (Figure 3). Pancreatic lesions in the mid-body are best approached through the lesser curvature, whereas

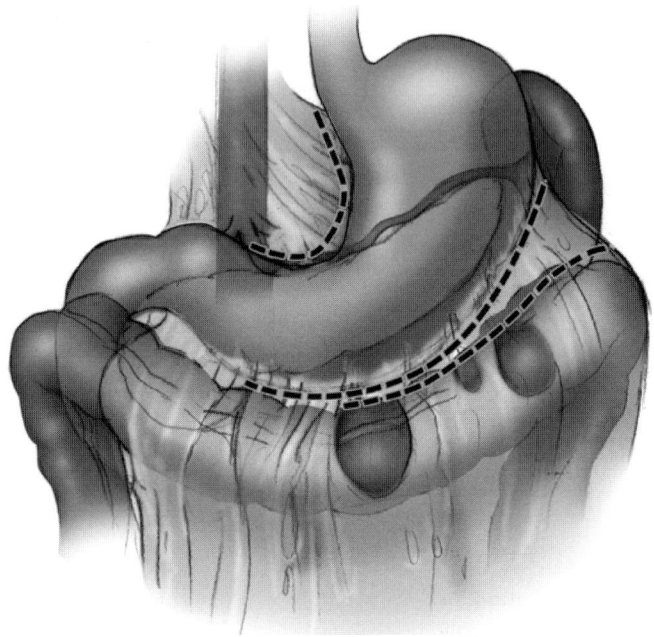

Figure 3. Dissection planes to enter the lesser sac space to expose the pancreas.

more distal lesions are best approached by dividing the gastroepiploic omentum along the greater curvature (while preserving the gastroepiploic arcade to the stomach). Care must be taken to avoid transecting the short gastric arteries to preserve the spleen. After the stomach is retracted cranially and to the patient's right, the pancreas is visualized (Figure 4). If necessary, a laparoscopic ultrasound may be employed to locate the tumor intraoperatively by applying it directly on the anterior surface of the gland. This may facilitate determining a transection site with an appropriate surgical margin from the pathology without unnecessarily taking too much of the pancreatic parenchyma. Ultrasound is also helpful for identifying the major blood vessels for pathology located in the body and neck of the gland. The inferior border of the pancreas is first exposed by opening the fatty tissue plane between the root of the transverse mesocolon and the anterior fascia of the pancreas (Fredet's fascia). The gland is then mobilized anteriorly in a focal area and the splenic artery and vein are identified, if possible. This transection site should be at least 1 cm proximal to the tumor in order to obtain an adequate margin. Selecting a relatively thin

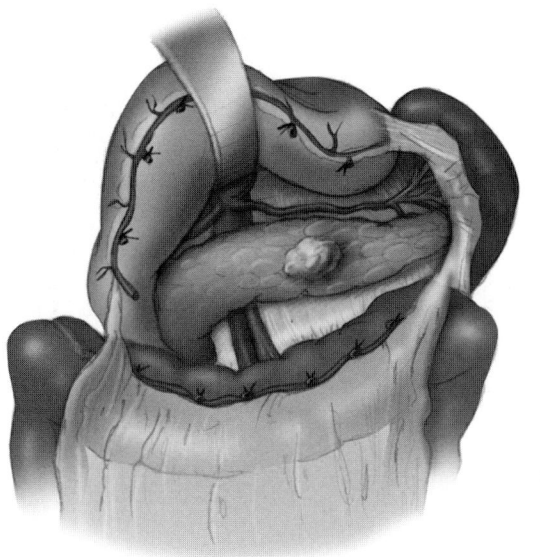

Figure 4. Cephalad retraction of the stomach to expose the pancreas (after dissecting/dividing the gastrocolic vessels).

portion of the gland is also technically helpful. Vessels incorporated in the pancreatic parenchyma are not dissected free; however, vessels which are already separate are divided independently of the parenchyma (Figure 5). The vessels are divided with an endoscopic linear stapler employing 2.0- or 2.5-mm linear staples if the vessels are free. The pancreatic parenchyma (with or without the splenic vein) is transected with 3.5-mm staples reinforced with a bioabsorbable buttress material. For thickened, inflamed, or fibrotic glands, as often seen in chronic pancreatitis, 4.8-mm linear staples are used, again with staple line reinforcement. An alternative approach is to divide some of the gland parenchyma with an electrosurgical device prior to stapling. The pancreatic staple line is then examined for staple line dehiscence. If dehiscence is present, the pancreatic staple lines are oversewn. If there is back-bleeding from the splenic artery and vein, endoscopic clips are used as necessary. After obtaining hemostasis, the gland is then dissected from the retroperitoneum in a medial to lateral direction with the splenic artery and vein embedded in the pancreas (Figure 6). The gland is then accessed from the left lateral aspect of the pancreas and the splenic vessels are divided again as far from the hilum as possible. Care is

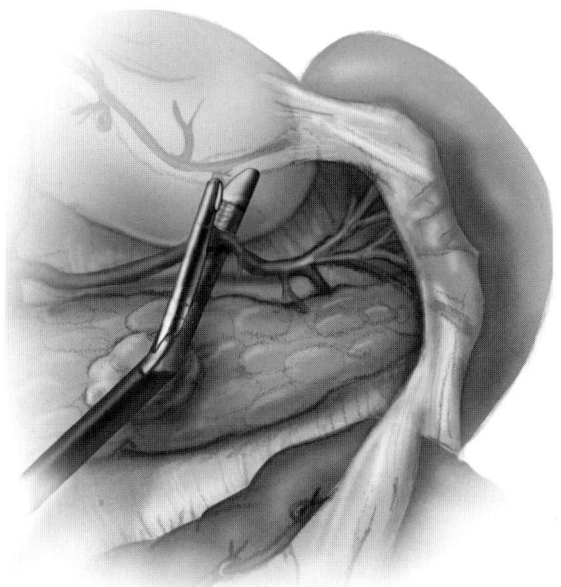

Figure 5. Division of the splenic artery (separate from the pancreatic parenchyma).

taken to preserve the short gastric vessels as well as potential collateral vessels from the omentum and splenic flexure of the colon, if possible. The resected pancreatic segment is then placed in an Endo-bag and removed from the abdomen. The pancreatic stump is re-examined and fibrin sealant may be applied to minimize the risk of a pancreatic leak and a single Blake drain is placed into the retroperitoneal space adjacent to the pancreatic stump. The port sites are closed in standard fashion.

If splenectomy needs to be performed, this can be carried out in a lateral-to-medial direction (spleen first) or medial-to-lateral direction (pancreas first). The former approach is preferred for lesions at the tail of the pancreas whereas the latter approach is preferred for lesions involving the body of the pancreas. In either approach, the splenic vessels along with the pancreas are transected just right of the tumor. The splenic attachments to the stomach, colon, and the retroperitoneum are taken down before removing the spleen and the pancreas together or individually. The umbilical port site may need to be extended in order to remove the specimen(s) in one piece. For the lateral-to-medial approach, turning the patient from supine to right decubitus position on the table facilitates exposure.

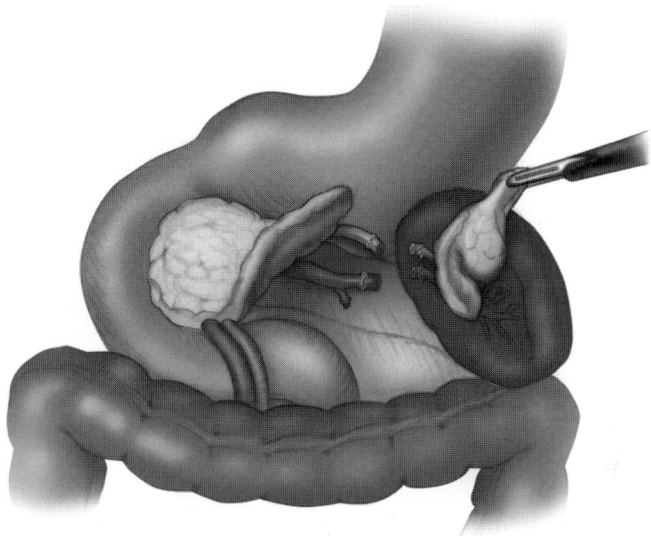

Figure 6. Medial–to–lateral dissection of the distal pancreatectomy specimen (after en-bloc resection of the pancreas along with its vessels).

OPEN DISTAL PANCREATECTOMY

Patient Positoning and Preparation

After induction of adequate anesthesia and endotracheal intubation, a foley catheter is placed and the patient is positioned in a supine position with both arms out. Sequential compression devices are placed on each leg for DVT prophylaxis. The abdomen is then prepped and draped in sterile fashion. The surgeon stands on the patient's right side and the assistant stands on the patient's left side.

Incision and Exposure

The surgery can be performed through a left subcostal incision or an upper midline incision. Abdominal retractors are needed to obtain the appropriate exposure. Once the lesser sac is entered, the stomach is retracted in a cephalad direction to expose the anterior surface of the pancreas. Additional retraction may be needed as the dissection is carried towards the left upper quadrant toward the splenic hilum.

Surgical Technique

The surgical technique for the open approach is exactly like the laparoscopic technique except an intraoperative ultrasound is less likely to be needed given that tactile sensation may be used to identify the location of the tumor;

POSTOPERATIVE CARE

Nasogastric tube is removed immediately after the operation. The foley may be kept in overnight, especially if an open approach was employed. Patients are started on clear liquids on postoperative day 1 and are advanced to a regular diet as tolerated. The fluid from the Blake drain is sent for amylase assessment when the patient is eating a regular diet. If the amylase level is elevated, the drain is kept in place until the patient is seen in clinic for their follow-up appointment in 1–2 weeks. The drain output is assessed at that time and if the output is minimal (<30 ml per 24 hours), the drain is pulled out. Of note, the definition of a pancreatic leak/fistula that is generally accepted by most surgeons is a fluid amylase level 3–5 times greater than the serum amylase level on postoperative day 5.

PANCREAS-RELATED COMPLICATIONS

When comparing the largest series on laparoscopic distal pancreatectomy and open pancreatectomy, the incidence postoperative complications appear to be similar.[5,14] Overall complication rate from laparoscopic pancreas surgery was reported to be 31% based on the large multicenter European study.[5] Pancreas-related local complications are more common than non-pancreas–related complications. Pancreatic leaks and fluid collection are quite common after pancreas surgery and the rate at which this complication occurs vary widely across literature from 0% to 50%, with a mean pancreatic fistula rate of 13% in open distal pancreatectomies (3.5–26%).[5] The largest study on open distal pancreatectomy with 235 patients from Johns Hopkins with a reported 5% fistula rate.[14] This large variation in the pancreatic fistula rate may be due to the discrepancy in reporting as well as defining what is and what is not a fistula. The fistula rate in laparoscopic distal pancreatectomy literature is similar to the data obtained from the open series. Park and Heniford reported one of the largest single institution series of laparoscopic distal pancreatectomies in 25 patients and they had one patient

Table 2. Methods of minimizing pancreatic fistula rate after pancreas surgery.

Techniques	Data
Oversewing the pancreatic stump.	4% pancreatic fistula rate in 25 patients undergoing laparoscopic distal pancreatectomy by routinely performing this technique.[2]
Using Bioabsorbable SeamGuard as a staple line reinforcement.	Unpublished data from Brent Matthews' group show a decrease in the fistula rate from 24% to 11% by routinely performing this technique.
Transecting the pancreas using an ultrasonic scalpel.	A porcine animal study from Johns Hopkins suggests that ultrasonic scalpel may be superior to stapling devices for laparoscopic pancreatic transection.[22] Vessels need to be identified and isolated first.
Selectively oversewing the pancreatic duct.	Failure to identify and selectively close the pancreatic duct was the only feature associated with an increased risk of pancreatic leak after open distal pancreatectomy.[23]
Transecting the pancreas using an ultrasonic scalpel and selectively oversewing the pancreatic duct.	Suzuki et al. reported a decrease in fistula rate from 26% to 4% by routinely performing these two techniques in combination.[24]
Transection of the pancreas exactly where the fine pancreatic branches from the splenic vessels were ligated (during splenic preservation).	Uranues et al. argue that this minimizes pancreatic ischemia and necrosis at the transaction line.[25]
Placement of an endoscopic pancreatic duct stent prior to distal pancreatectomy.	Abe et al. reported a 0% pancreatic fistula rate using this technique in nine patients.[26]
Using fibrin sealant to the pancreatic stump.	Although this technique is commonly used based on data from other GI surgeries,[27–28] a large retrospective study by Mabrut et al.[5] did not show any benefit.

(4%) with a pancreatic fistula that presented as a pseudocyst and required percutaneous drainage.[2] The multicenter study by Mabrut et al. reported a clinical pancreatic fistula rate of 17%.[5] There have been several studies analyzing techniques to minimize leak rates and below are some of the ways that different centers try to decrease the fistula rate (Table 2).

REFERENCES

1. Patterson EJ, et al. Laparoscopic pancreatic resection: single-institution experience of 19 patients. *J Am Coll Surg* 2001; 193(3):281–287.
2. Park AE, Heniford BT. Therapeutic laparoscopy of the pancreas. *Ann Surg* 2002; 236(2):149–158.
3. Fabre JM, et al. Is laparoscopic left pancreatic resection justified? *Surg Endosc* 2002; 16(9):1358–1361.
4. Fernandez-Cruz L, et al. Laparoscopic distal pancreatectomy combined with preservation of the spleen for cystic neoplasms of the pancreas. *J Gastrointest Surg* 2004; 8(4):493–501.
5. Mabrut JY, et al. Laparoscopic pancreatic resection: results of a multicenter European study of 127 patients. *Surgery* 2005; 137(6):597–605.
6. D'Angelica M, et al. Initial experience with hand-assisted laparoscopic distal pancreatectomy. *Surg Endosc* 2006; 20(1):142–148.
7. Dulucq JL, Wintringer P, Mahajna A. Laparoscopic pancreaticoduodenectomy for benign and malignant diseases. *Surg Endosc* 2006; 20(7):1045–1050.
8. Huscher CGS. Laparoscopic Whipple procedure. In: JL Cameron (ed). *Current Surgical Therapy*, Philadelphia, Elsevier Mosby. pp. 1266–1274. 2004.
9. Shoup M, et al. The value of splenic preservation with distal pancreatectomy. *Arch Surg* 2002; 137(2):164–168.
10. Aldridge MC, Williamson RC. Distal pancreatectomy with and without splenectomy. *Br J Surg* 1991; 78(8):976–979.
11. Benoist S, et al. Is there a role of preservation of the spleen in distal pancreatectomy? *J Am Coll Surg* 1999; 188(3):255–260.
12. Govil S, Imrie CW. Value of splenic preservation during distal pancreatectomy for chronic pancreatitis. *Br J Surg* 1999; 86(7):895–898.
13. Hutchins RR, et al. Long-term results of distal pancreatectomy for chronic pancreatitis in 90 patients. *Ann Surg* 2002; 236(5):612–618.
14. Lillemoe KD, et al. Distal pancreatectomy: indications and outcomes in 235 patients. *Ann Surg* 1999; 229(5):693–698; Discussion 698–700.

15. Warshaw AL. Conservation of the spleen with distal pancreatectomy. *Arch Surg* 1988; 123(5):550–553.
16. Sato Y, *et al.* Evaluation of splenic circulation after spleen-preserving distal pancreatectomy by dividing the splenic artery and vein. *Dig Surg* 2000; 17(5):519–522.
17. Killeen K, *et al.* CT Findings after Embolization for Blunt Splenic Trauma. *J Vasc Interv Radiol* 2001; 12:209–214.
18. Fecher A, Pappas T, Pryor A. splenic preservation during laparoscopic pancreatic tail resection. In *The Society for Surgery of the Alimentary Tract*. Chicago, Illinois. 2005.
19. de Buys Roessingh AS, *et al.* Follow-up of partial splenectomy in children with hereditary spherocytosis. *J Pediatr Surg* 2002; 37(10):1459–1463.
20. Lukish JR, *et al.* Spleen-preserving pancreatectomy for cystic pancreatic neoplasms. *Am Surg* 1999; 65(6):596–599.
21. Sheppard BC, Hunter JG. Laparoscopic pancreatic resections. In JL Cameron (ed). *Current Surgical Therapy*, Philadelphia, Elsevier Mosby. pp. 1261–1266. 2004.
22. Hanly EJ, *et al.* New tools for laparoscopic division of the pancreas: a comparative animal study. *Surg Laparosc Endosc Percutan Tech* 2004; 14(2):53–60.
23. Bilimoria MM, *et al.* Pancreatic leak after left pancreatectomy is reduced following main pancreatic duct ligation. *Br J Surg* 2003; 90(2):190–196.
24. Suzuki Y, *et al.* Randomized clinical trial of ultrasonic dissector or conventional division in distal pancreatectomy for nonfibrotic pancreas. *Br J Surg* 1999; 86(5):608–611.
25. Uranues S, *et al.* Laparoscopic resection of the pancreatic tail with splenic preservation. *Am J Surg* 2006; 192(2):257–261.
26. Abe N, *et al.* Preoperative endoscopic pancreatic stenting for prophylaxis of pancreatic fistula development after distal pancreatectomy. *Am J Surg* 2006; 191(2):198–200.
27. Bonanomi G, *et al.* Sealing effect of fibrin glue on the healing of gastrointestinal anastomoses: implications for the endoscopic treatment of leaks. *Surg Endosc* 2004; 18(11):1620–1624.
28. McCarthy PM, *et al.* Esophagogastric anastomoses: the value of fibrin glue in preventing leakage. *J Thorac Cardiovasc Surg* 1987; 93(2):234–239.

SURGICAL TECHNIQUES: ENUCLEATION PROCEDURES AND CENTRAL PANCREATECTOMY

48

Elisabeth Tracy* and
Theodore N. Pappas[†]

PANCREATIC ENUCLEATION

Indications

Enucleation is an acceptable alternative to standard anatomic pancreatic resections in patients with benign and low-malignant potential tumors of the pancreas. Lesions for which enucleation is appropriate include nonfuctioning pancreatic endocrine tumors, mucinous cystadenomas, solid pseudopapillary tumors, small branch-duct intraductal papillary mucinous tumors, and benign conditions such as cystic lymphangioma. Tumors involving the main pancreatic duct or adjacent vessels are not amenable to enucleation.

---

*Boston Children's Hospital, Boston, MA
[†]Division of General Surgery, Box 3479, Duke University Medical Center, Durham, NC 27710, Pappa001@mc.duke.edu

Preoperative Evaluation

Since enuclucleation is a nonanatomical resection, careful patient selection is a critical part of the preoperative evaluation. To be candidates for enucleation, lesions must be carefully characterized by preoperative imaging. Imaging should include a dedicated pancreatic CT scan as well as endoscopic ultrasound or intraoperative ultrasound. Enucleation is only appropriate for benign or low-grade malignant tumors with no evidence of adjacent organ invasion and which can be removed in their entirety. The lesion must be 2–3 mm away from the main pancreatic duct to be amenable to enucleation. On imaging, cystadenomas are typically multilobulated and are not in communication with the main pancreatic duct. Neuroendocrine tumors are hypervascular with a smooth, rounded appearance. Contraindications to enucleation include vascular involvement of the tumor (portal vein or hepatic artery involvement), or involvement of the main pancreatic duct.

In evaluating nonfuctioning pancreatic endocrine tumors, only tumors with low malignant potential should be considered for enucleation. These tumors should meet the following criteria: size <2 cm, no enlarged locoregional lymph nodes, and no distant metastastes. Enucleation for gastrinomas is controversial. Enucleation of gastrinoma in the head of the pancreas is reasonable given the morbidity of a formal resection. However, for gastrinomas in the body and tail, standard pancreatic resections may be associated with improved disease free survival since even small gastrinomas are malignant with nodal involvement as much as 80% of the time.[1,11–12]

Open Enucleation

Enucleation may be performed open or laparoscopically. In the open procedure, the lesser sac is opened and the head of the pancreas mobilized with a Kocher maneuver. The body and tail are carefully mobilized from the retroperitoneum by dissection in the avascular plane posterior to the pancreatic body and tail to allow for bimanual palpation and intraoperative ultrasound (IOUS). IOUS is helpful in identifying the tumor as well as its distance from the main pancreatic duct. It is also useful in ruling out multifocal disease within the pancreas in patients with multiple endocrine neoplasia-type 1.[1] Once the tumor is identified, care is taken not to violate the pseudocapsule during the resection. The parenchyma is divided and small vascular branches clipped or ligated. The main pancreatic duct is avoided to reduce the risk of postoperative fistula formation. Intraoperative frozen section is important for confirming the nature of the tumor and evaluating for negative magins. If any nodes are consistent with metastatic disease, a standard pancreatic resection with lymphadenectomy should be done instead of enucleation. Once the resection is complete, a drain is placed to monitor for pancreatic fistula during the postoperative period. Re-resection is indicated for incomplete resection, positive resection margins on final pathology, or presence of nodal metastases.

Laparoscopic Enucleation

Laparoscopic pancreatic enucleation has been described for insulinoma and nonfunctional endocrine tumors of the pancreas. From 1996–2008, enucleation has been reported in 11 studies each with 5–20 patients for a total of 101 patients.[2] The overall morbidity from these reports is 47% (48/101). The most common complication, as in the open procedure, is pancreatic fistula which has been reported in 29% of patients. There has been no reported mortality. While these reports show decreased intraoperative blood loss and decreased length of stay, large series with longer-term follow-up are lacking. At this point, the technical feasibility of the procedure has been established, but more data are needed to esablish safety and oncologic results.[1]

Complications

The most common complication of enucleation is pancreatic fistula, which occurs in 15–50% of patients (see Table 1).[3] Initial management of a suspected pancreatic fistula is bowel rest. If adequately drained by the intraoperatively placed drain, a low-output fistula (<200 ml/day) can be managed conservatively. If the fistulae persists greater than 2 weeks, nutrition should be initiated. Enteral feeding distal to the ligament of Trietz is as equally effective as TPN in reducing pancreatic exocrine secretions and has the advantage of a lower complication rate and cost.[13] Octreotide is a useful adjunct in managing high output fistulae to control the volume of drainage.

Fistulae that persist longer than 6 weeks will most likely fail conservative management and therefore require either operative or endoscopic intervention based on the patency of the main pancreatic duct. If the pancreatic duct is intact with a side fistula on MRCP, an ERCP with stenting of the main pancreatic duct may be sucessful in managing the fistula. If the pancreatic duct is disrupted on imaging or if the fistula persists despite

Table 1. Large series of patient outcomes after enucleation.

Report	Patients	Indications	Morbidity	Recurrence
Park et al., 1998[4]	30	Nonfunctioning endocrine tumors	Pancreatic fistula 15%	No recurrence
Talamini et al.,[5] 1998	10	Mucinous cystadenoma	Pancreatic fistula 50% (vs. 12% standard resection)	No recurrence
Boninsegna[11] et al., 2008 and Falconi et al. 2010	91	Insulinoma (65) Nonfunctioning endocrine tumors (26)	Pacreatic fistula 50% Reoperation 4%	One recurrence at 60 months, one patient developed liver metastases at 86 months
Crippa et al. 2009[9]	61	Insulinoma (22) Nonfunctional neuroendocrine (16) Epitheilial cyst (5), serous cystanedoma (5), mucinous cystadenoma (3), solid pseudopapillary tumors (3)	Pancreatic fistula 38% (clinically significant fistua in 23%) Reoperation 8%	No recurrence
Pitt et al., 2009[6]	37	Insulinoma (22) Nonfunctioning neuroendocrine (8) Gastrinoma (3) Glucogonoma (2)	Pancreatic fistula 38%	No recurrence

stenting, surgical management is indicated. Anastomosis of the fistula tract to a roux limb may be done if the the fistula tract is mature. Pancreatic body or tail leaks may be treated with distal pancreatectomy without the need for enteric anastomosis. More severe ductal diseases may require a pancreaticojejunostomy for adequate drainage.

Symptomatic pseudocysts that are detected later in the postoperative period also require intervention as well as imaging of the pancreatic duct. Endoscopic drainage may be attempted initially with surgical drainage reserved for persistent, symptomatic collections. Other complications, including exocrine insufficiency or new onset or worsening diabetes are lower with enucleation than standard pancreatic resections. In carefully selected patients, the rate of recurrence after enucleation is low, with several series reporting no local recurrence in follow up times up to 61 months.[1,4,5]

Outcomes

Enucleation has been associated with minimal perioperative mortality and morbidity and acceptable oncologic outcomes. Rates of recurrent disease remain low, comparable to standard resections in appropriately selected patients (see Table 1). For suitable head of the pancreas lesions, enucleation has been shown to have a decreased estimated blood loss, intraoperative time, and length of hospital stay compared with anatomic resection.[6]

CENTRAL PANCREATECTOMY

Indications

Central (or middle) pancreatectomy is a limited resection of the midportion of the pancreas which preserves the spleen, extrahepatic bile duct, and duodenum and spares more pancreatic parenchyma than a distal pancreatectomy or pancreaticoduodenctomy. Although central pancreatectomy was first described in by Guillemini and Bessot in 1957 for chronic pancreatitis, the modern surgical technique was described in 1984 by Dagradi and Serio for insulinoma.[1] Central pancreatectomy is associated with a lower incidence of endocrine or exocrine abnormalities and shorter length of stay than more extensive pancreatic resections. Central pancreactectomy is appropriate for patients with benign or low-grade malignant tumors not amenable to enucleation because of main pancreatic duct involvement, or location on the pancreatic neck or body. The most common indications for middle pancreatectomy are nonfuctioning pancreatic endocrine tumors (with size <2 cm, no vascular or peripancreatic invasion, no lymph node or liver metastases), cystic lymphangioma, and branch-duct IPMNs. Central pancreatectomy for main-duct IPMNs should be avoided because of the high rate of associated malignancy as well as potential for local recurrence. In one series, two of three patients with main-duct IPMNs who underwent central pancreatectomy had local recurrences while the overall local recurrence rate for central pancreatectomy was 3%. Central pancreatectomy may also be appropriate for resection of single, small pancreatic metastases or focal chronic pancreatitis.[7-8]

Preoperative Evaluation

Since central pancreatectomy is a less radical oncologic procedure, careful patient selection and preoperative workup is crucial to prevent tumor recurrence. Preoperative imaging, including a dedicated pancreatic protocol CT and endoscopic ultrasound, should confirm the diagnosis of the lesion and its benign or low-grade malignant potential of the tumor. While in most reports the patients undergoing central pancreatectomy are younger, with smaller lesions, and with more benign lesions than patients undergoing more extensive pancreatic resections, this technique can be applied to the elderly as well.

Open Technique

As with enucleation, exposure of the pancreas is obtained after entering the lesser sac. After the anterior face of the pancreas is exposed, a Kocher manuever is performed and then the pancreas is dissected free from the portal vein and superior mesenteric veins posteriorly. At this point, IOUS is helpful in (1) confirming the extent of the tumor, (2) excluding additional pancreatic lesions, and (3) evaluating the relationship between the tumors and pancreatic vessels as well as the main pancreatic duct. Once the tumor is identified, dissection is carried 1 cm from the tumor on both margins. The pancreas is then transected sharply or with a linear stapler. The transected head of the pancreas is oversewn, as is the pancreatic duct.

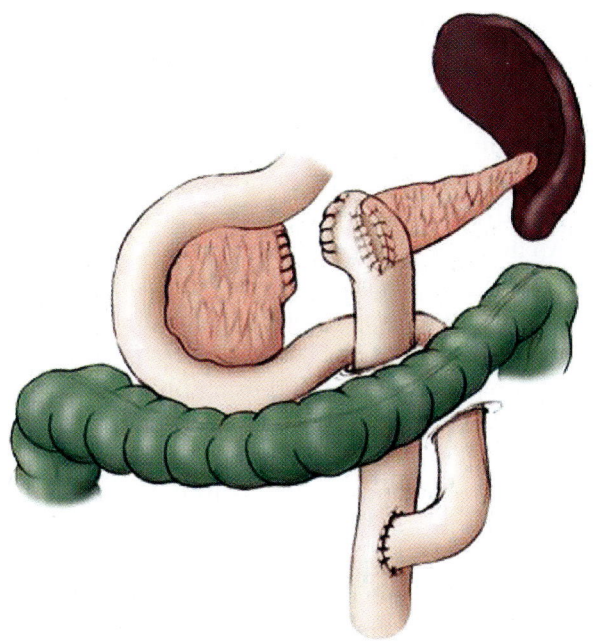

Figure 1. Reconstruction after central pancreatectomy.

The distal pancreatic stump is either oversewn or drained into a roux-en-y jejunal limb through the creation of an end-to-side pancreaticojejunostomy invagination of the pancreas into the jejunum or a two-layer duct-to-mucosal anastomosis (see Figure 1). Oversewing the tail remnant avoids an additional enteric anastomosis but has a leak rate of approximately 15–30%, with most leaks requiring intervention.[14]

An alternative reconstruction is pancreaticogastrostomy without creation of a roux limb. Others have described a double pancreaticojejunostomy of the proximal and distal stump to the same jejunal loop.[1] Intraoperative histological examination of the resected lesion to exclude a high-grade malignancy and examination of the two resection margins to confirm complete resection must be done. Enlarged lymph nodes encountered during exploration should be excised and sent for examination. Also, Crippa et al. argue that for endocrine tumors, peripancreatic nodes should routinely be sampled to avoid understaging patients.[1] Re-resection after central pancreatectomy is indicated for positive margins or lymph node involvement.

Laparoscopic Central Pancreatectomy

Since the fist laparoscopic central pancreatectomy in 2003, the procedure has been reported at several institutions. Trocars are placed subxiphoid, umbilical, and laterally in right and left upper quadrants. The body and tail of pancreas are exposed through a window in the gastrocolic ligament which is large enough to inspect from the gastroduodenal artery to the splenic hilum. An intraoperative ultrasound probe may be used at this point to identify the tumor. The pancreatic neck is then dissected free from the superior mesenteric vein and portal vein. A linear stapler may be used to transect the pancreas. A duct to mucosa pancreaticojejunostomy is then created (authors from one center reported using fibrin glue around the anastomosis).[10] In one series, the proximal end of the gland was anastomosed to the posterior wall of gastric body.[1] The resected portion of pancreas is placed in an endocatch bag and extracted through an enlarged trocar site.

Preliminary results from reported series include morbidity rates of 33%, consistent with the open approach as well as a reduced length of stay. As more centers gain experience with the approach, the data on the efficacy and safety of this approach will become more robust.

Complications

Since the central pancreatectomy requires the management of two pancreatic remnants, a common complication of the procedure is pancreatic fistula. Approximately 30% of patients undergoing central pancreatectomy develop pancreatic fistulae (the range from 12.5% to 40%). Although the fistula rate is high, the majority of pancreatic fistulae at high-volume centers are transient with little clinical impact (grade A fistula by the International Study Group on Pancreatic Fistula grading system). More clinically significant grades B and C fistulae have been shown in recent large series to occur at rates similar to extended left pancreatectomy.[9] Other complications include intra-abdominal abscess, splenic vein thrombosis with or without splenic infarction, pancreatitis, and delayed gastric emptying. Mortality in several large series ranges from 0% to 3%.

Outcomes

Central pancreatectomy has been reported to have a lower incidence of endocrine and exocrine insufficiency than more extensive pancreatic

Table 2. Complications of central pancreatectomy.

Complications of central pancreatectomy	Complication rates reported in major series[1,3,9–10]
Overall morbidity	27.5%–58%
Mortality	0%–3%
Pancreatic fistula — all	7.5%–50%
Clinically significant pancreatic fistula*	7.5%–30%
Reoperation	0%–5%
Endocrine insufficiency	2%–6%

*Clinically significant fistula (Grade B or C) only.

resections. Not only does central pancreatectomy spare more pancreatic parenchyma than larger resections, but the procedure also spares the pancreatic tail which is rich in islet cells. Rates for new onset diabetes and exocrine insufficiency were significantly lower for central pancreatectomy than for extended left pancreatectomy in a retrospective review of more than 150 cases at two high-volume institutions.[9] Local recurrence rates after central pancreatectomy range from 0% to 3% at experienced centers. Mortality rates also ranged from pancreatectomy range from 0% to 3%.

REFERENCES

1. Crippa S, Boninsegna L, Partelli S, *et al.* Parenchyma-sparing resections for pancreatic neoplasms. *J Hepatobil Pancreat Surg* 2010; 17(6):782–787.
2. Briggs CD, Mann DC, Irving GRB, *et al.* Systematic review of minimally invasive pancreatic resection. *J Gastrointest Surg* 2009; 13:1129–1137.
3. Aranha GV, Shoup M. Nonstandard pancreatic resections for unusual lesions. *AM J Surg* 2005; 189:223–228.
4. Park BL, Alexander HR, Libutti SK, *et al.* Operative management of iselt-cell tumors arising in the head of the pancreas. *Surgery* 1998; 124:1056–1061.
5. Talamini MA, Moesinger R, Yeo CJ, *et al.* Cystadenoma of the pancreas. Is enucleation an adequate operation? *Ann Surg* 1998; 227:896–903.
6. Pitt SC, Pitt HA, Baker MS, *et al.* Small pancreatic and periampullary neurodendocrine tumors: resect or enucleate? *J Gastrointest Surg* 2009; 13:1692–1698.
7. Suavenet A, Partensky C, Sastre B, *et al.* Middle pancreatectomy: a multi-institutional retrospective study of 53 patients by the French Pancreas Club. *Surgery* 2002; 132:836–843.

8. Hirono S, Yamaue H. Middle pancreatectomy for pancreatic neoplasms. *J Hepatobiliary Pancreat Sci* 2010; 17(6):803–807.
9. Crippa S, Bassi C, Warshaw AL, *et al.* Middle pancreatectoy: Indications, short- and long-ter operative outcomes. *Ann Surgery* 2007; 246:69–76.
10. Cunha A, Rault A, Beau C, *et al.* Laparoscopic central pancreatectomy: Single institution experience of six patients. *Surgery* 2007; 142:405–409.
11. Boninsegna L, Fanconi M, Zerba A, *et al.* Are atypical resections of the pancreas safe and effective in treating small pancreatic endocrine tumors? *JOP* 2008; 9(6):799–880.
12. Falconi M, Zerbi A, Crippa S, *et al.* Parenhyma-preserving resections for small nonfunctioning pancreatic endocrine tumors. *Ann Surg Oncol* 2010; 17(6): 1621–1627.
13. Voss M, Pappas T. Pancreatic fistula. *Curr Treatment Opt Gastroenterol* 2002; 5:345–353.
14. Wayne M, Neragi-Miandoab S, Kasmin F, *et al.* Central pancreatectomy without anastomosis. *World J Surg Oncol* 2009; 7:67.

SURGICAL TECHNIQUES: CHRONIC PANCREATIC PROCEDURES 49

John C. Haney* and
Eugene P. Ceppa[†]

INTRODUCTION

Chronic pancreatitis is a condition characterized by the progressive fibrosis and destruction of parenchyma leading to chronic pain and ultimately pancreatic exocrine and endocrine dysfunction. The chronic pain leads to nearly ubiquitous narcotic use and is the cause of significant impairment in quality of life. The natural history of the pain is ultimately resolution within two decades as the pancreas burns out. Improvement in this chronic pain is the indication for surgical intervention. As such, it is ultimately an entirely elective undertaking, and thus appropriate and thoughtful patient selection is paramount. Most patients will still experience some pain episodes after surgery, but with appropriate patient and procedure selection, surgery may yield excellent results with long-term improvement in pain and quality of life in three-quarter of patients.

---

*Duke University School of Medicine, Department of Surgery, Durham, North Carolina, USA
[†]Indiana University School of Medicine, Department of Surgery, Indianapolis, Indiana, USA

Approaches to the surgical management of pain in chronic pancreatitis can be categorized by resection of parenchyma or decompression and drainage of obstructed pancreatic ducts. Denervation procedures are of historical interest only, as they have proven ineffective.[1] Resection strategies offer the advantage of removing the inflammatory nidus. The main risk of resection, however, is the loss of valuable parenchyma, potentially hastening the onset of endocrine and exocrine dysfunction. As duct obstruction and luminal hypertension appear to play significant roles in pain mediation, drainage procedures promise improvement without loss of parenchyma, but may not adequately remove the inflammatory source. Within the last decade, the importance of the pancreatic head as the source of much chronic inflammatory pain has been increasingly recognized, and surgical practice has shifted in favor of local pancreatic head resections with or without additional drainage procedures.[2]

DRAINAGE PROCEDURES

Chronic inflammation of the pancreatic duct often results in structuring and stone formation with resultant upstream duct hypertension and dilation. Pain has been reproduced experimentally by elevating duct pressures, suggesting that duct obstruction plays a key role in chronic pain mechanisms. Conversely, chronic pain has also been improved by drainage of obstructed ducts. Enthusiasm for removal of obstructing calculi dates back to the turn of the century, and the defunctionalized limb of Swiss surgeon César Roux was used to decompress pancreatic pseudocysts since the 1920s. Catell initially described a Roux-en-Y pancreaticojejunostomy to decompress malignant obstruction in 1947 and in 1954 Duval and Zollinger described a caudal end-to-end pancreaticojejunostomy for chronic pancreatitis.[1] This initial attempt at focal drainage had a high rate of failure because of the nature of recurrent, segmental stenosis, the "chain of lakes" described by Puestow and Gillesby in 1958, leading them to describe a longitudinal decompression of the body with an invaginated pancreaticojejunostomy and distal tail resection. It was Partington and Rochelle in 1960 who modified the operation, creating a longitudinal anastomosis between incised pancreatic duct and jejunal limb that gives us the Puestow procedure as known today.[3] This procedure does not require tail resection and provides excellent decompression of the pancreatic body and tail. It provides excellent drainage of chronically obstructed ducts and thus pain relief, without loss of additional parenchyma. Early postoperative pain relief measures 80%. Within 3–5 years, however, up to 30% of patients have recurrence of pain.[1] The limitations of the procedure are twofold. First, the longitudinal decompression is increasingly difficult with smaller pancreatic ducts and thus really requires a significant level of duct dilation. Second, the procedure decompresses the body and tail but does not address the head of the pancreas. While decompressing the main pancreatic duct, it does not decompress the proximal duct of Wirsung or the uncinate and tributary ducts within the head of the pancreas. Over the last 2 decades, the importance of this pancreatic head inflammation in producing chronic symptoms has become increasingly realized. As we shall see later, it has been an appreciation for this role that has led to increasing enthusiasm for combined head resection and drainage procedures. Nevertheless, the modified Puestow longitudinal pancreaticojejunostomy provides excellent long-term outcomes in the appropriately selected patient, namely those with a grossly dilated pancreatic duct and no overt evidence of pancreatic head inflammation preoperatively.[4]

RESECTION PROCEDURES

While a drainage procedure reduces chronic pain by decompressing hypertensive pancreatic ducts, resection carries the promise of removing inflamed tissue altogether. The advantage is a permanent removal of the inflammatory nidus, while the obvious inherent risk, other than those of major pancreatic surgery in general, is the removal of otherwise functional parenchyma, hastening the onset of exocrine and endocrine insufficiency. The most obvious resection strategy is that of total pancreatectomy. This carries the predictable 85% improvement in pain, but obviously produces insufficiency 100% of the time, carrying the additional morbidity and mortality of a refractory form of diabetes. Complete loss of islet cells has the additional cost of the loss of glucagon signaling, creating an especially brittle diabetic state with high risk of hypoglycemia as well as the expected hyperglycemic state. In a series of 100 patients, over half of all deaths were due to hypoglycemia.[1] Autotransplantation of islet cells carried initial enthusiasm, but this technique has only proven effective in a very small number of centers, thus total pancreatectomy is rarely advisable.

Of the incomplete pancreatic resections, distal pancreatectomy remains the least morbid. With or without splenectomy, tail resection usually does not require anastomotic drainage of the distal body. While less morbid, distal pancreatectomy leaves the majority of the gland untreated, and does nothing to the pancreatic head that is often the inflammatory focus. Long-term pain relief is seen in 60% of patients. Initial enthusiasm for a subtotal (95%) distal pancreatectomy, leaving a swathe of parenchyma on the duodenum, was seen in the 1970s. Pain relief was approximately 80% at 6 years, but three-quarter of patients suffered early endocrine insufficiency and enthusiasm waned.[1]

The resection with the longest track record remains the classic pancreaticoduodenectomy as described by Allen Whipple of New York Hospital in 1935. With the advantage of removing an inflamed pancreatic head, the Whipple also leaves more parenchyma behind to provide function. Enthusiasm for pancreaticoduodenectomy for all indications increased in the 1970s with refinements of technique and reduction in morbidity and mortality. Anastomotic leak from the pancreaticojejunostomy remains the major cause of morbidity, but with improvements in technique leak rates are generally 6–20%. Pain relief of 71–89% at 6 years may be expected. While mortality is now less than 5%, the operation remains morbid with rates of 40%.[1]

Recognition of the importance of the inflamed pancreatic head and the morbidity of a formal pancreaticoduodenectomy led to a search for duodenal-sparing pancreatic head resections. In 1972, Hans Beger of the University of Berlin excised the central portion of the pancreatic head while leaving the ampulla intact. The critical components to the Beger operation include division of the pancreatic neck over the portal vein, preservation of the posterior branch of the gastroduodenal artery, and the preservation of a small rim of pancreatic tissue along the duodenum. Preservation of the posterior branch of the GDA is critical as it supplies blood to the remaining duodenum and the intrapancreatic bile duct. Reconstruction is performed with an end-to-end pancreaticojejunostomy to the distal pancreas and an end-to-side pancreaticojejunostomy to the remnant pancreas along the duodenum. The common bile duct may be decompressed via the Roux limb if needed (50% of the time). The distal pancreaticojejunostomy may be extended longitudinally if needed for obstruction of the duct within the body (10% of the time). Dr. Beger first published his series in 1980 and updated it in 1997 with 380 patients.[5] Pain control at 6 years was seen in 88%. The primary risks include anastomotic leak and duodenal ischemia, but morbidity remains lower than that of formal pancreaticoduodenectomy at 15–25%. Most importantly, because of the limited parenchymal resection, endocrine and exocrine functions were preserved and long-term rates of insufficiency mirror that of chronic pancreatitis alone.

While the Beger procedure represents an improvement on the Whipple in terms of morbidity and endocrine insufficiency, it remains a technically complicated resection requiring division of the pancreatic neck above the portal vein with preservation of posterior vascular structures. In an effort to improve upon the morbidity and recognizing the importance of decompressing a dilated pancreatic duct, in 1987, Charles Frey described the local resection of the pancreatic head with preservation of the pancreatic neck and posterior capsule and the inclusion of a lateral pancreaticojejunostomy.[6] The Frey procedure excavates the pancreatic head while preserving the posterior capsule, thus reducing the risk to vascular structures posterior to the gland. The ducts of Wirsung and Santorini are both decompressed in continuity with an opened dorsal duct, anastomosed longitudinally to a Roux limb of jejunum. Subsequent modifications have altered the extent of the longitudinal pancreaticojejunostomy as determined by the degree of dilation within the duct.[7] Long-term results from the Frey procedure show similarly pain relief with the predictable reduction in morbidity from both parenchymal preservation and limited resection. Morbidity from a Frey procedure has been estimated at 16% compared to 25% for the Beger and 40% from the Whipple procedures.[1]

Over the past decade, a number of reports on the long-term outcomes of the various resection techniques have been published, and a number of prospective, randomized trials have compared two or more.[8] The primary conclusion is that the long-term pain control rates are similar, with all producing effective relief in approximately 80% of patients, likely because all three address the role of the inflamed pancreatic head. The incidence of long-term pancreatic insufficiency remains high mirroring the natural history of the disease; all three techniques spare parenchyma and thus do not see the increase in early insufficiency of the subtotal or total pancreatectomies that make them ill-advised. While all three may be performed with acceptably low mortality, the morbidity does vary as described. The Whipple remains the most morbid at 40%, decreasing to 25% for the Beger and 16% for the Frey.[1] With similar long-term results, the choice of procedure has thus become highly individualized, but the data do suggest that the Frey remains a somewhat safer and less morbid procedure.

CONCLUSIONS

Surgical intervention for chronic pancreatitis is driven primarily by a desire for pain control. The natural history of chronic pancreatitis pain is that of resolution secondary to pancreatic burnout; thus, surgical intervention is ultimately an elective intervention intended to improve quality of life and reduce narcotic dependence. As such, patient selection and patient education are important prior to intervention. Surgical interventions may be classified by those that decompress hypertensive, obstructed ducts and those that resect inflammatory tissue. Resection offers the promise of improved control of the inflammatory nidus but is balanced by the loss of functional parenchyma and the risk of accelerating the rate of pancreatic insufficiency, especially that of brittle diabetes. The importance of the inflamed pancreatic head as a nidus for chronic inflammation and pain has been realized over the past 2 decades, resulting in the emergence of local resection strategies that remove the pancreatic head but minimize further loss of parenchyma and simplify resection to reduce morbidity. Long-term pain control from any head resection appears to be both highly successful (over 80%) and equal among resection strategies. The Frey procedure with its preservation of the posterior pancreatic capsule has emerged as the least morbid, yet a decision of which procedure is preferred should be based on the patient's burden of disease and surgeon's experience.

Preoperative imaging characteristics, then play a critical role in operative selection. Specifically, the location of inflammatory tissue relative to the gastroduodenal artery and the level of pancreatic ductal dilation are the crucial aspects. Drainage procedures, namely the modified Puestow longitudinal pancreaticojejunostomy, have a role for patients with a grossly dilated pancreatic duct without evidence of an inflammatory head mass. Distal pancreatectomy may be indicated in rare instances in which the disease appears limited to the tail. A formal Whipple pancreaticoduodenectomy remains the procedure of choice when there is concern for a potentially malignant mass lesion within the head. For patients with a significant inflammatory component within the head, the Frey procedure has emerged as the treatment of choice, offering local resection of the inflamed head with the lowest morbidity. The extent of the longitudinal decompressive pancreaticojejunostomy is determined by the degree of dilation within the duct. With appropriate patient and procedure selection, long-term pain relief can be achieved in greater than 80% of patients with acceptably low morbidity.

REFERENCES

1. Andersen DK, Frey CF. The evolution of the surgical treatment of chronic pancreatitis. *Ann Surg* 2010; 251(1):18–32.
2. Bachmann K, Izbicki JR, Yekebas EF. Chronic pancreatitis: modern surgical management. *Langenbecks Arch Surg* 2011; 396(2):139–149.
3. Partington PF, Rochelle RE. Modified Puestow procedure for retrograde drainage of the pancreatic duct. *Ann Surg* 1963; 152:1037–1043.
4. Ceppa EP, Pappas TN. Modified puestow lateral pancreaticojejunostomy. *J Gastrointest Surg* 2009; 13(5):1004–1008.
5. Beger HG, Schoenberg MH, Link KH, *et al.* [Duodenum-preserving pancreatic head resection—a standard method in chronic pancreatitis]. *Chirurg* 1997; 68(9):874–880.
6. Frey CF, Smith GJ. Description and rationale of a new operation for chronic pancreatitis. *Pancreas* 1987; 2(6):701–707.
7. Ho HS, Frey CF. The Frey procedure: local resection of pancreatic head combined with lateral pancreaticojejunostomy. *Arch Surg* 2001; 136(12):1353–1358.
8. Strate T, Taherpour Z, Bloechle C, *et al.* Long-term follow-up of a randomized trial comparing the beger and frey procedures for patients suffering from chronic pancreatitis. *Ann Surg* 2005; 241(4):591–598.

SURGICAL TECHNIQUES: PANCREAS TRANSPLANTATION 50

Errol L. Bush, Kadiyala V. Ravindra
and Bradley H. Collins

HISTORY/TRENDS/DATA

The first successful human pancreas transplant was performed in 1966 by Drs. Kelly and Lilllehei at the University of Minnesota. Because of advances in surgical techniques, organ preservation, post-transplant antibiotic prophylaxis, and immunosuppression agents, pancreas transplantation is an accepted treatment for Type 1 diabetics who are otherwise medically suitable. Unlike islet cell transplantation, whole organ pancreas transplantation is "curative" as patients enjoy normalization of glucose tolerance by testing as well as normal HgbA1c levels. According to the most recent Organ Procurement and Transplantation Network (OPTN) data, some 24,332 pancreas transplants have been performed in the United States since 1988, with 1,178 of those performed in 2010.[1] Five- and ten-year pancreatic allograft survival is 73% and 55%, respectively.[2]

As organ transplantation, in general, has become more successful and readily available. The most significant problem faced by transplant professionals during the last couple of decades has been the shortage of organs. The problem is no different for Type 1 diabetics desiring pancreas transplantation. There are approximately 2 million Type 1 diabetics in the

United States; however, only 1200 pancreas transplants were performed in 2010.[1] There were almost 8000 deceased donors during the same year; however, most were not suitable pancreas donors. In an effort to increase the organ donor pool, partial pancreatic allografts from living donors have been transplanted; however, these procedures are rare. Islet cell transplantation would further exhaust the deceased donor pool as each recipient requires the islets of more than one donor to achieve insulin independence. This chapter will focus on a discussion of the techniques of pancreas transplantation utilizing organs from deceased donors.

ANATOMY/FUNCTION

The pancreas lies in the retroperitoneum, is posterior to the stomach, and can be visualized at the base of the lesser sac. The head of the pancreas is nestled within the c-loop of the duodenum, and the tail is enclosed by the hilum of the spleen. Given this intricate relationship with foregut organs, it receives a dual blood supply from branches of both the celiac and superior mesenteric arteries. While the pancreas has both exocrine and endocrine functions, transplantation is indicated for restoration of endocrine function in Type 1 diabetics (i.e. endogenous insulin production by the β-cell component of islets of Langerhans). Some centers offer pancreas transplantation to type 2 diabetics; however, a lack suitable donors has limited the expansion of pancreas transplantation into this population of patients. Whole organ pancreas transplantation maintains normoglycemia in a physiologic fashion that is not possible with the current methods of exogenous insulin administration (intermittent subcutaneous injections or continuous pump infusions into the subcutaneous tissues) and secondarily improves quality of life while preventing or halting some of the secondary complications of diabetes.[3]

TRANSPLANTATION

Recovery

In general, selection of a suitable deceased donor for pancreas recovery is similar to that of other solid organs. A history of diabetes is a contraindication, although postmortem hyperglycemia or hyperamylasemia are often a result of the donor's critical care management or the stress-response to injury and should therefore prompt greater investigation into potential donor suitability. In general, deceased pancreas donors are less than 50 years of age as with aging, the pancreas undergoes senescence and its parenchyma is naturally replaced by fat and fibrosis. The pancreas from a donor who has died secondary to trauma with an associated injury to the pancreas or duodenum is usually considered nontransplantable.

Once a suitable donor has been identified and the appropriate consent has been obtained, a laparotomy is performed for organ exposure. Although incisions may vary based on the organs intended for recovery or surgeon's preference, in general, a generous midline incision with or without a periumbilical cruciate extension is utilized. The livers of virtually all pancreas donors are utilized for transplantation, so dissection is performed taking into account the anatomic needs of both recovery teams. The lesser sac is entered, and the pancreas is visualized and palpated for anatomic evaluation and texture. Much of the success of pancreas transplantation is the result of minimizing postoperative pancreatitis and organ edema; therefore, meticulous dissection is of upmost importance.

The duodenum is instilled with antibiotic solution via a nasogastric tube to reduce the risk of bacterial contamination and is divided proximally and distally with a stapling device before being freed medially to the aorta via the Kocher maneuver. The spleen is mobilized medially along with the pancreatic tail. This dissection is performed carefully noting the course of the splenic artery toward the celiac trunk. Exposure and dissection of the celiac artery and its branches ensue. Just inferior to the pancreatic margin, the superior mesenteric vessels are dissected, ligated and divided. After systemic heparinization, the infrarenal aorta is cannulated and occluded distally. The supraceliac aorta is then clamped, and the aorta is perfused in the retrograde direction with cold preservation solution. The pancreas, duodenum, and spleen are removed *en bloc* by dividing the superior mesenteric and splenic arteries near their origins and the portal vein a couple of centimeters distal to the insertion of the splenic vein. Some surgeons prefer to explant the liver and pancreas as a block and then separate the organs on the back table. In order to facilitate implantation, arterial reconstruction is necessary, therefore, a "Y"-segment of common iliac artery is recovered with adequate length distal to the bifurcation of the external and internal iliac segments. The pancreas and blood vessels are placed in a transport approved container where they are maintained at 4°C in preservation solution.

Back-Table Preparation

Recovery of the pancreas can be challenging, and it is imperative that the transplanting surgeon visually inspects the organ prior to incising the recipient, especially when the organ is recovered by another transplant team. Missed trauma or recovery injuries usually result in morbidity and occasionally mortality in the recipient. Allograft dysfunction results from the use of pancreases containing parenchyma infiltrated with fat or fibrosis. Pancreas transplantation should be considered an elective operation, so organs with any signs of damage or abnormality should be discarded.

Care is taken to minimize cold ischemia time to less than 12 hours with 24 hours considered the upper limit. This is accomplished by careful timing of the donor operation, as well as simultaneous back table graft preparation and recipient laparotomy by separate surgical teams to minimize implantation time. The back table work is performed at 4°C in a bath of preservative solution and begins with an inspection of the graft for injuries or aberrant anatomy not recognized during the recovery. If the pancreas is deemed suitable for implantation, splenectomy is performed, and the duodenum is shortened around the pancreatic head with a stapling device. The mesenteric root on the back side of the pancreas is secured with a running suture or a staple line. The pancreatic head and neck are supplied by branches of the superior mesenteric artery and the body and tail are fed by branches of the splenic artery. The superior mesenteric and splenic arteries are short in the dissected specimen and would be difficult to anastomose to the donor's target vasculature; therefore, the vessels are "lengthened" by use of the donor's iliac arterial Y graft. The external and internal iliac branches are sewn to the splenic and superior mesenteric arteries of the pancreas. Arterial inflow to the entire pancreas then can be accomplished readily by a single anastomosis.

Implantation

Most patients who undergo pancreas transplantation receive a concomitant kidney transplant. In general, these operations are performed via a midline incision, although bilateral retroperitoneal incisions have been utilized. In either case, ease of implantation dictates placement of the pancreas on the right side and the kidney on the left. Isolated pancreas transplantion may be performed by either approach, although a midline laparotomy is preferred.

Prior to implantation, consideration of operative technique should be given. Options include differences in graft positioning, management of exocrine output, and venous drainage of the allograft. The choices take into account anatomic variations and surgeon preference. The advantages of a midline incision include access to both sets of iliac vessels which is important in diabetics who often have premature atherosclerosis which can limit anastomotic targets. The pancreas is oriented in the peritoneal cavity with the head and attached duodenum pointing in the cephalad or caudal direction. In general, the venous anastomosis is performed first. The choice of venous target may have some mild physiologic effects in the early postoperative period. In the normal physiologic state, the pancreas "senses" blood glucose on the arterial side and releases insulin into the portal circulation where its concentration is decreased by 50% during first pass metabolism by the liver. Some centers mimic this scenario by anastomosing the donor's portal vein to the recipient's superior mesenteric vein (portal venous drainage). For ease of implantation, most centers utilize the systemic venous drainage technique by performing the donor portal vein anastomosis to the inferior vena cava or right common iliac vein in the recipient. Initially, recipients are hyperinsulinemic; however, this is short-lived and physiologically insignificant as recipients are rarely hypoglycemic, even in the early postoperative period. Arterial inflow is established by anastomosing the pancreatic arteries reconstructed with the iliac artery Y graft to the recipient's common iliac artery. The presence of dense atherosclerosis in the recipient may require the surgeon to use some degree of improvisation in establishing arterial supply to the graft.

In addition to its endocrine properties, the pancreas has important exocrine functions. Once the pancreas is successfully transplanted, the stapled donor duodenum begins to fill with effluent from the pancreatic duct. This output is usually diverted into the recipient's gastrointestinal tract, either the jejunum or ileum. The exact location is often determined by the loop of small intestine that is most closely apposed. For those centers that still use the bladder to manage the exocrine output of the pancreas, the caudal orientation facilitates anastomosis to the bladder. Although bladder drainage allows measurement of urine amylase level trends that may correlate with rejection, most transplant surgeons believe that the complications far outweigh any potential advantages. These include chronic, symptomatic metabolic acidosis due to the loss of bicarbonate-rich exocrine secretions in the urine. Other long-term complications of bladder drainage include recurrent urinary infections, hematuria, bladder stones, and urethral transection. Ultimately, a significant proportion of bladder-drained pancreases are converted to enteric drainage. The intestinal mucosa is better equipped to withstand the caustic exocrine output of the pancreas. While there is low *operative* risk associated with both enteric and bladder drainage, the systemic consequences of a leaking intraperitoneal enteric anastomosis are more severe than a pelvic bladder anstomosis leak that is usually confined to the pelvis and can often be treated nonoperatively (percutaneous drainage and prolonged bladder catheterization). The risk of anastomotic leak is sufficiently low that most centers employ the enteric anastomotic technique.

Postoperative Complications

Pancreatic function is monitored postoperatively by serial serum glucose levels which should normalize quickly in the presence of a well-functioning graft. Hyperglycemia (>200 mg/dL) should prompt expeditious assessment of the allograft by ultrasound and specifically, Doppler interrogation of the vasculature. The most common cause of early graft loss is vascular thrombosis, usually on the venous side. It is heralded by acute hyperglycemia following a period of euglycemia. Thrombosis of the donor portal vein can be due to edema of the graft, redundancy or twisting of the vein, or hypercoagulability. Arterial thrombosis is usually the result of a technical complication. Thrombosed grafts are rarely salvaged, and explantation is necessary. Some centers use systemic heparinization in an effort to prevent this devastating complication.

Acute cellular rejection is prevented by the use of agents that suppress the immune system. The state of immunosuppression can be induced preoperatively by corticosteroids and antibody preparations targeting T cells. Most centers use a three-agent regimen for maintenance immunosuppression: (1) calcineurin inhibitor (tacrolimus or cyclosporine, (2) antimetabolite (mycophenolate mofetil), (3) corticosteroids. Rejection of the pancreatic allograft is usually asymptomatic, and serum studies (amylase, lipase, etc.) are nonspecific. Hyperglycemia is such a late sign of pancreatic rejection that treatment is usually unsuccessful. Patients who undergo simultaneous pancreas and kidney transplantation from the same deceased donor have a lower rate of graft loss due to rejection than those who receive pancreas grafts alone because the renal component can serve as a marker for rejection. One would expect that those patients who have rejection of the pancreas will also develop rejection of the kidney that will be signified by an increase in serum creatinine, prompting percutaneous biopsy of the kidney. A high index of suspicion should be maintained for patients who receive isolated pancreas allografts. If rejection is suspected, percutaneous biopsy by ultrasound or computed tomography guidance is indicated.

REFRENCES

1. http://optn.transplant.hrsa.gov/, February 18, 2011.
2. 2009 OPTN/SRTR Annual Report: Transplant Data 1999–2008, http://optn.transplant.hrsa.gov/ar2009/.
3. Lerner SM. Kidney and pancreas transplantation in type 1 diabetes mellitus. *Mount Sinai Journal of Medicine* 2008;75:372–384.

INDEX

aberrant artery 6
aberrant hepatic arteries 6
aberrant left hepatic artery 8
abnormal pancreaticobiliary junction 335
abscess 27
accessory 6
accessory right hepatic artery 7
acinus 15
ACTHoma 514
acute 160
acute liver and chronic liver disease 171
acute liver disease 165
acute liver failure 159, 161
acute pancreatitis 429, 557–560, 562, 566, 569
Acute Pancreatitis Classification Working Group 446
adenoma 25, 26
adenosine 10
allograft rejection 538, 541, 544
ampulla of Vater 14
ampullary adenocarcinoma 491, 492, 497, 508
ampullary carcinoma 492, 502
angiography 25, 26, 30, 32
annular pancreas 431
anomalies of the gallbladder 12
Atlanta classification 439

Atlanta symposium 438, 446
autoimmune pancreatitis 460

Balthazar CT severity index 448
Beger 634
benign lipomatous tumors 68
bile duct 14
bile duct adenoma 65, 70
bile duct injury 377–379, 382
biliary obstruction 558, 566, 573, 596, 592
biliary stenting 594
bilobar gallbladders 12
bladder drainage 540, 541, 543, 544
Budd-Chiari syndrome 4

Calot triangle 7
canaliculi 11
Cantlie's line 4
carcinoid 514
carcinoma 491
Caroli's disease 336
caudate 254–256, 258
caudate lobe 4, 9, 12
cavernous hemangioma 24
celiac node 16, 17
celiac plexus 564
central pancreactectomy 625, 628

central vein 14, 15
Child-Pugh classification 80
cholangiocarcinoma 31, 491, 493, 498, 500, 503
cholangitis 312, 318–320
cholecystectomy 305–309
cholecystojejunostomy 602
choledochal cysts 333
choledochoceles 337
choledochojejunostomy 599, 600
choledocholithiasis 311–313, 316, 320, 385
chromogranin, synaptophysin, or neuron-specific enolase 512
chronic liver disease 159, 160, 167–171
chronic liver failure 160
chronic pancreatitis 428, 457, 557, 558, 560, 562–564, 567, 569
cisterna chyli 17
clinical islet transplantation 546
CLM 91, 93, 94, 96–99, 102, 105, 106
common bile duct (CBD) 7, 14, 256, 258–261
common bile duct (CBD) exploration 385–387, 390
common bile duct stones 313
common hepatic artery 6
common hepatic duct (CHD) 11, 14, 256–260
computed tomography 22
congenital diverticulum of the gallbladder 12
cords 14
coronary 16
coronary vein 9
cyst 22, 23

cystadenoma 23
cystic artery 8
cystic duct 7, 14, 256, 260, 261
cystic duct remnant 306
cystic neoplasms 469–471, 474–476, 478, 485, 488
cystic pancreatic lesion 423, 425
cystic plate 12

deceased donor 537, 539, 544, 545
deep system 16, 17
distal bile duct cholangiocarcinoma 508
distal pancreatectomy 607
distal pancreatectomy with en bloc splenectomy 608
distal pancreatectomy with splenic preservation 608
duct of Santorini 414
duct of Wirsung 414
ductus venosus 9
duodenal adenocarcinoma 491, 493, 498, 508
duodenal carcinoma 500
duodenal stenting 594
duodenum 14

Edmonton trial 546, 550, 552
embolization 191–196
endoscopic retrograde cholangiopancreatography (ERCP) 267, 268, 338, 385, 431, 557–560, 562, 564, 565, 573, 574
endoscopic ultrasonography 432
enteric drainage 544
enucleation 621, 622

Index

epiploic foramen of Winslow 6
EUS 557, 562, 564–566, 568, 572–574
extrahepatic bile duct 14

falciform ligament 16
fenestrated endothelium 15
Fibrolamellar HCC 85
focal nodular hyperplasia (FNH) 26, 27, 71
Frey 635
fulminant hepatic failure 161, 162, 165–167
fulminant liver failure 159
functional anatomy 4, 5

gallbladder 12, 273–278
gallbladder cancer (GBC) 323–331
gastric outlet 592
gastrinoma 514, 516, 517
gastroduodenal (GDA) artery 6
gastrojejunostomy 599, 600
Glissonian sheath 11
glucagonoma 514, 518
GOO 598

hammartomas, and inflammatory pseudotumors 65
HAP 8
hemangioma 66
hemangioma, fibroma, lipoma, angiomyolipoma, and lymphangioma 65
Henle trunk 414
hepatectomy 92, 93, 96–99, 101, 102, 104, 106
hepatic arterial buffer response 10

hepatic arterial infusion therapy 209, 210
hepatic arteriole 15
hepatic artery 6, 11, 15
hepatic artery, portal vein 14
hepatic artery proper 6, 7
hepatic duct 7
hepatic nodes 16, 17
hepaticojejunostomy technique 379–382
hepatic vein 10, 14
hepatocellular adenoma (hepatic adenoma) 65, 69
hepatocellular carcinoma (HCC) 21, 29, 30, 77
hepatocytes 11, 14
hepatoduodenal ligament 6
HIDA 266, 267
hypoglycemic unawareness 534, 536, 537

image 264
imaging 21, 22, 25, 27, 29, 30, 263
immunosuppression 536, 537, 540, 546, 548, 551
inferior mesenteric vein 9
inflammatory pseudotumor 74
insulinoma 514, 515
intestinal trunk 16
intraductal papillary mucinous neoplasm 425
intrahepatic cholangiocarcinoma (ICC) 77, 86
Islet cell tumors 428
islet transplantation 535, 546–549, 551–553

isolated hepatic perfusion   209, 211
IVC   10

Kupffer cells   15

laparoscopic bile duct exploration   386
laparoscopic CBD clearance,   386
laparoscopic CBD exploration   385, 389, 388
laparoscopic central pancreatectomy   628
laparoscopic cholecystectomy   369
laparoscopic enucleation   623
laparoscopic gastrojejunostomy   595
left hepatic artery   8, 9
left hepatic duct (LHD)   11, 14, 254, 256, 258–260
left hepatic vein   11
left lateral segmental   9
left lobe   16
left medial segment   9
left portal vein   9
liver   91, 93–106, 191–196
liver dysfunction   160, 163
liver failure   160
liver histology   14
living donor   537, 538, 544, 549
lobectomy   5
lobule   14
lymphatics of the liver   16
lymphatic system   16

magnetic resonance cholangiopancreatography   432
malignant degeneration   336
median scissura   11

MEN-1   511, 512, 515–517
mesenchymal hamartoma   74
metastases   21, 24, 28, 429
Milan criteria   83
MRCP   269–271
MRI   431
mucinous cystadenocarcinomas   424
mucinous (macrocystic) adenomas   424
Multidetector CT   419

necrosectomy   447, 451–453
necrotizing   449
necrotizing pancreatitis   435–438, 443, 445, 446, 450, 454
neurofibromatosis   511
nociception   461
nodular regenerative hyperplasia (NRH)   65, 73

obstruction   592
pancreas divisum   416
open enucleation   622
open gastrojejunostomy   596

pancreas   546
pancreas transplantation   534–539, 542, 545, 548, 553
pancreatic adenocarcinoma   427, 491, 500, 508
pancreatic cystosis   426
pancreatic divisum   430, 460
pancreatic fistula   618
pancreatic leaks   616
pancreatic lymphoma   429
pancreatic necrosis   558, 566, 569, 570

pancreaticobiliary maljunction 335
pancreaticoduodenectomy 500, 505, 577, 579, 581–589, 634
pancreaticojejunostomy 632
pancreatic splenosis 428
pancreatitis 449, 560
pars umbilicus 9
percutaneous hepatic perfusion 209, 213
periampullary 491
periampullary adenocarcinoma 495
periampullary carcinoma 491, 495, 500, 507
pericardia lymph nodes 16
porta hepatis 11, 14, 16, 17
portal pedicles 11
portal scissurae 4
portal triad 6, 11, 14
portal vein 6, 7, 9, 11
postcholecystectomy 305, 306, 308
postcholecystectomy syndrome 305–308
Ppoma 514
PRSS1 461
pseudocyst 429, 562, 563, 565–569
PTC 268, 269
Puestow 632

Ranson 437
Ranson's criteria 437, 448
Ranson's Score 449
recurrent stones 308
"replaced" right hepatic artery 7
replacing artery 6
retained stones 308
right and left hepatic arteries 6

right and left hepatic ducts 255, 256
right gastric artery 6
right hepatic artery 7–9
right hepatic duct (RHD) 11, 14, 255–260
right hepatic vein 11
right scissura 11
right triangular ligaments 16

scissura 4
sectors 4
segmentectomies 5
segments 4
serous (microcystic) adenoma 424, 426
simple cysts 66
sinusoids 6, 14
somatostatinoma 514, 519
space of Disse 15
sphincter of Oddi 561
sphincter of Oddi dysfunction 308, 309, 558, 560
Spink1 461
splanchnicectomy 603
splenectomy 614
splenic and superior mesenteric veins 9
split liver transplantation 18
stricture 305, 309
superficial 16
superficial system 16
superior mesenteric and splenic veins 9
superior mesenteric artery 7
supraduodenal artery 6

technetium sulfur colloid scan 27
the focal nodular hyperplasia 65

thoracic duct   16, 17
thoracoscopic splanchnicectomy   604
transabdominal ultrasound   432
transcystic   385
transcystic laparoscopic CBD exploration   389
transplantation   546
trisegmentectomies   18
tropical pancreatitis   460
TRP channels   461
true, epithelial-lined pancreatic cysts   425
trypsin   459

T-tube   387
tuberous sclerosis   511
tumor   191–196

ultrasound   21, 25, 32, 264, 265
ursodeoxycholic acid   308

video-assisted retroperitoneal debridement (VARD)   452, 453
VIPoma   514, 518
Von Hippel–Lindau   511, 512, 515

Whipple   579, 583, 586